Manual of Pediatric Therapeutics

Sixth Edition

Department of Medicine
Children's Hospital, Boston

Edited by John W. Graef, M.D.
Chief, Harvard Pilgrim Health
Care Services
at Children's Hospital, Boston

Editorial Board

Nancy C. Andrews, M.D., Ph.D.
Shari Nethersole, M.D.
Cedric J. Priebe, M.D.
Richard A. Saladino, M.D.
Elizabeth R. Woods, M.D., M.P.H.
Gregory J. Young, M.D.

Cathryn J. Lantigua, Editorial Assistant

Foreword by Frederick H. Lovejoy, Jr. M.D.
Associate Physician-in-Chief
Children's Hospital, Boston

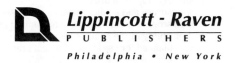

Lippincott - Raven
PUBLISHERS
Philadelphia • New York

Acquisitions Editor: Paula Callaghan
Manufacturing Manager: Dennis Teston
Production Manager: Maxine Langweil
Production Editor: Kimberly Swan
Cover Designer: Jeane Norton
Indexer: Jayne Percy
Compositor: Compset
Printer: R.R. Donnelley

R J
5 2
M 3 6
1 9 9 7

Printed in the United States of America

9 8 7 6 5 4 3 2 1

Library of Congress Cataloging-in-Publication Data

Manual of pediatric therapeutics / Department of Medicine, The
    Children's Hospital, Boston ; edited by John W. Graef ; foreword by
    Frederick H. Lovejoy. — 6th ed.
        p.   cm.
    Includes bibliographical references and index.
    ISBN 0-7817-1555-5
    1. Children—Diseases—Treatment—Handbooks, manuals, etc.
  I. Graef, John W., 1939–   . II. Children's Hospital (Boston,
  Mass.). Dept. of Medicine.
    [DNLM: 1. Therapeutics—in infancy & childhood.   WS 366 M294
  1997]
  RJ52.M36   1997
  615.5′42—dc21
  DNLM/DLC
  for Library of Congress   97-1436
                                                                CIP

To David Gordon Nathan, M.D.,
Physician-in-Chief, 1986–1995.
Clinician, scientist, teacher, statesman,
mentor, a man for all seasons, his
patients came first.

Contents

Foreword

Pressures for efficiency in care and education make the *Manual of Pediatric Therapeutics* of increasing importance and value. Well-packaged information that is current, accessible, and briefly stated is tremendously useful to the student, resident, nurse, and practitioner.

Dr. John Graef and his talented editorial board, including Drs. Nancy Andrews, Shari Nethersole, Cedric Priebe, Richard Saladino, Elizabeth Woods, and Gregory Young, have accomplished this task in a marvelously effective manner. Dr. Graef's broad knowledge of pediatrics and his vast experience as an editor have resulted in selection of information that is both pertinent and useful. The sixth edition has significant changes over the previous edition. All chapters are updated. New chapters on the Delivery of Pediatric Care, Dermatology, Musculoskeletal Disorders, and Developmental Disabilities have been added.

The Department of Medicine and Children's Hospital take great pride in this important manual, first published in 1970 under the leadership of Dr. Graef's mentor, Dr. Thomas Cone. The manual's multiple contributors, many trainees of our four chiefs, Drs. Charles Janeway, Mary Ellen Avery, David Nathan, and now Philip Pizzo, have all added immeasurably to its value. The sixth version is a fine successor to the previous edition. We are all deeply grateful to Dr. John Graef for his commitment to this task and to his editorial assistant, Ms. Cathy Lantigua, for her great skill and dedication to this edition.

Frederick H. Lovejoy, Jr., M.D.

Preface

One of the special satisfactions that comes with editing six editions of the *Manual of Pediatric Therapeutics* is working with the extraordinarily talented and able faculty who have participated in the preparation of each edition. Over the years, many have gone on to outstanding careers in academic medicine, some in areas far afield of the one for which they contributed material to the book. My good friend and colleague, Dr. Robertson Parkman, now Chief of Research Immunology and Professor of Pediatrics at the University of Southern California, comes to mind. In 1970, he contributed the chapter on newborn medicine in the first edition of the *Manual* but has since gone on to the field of bone marrow transplantation of which he is widely noted as one of the world's experts. In the same edition, Dr. Ralph Lopez wrote the chapter on fluid and electrolytes but went on to a successful career in adolescent medicine. Harvey Cohen, Lewis First, Margaret Hostetter, Fred Ledley, Jeffrey Lipton, Fred Lovejoy, Georges Peter, and Philip Pizzo among many others all contributed chapters or editorial work to the *Manual* early in their careers. To say that I have taken pride in what small role their participation in this book may have played in their thoughts as future educators and leaders in pediatric medicine is an understatement.

The current group of authors and editors is no exception. Drs. Andrews, Nethersole, Priebe, Saladino, Woods, and Young include three former Chief Residents, a Howard Hughes Investigator and two superb general pediatricians. Each has brought a unique perspective. Their selection of authors has once again produced an edition which, we hope, contains the most current thinking in each field.

The format of the manual has been changed slightly. It has been divided into three sections instead of two. The first section is meant to address principles of managing well children and includes the new chapter on Delivery of Pediatric Care which, for the first time, discusses such topics as telephone management and home care as well as the nuts and bolts of such difficult subjects as managing the dying patient. Also, our "well child" chapter now contains three subsections each devoted to one of the three main age groups of our specialty namely, infancy, childhood and adolescence. The next major section contains chapters devoted to acute care of ill children and includes such broad categories as Emergency and ICU Care, Antibiotics and Infectious Disorders, Poisonings, Managing the Sick Newborn, and Fluid and Electrolytes. The third and largest section is devoted to more traditional "organ system" topics. All chapters have been updated and revised. In addition to the new chapter on the Delivery of Pediatric Care, new chapters on Musculoskeletal Disorders and Developmental Disabilities[1] have been added and one former chapter on Dermatology has been restored.

The most difficult part of my job is not deciding what to include but what to

---

[1]We note with sadness the untimely death of our friend and colleague, Marilynn Haynie, who co-authored the chapter on Developmental Disabilities. Her passion for the care of disabled patients is a living inspiration to us all.

exclude. To provide space for new chapters requires reduction of others. All chapters either remained the same size or were cut slightly albeit with reluctance and the possible loss of a few friends. All topics have been chosen and are discussed with the general pediatrician or pediatric nurse practitioner in mind. As in our previous editions, few topics are included for which there is no therapeutic recommendation. It remains for you, our readers, to tell us whether we succeeded in striking the balance in content we strive for.

Finally, this edition would have been impossible without the invaluable assistance of our Editorial Assistant, Cathy Lantigua. Cathy assembled all the manuscripts, kept our authors and editors on track (even me) and maintained constant communication with our publisher(s) as the book progressed. The final product is a synthesis of the efforts of our expert authors, our superb Editorial Board and Cathy's extraordinary diligence. We hope you will find it helpful in the management of your patients.

John W. Graef, M.D.

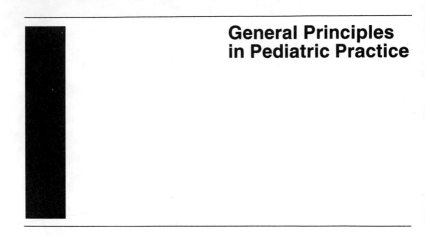

General Principles
in Pediatric Practice

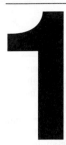

Caring for Children

John W. Graef

Pediatrics is organized around the relationship of a child's health and risk of illness to his or her growth and development. Stages of biologic and social development and the particular risks of disease associated with those stages are presented in Table 1-1.

I. Advocacy. Because of the age and vulnerability of pediatric patients, pediatricians have a special role as advocates. Historically, it has been shown that the needs of children may suffer when they require the expenditure of scarce public resources. If denial of full opportunity is true for healthy children, it is doubly true for disabled children with special needs (see Chap. 21). Because of the respect earned by pediatric physicians, it behooves them to speak out on public issues that affect children.

II. Counseling. It is the pleasant lot of the pediatrician to reassure patients and families that for the majority of illnesses, growing children need only be supported with a medical safety net should the illness be atypical or severe.

To accomplish effective reassurance, the pediatrician must make time available to hear patients' questions completely and supply information in an understanding and understandable manner. It is useful to ask that information be repeated back and confirmed to avoid confusion about what was said. Counseling is best heard when patients do not fear that the pediatrician has another agenda such as avoiding an inconvenient patient visit or encouraging an unnecessary visit. It is helpful to begin a conversation by offering to examine the child if the patient wishes but encouraging parents that they may be empowered by counseling to manage the child effectively. The ready availability of pediatric care, particularly at night or on weekends, may go a long way toward reassuring parents that help is near should they need it.

III. Coping with pediatric illness

  A. Patients. When they first enter pediatric practice, few pediatricians fully appreciate the emotional impact of pediatric illness either on children, parents, or physicians. Some of the interaction between pediatricians and sick children involves maneuvers and procedures that can be frightening or painful for children and may add to their distress as well as that of the parents. Yet the resiliency of children and their ultimate loyalty and affection for pediatric caretakers tells us that an honest, caring, and gentle approach to patients will overcome much of the initial adversity felt when physical discomfort occurs as a necessary part of evaluation and treatment.

  B. Parents. Occasionally, well-meaning parents may attempt to discourage necessary but invasive interventions such as lumbar punctures or even tuberculin skin tests to "protect" their children from unwanted physical or psychological trauma. In responding, pediatricians should not permit the issue to be one of control and the parents' refusal to "cooperate" should not be seen as an affront. Their fears must be addressed, and a patient, sympathetic, firm, but flexible response likely will be effective in winning them over. Rarely is any procedure so emergent that parents cannot be permitted time to grasp its importance and to steel themselves to their child's suffering. It may also be that proposed procedures are not absolutely essential to the child's treatment but part of a protocol. Clinical judgment permits flexibility in determining the priority and need for interventions. Pediatricians must also recognize and place in perspective their own distaste for performing necessary procedures. Not all physicians are comfortable or adequately skilled in inva-

3

Table 1-1. Health risks by age group

Age	Name of stage	Health risks
Conception	Prenatal	Maternal infection, parental age, environmental exposures, maternal substance abuse, malnutrition, endocrine or cardiovascular disorder, trauma during pregnancy
0–2 days	Perinatal	Congenital anomaly or infection, respiratory immaturity or obstruction, gastrointestinal or genitourinary obstruction, pH incompatibility, metabolic defect
2–30 days	Neonatal	Respiratory or cardiovascular defect; inability to feed; gastrointestinal obstruction; infection of the lung, central nervous system, or genitourinary system; metabolic defect; hepatitis or hepatic obstruction
1–6 months	Infancy	Malnutrition and/or food intolerance, infection, cardiovascular or metabolic defect
6–24 months	Toddler	CNS disability, seizure disorders, respiratory infections (otitis), malabsorption disorders, ingestions, lead poisoning, accidents, child abuse, early reactive airway disease, dehydration with diarrheal illness, neuroblastoma
2–5 years	Preschool	Respiratory infections, asthma, inflammatory bowel disease, nephrotic syndrome, vasculitis, accidents, sexual abuse, leukemias
5–10 years	School	Group A streptococcal illness, ADDH, accidents, JRA, IDDM, sexual abuse, allergies, nephritis, peripharyngeal abscesses, asthma
10–13 years	Puberty	Delayed or premature sexual development, acting-out behaviors, accidents, changes in IDDM, asthma, exacerbation of latent tuberculosis, sexual abuse, early substance abuse, sinusitis
13–18 years	Adolescence	Accidents, Crohn's disease, substance abuse, asthma, migraine, pancreatitis, lymphomas, violence, date rape, sexually transmitted disease, pregnancy, infectious mononucleosis

ADDH = attention deficit disorder with hyperactivity; JRA = juvenile rheumatoid arthritis; IDDM = idiopathic diabetes mellitus.

sive procedures; each must be willing to enlist colleagues or physician extenders as appropriate, understanding that patients and parents will ultimately appreciate this step.

   C. Follow-up. Once a treatment plan has been accomplished, follow-up and continuity of care should be assured. Parents appreciate follow-up visits and telephone checks, which demonstrate continuing interest in the welfare of their child. Children with acute exacerbations of chronic disease need the ongoing supervision of monthly or quarterly visits even in the absence of acute symptoms. Support provided by documentation for schools and other caretakers is important to the overall care of the child.

IV. The pediatric consultation. Pediatricians may be asked to consult with colleagues from other medical specialties, other pediatric providers, or other pediatricians. The following guidelines may be helpful.

   A. Respond as soon as possible. A colleague seeking consultation is usually in need of prompt assistance. If necessary, and with notification, a suitable substitute should be offered.

B. Determine what questions need your help and respond specifically to them.

C. Your colleague has asked for help, not replacement. Explain the limits of your role to patients and parents at the onset and maintain those limits through follow-up.

D. Successful consultation is best accomplished by meticulous attention to detail. You may not have more knowledge than a requesting colleague, but may have more time.

E. Do not comment on a colleague's management in the presence of the patient or parents. Such comments are frequently misunderstood or blown out of proportion.

F. Provide the requesting colleague with information. Do not attempt to dictate patient care.

G. Discuss your findings with the requesting colleague and ask for her or his permission *before* discussing them with patient and family. Medical practice is, at best, inexact. Part of good medical judgment is knowing when to ask for help. Consultation provided in a prompt and helpful manner assures a patient of an extra measure of knowledge and concern, with the added benefit of enhancing the knowledge of all participants.

V. Death of a child. The strongest of all grief reactions occurs when parents have lost a child. When a child has a fatal disease, the parents and immediate family face the loss of all their expectations for the child and an extended period of sadness. What health professionals do during this period is usually based on their own feelings as well as on assumptions that arise from customs, traditions, state and hospital health rules, and even research interests. Thoughtful and caring medical personnel can share and help to lighten the family's burden. (See Chap. 2, pp. 13–14, Chap. 22 p. 559 for specific recommendations.)

There is nothing wrong with feeling a sense of loss at the death of a patient or with the need to grieve, but it is the physician's hard task to put his or her own grief aside until the needs of the parents and family have been met.

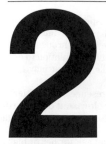

Delivery of Pediatric Therapy

Cedric J. Priebe

The physical, economic, legal, and cultural contexts of pediatric therapy strongly impact its delivery. The nature of all such settings and processes is established by local history and policy. Those presented here are generalizations of delivery models adapted partly from the Medical Staff Bylaws and House Officer's Manual of Children's Hospital, Boston.

I. Settings for pediatric care

A. The hospitalized patient. Pediatric hospitalization rates and average lengths of stay (ALOS) have seen a dramatic decline in the past decade. Admission to children's hospitals or to the pediatric wards of general hospitals, however, remains a crucial setting for the diagnosis and care of the severely ill child.

1. **The pediatric ward.** The pediatric ward setting fosters multidisciplinary care teams capable of managing a variety of complex medical and social problems. These teams include general pediatricians and specialists, pediatric nurses and nurse practitioners, physical therapists, respiratory therapists, nutritionists, activities therapists, and social workers. Rounds on admitted patients should be made at least daily on stable, long-term patients, and at least twice a day on patients who are acutely ill. The primary care pediatrician may function as attending physician or as a consultant to a hospital-based pediatrician or subspecialist attending physician. The care of children with complex medical problems frequently involves extended conversations among the care team and with parents. These interactions are sometimes best conducted at formally scheduled team and family meetings.

2. **The neonatal and pediatric intensive care unit** (see Chaps. 6 and 7).

3. **The delivery room** (see Chap. 6).

4. **The newborn nursery.** Full-term infants, with no complications, born to healthy mothers are now being discharged from the hospital on the first or second postdelivery day. Given this constraint, the following goals of newborn care should be met (see Chap. 3).

   a. Newborns should be examined within 24 hours of delivery or sooner if the obstetric or nursing staff expresses any concern, or if significant risk factors for infection are present.

   b. Neonatal metabolic and genetic screening should be obtained according to state health policy.

   c. Parents should be educated on feeding techniques and schedules, use of the car seat, and need to observe for jaundice.

   d. A trusting relationship between parents and pediatrician should be established.

   e. Vital statistics from the delivery and nursery course should be communicated to the primary care pediatrician.

B. The ambulatory patient

1. **Private office, health center, and clinic.** General pediatric therapy is predominantly delivered in the ambulatory setting and is maximized by a continuing relationship between primary care providers and families over time. Clearly established lines of authority and job descriptions for physician, nursing, and business staff ensure smooth flow of patient services.

2. Emergency departments. If at all possible, parents are encouraged to contact their pediatrician before taking their children to an emergency room. Most health maintenance organizations (HMOs) will not approve payment for the nonurgent use of the emergency room (ER) unless authorized by the primary care pediatrician. Unless a life-threatening emergency precludes involvement by the primary care pediatrician, the pediatrician should alert the ER staff of the expected patient. Depending on the ER's staffing for pediatric emergencies, the pediatrician may be required to assist in ER care.

3. Home care. The coordination and supervision of home medical care by the pediatrician is particularly crucial for the chronically ill and medically complex child. Physician orders are usually required for access of home care services. Many health insurance plans *require* that the primary care physician make the referral for home care services.

III. Compensation

A. Indemnity insurance. Traditional health insurance is purchased from third-party insurers by employers as a group benefit or by individuals. Some large employers provide self-insurance plans to their employees. Indemnity insurance plans reimburse pediatricians on a usual, customary, and reasonable fee-for-service basis for visits and procedures covered in the policy agreement. Health supervision services are frequently *excluded*. In addition, the following features may apply.

1. Annual deductibles.

2. Maximum benefits.

3. Excludable conditions or procedures.

4. Preadmission authorizations.

5. Utilization review.

B. Managed care systems combine delivery and financing in one system, attempting to control costs and quality through such measures as preventive services, quality assurance, utilization review, and appropriate financial incentives. A member's ability to "self-refer" is restricted or eliminated. Physicians may be restricted from participating by the managed care system's professional or economic credentialing requirements, or both. Providers may assume some level of financial risk by accepting capitated compensation (fixed payment per member per unit time, usually monthly) for a defined group of services.

1. Preferred provider organization (PPO). A designated panel of physicians and institutions is contracted to provide care at a significant discount from usual, customary, and reasonable fee schedules. Members may access providers outside the PPO with increased copayment or higher deductibles. Although there is no formal risk-sharing arrangement, there is a strong emphasis on utilization review.

2. Health maintenance organization (HMO). A federally qualified organization of physicians, hospital facilities, and other health care providers under contract to provide comprehensive health care to members. In most HMOs, a significant emphasis is placed on prevention.

a. Staff model HMO: physicians as salaried employees.

b. Group and network model HMO: contract of HMO with a single multispecialty medical group or with a network of many primary and multispecialty medical groups.

c. Independent practice association (IPA) model HMO: contracts between HMO and office-based physicians. Practices are reimbursed either on a discounted fee-for-service or capitated basis according to a prearranged contract incorporating mechanisms that act to place the physician at financial risk for extraordinary hospitalization or subspecialty service costs for members.

C. Integrated delivery system (IDS). A complete provider entity that includes physicians, ancillary services (laboratory and imaging), and secondary and tertiary care hospitals. These systems attempt to provide a complete range of medical care to members on a capitated basis. Primary care practices may be acquired by such a system and/or enter long-term employment or independent service contracts.

D. Government programs
1. **Medicaid.** Each state establishes its own Medicaid regulations within federal guidelines. Eligibility is usually based on family size and income relative to the federal poverty level. Medicaid cards stating dates of eligibility are issued by local health and human services departments. The Early and Periodic Screening, Diagnosis, and Treatment (EPSDT) program within Medicaid covers routine health supervision services provided by qualified physicians.
2. **CHAMPUS.** The Civilian Health and Medical Program of the Uniformed Services covers care provided by civilian physicians and hospitals to active-duty and retired military dependents whose needs cannot be met by the Uniformed Services Pediatrics Program. Reimbursement is fee-for-service. Health supervision visits and immunizations are covered only for the first 2 years of life. Families are responsible for a yearly deductible and a 20% copayment for sick visits.

E. Direct payment. Patients and families without indemnity insurance and income above Medicaid eligibility levels are billed directly for medical services. Pools of municipal, institutional, and philanthropic funds are sometimes available to defray out-of-pocket costs to families for pediatric care.

III. Documentation
A. General guidelines for medical record entries
1. Include date and time of entry.
2. Use black ink and write legibly.
3. Sign all entries with legible printing of name and professional designation.
4. Use abbreviations only when approved by the facility.
5. Record all significant events, as well as anticipated events that did not occur, such as missed appointments or doses.
6. Record all therapeutic interventions and the patient's response.
7. Make objective rather than subjective statements; state facts rather than conclusions.
8. Limit to clinically relevant material.
9. Never delete, physically damage, or alter any previous entry.
10. Addenda should be date and time stamped, signed, and cross-referenced to the original entry.

B. Components of the pediatric medical record
1. **Acute care record**
   a. Admission history and physical assessment.
   b. Nursing flowsheets.
   c. Progress notes.
   d. Procedure notes.
   e. Doctor's orders.
   f. Discharge summary.
2. **Ambulatory record**
   a. Problem lists.
   b. Immunization history.
   c. Health supervision screens.
   d. Well-child visit notes.
   e. Urgent care visit notes.
   f. Telephone triage and consultation.
   g. Medications and prescription refills.
   h. Correspondence
      (1) Letters to and from specialists.
      (2) Letters to airlines.
      (3) Letters to utilities.
3. **Abstractions of the medical record.** The pediatrician is frequently called on to provide documentation of a patient's health status, including physical examination, immunization record, screening tests, current medications, and activity limitations. Such documentation is often required for the child's enrollment in school, participation in recreational activities, or receipt of public assistance. Attention must be given to the confidentiality of sensitive medical information in the completion of these required forms.

a. School and camp forms.
b. Enrollment forms for Women, Infants and Children (WIC) nutritional assistance program.
c. Disability claim forms.

C. Medical orders. Medical orders are the physician's communication and documentation of instructions to the nursing, pharmacy, and laboratory staff concerning the care and treatment of a particular patient. Although medical orders are the legal responsibility of the physician, the nurse's input in the formulation of medical orders is essential. Orders should be discussed and verified by the patient's nurse at the time they are written. All standing orders on admitted patients should be reviewed and/or rewritten at intervals determined by hospital policy, usually 48 hours.

1. Written orders. The following are recommendations for handwritten orders.
   a. Entries should be clear and legible, with special attention to dosage amounts and decimal points.
   b. Each page of orders should be correctly labeled with the patient's identifier.
   c. Each order is preceded by the **date** and **time** of entry and followed by the ordering physician's signature, **printed name,** and other clearly legible identifiers.
   d. Orders entered by medical students require cosignature by the supervising physician.
   e. Incorrect entries discovered *before* signature are stricken by drawing a single line through the error with the word *error* written and initialed nearby.
   f. Changes to orders *after* signature are transacted by a separate order to *cancel* and *replace* the prior order with the correction.

2. Voice orders. Physicians' duties occasionally require transcription of voice or telephone orders by nursing staff. Such orders are valid for a period limited by institutional policy and must be cosigned by the ordering physician within a certain period, usually 24 hours or less.

3. Computerized orders. Computerized hospital information systems offer rapid communication of orders and immediate decision aids to the ordering physician; they also can facilitate monitoring of resource utilization. Special considerations inherent in computerized order management systems include the accessibility and ease of use by clinicians, the handling of updates and corrections with audit trails, and the ability to adapt orders to circumstances unique to pediatrics.

4. Order format. Medical orders for admitted patients generally address the following areas.
   a. Identify physician and/or physician groups responsible for the patient.
   b. Diagnosis or reason for hospitalization.
   c. Condition: critical, serious, guarded, fair, or satisfactory.
   d. Allergies to medications.
   e. Infectious exposures.
   f. Infectious isolation or precautions
      (1) Complete/respiratory precautions.
      (2) Mask within 3 ft.
      (3) Gown and gloves for contact.
      (4) Universal precautions.
   g. Permitted activities.
   h. Monitoring.
      (1) Frequency of vital signs and weight.
      (2) Use of monitoring devices.
      (3) Measurement of intake and output.
   i. Diet. Define an enteral diet appropriate for age, caloric needs, and any special problems of velopharyngeal coordination, absorption, or transit time.
   j. Intravenous fluids or parenteral nutrition.
   k. Diagnostic tests. List all tests with dates, times, and frequencies of performance.

l. **Drugs.** Include generic drug name, preparation, dose amount, route, frequency, and duration of administration. Most institutions restrict drug utilization to a formulary of preparations and brands. Orders for nonformulary drugs in special circumstances require justification. Orders for oxygen therapy should be explicit as to means of administration and inspired oxygen concentration (FiO_2).

m. **Therapies.** Respiratory, physical, and/or occupational therapy are ordered with definition of type, frequency, and goals of treatment.

IV. **Consultations and referrals.** Pediatricians function within the medical community as peers, consultants, and referral sources. Careful management of these relationships is key to providing sound pediatric therapy.

A. **Consultations.** Pediatricians may be asked to consult with colleagues from other medical specialties (e.g., surgery, internal medicine), other pediatric providers (e.g., family practitioners, child psychologists), or other pediatricians. The following guidelines may be helpful.

1. Respond as soon as possible. If necessary, a substitute consultant should be offered.

2. Determine what questions require your assistance and respond *specifically* to them.

3. Explain to the patient and parents the limits of your role as consultant to, not replacement of, the requesting physician, particularly if the consultation requires follow-up.

4. Successful consultation is best accomplished by meticulous attention to detail. Do not assume that you have more knowledge than a requesting colleague. You may, however, have more time. Frequently, the answer to a clinical dilemma lies in elucidation of historical details or an overlooked physical finding.

5. Do not comment on a colleague's management in the presence of the patient or parents.

6. The best consultation provides the requesting colleague with information or opinion, or both, on which to base clinical decisions.

7. Discuss your findings with the requesting colleague and ask for permission *before* sharing them with the patient and family.

B. **Referrals.** As primary care provider, the pediatrician functions within limits of time, expertise, and training. If the needs of patients exceed these limits, referrals to specialists are necessary. While parents and patients greatly appreciate referral to another highly qualified provider of specialized care or service, pediatricians are increasingly called on to mediate the patient's contact with secondary and tertiary services.

1. **Pediatric subspecialties.** Pediatricians should be familiar with local and regional practitioners of medical and surgical pediatric subspecialties, as well as dentists, psychologists and psychiatrists, podiatrists, occupational and physical therapists, and speech and language therapists.

2. **Community services.** Pediatricians should be aware of state and federal laws that influence the access of children to educational and health services. For example, Public Law 99-457, the Education of the Handicapped Amendments of 1986, requires early intervention services and preschool programs for infants, toddlers, and preschoolers with handicaps.

3. **Visiting nurse services.** The continuation or monitoring of medical care at home requires participation of home visiting nurse services.

4. **Social services.** While some pediatric primary care practices offer social service counseling to patients and families, pediatricians should also be aware of community-based services that address these needs, including private social work practitioners. In addition, the pediatrician should be aware of state regulations on mandatory reporting of suspected physical or sexual child abuse.

5. **National organizations.** For the parents and family of children with chronic diseases or conditions, referral to a national or regional organization may provide significant education and empowerment (Table 2-1).

Table 2-1. National and regional community services organizations and resources for parents and children

Education
Council for Exceptional Children Information Service (Reston, VA)
Human Resources Center (Albertson, NY)
National Association of Private Schools for Exceptional Children (Bethesda, MD)

Legal Aid
Children's Defense Fund (Washington, DC)
Disability Rights Center (Washington, DC)
Legal Services Corporation (Washington, DC)

Environment/Travel
Adaptive Environments Center, Massachusetts College of Art (Boston, MA)
Architectural Barriers and Compliance Board (Washington, DC)
Society for the Handicapped (Brooklyn, NY)

Advocacy Groups/Informative
American Coalition of Citizens with Disabilities (Washington, DC)
American Foundation for the Blind (New York, NY)
Association for Children with Birth Defects (Orlando, FL)
Association for Retarded Citizens of the United States (Arlington, FL)
Association for the Severely Handicapped (Seattle, WA)
Downs Syndrome Congress (Chicago, IL)
Epilepsy Foundation of America (Landover, MD)
Foundation for Children with Learning Disabilities (Washington, DC)
Muscular Dystrophy Association (New York, NY)
National Association of the Deaf (Silver Springs, MD)
National Easter Seal Society (Chicago, IL)
National Society for Autistic Children (Washington, DC)
Orton Dyslexia Society (Baltimore, MD)
Spina Bifida Association of America (Chicago, IL)
United Cerebral Palsy Association (New York, NY)

Directories/Data Bases
Accent on Information: Computerized Retrieval System (Bloomington, IL)
Directory for Exceptional Children (Sargent Publishers, Boston)
Directory of Educational Facilities for the Learning Disabled (Association for Children with
    LD, Pittsburgh, PA)
Directory of Learning Resources for the Handicapped (Croft Net Publishers, Waterford, CT)
National Directory of Children and Youth Services (CPR Services, Washington, DC)
National Rehabilitation Information Center Data Base (Washington, DC)

Family Support Groups
Parents Campaign for Handicapped Children and Youth (Washington, DC)
Sibling Information Network, University of Connecticut (Storrs, CT)

Recreation/Arts
American Dance Therapy Association (Columbia, MD)
National Association for Music Therapy (Washington, DC)
National Association of Sports for the Cerebral Palsied (New York, NY)
National Committee on Arts for the Handicapped (Washington, DC)
National Wheelchair Athletic Association (Colorado Springs, CO)
North American Riding for the Handicapped (Ashburn, VA)
Special Olympics (Washington, DC)
US Association for Blind Athletes (Beach Haven, NJ)
US Deaf Skiers Association (Simmsbury, CT)

Day Care/Respite Care
Children's Aid Society (New York, NY)
Project Head Start, Office of Health and Human Services (Washington, DC)

V. The dying patient
  A. Do not resuscitate orders. Cardiopulmonary resuscitation (CPR) should be initiated in the event of sudden or impending respiratory or cardiac arrest unless a properly executed order to the contrary has been given. The following outline addresses situations in which "do not resuscitate" (DNR) orders may be appropriate and offers a method for their conduct.
   1. Determination of appropriateness of DNR orders. CPR may be withheld from some patients who are terminally ill and imminently dying, or whose illness or injury is irreversible, and irreparable, or for whom continuous advanced life support would entail prolonged, unrelieved pain or discomfort.
   2. Role of patient and parents. A DNR order requires concurrence of the patient, family, or legal guardian. For older minor patients, it may be both appropriate and helpful to discuss the proposed order with them and their parent or guardian. Some patients under 18 years old are legally competent, and the law will not recognize parental consent as binding. Patients over 18 are generally recognized as legally competent except where cognitive delay or other factors render them incompetent. For an individual patient or parent to make an informed decision, he or she must understand the nature of the patient's illness, the likely prognosis with and without treatment, the purpose of the DNR order, and its expected consequences.
   3. Documentation
      a. Progress notes. When discussion among the care team, family, and possibly the patient results in adoption of a DNR status for the patient, the attending physician should document the following in the *progress notes* section of the patient record.
         (1) *Why* and *how* the initial question of DNR orders was raised.
         (2) The decision-making process that was followed, including
            (a) Professional staff involvement.
            (b) Role of parents and patient.
            (c) Data on which decision is based.
         (3) Summary and updates of planning process and decisions.
         (4) Summary of conversations with the patient and parents.
      b. The DNR order. Many institutions have successfully implemented a standardized DNR order format. The order must be signed by the attending physician and nurse and **must be renewed weekly.** The hospital care team is responsible for ensuring that all pertinent caregivers who will be providing care, or who will assume care, are aware of the DNR order status and should be involved in future discussions to ensure continuity and consensus.
   4. Revocation of a DNR order. The individual patient, parent, or guardian who originally concurred with the DNR order may revoke it *at any time.* Any member of the health care team or family may request that the DNR order be reevaluated. Discontinuation of a DNR order should be noted in the appropriate place in the patient orders and explained in the progress notes.
   5. Reassessment of DNR orders before anesthetic and surgical procedures. Due to special circumstances during general anesthesia, when cardiac or respiratory arrest is likely to be reversible and procedures that might be viewed as "resuscitation" are often necessary, DNR orders should be suspended during intraoperative and immediate postoperative periods. The anesthesiologist, in conjunction with the patient's other attending physicians, is responsible for discussing the suspension or continuation of DNR orders during anesthesia and surgery.
  B. Determination of death. With certain qualifications applicable to neonates, the following general guidelines for the determination of irreversible coma, derived from the President's Commission for the Study of Ethical Problems in Medicine (Guideline for the determination of death. *JAMA* 245:2184, 1981), can be used to determine brain death in children.
   1. An individual with *irreversible cessation* of circulatory and respiratory function is **dead.**

    a. *Cessation* is recognized by appropriate clinical examination to disclose the absence of responsiveness, heartbeat, or respiratory effort.

    b. *Irreversibility* is recognized by persistent cessation of circulatory and respiratory functions during an appropriate period of observation or trial of resuscitative therapy.

2. An individual with *irreversible cessation* of all functions of the entire brain, including the brainstem, is **dead.**

    a. *Cessation* in this case is recognized when evaluation discloses both the absence of cerebral function and brainstem functions.

        (1) Deep coma, or cerebral unresponsivity, may require the use of confirmatory studies such as EEG or brain flow study. True decerebrate or decorticate posturing or seizures are inconsistent with brain death.

        (2) Brainstem testing requires the careful assessment of papillary light, corneal, oculocephalic, oculovestibular, oropharyngeal, and respiratory (apnea) reflexes. Peripheral nervous system activity and spinal cord reflexes may persist after death.

           (a) **Apnea testing** can be employed to assess the presence of brainstem function. Mechanical ventilation with pure oxygen or oxygen and carbon dioxide mixture is given for 10 minutes before mechanical ventilation is suspended and a passive flow of oxygen is delivered. A 10-minute period is usually sufficient to attain an arterial carbon dioxide tension ($PaCO_2$) greater than 60 mm Hg at which respiratory effort should be stimulated. Testing of arterial blood should confirm this level of hypercarbia. Spontaneous breathing effort indicates that part of the brainstem is functioning.

    b. *Irreversibility* of the cessation or brain functioning requires all of the following to be true:

        (1) The cause of the coma is established and is sufficient to account for the loss of brain functions.

        (2) The possibility of recovery of any brain function is excluded.

        (3) The cessation of all brain functions persists for an appropriate period of observation or trial of therapy. In well-established, irreversible conditions that cause cessation of brain function, a period of 12 hours of observation without brain function is usually sufficient. Anoxic brain injury and other potentially reversible conditions, such as drug intoxication, hypothermia, or shock, may require longer periods of observation. The use of the following confirmatory tests may allow earlier confirmation of irreversibility.

           (a) **Electrocerebral silence documented by EEG** verifies irreversible loss of cortical functions, except in patients with drug intoxication or hypothermia.

           (b) **Four-vessel intracranial angiography** can confirm the absence of circulation to the entire brain. Complete cessation of circulation of the normothermic adult brain for more than 10 minutes is incompatible with survival of brain tissue.

           (c) **Cerebral perfusion studies** such as radioisotope bolus cerebral angiography and gamma camera imaging with radioisotope cerebral angiography do not adequately assess brainstem perfusion.

C. Managing pediatric death and bereavement. The strongest of all grief reactions occurs when a parent loses a child. The ability of the medical team to facilitate grieving can make a significant difference in the family's experience of their loss and future attitudes towards illness and death. (see also Chap. 1, p. 5)

1. Grief reaction stages. The time course of the grief process is usually 6 to 12 months.

    a. Shock: denial and disbelief.

    b. Suffering: the acute mourning reaction

        (1) Somatic distress.

        (2) Preoccupation with the image of the deceased.

(3) Feelings of guilt.
(4) Feelings of hostility.
(5) Breakdown of normal patterns of conduct.
  c. **Resolution:** acceptance of loss, return to well-being, awareness of having grieved.
2. Normal differences in grieving
  a. One or both parents may act as a "manager" who may avoid the reality of the child's death, increase their involvement outside the home, and reject professional support.
  b. Mothers may be more expressive or more withdrawn, may feel more acutely separated, and may not want to burden other family members.
  c. Surviving siblings over 10 years old are generally able to understand that death is inevitable and irreversible. They are able to resolve the problem of loss, and do substantially better when they are included in the grief process. Children younger than 10 years of age lacking this level of understanding may assume responsibility for a sibling's death or engage in magical thinking about the death.
  d. Physical displays of grief vary with a family's cultural and religious background.
3. Strategies around the time of death
  a. Try to anticipate
    (1) Provide consistent information.
    (2) Avoid notification by telephone if at all possible.
  b. Encourage parents to hold the infant or child after death and allow them time alone.
  c. Reinforce their role in their child's life.
  d. Discuss the technical aspects of death in simple terms.
  e. Offer a postmortem examination, stressing its importance and recognizing its limitations (see sec. **E** below).
  f. Encourage a funeral, particularly for deceased newborns.
  g. Anticipate grief reactions and reassure that these feelings are normal.
  h. Establish expectation of continuing contact with the family.
    (1) Telephone contact in the first few days.
    (2) At 4 to 8 weeks, scheduled meeting with the primary team to review hospital course, postmortem results, and grieving process. Anticipate difficulties with anniversaries. Discuss genetic counseling and future pregnancies.
    (3) Telephone contact at 1 year.
D. Organ donation
  1. The disparity between the supply and demand for donor organs remains the major constraint in pediatric solid organ transplantation.
  2. Identification of the potential organ donor
    a. The single indisputable requirement for organ donation is a declaration of brain death (see sec. **B** above).
    b. The determination of brain death must be independent of the transplantation process.
    c. Local organ procurement agencies should be contacted and can provide trained personnel to respond to questions of medical team and family regarding organ donation.
  3. Contraindications for organ donation
    a. Absolute contraindications
      (1) Infectious diseases
        (a) Human immunodeficiency virus
        (b) Hepatitis B
        (c) Untreated systemic viral or bacterial disease
      (2) Systemic lupus erythematosus or other collagen vascular diseases.
      (3) Congenital metabolic disorders.
      (4) Sickle cell or other hemoglobinopathies.
      (5) Malignancies (except those confined to the central nervous system).

b. Relative contraindications

(1) Refractory hypotension.

(2) Bacterial infection localized to the central nervous system and/or adequately treated.

(3) Diabetes mellitus.

(4) Hypertension requiring treatment.

(5) Extensive burns.

(6) Central nervous system malignancy.

(7) Disseminated intravascular coagulopathy.

(8) Positive cytomegalovirus titer (if recipient is CMV negative).

4. Maintenance of optimal organ function of potentially transplantable organs, including kidneys, heart, lungs, liver, and pancreas, requires consideration of the following conditions in the brain-dead organ donor with beating heart.

a. Temperature instability. Environmental control and minimization of heat loss are recommended to maintain the donor's core body temperature above 33°C.

b. Cardiopulmonary arrest occurs in a significant number of brain-dead organ donors during the maintenance phase, resulting from

(1) Dehydration related to the use of osmotic agents and diuretics used in the treatment of cerebral edema.

(2) Exogenous fluid losses related to central diabetes insipidus.

(3) Loss of peripheral vasomotor tone related to autonomic nervous system dysfunction.

(4) Myocardial dysfunction.

c. Hemodynamic instability

(1) Hypertension related to cerebral edema may require adrenergic blocking agents (see Chap. 9, sec. VI, pp. 298 ff.).

(2) Hypotension requires intravascular volume infusions and vasopressor agents. In pediatric organ donors with refractory shock, adrenal insufficiency should be suspected (see Chap. 13, sec. VI, A, p. 396–7).

d. Respiratory instability (see Chap. 7)

(1) Because ventilation requirements are minimal in the brain-dead organ donor, excessive ventilator pressures should be avoided.

(2) Supplemental oxygen may be required to maintain adequate tissue oxygenation.

(3) Pulmonary edema related to fluid overload or other perimortem causes that result in a significant oxygenation defect can exclude lung donation.

e. Fluid and electrolyte imbalance (see Chap. 4)

(1) Central venous or pulmonary artery pressure catheters, or both, may be needed.

(2) Manage hydration according to expected maintenance, calculated deficit, and measured ongoing losses.

(3) Vasopressin replacement is recommended if urinary fluid losses due to diabetes insipidus are suspected. An initial infusion rate of 2 mU/hr may need to be increased to maintain effect. (see also pp. 391–2)

(4) Minimal cerebral glucose metabolism requires close observation for glycosuria and may necessitate insulin infusion.

(5) Bowel ischemia may result in significant gastrointestinal fluid losses.

(6) Hypocalcemia is frequently seen after extensive resuscitation efforts.

(7) Transfusion of blood products should be avoided if possible.

E. Postmortem examination

1. As an opportunity to discuss the disease process that resulted in death, the postmortem examination offers great benefits to families and care team. It

a. Facilitates the processing of grief by surviving family members.

b. Provides information pertinent to the health of family members, future pregnancies, and other patients with similar conditions.

c. Provides confirmation or refutation of pathophysiologic assumptions made before death.

2. Autopsy permission

a. Before discussing postmortem examination with next of kin, it is important to verify that the patient's death does not require notification of the Medical Examiner (see sec. **F** below).

b. In cases declined by the Medical Examiner and those that do not require Medical Examiner notification, the performance of a postmortem examination should be offered to the appropriate family member. If closest relations to the deceased patient are not present at the time of death and neither such persons nor the patient before death have expressed contrary inclination, permission may be obtained from

   (1) A spouse.

   (2) An adult son or daughter.

   (3) Either parent; if possible, both parents should give permission.

   (4) An adult sibling.

   (5) The guardian of the patient.

F. Medical examiner notification. Laws requiring notification of the Medical Examiner of the time, place, manner, circumstances, and cause of certain deaths are set at the state and local levels. Generally, the following deaths should be reported.

1. All cases of dead-on-arrival.
2. Death within 24 hours of admission.
3. Death of a patient admitted unconscious who never regained consciousness.
4. Death during surgery or any therapeutic or diagnostic procedure.
5. Death that is sudden and unexpected.
6. Death related to any kind of trauma including motor vehicle accidents.
7. Death related to an abortion.
8. Death related to a traumatic or unattended home delivery.
9. Death related to an occupational injury.
10. Death related to physical or sexual abuse.
11. Death related to malnutrition.
12. Death related to any chemical agent including poisons or drugs.
13. Death related to electrical or thermal injury.
14. Death due to drowning.

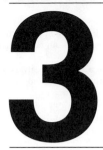

Principles of Normal Newborn, Well-Child, and Adolescent Care

Shari Nethersole, Sara Foreman, and Charles F. Simmons

I. **General assessment and management of the healthy newborn**
   A. **Physical examination of the newborn.** At birth, more information is obtained from the general overall visual and auditory appraisal of a naked infant than from an exhaustive system-by-system examination.

   On initial examination, four categories are of the utmost importance: **cardiorespiratory status;** the **presence of congenital anomalies;** the **effects of gestation, labor, delivery, and maternal medications;** and **signs of infection or other systemic disease.** A fretful infant should be quieted with a nipple. A useful sequence of examination is as follows.
   1. **Respiratory**
      a. Evaluation includes color, presence of acrocyanosis (quite common in the first 24–48 hours of life), and respiratory rate (normal 40–60 and often periodic).
      b. Retractions, nasal flaring, and respiratory grunting are abnormal in the absence of crying.
   2. **Cardiac**
      a. Evaluation includes the position of maximal impulse, palpation of femoral or dorsalis pedis pulses, and auscultation of the heart for rate (generally 120–160 beats per minute; occasionally <100 in term or postterm infants at rest), rhythm, and presence of murmurs.
      b. Because of rapid alterations in systemic and pulmonary pressures, **murmurs,** especially in the first 24 hours of life, usually do not reflect the presence of significant heart disease.
      c. Distant heart sounds, especially if accompanied by respiratory distress, may be secondary to pneumomediastinum or pneumothorax.
   3. **Abdomen**
      a. Observe for asymmetry (including the musculature), masses, and fullness.
      b. Bowel sounds may or may not be present.
      c. Palpate with gentle pressure to determine the size of the liver (may extend 2.5 cm below the right costal margin) or spleen (generally, at most, a tip may be palpable). Palpate *deeply* for both kidneys.
   4. **Genitalia and rectum**
      a. In boys, observe for presence of both testes, and normal placement and patency of the urethral orifice and anus. The testes should be similar in size and should not appear blue through the scrotum (a sign of torsion). Hydroceles are common.
      b. In girls, in addition to observing for anal patency, one should search for interlabial masses; mucosal vaginal tags are normal. A **mucoid vaginal discharge** (occasionally blood streaked) is often noted.
   5. **Skin**
      a. Jaundice in the first day of life is abnormal and an investigation for the cause should ensue (see Chap. 6). Mild jaundice on subsequent days is common.
      b. Common findings are
         (1) Milia (tiny yellow papules, representing blocked sebaceous glands, usually found on the nose and cheeks).

    (2) Mongolian spots (bluish, often large, patches most commonly found on back, buttocks, or thighs of infants of Asian or black background).

    (3) Erythema toxicum (papular or vesicular lesions on an erythematous base, seen on the torso and limbs).

    (4) Pustular melanosis (small, superficial pustules that easily rupture, leaving hyperpigmented macules and seen most commonly in black infants).

6. Extremities, spine, and joints

    a. Observe for anomalies of the digits, hand creases, structural abnormalities (especially in the sacral area), hip dislocation, and positional deformities.

    b. The clavicles should be palpated to detect fractures.

7. Head, neck, and mouth

    a. Inspect for cuts, bruises, caput, cephalohematoma, mobility of suture lines, and skull molding.

    b. Measure the head circumference from occiput to midbrow—generally 31 to 36 cm at term (Fig. 3-1).

    c. Observe for neck flexibility and asymmetry.

    d. Inspect for cleft palate.

8. Neurologic examination. Observations for neurologic status can usually be made concurrently while handling the baby for the preceding examinations. Observe for tone, activity, symmetry of the extremities and facial movements,

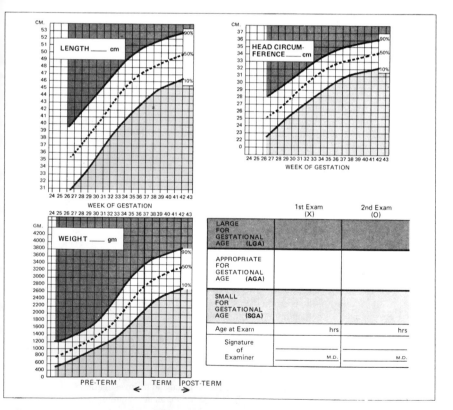

Fig. 3-1. Classification of newborns based on maturity and intrauterine growth. (Adapted from LC Lubchenco, C Hansman, E Boyd. *Pediatrics* 37:403, 1966; and FC Battaglia, LC Lubchenco. *J Pediatr* 71:159, 1967. Copyright © 1978, Mead Johnson & Co, Evansville, IN.

alertness, consolability, and reflexes, including the Moro, suck, root, grasp, and plantar reflexes.

9. **Eye examination.** (Periorbital edema in first few days of life may interfere.)
    a. Usually, the presence of cataracts and tumors can be largely ruled out by elicitation of the *red reflex.*
    b. Scleral hemorrhage (very common) and pupillary size and shape can be assessed.
    c. All infants should have received prophylaxis for bacterial conjunctivitis with topical ophthalmic ointments—tetracycline 1%, erythromycin 1%, or silver nitrate 1%.
10. The **discharge examination** should include attention to overall appearance, cardiac status (cyanosis, congestive heart failure, or new murmur), abdomen (masses), skin (jaundice, pustules), cord (infection), and circumcision wound. Additionally, feeding, amount of weight loss, and stool/urine output should be reviewed. Maternal preparation should be assessed and medical follow-up established.

B. **Nursery care**
1. **Temperature control.** Heat loss may be minimized by placing an infant in a neutral thermal environment, the thermal condition at which heat production is minimal yet core temperature is within normal range. **Hypothermia can produce apnea, hypoxemia, hypoglycemia, and acidosis.** In the healthy infant, the skin should be dried, wet towels removed, and the infant wrapped. Examination in the delivery room should be performed under a radiant warmer with a skin probe, keeping the skin temperature at 36.5°C (97.7°F). Appropriate clinical judgment will determine need for radiant warmer, isolette, or open crib.
2. **Feeding and nutrition.** Growth requirements for full-term neonates are 90 to 120 kcal/kg/day. The protein requirement is 2 to 3 g/kg/day. Fat should make up 30 to 50% of caloric intake, protein 7 to 15%, and carbohydrate 30 to 65%.
    a. **Breast feeding**
        (1) Breast milk is of proved nutritional, immunologic, and emotional value for the feeding of the full-term and preterm infant, and should be encouraged for all full-term and most preterm infants.
        (2) Human milk contains antimicrobial components not found in infant formulas: immunoglobulins, leukocytes, lactoferrin, the third component of complement in colostrum, and lysozymes. **In areas in which sanitation is poor, the use of nonhuman milk formulas has been clearly associated with increased infant mortality from infection.**
        (3) Fostering successful breast feeding
            (a) Both the obstetrician and the pediatrician should discuss and encourage nursing prenatally with the mother.
            (b) Experienced nursing mothers should be available to discuss the satisfaction and techniques of breast feeding with expectant mothers.
            (c) Obstetric ward and neonatal unit practices should support successful nursing including
                (i) Decreasing the amount of sedation or anesthesia given to mothers.
                (ii) Encouraging the mother to nurse the infant immediately after delivery, if possible.
                (iii) Encouraging "rooming in" to avoid separation of mother and infant.
                (iv) Having infants fed on demand rather than on a rigid schedule.
                (v) Discouraging the routine use of "supplemental" water or formula by nursery personnel, unless absolutely necessary.
    b. **Formula feeding for full-term infants.** A number of commercially available formulas are adequate (Table 3-1). Those based on cow's milk

Table 3-1. Human milk and formula composition

Formula (distributor)	kcal/30 ml	Protein (g/dl)	Fat (g/dl)	Carbohydrate (g/dl)	Minerals (mg/dl)			Electrolytes (mEq/dl)			Vitamins (IU/dl)			Folate (mg/dl)	Osmolality (mOsm/kg)	Renal solute load (mOsm/liter)[b]
					Ca	P	Fe[a]	Na+	K+	Cl−	A	D	E			
Breast milk (composition varies)	20–22	1.1	4.5	7.1	33	15	0.03	0.8	1.4	1.1	250	2.2	0.18	5.0	290–300	75
Standard cow's milk–based formulas																
Similac 20 (Ross)	20	1.5	3.6	7.2	51	39	0.15 (1.2)	0.8	1.9	1.3	203	41	2.0	10	300	100
Enfamil (Mead Johnson)	20	1.5	3.8	6.9	46	32	0.11 (1.3)	0.8	1.8	1.2	210	41.5	2.1	10.5	300	98
Similac 24 (Ross)	24	2.2	4.3	8.5	73	56	0.18 (1.5)	1.2	2.7	1.9	244	49	2.4	12	380	146
Enfamil 24 (Mead Johnson)	24	1.8	4.5	8.3	56	38	0.13 (1.5)	1.0	2.2	1.4	251	50	2.5	13	360	117
Soy formulas																
Isomil (Ross)	20	1.8	3.7	6.8	71	51	1.2	1.4	1.9	1.2	203	41	2.0	10.0	240	116
Prosobee (Mead Johnson)	20	2.0	3.6	6.8	63	50	1.3	1.0	2.1	1.6	208	41.5	2.1	10.5	200	127

Preterm formulas[c]

Similac Special Care (Ross)	24	2.2	4.4	8.6	146	73	0.3 (1.5)	1.5	2.7	1.9	552	122	3.2	30	300	149
Enfamil Premature (Mead Johnson)	24	2.4	4.1	8.9	134	68	0.2	1.4	2.3	2.0	970	220	3.7	29	300	153

Specialized formulas

Pregestimil (Mead Johnson)	20	1.9	3.8	6.9	63	42	1.3	1.4	1.9	1.6	250	51	2.5	10.5	320	125
Nutramigen (Mead Johnson)	20	1.9	2.6	9.1	63	42	1.3	1.4	1.9	1.6	208	42	2.1	10.5	320	125
Portagen (Mead Johnson)	20	2.4	3.2	7.8	63	48	1.3	1.6	2.2	1.6	530	53	2.1	10.5	220	152
Similac PM 60/40 (Ross)	20	1.6	3.8	6.9	38	19	0.15	0.7	1.5	1.1	203	41	2.0	10.0	280	96
Similac 27 (Ross)	27	2.5	4.8	9.6	82	64	0.2	1.4	3.1	2.1	274	55	2.7	14.0	430	164

Ca = calcium; P = phosphorus; Fe = iron; Na$^+$ = sodium; K$^+$ = potassium; Cl$^-$ = chloride.

[a]In instances in which high and low Fe formulations are available, the low Fe value appears.

[b]Estimated renal solute load = [protein (g) × 4] + [Na(mEq) + K(mEq) + Cl(mEq)].

[c]20 kcal/30 ml formulations are also available.

Source: JP Cloherty, AR Stark (eds). *Manual of Neonatal Care* (3rd ed). Boston: Little, Brown, 1991. Pp 538–539.

(e.g., Similac, Enfamil) are the usual formulas for full-term infants under most circumstances. For special circumstances other formulas may be needed.

(1) Soy-based formulas should be reserved for special situations, such as a strong history of cow's milk intolerance.

(2) For most industrialized countries, the practice of boiling water for preparation of powdered or concentrated infant formula is not necessary and may inadvertently concentrate nonbiologic impurities from the cooking vessel itself.

c. **Supplements (vitamins, iron) for full-term infants. All newborns should receive vitamin K** (vitamin K oxide, 1.0 mg IM; 0.5 mg IM if <1,500 g) at birth.

(1) **Breast-fed infants**

(a) There is no conclusive evidence that healthy, breast-fed infants of well-nourished mothers require vitamin supplementation **provided** that sunlight exposure is adequate for vitamin D synthesis (see p. 48).

(b) The use of iron supplements in breast-fed infants is controversial.

(2) **Formula-fed infants.** Formulas usually contain adequate vitamins (1 qt formula/day). Only iron-fortified formula should be used, *not* "low-iron" formula. If low-iron formula is used, iron supplementation after 8 weeks of age may be necessary (2 mg/kg/day elemental iron).

d. **Special nutritional needs of the well low-birth-weight infant**

(1) **Nutritional requirements.** Daily caloric requirements for premature infants are 50 to 100 kcal/kg/day by 3 days of age and 110 to 150 kcal/kg/day during later growth.

(2) **Formulas for premature infants.** The caloric, protein, and calcium requirements for premature infants are somewhat higher than those for term infants.

(a) **Breast milk.** Premature infants should receive breast milk whenever possible. Appropriate supplementation can be provided by adding milk fortification (Human Milk Fortifier or Natural Care; Table 3-2) to adjust caloric density to 24 kcal/oz.

(b) **Formula feeding.** Modified formulas (e.g., Special Care or Enfamil Premature) are acceptable alternatives to breast milk. These have higher whey-casein and calcium-phosphorus ratios, and are supplied in kcal/oz concentrations (see Table 3-1). Increased caloric content may be achieved by use of carbohydrate or fat supplements (Table 3-3).

(3) **Fluid requirements of premature infants.** Fluid intake of low-birth-weight infants should increase from 75 ml/kg/day on day 1 to approximately 150 ml/kg/day after day 5 (see Chaps. 4 and 6, p. 213).

(4) **Feeding techniques.** Coordinated sucking and swallowing may not mature until 34 to 35 weeks' gestational age. Direct breast feeding can be attempted but may not be successful. Such infants can be fed using smaller/softer nipples.

(a) **Gavage feeding.** For infants who are too immature for oral feedings, enteral feedings can be administered by gavage.

(b) **Intravenous supplementation**

(i) If the infant is under 1,500 g, start an IV line with 10% dextrose in water (D/W) at 75 to 100 ml/kg/day. Decrease this IV fluid supplement as gavage volume increases until gavage feedings exceed 100 ml/kg/day.

(ii) Electrolyte supplementation may be necessary if IV support is required beyond the first day.

(5) **Keep gastric intake below 200 ml/kg/day to avoid aspiration.** Infants who need to suck in excess of their appetite can be appeased with pacifiers, which also appear to improve gastric motility.

Table 3-2. Oral dietary supplements

	Supplements		Human milk (dl)* (approximate value)	
Nutrient	Enfamil Human Milk Fortifier (Mead Johnson) per 4 packets	Similac Natural Care (Ross) per dl	Plus 4 packets Enfamil HMF (Mead Johnson) per dl	Diluted 1:1 with Natural Care (Ross) per dl
Energy (kcal)	14	81	81	77
Protein (g)	0.7	2.2	1.73	1.6
Fat (g)	<0.1	4.4	4.0	4.2
Carbohydrate (g)	2.7	8.6	9.9	7.9
Minerals				
Calcium (mg)	90	171	118	100
Phosphorus (mg)	45	85	59	50
Magnesium (mg)	—	10	3.5	6.8
Sodium (mEq)	0.3	1.5	1.1	1.1
Potassium (mEq)	0.4	2.7	1.8	2.0
Chloride (mEq)	0.5	1.1	1.7	1.5
Zinc (mg)	0.71	1.9	0.83	0.7
Copper (μg)	80	203	105	114
Manganese (μg)	9	10	9.4	5.3
Vitamins				
A (IU)	780	552	1,003	388
D (IU)	210	122	212	62
E (IU)	3.4	3.2	3.6	1.7
K (IU)	9.1	10	9.3	5.1
Thiamine (μg)	187	203	208	112
Riboflavin (μg)	250	503	285	269
Niacin (μg)	3,100	4,060	3,220	2,105
Pantothenate (μg)	790	1,543	970	862
Pyridoxine (μg)	193	203	213	112
Biotin (μg)	0.81	30	1.2	15.2
Vitamin B_{12} (μg)	0.21	0.45	0.25	0.25
Vitamin C (mg)	24	30	28	17
Folate (μg)	23	30	28	18

*Milk-based and soy-based infant formulas for feeding infants in the hospital. Ross Laboratories, Columbus, OH, 1989.
Source: JP Cloherty, AR Stark (eds). *Manual of Neonatal Care* (3rd ed). Boston: Little, Brown, 1991. P 540.

    (6) Close monitoring
        (a) Follow serum glucose carefully, starting at birth, at 1 and 2 hours of age, and then before feeds until the infant's condition is stable. Hypoglycemia can result if the IV supplement stops abruptly.
        (b) Monitor urine specific gravity, skin turgor, body weight, serum and urine osmolarity, and electrolyte concentrations as necessary.
    (7) Supplements
        (a) Calories. Caloric concentration of formula should not exceed 30 calories/oz. A caloric concentration of 24 calories/oz is usually sufficient (see Tables 3-1 and 3-3).

Table 3-3. Oral dietary supplements available for use in infants

Nutrient	Product	Source	Energy content
Fat	MCT oil (Mead Johnson)	Medium-chain triglycerides	8.3 kcal/g 7.7 kcal/ml
	Corn oil	Long-chain triglycerides	9 kcal/gm 8.4 kcal/ml
Carbohydrate	Polycose (Ross)	Glucose polymers	4 kcal/g 8 kcal/tsp (powder) 2 kcal/ml (liquid)
Protein	Casec (Mead Johnson)	Calcium caseinate	3.7 kcal/g 5.8 kcal/tsp
	Promod (Ross)	Whey concentrate	4.2 kcal/g 5.7 kcal/tsp

Source: JP Cloherty, AR Stark (eds). *Manual of Neonatal Care* (3rd ed). Boston: Little, Brown, 1991. P 543.

> (i) **Carbohydrates.** Glucose polymer (Polycose) provides 8 kcal/tsp (powder) or 2 kcal/ml (liquid).
> (ii) **Fat.** Medium-chain triglyceride (MCT) oil provides 7.7 calories/ml.
>
> (b) **Vitamins.** Vitamin supplementation is begun as soon as the infant is receiving full volume feedings.
> > (i) Vitamin supplementation is needed for preterm babies in order to meet recommended intakes, particularly with respect to vitamin D (400 IU/day) and folate (50–65 μg/day).
> > (ii) Liquid drop preparations currently available in the United States for infants contain either vitamins A, C, and D or vitamins A, C, D, thiamine, riboflavin, niacin, B_6, B_{12}, and E. Folate is not included because it is relatively unstable in solutions.
>
> (c) **Calcium.** Supplemental calcium (150 mg/kg/day elemental calcium is the recommended total daily consumption) may be necessary because formulas commonly used for full-term infants contain approximately 44 to 53 mg/dl calcium. Premature infant formulas (see Table 3-1) contain sufficient calcium such that supplementation is rarely necessary.

(8) Infants who are unable to tolerate oral gavage feedings need parenteral nutrition (see Chap. 11).

II. **Anticipation of common problems** (see also Chap. 6)

A. **Premature infants** (under 37 weeks' gestation)

1. **Thermal regulation.** Premature infants experience more rapid heat loss than do term infants. Management usually requires an overhead radiant warmer or a closed incubator for infants less than 1,800 g.

2. **Respiration.** Many healthy premature infants have **transient tachypnea** from delayed resorption of fetal lung fluid. This may be distinguished from hyaline membrane disease or pneumonia, which would require immediate aggressive treatment (see Chap. 6).

3. **Apnea.** Significant **apnea** will occur in 5 to 10% of 33- to 34-week-old infants. The rate is higher for less mature prematures. All infants younger than 34 to 35 weeks old should be monitored until they are apnea free for up to 5 days.

4. **Cardiovascular.** Careful computation of fluids is essential. Inadvertent fluid overload can promote patent ductus arteriosus.

5. **Hematologic.** Anemia is common, both iatrogenic and physiologic (nadir at 4–6 weeks). This should be monitored. Treatment is described in Chapter 6.

      6. Hyperbilirubinemia, hypoglycemia, hypocalcemia, and hyponatremia are common.
  B. Small-for-gestational-age (SGA) infants (birth weight below the 10th percentile for gestational age; see Fig. 3-1)

    1. During **pregnancy,** identification, evaluation, and monitoring of fetal growth and well-being are essential. Possible causes of intrauterine growth retardation should be investigated. A standard workup includes a review of obstetric causes, examination for identifiable syndromes, and laboratory evaluation for congenital infection (particularly cytomegalovirus). Examination of the placenta is frequently useful.

    2. At delivery, anticipate possible fetal distress, perinatal depression, meconium aspiration, hypoxia, and heat loss.

    3. In the newborn, monitor for hypothermia, polycythemia, hypoglycemia, and hypocalcemia.

    4. Leukopenia, neutropenia, and thrombocytopenia are often seen in infants born to *hypertensive* mothers.

    5. SGA infants should receive early feeds.

  C. Large-for-gestational-age (LGA) infants (birth weight over the 90th percentile for gestational age; see Fig. 3-1). These infants are at high risk of **birth trauma,** including clavicular fractures, brachial plexus injuries, and perinatal depression. **Hypoglycemia** and **polycythemia** should be anticipated.

  D. Postmature infants (gestation over 42 weeks). These infants are unusually susceptible to **placental insufficiency.** As a result, fetal distress, meconium aspiration, and neonatal hypoglycemia occur more frequently.

    1. Management during pregnancy includes careful estimation of fetal gestational age by dates and ultrasound. Monitoring of fetal well-being should start at 41 weeks and especially during labor.

    2. Affected infants should receive early feeds and monitoring for hypoglycemia and polycythemia.

  E. Common signs and symptoms. Newborns manifest illness in a limited number of signs and symptoms. These should prompt evaluation for specific illnesses detailed in Chapter 6.

    1. Respiratory distress. Most infants have some tachypnea during the first minutes of life. Infants with sustained tachypnea, audible grunting, retracting, or flaring should be evaluated.

    2. Cyanosis. Cyanosis in the context of respiratory distress is an emergency. Other causes of cyanosis are
      a. Polycythemia.
      b. Hypothermia.
      c. Apnea, choking, or airway obstruction.
      d. Cyanotic congenital heart disease.

    3. Apnea. Apnea in term infants is a serious symptom. Apnea in prematures is common but should be evaluated with the first episode. Causes include
      a. Infection (systemic or meningitis).
      b. Central nervous system (malformation, bleed, or infection).
      c. Respiratory obstruction (aspiration, anatomic).

    4. Lethargy. Sleepiness in newborns is common, but marked lethargy should prompt evaluation for
      a. Sepsis or meningitis.
      b. Metabolic disturbances.
      c. Neurologic insults.

III. General principles of well child and adolescent care. The chief functions of well child and adolescent care are **health assessment, prevention, screening,** and **triage.** As part of this, providers need to take the time to

Establish a relationship of trust and open communication.
Gain an understanding of the child's cultural, ethnic, religious, and socioeconomic background.
Inquire about the child's environment.

Detect stresses that affect the family.
Determine risks of genetically transmitted diseases.
Detect early disease by a history, physical examination, and screening tests.
Detect early developmental and behavioral problems and monitor their remediation.
Provide health maintenance (i.e., immunizations, information on nutrition).
Provide appropriate counseling and anticipatory guidance.
Provide referral with specific documentation to specialists when knowledge, time, or diagnostic resources are insufficient for appropriate management.
Provide prompt follow-up and coordination of specialty care as needed.
Provide advocacy for the patient and family as needed when other caretakers are involved.

A. Frequency of visits. The American Academy of Pediatrics (AAP) has made recommendations for the minimum number of health supervision visits that all children should have. The recommendations are visits at 1 to 2 weeks, 2 months, 4 months, 6 months, 9 months, 12 months, 15 months, 18 months, 2 years, 3 years, 4 years, and 5 years, with visits every 2 years thereafter. (Some providers combine the 9-month and 12-month visits.) Table 3-4 shows the recommended schedule and care guidelines. Increased visit frequency is recommended for parents with a particular need for guidance or education, those who come from a disadvantaged social or economic environment, and patients with perinatal disease, congenital defects, or acquired illness of a chronic nature.

The American Medical Association (AMA) published *Guidelines for Adolescent Preventive Services* (GAPS) in 1992, which provides a set of recommendations to help direct practitioners in the care of teens (Table 3-5). GAPS recommends annual preventive services visits for adolescents from ages 11 to 21 to screen for high-risk behaviors and to promote healthy lifestyles, including fitness, diet, and injury prevention. Physical examinations should be performed during early (11–14 yr), middle (15–17 yr), and late (18–21 yr) adolescence unless more frequently warranted by symptoms and need for sports or camp physical examinations. Sexually active females require **at least annual gynecologic assessments** for Papanicolaou (Pap) and sexually transmitted disease (STD) screening regardless of age.

B. Goals of health maintenance visits
  1. Assess growth and development
    a. Height and weight charts. Height and weight should be plotted at each well child visit on a National Center for Health Statistics (NCHS) growth chart (Figs. 3-2 through 3-5). It should be kept in mind that these charts are normed for American-born children and may not be valid for specific ethnic or racial groups. Head circumference should be recorded for at least the first 12 months of life. The NCHS charts include a graph of the weight-to-height ratio, which can be helpful in judging whether a child is underweight or overweight for height. Sequential measurements are much more useful than single determinations of weight and height in giving an overall picture of the child's growth pattern. When in doubt, incremental growth charts should be used.
    b. Simple **screening tests,** such as the Denver Developmental Screening Test (DDST; Fig. 3-6), can be used to detect infants who require further evaluation for possible delays in gross motor, fine motor, language, and social skills. The abbreviated revised DDST is a more efficient screen that requires only 5 to 7 minutes to administer. Table 3-6 summarizes usual ages of attainment of developmental milestones.
  2. Screening. Because parents often notice abnormalities before they become evident to the pediatrician, *the best screening test is a good history.*
    a. Simple testing includes visual and hearing acuity and tuberculosis skin tests.
    b. Simple laboratory tests include screens for anemia, lead poisoning, and pyuria. Guidelines for appropriate times for these screens are suggested by the AAP (see Table 3-4).

3. **Physical examination.** Physical examination serves to verify normalcy for the parent's benefit, and to pick up abnormalities that may not have been previously noted. Examples include strabismus, heart murmurs, abdominal masses, orthopedic anomalies (e.g., internal tibial torsion, developmental dysplasia of the hip), hypertension, and dental problems.

4. **Immunizations.** The AAP and the Advisory Committee on Immunization Practices (ACIP) have recommended a schedule for routine active immunization of normal infants and children. This schedule allows for some variability in the timing of certain immunizations, while encouraging immunization as early in life as the vaccines can have efficacy (Table 3-7). This schedule is appropriate for premature and low-birth-weight infants with the exception that oral polio vaccine (OPV) should always be given after discharge from the hospital (see sec. **c.(1)** below). Table 3-8 includes a schedule for primary immunization of children not immunized in infancy. In children more than 6 years of age, the adult-type diphtheria tetanus (Td) vaccine is preferred over the diphtheria-pertussis-tetanus (DPT) vaccine. Because recommendations are often revised, one should consult the *Morbidity and Morality Weekly Reports* or the AAP's *Report of the Committee on Infectious Diseases* (The Redbook) for the most current information.

   a. **Informed consent.** The AAP has emphasized the importance of providing patients and parents with benefit and risk statements about vaccines in lay terminology. The Centers for Disease Control (CDC) has developed "vaccine information sheets," which are available from the immunization divisions of state health departments. Current recommendations from the AAP state that *parents' signatures on a form are not as important as making sure the information is understood and consent given.* Consent should be documented in the medical record.

   b. **Scheduling—other considerations**
      (1) **Acute febrile illness.** Postpone immunization; **do not postpone** for minor illnesses such as upper respiratory infections or nonfebrile otitis media.
      (2) **Unknown immunization status.** Consider child susceptible and immunize.
      (3) **Lapse in routine immunization schedule.** This does not interfere with immune response. It is unnecessary to repeat doses. **Do not give any reduced dosages,** as this may induce inadequate immune response.
      (4) **Prior anaphylactoid reaction** to same or related vaccine. Defer immunization until skin testing is performed.

   c. **Contraindications to live virus vaccines** (trivalent oral polio vaccine [TOPV], measles-mumps-rubella, varicella)
      (1) **Immunodeficiency.** Patients infected with human immunodeficiency virus (HIV) should receive measles-mumps-rubella (MMR) vaccine, as the risk of measles is thought to outweigh the risks of the vaccine. Varicella vaccination is currently not recommended in immunocompromised children, including children with HIV. Use of varicella vaccine in healthy children living in a household with immunocompromised individuals is recommended. Immunodeficient patients or children living in a household with an immunodeficient person can be given killed polio vaccine (IPV), rather than TOPV.
         Hospitalized children should not be given OPV because of the possibility of transmission of the vaccine virus to an immunosuppressed person.
      (2) **Immunosuppressed individuals,** including those receiving radiation therapy, steroids, or antimetabolites. Children receiving alternate-day steroids at low to moderate doses or those on short-term steroids (i.e., asthmatics) can be immunized.
      (3) **Pregnancy.** Pregnant women should **not** receive live viral vaccines. However, it is permissible to give live vaccine to a household contact of a pregnant woman.

Table 3-4. Recommendations for Preventive Pediatric Health Care[a]

	Newborn	2–4 d[b]	By 1 mo	2 mo	4 mo	6 mo	9 mo	12 mo	15 mo	18 mo	24 mo	3 yr	4 yr	5 yr	6 yr	8 yr	10 yr
	Infancy								Early childhood					Middle childhood			
History																	
Initial/interval	•	•	•	•	•	•	•	•	•	•	•	•	•	•	•	•	•
Measurements																	
Height and weight	•	•	•	•	•	•	•	•	•	•	•	•	•	•	•	•	•
Head circumference	•	•	•	•	•	•	•	•	•	•	•						
Blood pressure												•	•	•	•	•	•
Sensory screening																	
Vision	S	S	S	S	S	S	S	S	S	S	S	O	O	O	S	S	O
Hearing[c]	S/O	S	S	S	S	S	S	S	S	S	S	O	O	O	S	S	O
Developmental/behavioral assessment	•	•	•	•	•	•	•	•	•	•	•	•	•	•	•	•	•
Physical examination	•	•	•	•	•	•	•	•	•	•	•	•	•	•	•	•	•

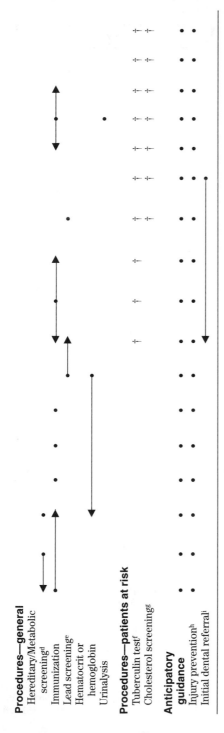

Procedures—general
Hereditary/Metabolic screening[d]
Immunization
Lead screening[e]
Hematocrit or hemoglobin
Urinalysis

Procedures—patients at risk
Tuberculin test[f]
Cholesterol screening[g]

Anticipatory guidance
Injury prevention[h]
Initial dental referral[i]

• = to be performed; † = to be performed for patients at risk; S = subjective, by history; O = objective, by a standard testing method; ←•—▶ = the range during which a service may be provided, with the dot indicating the preferred age.

[a]These guidelines are for the care of children who are receiving competent parenting, who have no important health problems, and whose growth and development are satisfactory. They represent a consensus by the Committee on Practice and Ambulatory Medicine in consultation with the American Academy of Pediatrics.

[b]For newborns discharged in less than 48 hr after delivery.

[c]Some experts recommend objective appraisal of hearing in the newborn period. The Joint Committee on Infant Hearing has identified patients at significant risk for hearing loss. All children who meet these criteria should be objectively screened. See the Joint Committee on Infant Hearing 1994 Position Statement.

[d]Metabolic screening (e.g., thyroid, hemoglobinopathies, phenylketonuria, galactosemia) should be done according to state law.

[e]Blood lead screen per AAP statement "Lead Poisoning: From Screening to Primary Prevention" (1993).

[f]Tuberculosis testing per AAP statement "Screening for Tuberculosis in Infants and Children" (1994). Testing should be done on recognition of high risk factors. If results are negative but the high-risk situation continues, testing should be repeated on an annual basis.

[g]Cholesterol screening for high-risk patients per AAP "Statement on Cholesterol" (1992).

[h]From birth to age 12, refer to AAP's injury prevention program (TIPP) as described in "A Guide to Safety Counseling in Office Practice" (1994).

[i]Earlier initial dental evaluations may be appropriate for some children. Subsequent examinations as prescribed by dentist.

Source: Modified from Committee on Practice and Ambulatory Medicine, AAP. Recommendations for preventive pediatric health care. *Pediatrics* 96:373–374, 1995.

Table 3-5. Summary of GAPS preventive services

Service	Frequency
Health Guidance	
Parenting	Early adolescence (11–14 yr), Middle adolescence (15–17 yr)
Adolescent development	Annually
Safety practices	Annually
Diet and fitness	Annually
Healthy lifestyles (sexual behavior, smoking, alcohol and drug use)	Annually
Screening	
Hypertension	Annually
Hyperlipidemia	Early adolescence, if at risk;[a] late adolescence
Eating disorders	Annually
Obesity	Annually
Tobacco use	Annually
Drug and alcohol use	Annually
Sexual behavior	Annually
Sexually transmitted diseases (STDs)	
Gonorrhea	Annually, if sexually active
Chlamydia	Annually, if sexually active
Genital warts	Annually, if sexually active
Syphilis	If at high risk[b]
HIV infection	Offer test, if at high risk[b]
Cervical cancer	Annually, if sexually active; ≥age 18 yr
Depression/suicide risk	Annually
Physical, sexual, or emotional abuse	Annually
Learning problems	Annually
Tuberculosis (TB)	If at high risk[c]
Immunizations	Appropriate for age

GAPS = Guidelines for adolescent preventive services.
[a]High risk if there is a family history of hyperlipidemia, family history of cardiovascular disease, or if family history is unknown.
[b]High risk is having had more than one sexual partner in the past 6 months, having exchanged sex for drugs, being a male who has engaged in sex with other males, having used IV drugs, having had other STDs, having lived in an area that was endemic for the infection, or having had a sexual partner who is at risk for the infection.
[c]High risk is those who have been exposed to active TB, have lived in a homeless shelter, have been incarcerated, have lived in an area endemic for TB, or who are currently working in a health care setting.
Source: Modified from *Guidelines for Adolescent Preventive Services, Recommendations Monograph*, 2nd ed, American Medical Association, p. 2, 1995.

    d. Contraindications to pertussis vaccine (see also sec. **e.(1)**). Currently, these apply to both whole-cell pertussis vaccine (DTP) and acellular pertussis vaccine (DTaP).
        (1) Evolving neurologic disorders (e.g., infantile spasms, uncontrolled epilepsy, progressive encephalopathy).
        (2) Personal history of seizure—begun recently or not well controlled; this does **not** include a family history of seizures.
        (3) Neurologic conditions that predispose to seizure or neurologic deterioration (e.g., metabolic and degenerative disease, tuberous sclerosis).
    e. Common side effects of vaccines. Parents should be advised that side effects may occur, but that the incidence and severity of these side effects

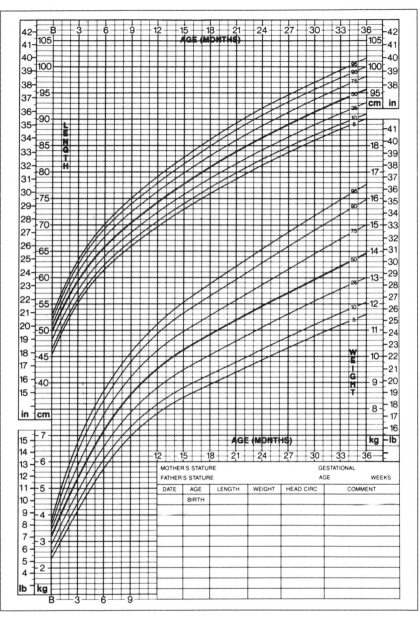

Fig. 3-2. Physical growth of girls from birth to 36 months of age. NCHS percentiles. (Adapted from PVV Hamill et al. Physical growth: National Center for Health Statistics percentiles. *Am J Clin Nutr* 32:607, 1979. Data from the Fels Research Institute, Wright State University School of Medicine, Yellow Springs, OH. © 1982 by Ross Laboratories, Columbus, OH.)

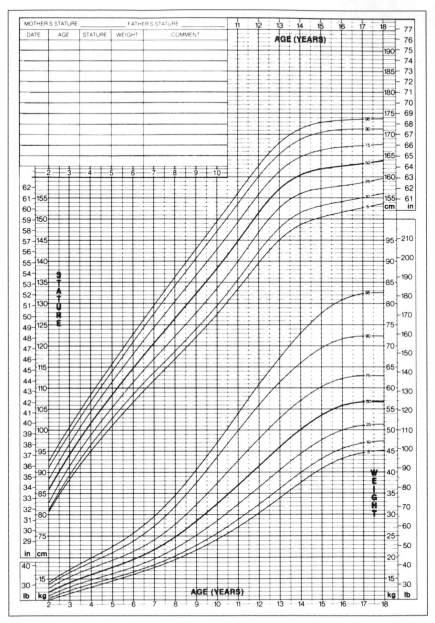

Fig. 3-3. Physical growth of girls from 2 to 18 years of age. NCHS percentiles. (Adapted from PVV Hamill et al. Physical growth: National Center for Health Statistics percentiles. *Am J Clin Nutr* 32:607, 1979. Data from the National Center for Health Statistics, Hyattsville, MD. © 1982 by Ross Laboratories, Columbus, OH.)

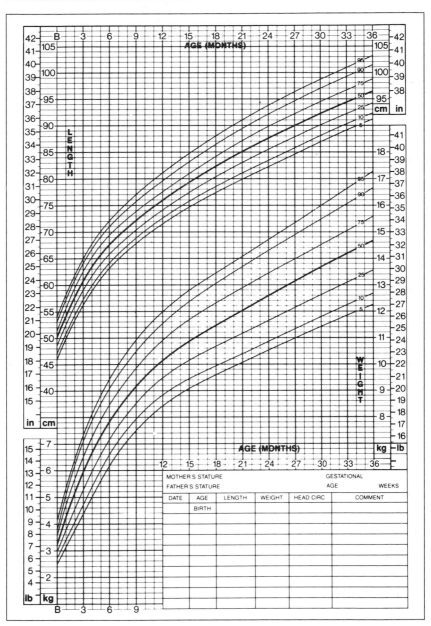

Fig. 3-4. Physical growth of boys from birth to 36 months of age. NCHS percentiles. (Adapted from PVV Hamill et al. Physical growth: National Center for Health Statistics percentiles. *Am J Clin Nutr* 32:607, 1979. Data from the Fels Research Institute, Wright State University School of Medicine, Yellow Springs, OH. © 1982 by Ross Laboratories, Columbus, OH.)

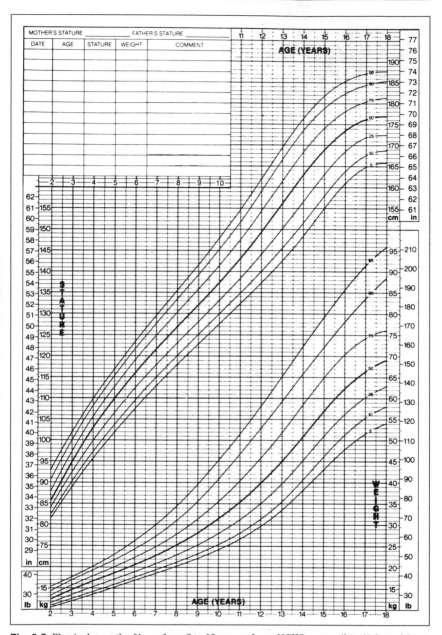

Fig. 3-5. Physical growth of boys from 2 to 18 years of age. NCHS percentiles. (Adapted from PVV Hamill et al. Physical growth: National Center for Health Statistics percentiles. *Am J Clin Nutr* 32:607, 1979. Data from the National Center for Health Statistics, Hyattsville, MD. © 1982 by Ross Laboratories, Columbus, OH.)

are far exceeded by the risks and damages of the diseases against which vaccines afford protection.

(1) **Pertussis** (symptoms occur within 48–72 hours of injection). Local reactions include pain, and redness and swelling. Systemic side effects include fever greater than 38°C, as well as fretfulness or irritability. Rare, more serious side effects can occur and these may contraindicate further vaccination with pertussis.

   (a) The following adverse events would contraindicate further vaccination with DTP or DTaP:

   (i) Encephalopathy within 7 days.

   (ii) An allergic (anaphylactic) reaction to vaccine.

   (b) The following adverse events would contraindicate further vaccination with DTP, but vaccination with DTaP may still be warranted, depending on risk of exposure:

   (i) Seizure with or without fever, within 3 days.

   (ii) Persistent inconsolable crying for 3 or more hours or an unusual, high-pitched cry, within 48 hours.

   (iii) Shocklike state (hypotonic-hyporesponsive episode), within 48 hours.

   (iv) Temperature of 40.5°C (104.9°F) or greater, unexplained by another cause, within 48 hours.

(2) **MMR.** A temperature of 39.4°C (103°F) or more may develop between the sixth and tenth day after vaccination and last 1 to 2 days. Transient rashes and arthralgias may occur.

(3) *Haemophilus influenzae* **type B (Hib).** Mild local reactions (erythema or swelling) may occur and usually resolve within 24 hours. Systemic reactions are rare.

(4) **TOPV.** Minute risks of producing poliomyelitis.

(5) **IPV.** Mild local reactions only.

(6) **Hepatitis B.** Minor local reaction and low-grade fever for 24 hours.

(7) **Varicella.** Minor local reaction; a mild vesicular rash may develop within one month of immunization.

f. **Acellular pertussis vaccines.** The Food and Drug Administration (FDA) has approved an acellular pertussis vaccine combined with diphtheria and tetanus toxoids (DTaP). This vaccine can be given for **any** of the five childhood doses, starting at 2 months. Children who receive acellular pertussis vaccine experience fewer and milder local and systemic side effects than those who receive the whole-cell (DTP) vaccine. For this reason, the acellular vaccine is preferred if available. DTaP can be used to complete the immunization schedule for infants and children who received DTP in their primary immunization schedule.

g. **Natural immunity.** Children who have incurred the natural disease of pertussis, measles, mumps, varicella, or rubella develop lifelong immunity and do not need to receive the vaccine. However, receipt of the vaccine when prior immunity to these diseases exists will cause no problem. Infection with *H. influenzae* B in immunized children less than 24 months of age **does not confer immunity and these children should be immunized.**

h. There are no known problems with the **simultaneous administration** of DTP or DTaP, TOPV or IPV, MMR, hepatitis A, hepatitis B, HIB, and varicella. They should be given at different sites and should not be mixed in the same syringe unless approved by the Food and Drug Administration (FDA). Some polyvaccine products have recently been approved (e.g., DTP-Hib, DTaP-Hib, and Hib-hepatitis B).

i. The use of the Hib vaccine conjugated with diphtheria toxoid alone does not produce immunity to diphtheria. Routine immunizations with DTP must be done. Children not immunized as infants should receive Hib vaccine when first seen up until the age of 5 years. Revaccination is not

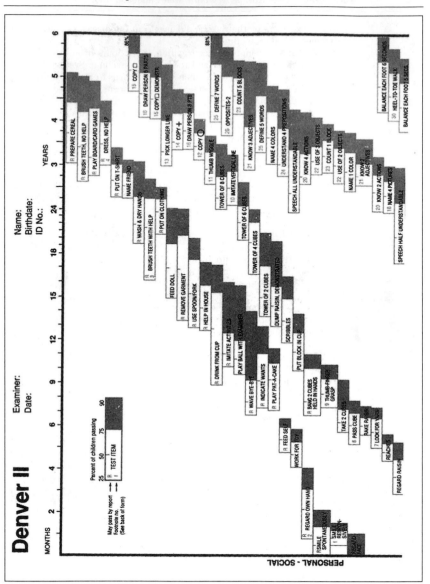

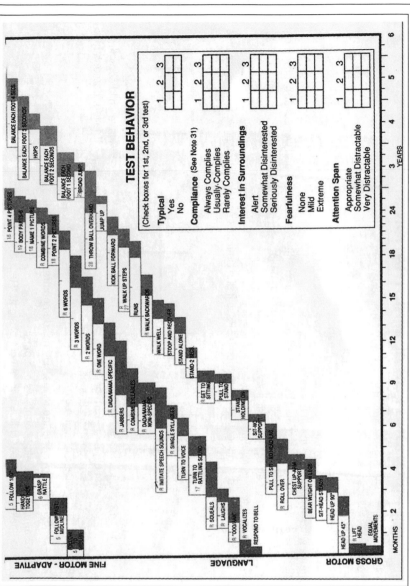

Fig. 3-6. Denver Developmental Screening Test. © 1969, 1989, 1990 by WK Frankenburg and JB Dodds. © 1978 by WK Frankenburg.

DIRECTIONS FOR ADMINISTRATION

1. Try to get child to smile by smiling, talking or waving. Do not touch him/her.

2. Child must stare at hand several seconds.

3. Parent may help guide toothbrush and put toothpaste on brush.

4. Child does not have to be able to tie shoes or button/zip in the back.

5. Move yarn slowly in an arc from one side to the other, about 8" above child's face.

6. Pass if child grasps rattle when it is touched to the backs or tips of fingers.

7. Pass if child tries to see where yarn went. Yarn should be dropped quickly from sight from tester's hand without arm movement.

8. Child must transfer cube from hand to hand without help of body, mouth, or table.

9. Pass if child picks up raisin with any part of thumb and finger.

10. Line can vary only 30 degrees or less from tester's line.

11. Make a fist with thumb pointing upward and wiggle only the thumb. Pass if child imitates and does not move any fingers other than the thumb.

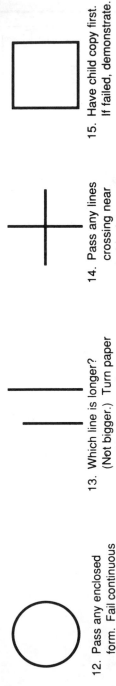

12. Pass any enclosed form. Fail continuous round motions.

13. Which line is longer? (Not bigger.) Turn paper upside down and repeat. (pass 3 of 3 or 5 of 6)

14. Pass any lines crossing near midpoint.

15. Have child copy first. If failed, demonstrate.

16. When giving items 12, 14, and 15, do not name the forms. Do not demonstrate 12 and 14.

16. When scoring, each pair (2 arms, 2 legs, etc.) counts as one part.

17. Place one cube in cup and shake gently near child's ear, but out of sight. Repeat for other ear.

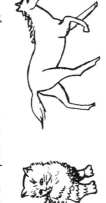
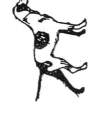
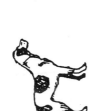
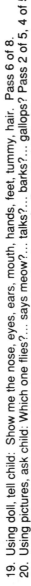

18. Point to picture and have child name it. (No credit is given for sounds only.) If less than 4 pictures are named correctly, have child point to picture as each is named by tester.

19. Using doll, tell child: Show me the nose, eyes, ears, mouth, hands, feet, tummy, hair. Pass 6 of 8.
20. Using pictures, ask child: Which one flies?... says meow?... talks?... barks?... gallops? Pass 2 of 5, 4 of 5. Ask child: What do you do when you are cold?... tired?... hungry?   Pass 2 of 3, 3 of 3.
21. Ask child: What do you do when you are cold?... tired?... hungry?   Pass 2 of 3, 3 of 3.
22. Ask child: What do you do with a cup? What is a chair used for? What is a pencil used for? Action words must be included in answers.
23. Pass if child correctly places and says how many blocks are on paper. (1, 5).
24. Tell child: Put block on table; under table; in front of me, behind me. Pass 4 of 4. (Do not help child by pointing, moving head or eyes.)
25. Ask child: What is a ball?... lake?... desk?... house?... banana?... curtain?... fence?... ceiling? Pass if defined in terms of use, shape, what it is made of, or general category (such as banana is fruit, not just yellow). Pass 5 of 8, 7 of 8.
26. Ask child: If a horse is big, a mouse is ___? If fire is hot, ice is ___? If the sun shines during the day, the moon shines during the ___? Pass 2 of 3.
27. Child may use wall or rail only, not person. May not crawl.
28. Child must throw ball overhand 3 feet to within arm's reach of tester.
29. Child must perform standing broad jump over width of test sheet (8 1/2 inches).
30. Tell child to walk forward, ⇔⇔⇔➔ heel within 1 inch of toe. Tester may demonstrate. Child must walk 4 consecutive steps.
31. In the second year, half of normal children are non-compliant.

OBSERVATIONS:

Fig. 3-6. (continued)

Table 3-6. Usual ages of attainment of developmental milestones

1 mo	GM	Head up in prone	9 mo	GM	
	FM			FM	Objective constancy
	LAN	Social smile (6 wk)			Bangs cubes together
2 mo	GM	Chest up in prone			Rings bell for fun
	FM	Follows across midline		LAN	Gesture games
	LAN	Coos	10 mo	LAN	"Dada" (discriminately)
3 mo	GM	On elbows in prone	11 mo	FM	Plucks pellet
	FM	Follows in a circle		LAN	First word (other than
		Blinks to visual threat			ma/da)
	LAN		12 mo	GM	Walks independently
4 mo	GM	Up on wrists in prone		FM	Places pellet in bottle
		Rolls prone to supine			Voluntary release
	LAN	Orients to voice (E)			Marks with a crayon
		Laughs out loud (4.5)		LAN	Immature jargon
5 mo	GM	Rolls supine to prone			Imitates squeezing a
		Transfers		P/S	doll (E)
	FM	Pulls down ring			Drinks from a cup
	LAN	Orients to sound (E)			Assists with dressing
6 mo	GM	Sits (unsupported)	15 mo	GM	Runs
	FM	Unilateral reach		FM	Dumps pellet from
	LAN	Babbles			bottle
7 mo	GM	Comes to sit (7.5)		LAN	Directed pointing
	FM	Attempts pellet			4–6 words
	LAN		18 mo	FM	Scribbles spontaneously
8 mo	GM	Crawls; pulls to stand			Uses tools
	FM	Attains pellet			3-cube tower
		Inspects bell		LAN	3 body parts
	LAN	Understands "no"			Parallel play
		"Dada" (indiscriminate)			Domestic imagery
					7- to 20-word vocabulary
					Mature jargon (16 mo)
				P/S	Uses spoon
			21 mo	LAN	2-word phrases
					50-word vocabulary
					Points to pictures (E)
				FM	3-cube train
			24 mo	LAN	2-word sentences

FM = fine motor/problem solving; GM = gross motor; LAN = language; P/S = personal/social. Gross motor and personal social milestones are historical. Fine motor/problem solving are elicited. Language milestones are historical save where noted by examiner (E).
Source: Reprinted with permission from R Dershewitz (ed). *Ambulatory Pediatric Care*. Philadelphia: Lippincott, 1988.

presently recommended if a dose of the vaccine has been received on or after 15 months of age.

j. **Pneumococcal vaccine.** A 23-valent vaccine containing polysaccharide antigens from the serotypes that cause nearly 100% of pneumococcal bacteremia and meningitis in children is available. Infants or toddlers may have a poor or unpredictable antibody response; hence, the vaccine is not recommended for children under 2 years of age. **High-risk children** with sickle cell disease, functional or anatomic asplenia, or nephrotic syndrome, and those about to undergo cytoreduction therapy for Hodgkin's disease, should be vaccinated.

k. Hepatitis B vaccine. Two recombinant vaccines (Recombivax HB and Energix-B) are licensed and produced in the United States. They induce more than 90% protection against hepatitis B virus (HBV) infection, and adverse effects are minimal, consisting primarily of soreness at the injection site. Current recommendations state that the highest priority should be immunization of high-risk children and all infants, followed by immunization of adolescents living in high-risk areas, and all adolescents. A summary of recommendations follows.

   (1) Routine serologic screening of all pregnant women for hepatitis B surface antigen (HBsAg) should continue.

   (2) All newborn infants should be immunized with HBV vaccine. The appropriate doses are listed in Table 3-9.

   (a) For infants born to **HBsAg-negative mothers:** Administer first dose to newborn (0–2 days) before discharge from the hospital; administer second dose at 1 to 2 months of age, followed by the third dose at 6 to 18 months of age. Infants who did not receive a dose of vaccine at birth should receive three doses by 18 months of age. The minimal interval between the first two doses is 1 month and between the second and third doses is 4 months. An alternative schedule of immunizations at 2, 4, and 8 to 18 months of age, although not preferred, is acceptable, *provided the infant's mother is HBsAg negative.*

   (b) Infants born to **HBsAg-positive women** must be immunized at or shortly after birth and should receive one dose of hepatitis B immune globulin (HBIG) *as soon as possible after birth.* The second dose should be administered at 1 month and the third dose at 6 months. These infants should have their serologic status checked at 9 months of age. If their anti-HBs titer is less than 10 mIU/ml, they can receive up to two more doses of vaccine.

   (c) If the mother's **HBsAg status is unknown** at the time of delivery, the infant should be immunized at birth with the dose of vaccine recommended for infants born to HBsAg-positive mothers. The mother should be screened as soon as possible to determine the need for HBIG if she is HBsAg positive.

   (3) Older children, adolescents, and adults at increased risk of HBV infection (Table 3-10) should be immunized with HBV vaccine.

   (4) Routine immunization of all adolescents against HBV should be implemented when feasible.

l. Varicella vaccine. A live, attenuated varicella vaccine has been approved by the FDA. Both seroconversion rates and protective efficacy were greater than 95% when the vaccine was administered to healthy children. The current recommendation of the AAP and ACIP is that all children be immunized between 12 and 18 months of age, if they have no reliable history of varicella. Children ages 18 months to 13 years who have not been immunized and who lack a reliable history of the disease should also be immunized. Healthy adolescents past their thirteenth birthday who have not been immunized and who lack a history of infection should be given two doses of the vaccine 4 to 8 weeks apart.

m. Influenza vaccine. Yearly preparations of influenza vaccine should be administered to all children and adolescents who have cardiac or pulmonary disorders, who are immunosuppressed, or have debilitating chronic diseases.

n. Hepatitis A vaccine. An effective hepatitis A vaccine has recently been licensed for individuals 2 years of age and older. Three doses are required for children from 2 to 18 years of age. The second dose is given 1 month after the first, and the third dose 6 to 12 months later. Though universal immunization of children may be recommended in the future, current CDC recommendations are for immunization of travelers to endemic areas and mem-

Table 3-7. Recommended childhood immunization schedule, United States, January–December 1997

Vaccine	Birth	1 mo	2 mos	4 mos	6 mos	12 mos	15 mos	18 mos	4–6 yrs	11–12 yrs	14–16 yrs
Hepatitis B[2,3]	Hep B-1	Hep B-2			Hep B-3					Hep B[3]	
Diphtheria, Tetanus, Pertussis[4]			DTaP or DTP	DTaP or DTP	DTaP or DTP		DTaP or DTP[4]		DTaP or DTP	Td	
H. influenzae type b[5]			Hib	Hib	Hib[5]	Hib[5]					
Polio[6]			Polio[6]	Polio			Polio[6]		Polio		
Measles, Mumps, Rubella[7]						MMR			MMR[7] or MMR[7]		
Varicella[8]							Var			Var[8]	

Note: Vaccines[1] are listed under the routinely recommended ages. Bars indicate range of acceptable ages for vaccination. Shaded bars indicate *catch-up vaccination:* at 11–12 years of age, hepatitis B vaccine should be administered to children not previously vaccinated, and Varicella vaccine should be administered to children not previously vaccinated who lack a reliable history of chickenpox. Approved by the Advisory Committee on Immunization Practices (ACIP), the American Academy of Pediatrics (AAP), and the American Academy of Family Physicians (AAFP).

[1] This schedule indicates the recommended age for routine administration of currently licensed childhood vaccines. Some combination vaccines are available and may be used whenever administration of all components of the vaccine is indicated. Providers should consult the manufacturers' package inserts for detailed recommendations.

[2] Infants born to HBsAg-negative mothers should receive 2.5 µg of Merck vaccine (Recombivax HB) or 10 µg of SmithKline Beecham (SB) vaccine (Energix-B). The 2nd dose should be administered ≥ 1 month after the 1st dose.

Infants born to HBsAG-positive mothers should receive 0.5 ml hepatitis B immune globulin (HBIG) within 12 hrs of birth, and either 5 µg of Merck vaccine (Recombivax HB) or 10 µg of SB vaccine (Engerix-B) at a separate site. The 2nd dose is recommended at 1–2 mos of age and the 3rd dose at 6 mos of age. Infants born to mothers whose HBsAg status is unknown should receive either 5 µg of Merck vaccine (Recombivax HB) or 10 µg of SB vaccine (Engerix-B) within 12 hrs of birth. The 2nd dose of vaccine is recommended at 1 mo of age and the 3rd dose at 6 mos of age. Blood should be drawn at the time of delivery to determine the mother's HBsAG status; if it is positive, the infant should receive HBIG as soon as possible (no later than 1 wk of age). The dosage and timing of subsequent vaccine doses should be based upon the mother's HBsAG status.

[3] Children and adolescents who have not been vaccinated against hepatitis B in infancy may begin the series during any childhood visit. Those who have not previously received 3 doses of hepatitis B vaccine should initiate or complete the series during the 11–12 year-old visit. The 2nd dose should be administered at least 1 mo after the 1st dose, and the 3rd dose should be administered at least 4 mos after the 1st dose and at least 2 mos after the 2nd dose.

[4] DTaP (diphtheria and tetanus toxoids and acellular pertussis vaccine) is the preferred vaccine for all doses in the vaccination series, including completion of the series in children who have received ≥1 dose of whole-cell DTP vaccine. Whole-cell DTP is an acceptable alternative to DTaP. The 4th dose of DTaP (DTaP) may be administered as early as 12 months of age, provided 6 months have elapsed since the 3rd dose, and if the child is considered unlikely to return at 15–18 mos of age. Td (tetanus and diphtheria toxoids, absorbed, for adult use) is recommended at 11–12 years of age if at least 5 years have elapsed since the last dose of DTP, DTaP, or DT. Subsequent routine Td boosters are recommended every 10 years.

[5] Three *H. influenzae* type b (Hib) conjugate vaccines are licensed for infant use. If PRP-OMP (PedvaxHIB [Merck]) is administered at 2 and 4 mos of age, a dose at 6 mos is not required. After completing the primary series, any Hib conjugate vaccine may be used as a booster.

[6] Two poliovirus vaccines are currently licensed in the US: inactivated poliovirus vaccine (IPV) and oral poliovirus vaccine (OPV). The following schedules are all acceptable by the ACIP, the AAP, and the AAFP, and parents and providers may choose among them:

1. IPV at 2 and 4 mos; OPV at 12–18 mos and 4–6 yr
2. IPV at 2, 4, 12–18 mos, and 4–6 yr
3. OPV at 2, 4, 6–18 mos, and 4–6 yr

The ACIP routinely recommends schedule 1. IPV is the only poliovirus vaccine recommended for immunocompromised persons and their household contacts.

[7] The 2nd dose of MMR is routinely recommended at 4–6 yrs of age or at 11–12 yrs of age, but may be administered during any visit, provided at least 1 month has elapsed since receipt of the 1st dose and that both doses are administered at or after 12 months of age.

[8] Susceptible children may receive Varicella vaccine (Var) at any visit after the first birthday, and those who lack a reliable history of chickenpox should be immunized during the 11–12 year-old visit. Children ≥ 13 years of age should receive 2 doses, at least 1 mos apart.

Table 3-8. Recommended immunization schedules for children not immunized in the first year of life

Recommended time/age	Immunization(s)[a,b]	Comments
Younger than 7 yr		
First visit	DTP or DTaP, Hib, HBV, MMR, OPV	If indicated, tuberculin testing can be done at same visit If child is 5 yr of age or older, Hib is not indicated
Interval after first visit		
1 mo	DTP or DTaP, HBV	OPV can be given if accelerated poliomyelitis vaccination is necessary, such as for travelers to areas where polio is endemic
2 mo	DTP or DTaP, Hib, OPV	Second dose of Hib is indicated only in children whose first dose was received when younger than 15 mo
≥8 mo	DTP or DTaP, HBV, OPV	OPV is not given if the third dose was given earlier
4–6 yr (at or before school entry)	DTP or DTaP, OPV	DTP or DTaP is not necessary if the fourth dose was given after the fourth birthday; OPV is not necessary if the third dose was given after the fourth birthday
11–12 yr	MMR	At entry to middle school or junior high school
10 yr later	Td	Repeat every 10 yr throughout life
7 yr and older[c,d]		
First visit	HBV,[e] OPV, MMR, Td	
Interval after first visit		
2 mo	HBV,[e] OPV, Td	OPV can also be given 1 mo after the first visit if accelerated poliomyelitis vaccination is necessary
8–14 mo	HBV,[e] OPV, Td	OPV is not given if the third dose was given earlier
11–12 yr	MMR	At entry to middle school or junior high
10 yr later	Td	Repeat every 10 yr throughout life

DTP = diphtheria, tetanus, pertussis; Hib = *Haemophilus influenzae* type b; HBV = hepatitis B virus; MMR = measles-mumps-rubella; OPV = oral polio vaccine; DTaP = diphtheria, tetanus, acellular pertussis.

[a]If all needed vaccines cannot be administered simultaneously, priority should be given to protecting the child against those diseases that pose the greatest immediate risk. In the US, these diseases for children younger than 2 yr usually are measles and *Haemophilus influenzae* type b infection; for children older than 7 yr, they are measles, mumps, and rubella.

[b]DTP or DTaP, HBV, Hib, MMR, and OPV can be given simultaneously at separate sites if failure of the patient to return for future immunizations is a concern.

[c]If person is 18 yr or older, routine poliovirus vaccination is not indicated in the US.

[d]Minimal interval between doses of MMR is 1 mo.

[e]Priority should be given to hepatitis B immunization of adolescents.

Source: Committee on Infectious Diseases, American Academy of Pediatrics. *1994 Redbook.* P. 24.

Table 3-9. Recommended dosages of hepatitis B vaccines[a]

Patients	Vaccine[b,c]			
	Recombivax HB[d] dose: μg	(ml)	Energix-B[e,f] dose: μg	(ml)
Infants of HBsAg-negative mothers and children < 11 yr	2.5	(0.5)[g]	10	(0.5)
Infants of HBsAg-positive mothers (HBIG [0.5 ml] should also be given)	5	(0.5)[h] (1.0)[g]	10	(0.5)
Children and adolescents 11–19 yr	5	(0.5)[h]	20	(1.0)
Adults ≥ 20 yr	10	(1.0)[h]	20	(1.0)
Dialysis patients and other immunosuppressed adults	40	(1.0)[i]	40	(2.0)[j]

[a]Heptavax-B (Merck, West Point, PA), a plasma-derived vaccine, is also licensed but no longer produced in the US.
[b]Vaccines should be stored at 2°–8°C. Freezing destroys effectiveness.
[c]Both vaccines are administered in a 3-dose schedule.
[d]Merck, West Point, PA.
[e]The Food and Drug Administration has approved this vaccine for use in an optional 4-dose schedule at 0, 1, 2, and 12 mo.
[f]SmithKline Beecham, Philadelphia, PA.
[g]Pediatric formulation.
[h]Adult formulation.
[i]Special formulation for dialysis patients.
[j]Two 1.0-ml doses given at one site in a 4-dose schedule at 0, 1, 2, and 6–12 mo.
Source: Committee on Infectious Diseases, American Academy of Pediatrics. *1994 Redbook.* P. 229.

bers of high risk groups (Alaskan natives, Native Americans, homosexual men, IV drug users, day care center employees, and military personnel).
   o. **Poliovirus vaccines.** Given the eradication of wild-type poliovirus from the Western hemisphere since 1994, and the small but real risk of vaccine-associated paralytic polio, the AAP has approved a sequential IPV/OPV schedule for use in the United States (first two doses IPV, next two doses OPV). OPV still should only be used in countries with continued or recent circulation of wild-type poliovirus and occurrence of paralytic poliomyelitis, and for those countries in which the increased cost of IPV and its administration make its use impractical (AAP recommendation, November 1996).
5. **Anticipatory guidance.** A well-child visit is incomplete without adequate time for anticipatory guidance. The AAP has issued two companion manuals, *Guidelines for Health Supervision* and *Health Supervision Visit*, which address anticipatory guidance for each visit. In summary, visits include the following:
   a. **Newborn visit** (1–2 weeks): reassurance that adequate weight gain is occurring and that the baby is otherwise healthy. Encouragement is also provided. Guidance is offered for possible symptoms of colic.
   b. **2-month visit:** reassurances that breast milk or formula without additional foods supplies adequate nutrition (see p. 49).
   c. **4-month visit:** introduction of solids (see Sec. **IV.A.1.c**). Accident prevention—baby becoming mobile (Table 3-11). Teething (see p. 50).
   d. **6-month visit:** review of developmental milestones reached or soon to be reached; sitting without support, holding objects, babbling. Accident prevention (see Table 3-11). Supply Poison Control Center telephone number and possibly ipecac sample.

Table 3-10. Persons who should receive hepatitis B immunization

All infants. Infants of HBsAg-positive mothers require postexposure immunoprophylaxis with HBIG and vaccine.
Infants and children at risk of acquisition of HBV by person-to-person (horizontal) transmission should be immunized by 6–9 mo of age.
Adolescents.* Special effort should be made to vaccinate those adolescents in the categories of high risk for hepatitis B virus (HBV) infection.
Users of intravenous drugs.
Sexually active heterosexual persons with more than 1 sex partner in the previous 6 mo or with a sexually transmitted disease.
Sexually active homosexual or bisexual males.
Health care workers at risk of exposure to blood or body fluids.
Residents and staff of institutions for developmentally disabled persons.
Staff of nonresidential child care and school programs for developmentally disabled persons if attended by a known HBV carrier.
Hemodialysis patients.
Patients with bleeding disorders who receive certain blood products.
Household contacts and sexual partners of HBV carriers.
Members of households with adoptees from countries where HBV infection is endemic who are HBsAg positive.
International travelers who will live for more than 6 mo in an area of high HBV endemicity and who otherwise will be at risk.
Inmates of long-term correctional facilities.

*Implementation can be initiated before children reach adolescence.
Source: Committee on Infectious Diseases, American Academy of Pediatrics. *1994 Redbook.* P. 234.

  e. 9- to 12-month visit: introduction of finger foods, increasing autonomy, accident prevention (see Table 3-11).
  f. 18-month to 2-year visit: discussion of temper tantrums, toilet training, and limit-setting techniques.
IV. Specific considerations
  A. Common management issues in infants and toddlers
    1. Feeding. The early discussion of variability in feeding patterns, both in quantity and quality, helps to allay future concerns.
      a. Breast feeding. Breast-feeding mothers often benefit from additional counseling by the physician, nurse, or, if available, lactation consultant to help with mechanics.
        (1) Feeding frequency should be determined by the baby's demand, usually every 2 to 3 hours during the first 2 to 3 weeks. While clinicians differ, we recommend that the duration of each feeding be 5 to 10 minutes per breast. The mother should alternate the breast on which the nursing is begun at each feeding to keep milk production and consumption fairly even. "Bubbling" or "burping" should be done at least between breasts or possibly more frequently as needed. Milk supply is low for the initial 2 to 5 days, and the new mother needs reassurance that her milk will "come in," that she should continue to put the baby to breast, and that the baby will be fine until that time.
        (2) Nipple soreness is a common early problem that may be helped by keeping initial feeding periods brief in the first 24 to 48 hours, using only water to cleanse nipples, and changing position to assure proper "latching on," which will minimize soreness and prevent cracking of nipples at pressure points.
        (3) Breast engorgement may begin 2 to 3 days postpartum and can be alleviated by a supportive bra, compresses (cool at first, warm if no relief), and oral analgesics.

Table 3-11. Accident prevention in childhood

Age and cause of morbidity	Prevention
0–6 mo	
Auto accidents	Use authorized car seat until child is 3 yr old; then use seat belts
Crib injuries	Be sure that crib meets consumer protection specifications; refrain from using pillow; avoid prone sleeping position
Burns/fire	Install smoke detector; lower water tank temperature to 120°F
6–12 mo	
Falls	Use childproof barriers for stairs and doors; have screens and locks on windows
Foreign body ingestions	Check toys for small removable parts and discard; keep floors clear of coins, buttons, nails, tacks, etc.
Shocks	Insert plastic covers into electric outlets
Pica	Remember that paint on walls and ceilings—and yard dirt—may contain lead
Crib injuries (from falling)	Ascertain that height from the mattress to the top of crib rail is 21 in. or more
12–24 mo	
Burns	Keep hot beverages away from table edge; use rear burners of stove whenever possible; keep matches out of reach
Ingestions	Keep all medicines, cleaners, and chemicals out of reach in a locked cabinet; have ipecac and the telephone number of the Poison Control Center on hand at home
Car accidents (as pedestrian)	Buy suitable toys—two wheelers, skateboards, rollerskates, and even some tricycles cannot be controlled by a typical toddler; supervise play near streets or have the child play in a fenced-in area
24–48 mo (same as for 12–24 mo)	
Burns/fire	Begin fire hazard education, especially fire escape route and "drop and roll"
School age	
Sports injuries	Maintain adult supervision in contact sports; buy appropriate protective equipment for contact sports

(4) Alveolar engorgement may occur on days 3 to 4 postpartum as the result of milk secretion unresolved by proper letdown and emptying. Treatment involves facilitating the letdown reflex by ensuring maternal comfort and the manual expression of enough milk to relieve some fullness.

(5) The breast-fed baby may require 2 and occasionally even 3 weeks to regain birth weight. **Inadequate weight gain** at 2 weeks is best assessed by observing the mother and infant during feeding. Usually, increasing the frequency of feeds and assuring that support systems are available to the mother so that she can get adequate physical and emotional rest will suffice. The weight should be rechecked within a few days.

(6) Jaundice is more likely to occur in the breast-fed baby than in the formula-fed infant. Jaundice from breast feeding generally occurs with the onset of the milk coming in and peaks at about 10 to 14 days of age. All other causes of jaundice should be excluded. If the bilirubin is high ($\geq$20), the mother should stop breast feeding for 12 to 48 hours. If the etiology of the jaundice is the milk, the bilirubin level will fall, even as much as 2 mg/dl in 12 hours. Breast feeding should then be reinstituted. Generally, the bilirubin does not rise to its previous high point. The mother should pump her breasts if an observation period is necessary, so that breast feeding will not be compromised when reinstituted. Since there are no reported cases of kernicterus associated with breast milk jaundice, breast feeding should never have to be discontinued on this basis.

(7) **Supplementation** with formula can be used after nursing is established (3–6 weeks), but the mother should understand that as suckling at the breast decreases, so will milk production. If the breast milk supply seems inadequate, formula can be offered *after* nursing to supplement; this still assures the suckling stimulus to continued milk production. Soy-based formula may be preferable to cow's milk for "mixed" feeding regimens.

(8) Breast milk pumping allows the woman who works outside the home to continue to provide breast milk for her infant. Breast milk can be refrigerated for 24 hours or frozen for up to 8 weeks. Pumping can be done 1 to 2 hours after feeding or from the alternate breast. Weaning should be done gradually to prevent painful breast engorgement. One breast milk feeding should be replaced at a time with a few days in between.

(9) **There has been some debate as to when** breast-fed infants should be **supplemented** with **fluoride drops. The current recommendations of the AAP are shown in Table 3-12.** There is also some disagreement over the necessity of **vitamin D.** Dark-skinned infants who are exclusively breast fed during the winter months are at highest risk for development of rickets. If given, the common preparations of multivitamins containing 400 IU/day in combination with 1,500 IU vitamin A and 50 mg vitamin C are generally used. Breast milk is adequate in all other nutritional requirements as the sole intake for the first 4 to 6 months of life. Contraindications to breast feeding are well discussed in J Cloherty, A Stark [eds]. *Manual of Neonatal Care.* Boston: Little, Brown, 1991.

b. **Formula feeding**
(1) A **cow's milk–based** formula containing iron (12 mg elemental iron/liter) is recommended for the first 9 to 12 months of life. Powdered or concentrated formula mixed with tap water is recommended for babies in communities with fluoridated water. There is no need to boil the water in most municipal water supplies. However, it is prudent to flush the water system by running tap water for 30 to 60 seconds to avoid adding accumulated impurities such as lead to formula.

Table 3-12. Fluoride supplementation*

	Water fluoride content (ppm)		
Age	<0.3	0.3–0.6	>0.6
Birth–6 mo	0	0	0
6 mo–3 yr	0.25	0	0
3–6 yr	0.50	0.25	0
6–16 yr	1.00	0.50	0

*Fluoride daily doses are given in milligrams.
Source: Committee on Nutrition, American Academy of Pediatrics. Fluoride supplementation for children: Interim policy recommendations. *Pediatrics* 95:777, 1995.

If ready-to-feed formula is used or bottled water is mixed with powder or concentrate, the infant may need to be supplemented with fluoride drops after 6 months of age (see Table 3-12).

(2) **Soy-based formulas** can be used initially for babies with a strong family history of atopic disease and as a supplement for breast feeding. Because all soy formulas currently contain iron, iron supplements are not needed.

(3) Most newborns require approximately 5 oz formula/kg/day, based on caloric needs of 100 calories/kg/day and formula caloric density of 20 calories/oz. Infants of any age rarely require more than 38 oz of formula per day, because caloric requirements decline with age and alternate food sources become available to the older infant.

(4) **Whole cow's milk** can be introduced between 9 and 12 months of age, provided that the infant is consuming one third of calories as supplemental foods that provide adequate sources of iron and vitamin C since 30 to 40% of dietary calories should be in the form of fat. Defatted cow's milk is **not recommended** in children less than 2 years of age.

c. **Introduction of solids**

(1) The timing of introducing solids varies widely. The most uniformly accepted age in the US is probably 3 to 6 months. This timing should be based on the attainment of developmental milestones, that is, adequate head control, loss of the tongue thrust, and some ability to express hunger and satiety. Some intake and growth factors can be considered: intake of formula greater than 32 oz/day, doubling of the birth weight, and/or an unacceptable increase in frequency of feedings.

(2) Iron-fortified cereals are recommended as the first solid foods. Fruits and vegetables in a blenderized or strained form are begun next. A 2- to 4-day period should separate the introduction of each new food to mark the occurrence of specific food intolerance or allergy.

(3) Although specific food intolerance or allergy is unusual during the first year of life, parents of infants with family histories of allergy might delay introduction of the more troublesome foods, that is, egg whites, citrus fruits, strawberries, chocolate, and fish. Delayed exposure has been shown to reduce sensitivity reactions.

(4) During the second half of the first year of life, infants begin to like "finger foods," which allow some independence in feeding (before the development of dexterity, it is still necessary to feed the baby with a spoon).

(5) After one year of age, parents should offer a varied diet including each of the major food groups. Periods of apparent decreased food intake may occur at 7 to 9 months, when the desire of babies to feed themselves begins; at 2 to 3 years, when there is a further need for independence; and at 5 to 6 years. In general, parents can be reassured during these periods by demonstrating the child's continued adequate weight gain on growth charts. *Forced feedings are never useful at any age.*

2. **Crying.** Parents need to understand that babies normally cry for as many as 4 hours per day. It takes time to understand babies' cries and what they mean. Parents also need reassurance that sometimes there is no discernible cause and allowing the infant to cry is acceptable.

a. The term **colic** is used loosely and includes moderate to severe and otherwise unexplained bouts of crying. It occurs in 10 to 15% of infants, starting by the age of 3 weeks and usually ending at 3 months.

(1) **Etiology.** There is no single cause. **Persistent** crying signals distress and should stimulate reasonable efforts for an explanation. The **typical pattern** is that of a usually calm and placid infant who suddenly screams, who draws knees up to abdomen, and who may pass flatus or feces. An episode can last for 10 minutes to 2 hours, and episodes occur more commonly in the late afternoon and early evening hours.

(2) Management

  (a) Hunger, swallowed air, milk intolerance, or an acute illness must be excluded.

  (b) Underfeeding and overfeeding should be discontinued. Air swallowing may be prevented by altering feeding and increasing burping techniques and frequency. If the infant is formula fed, enlarging the nipple holes may help improve flow of the formula.

  (c) **Listening and lending support are the cornerstones of management.** The baby who is often fussy and crying provokes anxiety and tension, and the parents need an outlet for their own concerns and feelings.

  (d) Holding a fussy infant with colic is recommended. Gentle rocking, holding the baby close to the body in a front pack, and using soothing words are helpful. Sometimes an automobile ride, if available, works wonders.

  (e) Parents need reassurance that allowing the infant to cry is an acceptable option if all soothing techniques have failed. This simple "giving of permission" may lessen parental anxiety and tension, resulting in a calmer infant.

  (f) When parents are especially tired or anxious, it is important to ask whether they are afraid of hurting the baby, and definite strategies for respite time may need to be established.

  (g) Sedative and anticholinergic drugs are ineffective, and the hazards of overdosage and toxicity are such that **use of these drugs is not recommended.** The use of simethicone drops as an antiflatulent has not been proved effective, but they are safe and acceptable on a trial basis.

  (h) Devices that attach to the crib and cause vibration are available and may be of benefit in selected infants.

  (i) Parents need to be reassured that they can ask to have their infant examined by their primary care provider. Often a reassuring visit may preclude an inappropriate emergency room visit in the middle of the night.

3. Teething

 a. General considerations

  (1) Teething is defined as the infant's reaction to the normal gingival inflammation that accompanies natural eruption of teeth. The symptoms that accompany the process begin from the first to the fifteenth month and may continue off and on into the third year of life.

  (2) Teething is probably never responsible for *significant* fever, rhinorrhea, rashes, or diarrhea.

  (3) The normal appearance at age 4 months of oral exploration and consequent salivation and drooling is frequently attributed to, but rarely due to, teething. A gingival inflammation that occurs with actual eruption of a tooth may produce an increase in this activity, as well as periods of irritability and "congestion."

  (4) The lower central incisors are generally the first teeth to erupt and usually do so at 6 to 7 months of age. For an appropriate chronology of deciduous tooth eruption, see Table 3-13.

 b. Management

  (1) Rubbing swollen gums or giving the infant a cold, hard object to bite may provide relief of discomfort.

  (2) Application of commercially available topical analgesics and gels at best provides limited and very transient relief.

  (3) When discomfort and irritability are clearly related to teething, acetaminophen or ibuprofen (for children over 6 months) may be useful.

Table 3-13. Chronology of eruption of deciduous teeth

Deciduous tooth	Mean age at eruption in mo ± (range)
Maxillary	
Central incisor	10 (8–12)
Lateral incisor	11 (9–13)
Canine	19 (16–22)
First molar	16 (13–19, boys; 14–18, girls)
Second molar	29 (25–33)
Mandibular	
Central incisor	8 (6–10)
Lateral incisor	13 (10–16)
Canine	20 (17–23)
First molar	16 (14–18)
Second molar	27 (23–31, boys; 24–30, girls)

Source: Adapted from JM Davis et al. *An Atlas of Pedodontics* (2nd ed). Philadelphia: Saunders, 1981.

4. Fever (see also Chap. 7, p. 238)
  a. General considerations
   (1) Most fevers in infants and children are caused by acute viral infection. Fever, unless exceptionally high—over 41.1°C (106°F)—does no specific harm to the patient. Indeed, there is evidence to suggest that fever may play a role in the natural body defenses against infection.
   (2) While the height of the fever does not necessarily correlate with the severity of its cause, the physician's concern should be aroused when patients fail to act and look better when less febrile. Further, the actual response to antipyretics in terms of a decrease in the degree of fever is not predictive of the seriousness of the infection.
   (3) Because of the increased risk of bacteremia, the presence of fever in an infant under 3 months of age should prompt the physician to see that child without delay.
   (4) In the neonatal period, a temperature below normal is probably of as much concern as an elevated temperature.
  b. Management
   (1) The treatment of temperature elevation should be aimed at making the patient comfortable. **The mere presence of fever does not always mandate treatment.** However, the child with a **history of febrile seizures** should have fever promptly treated.
   (2) Adequate hydration of the patient with oral fluids and increased ambient fluid content of the air may help prevent dehydration.
   (3) Exposure of the skin to the air by removal of clothing and active sponging of the body with tepid water promote heat loss. Alcohol or ice water should **never** be used for this purpose, since they cause a rapid lowering of the skin temperature, with resulting vasoconstriction and prevention of heat loss.
   (4) Antipyretics
     (a) Acetaminophen has both antipyretic and analgesic properties. Children's preparations are available in drops, syrup, chewable tablets, and suppositories. The dosage is 10 to 15 mg/kg q4h. At therapeutic dosages, acetaminophen should have no adverse effects. Acetaminophen intoxication may cause serious hepatic injury. For management of overdose, see Chapter 8, p. 271.

(b) Ibuprofen. Children's liquid preparations of ibuprofen are now available without prescription. It has antipyretic, analgesic, and anti-inflammatory properties.

(c) Aspirin, or acetylsalicylic acid, **is contraindicated in the routine management of pediatric fever.** Its side effects as well as possible association with Reye's syndrome when used in children with viral illness make it an unacceptable choice.

5. Vomiting and diarrhea (see also Chap. 11, p. 346)

a. General considerations. Vomiting and diarrhea are common symptoms. When the two occur together, the most common cause is viral gastroenteritis.

(1) Vomiting

(a) Causes of vomiting in infancy include overfeeding, infection, formula intolerance, reflux, intestinal obstruction, and increased intracranial pressure.

(b) In monitoring the adequacy of hydration (a major complication of vomiting along with electrolyte abnormalities), the physician should question the parents as to the frequency of urination, the degree of moistness of the mucous membranes, the presence or absence of tears with crying, and the child's activity level. The parental perception of how sick the child is between episodes of vomiting will help in determining how soon the child needs to be seen.

(c) Always be alert for **intestinal obstruction,** either partial or complete, or for **increased intracranial pressure** as causes of vomiting. This vomiting can often be *sudden* or *projectile*, or both, and not associated with feelings of nausea.

(d) Medicines such as theophylline and erythromycin can cause vomiting.

(2) Management of nonobstructive vomiting

(a) Initiate frequent (q30–60min) small (1–2 oz) amounts of easily digested clear fluids. The volume can be increased as the symptom decreases.

(b) Formula intolerance may be due to the sugar or to the protein in the formula. A change to a soy product that does not contain lactose or to a casein-based formula may be helpful.

(c) The assessment of improper feeding technique requires first-hand observation in the office and continuing follow-up by telephone.

(d) If vomiting is due to simple gastroenteritis in a child over 2 years of age, a **single** dose of an antiemetic such as prochlorperazine intramuscularly or per rectum may provide relief.

(3) Diarrhea

(a) Causes include local intestinal factors; viral, bacterial, and parasitic infections; antibiotics; inflammatory bowel disease; or extraintestinal infections, such as otitis media, pneumonia, and urinary tract infection.

(b) Important facts in the history include the general condition of the patient; presence of fever; number, consistency, and size of the stools; presence or absence of blood in the stool; and diarrhea in family members. When seeing a child with gastroenteritis, always **record a weight,** noting the clothing worn.

(c) Evaluate the state of hydration (skin turgor, mucous membranes, fullness of the fontanels, presence of tears), activity level of the child, and presence or absence of infection other than in the gastrointestinal tract.

b. Management

(1) Because most cases of gastroenteritis are caused by self-limiting viral infections, an initial period of dietary treatment is helpful, with daily telephone contact to follow the patient's progress. Initially (for the first 12–24 hours), clear liquids, such as oral electrolyte solutions, are given in small amounts if the child is vomiting.

(2) After 12 to 24 hours, when the vomiting has stopped and diarrhea alone is present, early refeeding with breast milk, a gradually strengthened soy-based formula, or lactase-treated cow's milk, in addition to the oral electrolyte solution, will prevent starvation stooling, and a deficit of protein and calories, and will stimulate repair of intestinal mucosa.

(3) After 24 to 48 hours, a bland diet (banana, rice cereal, applesauce, and unbuttered toast) can be introduced.

(4) Kaopectate and antispasmodics should not be used. Such medications make many parents lose sight of the importance of a restrictive, clear-fluid diet. Even with a decrease in the number of stools, continual fluid loss into the gut may persist.

6. Constipation (see also Chap. 11, p. 349)

a. Diagnosis

(1) Constipation may be diagnosed by history with the findings of fecal contents on abdominal or rectal examination. Abdominal pain may suggest it.

(2) Although constipation may accompany many syndromes, it more often represents too little free water in the diet, inadequate intake of high-residue food, disruption of the child's daily habits, or a painful anal fissure that causes withholding of the stool.

(3) Passing a daily stool does not exclude constipation as a problem. Large, hard, or painful stools, sometimes large enough to clog the toilet, are significant signs even if they occur daily by history. Conversely, infrequent stools, even once every 3 to 7 days, can be normal in breast-fed infants, and are even common in formula-fed infants.

b. Treatment. A stepwise approach follows.

(1) To assist the child under age 2 to pass a hard stool

   (a) Glycerine suppository.

   (b) Single dilation with a lubricated rectal thermometer or finger.

(2) To increase bulk and soften the stool

   (a) Increased intake of **free water.**

   (b) Natural dietary **lubricants** (e.g., prune juice, olive oil, tomatoes, and tomato juice).

   (c) High-residue foods (e.g., fruits and green vegetables). The addition of bran and whole grain products is optimal for lifelong dietary changes.

   (d) Pharmacologic stool softeners, such as dioctyl sodium sulfosuccinate (Colace), malt soup extract (Maltsupex), or senna concentrate (Senokot), may be useful. The dosage of stool softeners is as follows: age 1 month to 1 year, 1/2 tsp bid; age 1 to 5 years, 1 tsp bid; 5 to 15 years, 2 tsp bid. Large initial doses are essential; when the stools become soft, the dosage can be reduced. Regular daily dosage is continued for about 2 to 3 months and slowly reduced as bowel tone and regular bowel habits are reacquired. Relapses are common, and monthly follow-up visits are advisable until the problem is clearly resolved. Initially, Senokot, in particular, may produce cramping.

(3) To assist the child with anal fissures

   (a) A glycerine or bisacodyl suppository may be necessary (one only).

   (b) Soften the stool as described.

   (c) Sitz baths tid for small children.

(4) If anatomic lesions have been ruled out

   (a) Establish a pattern of bowel movement after meals (gastrocolic reflex) or at other times—but at the same time each day—by sitting the child on the toilet whether or not a bowel movement results.

(b) Be sure that emotional stress and anxiety have been carefully excluded as causes.

(5) If constipation persists and encopresis occurs, further medical and, possibly, psychiatric evaluation are indicated, and long-term management by the pediatrician is required (see Chap. 11, p. 349).

7. Coryza (upper respiratory infection)

a. General considerations

(1) The symptom of persistent mucous drainage from the nose is most often called a "cold" and is by far the most frequently encountered illness in pediatric practice.

(2) The illness is most often caused by a respiratory virus, produces a clear nasal discharge, and, when uncomplicated, lasts 3 to 5 days and disappears.

(3) Such viral infections may lower local resistance in the nose and throat, which can in turn lead to secondary bacterial invasion (e.g., otitis, sinusitis, pneumonia).

(4) Coryza can be due to excessively dry air or irritants such as allergens.

b. Management in the infant

(1) Remove mucus with a suction bulb. A 3-oz bulb is most efficient.

(2) Increase the humidity in the environment by using a cold mist humidifier or by placing a pan of water on the radiator.

(3) Thin nasal mucus with a few drops of saline solution made by dissolving 1 tsp salt in an 8-oz cup of water. Place two to three drops of the solution into one nostril at a time, wait 2 minutes, and then suction that nostril. This should be done before meals and before sleep as needed.

(4) If the discharge becomes purulent and is associated with fever, consider secondary infection such as otitis or sinusitis.

(5) Over-the-counter decongestants contain cardiotonic agents and should not be used in infants under 6 months of age. In any case their value remains unproven. A small amount of pseudoephedrine or phenylpropanolamine may be useful.

c. Management in the older child

(1) Treat as for the infant, except that gentle nose blowing can also be attempted.

(2) A vasoconstricting nose drop can be prescribed but should not be used chronically because of "rebound phenomenon," in which vasodilation and further edema of the turbinates can occur with repeated usage.

(3) Oral decongestants (sympathomimetics) have not been established as effective drugs; however, in some children they may relieve profuse coryza. The benefits must be weighed against the possible side effects of irritability and drowsiness. Occasionally, paradoxical hyperactivity may occur. Antihistamines have no place in treatment of viral coryza but can be useful in allergic rhinitis.

8. Cough

a. General considerations

(1) A cough is a reflex directed at clearing the upper and lower airway of irritating secretions or foreign material. Many parents have the misconception that cough itself is harmful and **must** be treated. An explanation can be offered of the usefulness and protective benefits of coughing in lieu of a prescription.

(2) Only in a few specific conditions (croup, asthma, perhaps foreign bodies, pertussis) do the characteristics of the cough itself help to make the diagnosis.

b. Management

(1) Treatment should be directed at the underlying cause, for example, infection, allergy, foreign body, irritants such as cigarette smoke.

(2) **Humidification** of an otherwise dry environment may be beneficial in enhancing expectoration. Parents should be asked about their heating system. Steam radiators, electric baseboard heat, forced hot air, and wood stoves are particularly drying.

(3) One may consider use of a dextromethorphan cough suppressant for the irritative cough that interferes with sleep. Dextromethorphan is a nonnarcotic analogue that, with adequate dosing, can be considered equipotent to codeine but without the narcotic side effects.

(4) Expectorants, though thought to increase the flow of respiratory tract secretions, have never been clinically proven to be more effective in decreasing sputum viscosity or easing expectoration over a placebo or simply good hydration. Thus, they should not be routinely recommended for pediatric usage.

9. **Sleeping habits** (see also Chap. 22, p. 551)
   a. **General considerations.** After the first few months of life, sleeping patterns are, in large part, learned responses. By 3 to 4 months of age, most babies have learned to sleep in an apparently uninterrupted stretch of 6 to 8 hours, generally at night if their feeding, bathing, and play time are scheduled in the daytime. By 7 to 12 months, babies should be accustomed to taking their long sleep period at the family's convenience, namely, at night.
   b. **Management**
      (1) It is best to remove the baby's crib from the parents' room by 3 to 6 months, so that the periodic awakening of most young infants at night does not escalate into a prolonged wakeful time.
      (2) After 6 to 9 months of age, the baby's waking at night, despite having been fed, tucked in, and diapered, needs to be handled with a resolute firmness and consistency, so that by experience the baby learns that there is a quiet time for *all* members of the family.
      (3) If the child cries on being placed in the crib at night after the bedtime routine (and is otherwise healthy), or awakens crying in the middle of the night as a means of getting attention or food, the parent should be encouraged to reassure the child with a minimal amount of physical contact (e.g., standing at the door to the room) or refreshment, or both. The parent should then leave the room and return after longer and longer intervals. This technique often allows the child to establish his or her own ability to fall back to sleep without any significant parental intervention.
      (4) Nightmares and night terrors (3–4 years of age) are common and need to be handled with reassurance and gentle comforting in the dimly lit bedroom. Frequent episodes should be investigated with regard to possible daytime environmental factors that might be precipitating these frightening nighttime dreams (see also Chap. 22). A child is not apt to remember being afraid in the setting of a night terror, whereas a nightmare is often remembered with vivid detail. Parents may be frustrated by their inability to comfort the child with a night terror, but should be reassured that their being there is sufficient support for the child (who will be less concerned than the parent the following morning). On the other hand, discussion of the nightmare with the child by the parent can be reassuring for both parties.
      (5) The young child should grow up with the firm conviction that he or she is to stay in his or her bed until morning. This is a safe habit and also allows the parents the privacy and comfort of their own bed and bedroom. Advise the parents to be firm about *not* allowing the child to come into the parents' bed. If the child must be comforted for a special reason, it should be done in his or her own room and bed.
      (6) Many children are able to give up their crib by 2 years of age, while some remain in cribs until almost 3. Do not advise parents to make the change too early, because they might be losing a "safe place" for the child at night. If a bed move is planned due to the arrival of a new sibling, that move should occur several weeks before or after the

arrival of the new baby so as not to convey to the child the sense of being "evicted" or "displaced" by the new family member.

10. Toilet training

   a. General considerations. All normal children will toilet train themselves. Most parents, however, have difficulty in waiting for this to happen. The parents can **help** the child achieve this goal and should think of it in this manner, not that they are actually training the child. Remind parents that there is no earthly way for them to keep their child from becoming toilet trained, but unfortunately they can do all sorts of things to delay the process.

   b. Management

   (1) The best time to start is between **18 months and 3 years** of age, which is the time when many children begin to train themselves. Before this age, they have to learn by association, coincidence, luck, and fleet parental feet. Children who voice their displeasure with a full diaper and are interested in watching others in the bathroom are usually ready to begin training.

   (2) Bowel control is much simpler for a child to master than control of urination because the former involves much less complicated muscle coordination and occurs far fewer times during the day. It might help to put the child on the potty or toilet just after a meal when the gastrocolic reflex occurs.

   (3) Urine training should begin when the frequency of urination decreases and the child begins to awaken dry after a nap, usually around 2 to 3 years of age.

   (4) Any child who *has been trained* and in whom *urinary or fecal incontinence* then develops should be evaluated.

11. Self-stimulation

   a. General considerations. What parents report as "self-stimulation" usually consists of the normal self-soothing habits of children that arise in early infancy. Such behaviors appear in two forms.

   (1) Rhythmic habits, including rocking, head rolling, and head banging. Appearing in the second half of the first year, these behaviors usually occur at times of fatigue, sleepiness, or frustration, and serve to comfort the child.

   (2) Genital exploration or manipulation. The extent of this behavior is directly correlated with age. In an infant or young child, genital manipulation is a manifestation of wholesome curiosity, while in the 3- to 6-year-old, it is an expression of a normal interest in sex. At this stage, genital stimulation should arouse no concern if the child is outgoing, sociable, and not preoccupied with the activity. Excessive stimulation usually indicates underlying high-level anxiety or family conflict, or may be a sign of emotional disturbance. In the latent stage, from 6 years to puberty, such behavior, in general, is suppressed naturally.

   b. Management

   (1) Management of concerns regarding rhythmic behavior is directed toward averting injury and reducing noise. No attempt should be made to discipline or restrain the young child once the behavior has started.

   (2) Management of concerns regarding masturbation is directed toward reassuring parents that masturbation is part of normal development. Parents should be advised that gently inhibiting or distracting the child is more appropriate than calling attention to the activity. **Attempts to suppress the activity, especially if punitive, can produce potentially damaging psychological sequelae.**

B. Common management issues in the school-aged child. Issues that frequently arise in elementary school children include headaches, abdominal pain, enuresis, and encopresis, and school avoidance. The first two topics are discussed on p. 57; the latter three in Chapter 22.

C. Common management issues in adolescents
 1. **Headache** (see also Chap. 20, p. 521)
   a. **General considerations.** Headache is a common complaint of children and adolescents, and repeated evaluations may be needed. Associated symptoms and signs that mandate evaluation are vomiting; hypertension; abnormal neurologic findings, including motor or visual abnormalities; nocturnal or early-morning awakening; new onset with rapid escalation; and frequent school absences.
     (1) Location and pattern of symptoms may suggest sinus infection, dental disorders, or systemic infection.
     (2) Poor vision is a rare cause of headache.
     (3) Muscle contraction/tension headaches are commonly felt as "pressure" or aching in the occipital or frontal area with a band-like sensation.
     (4) Migraine headaches are experienced as paroxysmal, throbbing or pounding, unilateral or bifrontal, temporal, or occipital pain. They are commonly associated with nausea, pallor, and photophobia. Positive family history and motion sickness are often seen in patients with migraines.
   b. **Management**
     (1) A complete history and physical examination with attention to a thorough neurologic examination, blood pressure measurement, and funduscopic examination are essential for evaluation of headache.
     (2) Attempts should be made to uncover any conflict or stress in an adolescent's life that may exacerbate headaches. Having the patient complete a pain diary for a few weeks to document severity and occurrence of headaches may be helpful.
     (3) Treatment for adolescents with normal neurologic examinations includes acetaminophen, nonsteroidal anti-inflammatory medications (ibuprofen, naproxen), biofeedback, and butalbital compounds (Fioricet or Esgic) or ergotamine compounds for episodic migraines in nonpregnant patients. Frequent follow-up with a primary care provider may assist a teenager in a stressful situation. Chronic prophylactic therapy for individuals is discussed in Chapter 20, p. 522.
 2. **Abdominal pain**
   a. **General considerations.** Adolescents often complain of diffuse, intermittent abdominal pain and a clear etiology is often not found. Chronic right upper quadrant or pelvic pain is more likely to be pathologic. Repeated follow-up may be needed to fully evaluate the problem.
     (1) Signs and symptoms that may indicate increased seriousness include weight loss, vomiting, diarrhea, visible and microscopic blood in the stool, sexual activity, and school absenteeism.
     (2) Differential diagnosis of chronic abdominal pain may include constipation, lactose intolerance, functional bowel problems, menstrual cramps, episodic mittelschmerz, pregnancy, inflammatory bowel disease, pelvic inflammatory disease (PID), other gynecologic disorders (see Chap. 14, pp. 418–25), and occasionally eating disorders or possible abuse history.
     (3) Adolescents can be vague historians and a written record by the patient of pain location and quality, and missed activities, can be helpful.
   b. **Management**
     (1) A complete history and physical examination including a rectal exam for blood in the stool can help to assess the seriousness of the complaint. If a rectal exam is needed in a female, a bimanual rectoabdominal examination in lithotomy position can also be performed to assess uterine and ovarian tenderness.
     (2) Laboratory tests, such as CBC, differential, erythrocyte sedimentation rate (ESR), stool for culture and ova and parasites, sickle cell

screen, liver function tests, urinalysis, amylase, and urine pregnancy test, should be tailored to the findings during history and physical examination.

(3) All sexually active adolescents with significant abdominal pain should have a pregnancy test and a pelvic examination to screen for STDs and PID.

(4) Constipation can be treated by encouraging fluids, increasing fiber in the diet, and establishing more regular bowel habits (often problematic in busy teens). Brief courses of mild stool softeners and laxatives may be effective for the initial management of constipation.

(5) Lactose intolerance is very common in the adolescent population and adjustment in diet to remove lactose-containing foods can be effective in eliminating pain.

3. Fatigue
a. General considerations
(1) Fatigue can indicate a variation of normal adolescent development or school phobia, insufficient sleep or disordered sleep schedule, anemia, depression, pregnancy, chronic infection, collagen vascular disease, or, very rarely, hematologic-oncologic etiologies. The ability of the adolescent to accomplish daily and weekend activities is a good test of severity of fatigue. Fatigue is a very common complaint in the growing teenager who is pulled in many directions by school, family, and peers.

(2) Chronic fatigue syndrome is a recently identified syndrome that includes more than 6 months of debilitating fatigue after an identifiable illness. Specific criterion have been developed (GP Holmes et al. Chronic fatigue syndrome: A working case definition. *Ann Intern Med* 108:387–389, 1988).

b. Management
(1) A complete history and physical examination including sleep patterns and environmental stressors are necessary for evaluation of fatigue.

(2) Tests such as CBC, differential, electrolytes, urinalysis, monospot, ESR, pregnancy, liver function, chest x-ray, antinuclear antibody (ANA), Lyme titers, and human immunodeficiency virus (HIV) may be needed to screen for various medical causes of fatigue and reduce the likelihood of serious etiologies. These tests should be carefully tailored to the history and physical examination or performed when symptoms of fatigue are severe and the etiology is unclear.

(3) Formal psychological screening for depression and school problems should be done in adolescents with debilitating fatigue.

(4) For those who suffer from chronic fatigue syndrome, multivitamins with iron, routine sleep-wake cycles with no napping, and daily exercises can sometimes improve symptoms.

(5) For severe symptoms, nonsteroidal anti-inflammatory drugs for pain and low-dose amitriptyline or other antidepressants can be useful in chronic fatigue syndrome, as can psychotherapy, biofeedback, and physical therapy.

4. Dysuria
a. General considerations
(1) Females: Dysuria in adolescents may indicate a gynecologic etiology or a urinary tract infection. Common causes of dysuria include STDs (gonorrhea, chlamydia, herpes), vaginitis (*Candida*, *Trichomonas*, bacterial vaginosis), urinary tract infections, and pregnancy.

(2) Males: Common causes include STDs. Urinary tract infections (UTIs) are extremely rare in males without a prior history of anatomic anomalies.

b. Management
(1) Females: A full history including sexual history is necessary.

(a) Nonsexually active teenagers should have a urinalysis, a urine culture, and an inspection of the vulva. Wet preps can be done with cotton swabs inserted into the vagina to rule out *Candida*.

(b) All **sexually active** females with dysuria that is not otherwise accompanied by hematuria, frequency and urgency, pyuria, or history of recurrent UTIs (Chap. 5, p. 121) should have a pelvic examination, including screening for STDs and wet preps. A pregnancy test, urinalysis, and urine culture should be performed. Positive urinary leukocytes and nitrates may indicate UTI while a friable cervix or purulent discharge on pelvic examination may indicate STD. A bimanual examination to assess uterine and adnexal tenderness and cervical motion tenderness can aid in the diagnosis of PID (Chap. 14, p. 129). Optimally, adolescents should be treated on the same day of the visit for dysuria (without abdominal pain) for suspected organisms to prevent progression to PID or pyelonephritis and return for reevaluation depending on culture results.

(2) Males: A careful history, including sexual activity, symptoms, and exposure to STDs, is necessary. Urinalyses showing leukocyte esterase on the first-catch urine (first 10–15 ml) is highly suggestive of an STD in sexually active males. Males can be screened for gonorrhea by placing a sample of unspun urine, urine sediment, urethral discharge, or urethral swab on Thayer-Martin agar. Screening for chlamydia can be performed by obtaining a urethral swab for culture or rapid test, although urine screening using polymerase chain reaction (PCR) or ligase chain reaction (LCR) for chlamydia looks promising. Most sexually active males with dysuria or pyuria, or both, should be treated at the first visit for at least presumptive chlamydia (p. 129). If facilities are available, a Gram's stain of urinary sediment or penile discharge to look for gram-negative intracellular diplococci (gonorrhea) can be helpful to direct the treatment (p. 128).

5. Television

a. General considerations

(1) The physician should include questions about the television habits of patients and their families in the general checkup.

(2) There is some evidence that watching violent scenes produces aggressive behavior in young people.

(3) Television advertisements may encourage conflict and confrontation between parent and child.

(4) Excessive television watching (>5 hours/day) is associated with obesity and decreased reading skill.

b. Management

(1) Parents should be encouraged to set limits on television viewing by their children and should monitor their own viewing habits.

(2) Excessive television viewing is potentially a mental and physical health hazard and can significantly compromise the child's functioning in school and in the social sphere. As for any health hazard, the key is prevention.

(3) Guidelines for television viewing can be obtained from the San Francisco Committee on Children's Television, Inc.; the American Academy of Pediatrics; or Action for Children's Television, Newton, Massachusetts.

(4) Decreasing television viewing to 2 hours or less per day is recommended.

6. Cigarettes

a. General considerations

(1) The pediatrician can influence behavior patterns and growth through repeated encounters with the child, and early and repeated discussions of drug issues, including cigarette smoking, may influence future usage patterns.

(2) Areas to be emphasized are the immediate bad effects of smoking. Discussion of the concrete negative effects, such as smell of clothing, discoloration of teeth, bad breath, and effect on exercise tolerance, associated with smoke is especially helpful in encouraging cessation in the teen population.

b. Management

(1) Physicians and nurses can obviously act as examples by not smoking and by not permitting smoking in their offices.

(2) Encourage abstaining from cigarettes.

(3) Encourage cessation in teenagers who have already started smoking by urging them to choose a quit date or to at least consider decreasing the quantity of cigarettes smoked.

(4) In heavy smokers (>1 pack/day), nicotine gum and nicotine patches can be helpful in avoiding withdrawal symptoms, although these methods should be used judiciously in the adolescent population, who may smoke while using the patch.

7. Other common management issues that should be included at adolescent visits include:

a. Depression/suicide. See Chap. 7, p. 245.

b. Drug and alcohol abuse. See Chap. 22, p. 557.

c. Sexuality. See Chap. 14, p. 425; Chap. 22, p. 556.

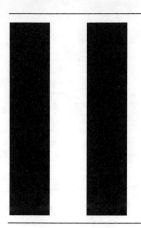

Acute Care

4

Fluid and Electrolytes

John T. Herrin

I. General principles
A. Renal function. The glomerular filtration rate (GFR) is low in infants and reaches an adult value at age 1 to 2 years. Other functions are similarly depressed (Table 4-1).

B. Fluid and volume physiology. At birth, total body water (TBW) constitutes 75 to 80% of the infant's weight and falls to 60% in childhood (see p. 64). There is rapid diuresis of 7% of TBW over the first few days of life.

1. **Body fluids.** Total body water comprises two major compartments.
   a. **Extracellular fluid (ECF)** constitutes 35 to 45% of body weight in infants and 20% in adults (15% interstitial and 5% intravascular).
   b. **Intracellular fluid (ICF)** constitutes 40% of body weight in both infants and adults.

2. **Regulatory mechanisms** independently control water and sodium balance to preserve osmolality and circulating volume.
   a. The **kidney** regulates water balance, osmolality, and the distribution of body water.
   b. **Principles**
      (1) **Tonicity** (osmolality) is conserved in preference to volume.
      (2) The kidneys provide better protection against **dilution** of body fluids than against **dehydration.**
      (3) Extracellular fluid volume is controlled by **sodium.**
   c. **Osmolality** is the number of osmotically active particles per 1,000 g water in a solution (units = mOsm/kg).
      (1) Extracellular fluid osmolality is higher than that of the ICF because of the contribution by plasma proteins.
      (2) Water flux follows ionic flux to equalize fluid concentrations.
      (3) Approximate osmolality can be calculated:

      $$\text{Osmolality} = 2(Na^+) + BUN/2.8 + glucose/18$$

      Solute excretion depends on the concentrating ability of the kidney. Maximal urine osmolality ranges from 1,200 mOsm/kg in the healthy child (600–700 mOsm/kg in the healthy infant), down to 300 mOsm/kg in the diseased kidney.

   d. **Volume** is regulated by numerous factors. Because the body's sodium content determines ECF distribution, maintenance of **total body sodium** is essential to volume regulation. **Angiotensin II** causes peripheral vasoconstriction and enhanced sodium reclamation by the proximal tubule. **Aldosterone** enhances active transport of sodium, which brings about passive water transfer, thereby restoring ECF volume. In addition, **antidiuretic hormone (ADH)** release augments water retention. Atrial-natriuretic factor increases sodium and water excretion.
   e. **"Third-space"** accumulations trap fluids and electrolytes outside their normal boundaries, thus decreasing effective circulating volume.

C. Electrolyte physiology
1. **Sodium (Na+).** 1 mEq = 23 mg; 1 g = 43.5 mEq; plasma concentration = 135–140 mEq/liter. **Note:** 1 g salt (NaCl) = 18 mEq Na+.

Table 4-1. Normal values of renal function*

Measurement	At birth	1–2 wk	6 mo–1 yr	1–3 yr	Adult
GFR (ml/min/m²)	15 ± 11	31 ± 15	45 ± 12	55 ± 13	68 ± 10
RPF (ml/min/m²)	51 ± 12	89 ± 20	203 ± 42	310 ± 70	354 ± 53
T_m PAH (mg/min/m²)		8 ± 1	30 ± 12	38 ± 11	46 ± 7
T_m glucose (mg/min/m²)		10 ± 12			196 ± 29

m² = body surface area in square meters; T_m = maximum rate of tubular reabsorption; PAH = para-aminohippurate; RPF = renal plasma flow.
*Mean ± SD.

    a. Na⁺ is the principal volume regulator. Normally, Na⁺ accounts for 90% of extracellular cationic osmolality.

    b. Although Na⁺ is principally distributed in the ECF, the true Na⁺ space is the TBW.

    c. Measurement of Na⁺ by flame photometer is artifactually depressed in hyperlipemic and hyperglycemic states. **Rule of thumb:** *Na⁺ is depressed 5 mEq/liter for every 200 mg/dl glucose concentration above 100 mg/dl.*

    d. Requirements for Na⁺ vary. A typical daily requirement is 40 to 60 mEq/m² or 1 to 3 mEq/dl water requirement.

    e. In the newborn, the Na⁺ and volume regulatory mechanisms are qualitatively similar to those of adults but quantitatively limited. Net excretion is limited by a relative concentrating defect (maximal urine osmolality approximately 600–700 mOsm/liter). Therefore, obligatory solute loads require extra free water for their elimination.

  2. Potassium (K⁺). 1 mEq = 39.1 mg; 1 g = 25.6 mEq; plasma concentration = 3.4–5.5 mEq/liter (may be higher in neonates).

    a. K⁺ is the principal cation of the ICF and contributes to the maintenance of intracellular tonicity and the cell membrane resting potential. The ICF contains 98% of the body K⁺.

    b. The proportion of K⁺ in the ECF is controlled by multiple factors. Measurement of serum K⁺ provides only an indirect assessment of total body K⁺ stores and may be misleading. **No practical estimate of K⁺ space can be given for therapeutic replacement purposes.**

    c. A typical daily K⁺ requirement is 30–40 mEq/m²/24 hr or 1 to 3 mEq/dl fluid. There is an obligatory K⁺ loss via the urine since the tubular resorption generally cannot lower U_{K^+} below 10 mEq/liter.

    d. A maximal intravenous dose of K⁺ is 1 mEq/kg/hr, preferably administered into a large vein via intravenous pump. Intravenous administration of K⁺ in concentrations greater than 40 mEq/liter often leads to phlebitis.

    e. The danger of an **abnormal serum K⁺** is exacerbated by change in serum calcium in the opposite direction.

    f. Hypokalemia occurring with renal tubular defects, starvation, chronic diarrhea or vomiting, diabetic ketoacidosis, hyperaldosteronism, chronic use of diuretics, or inadequate long-term IV replacement is usually accompanied by chloride depletion with metabolic alkalosis.

      (1) Symptoms include muscle weakness, cramps, paralytic ileus, decreased reflexes, lethargy, and confusion.

      (2) Acid urine in the presence of metabolic alkalosis (paradoxical aciduria) also indicates K⁺ depletion. Hypokalemic metabolic alkalosis is usually accompanied by a K⁺ deficit of at least 4 to 5 mEq/kg.

      (3) Cardiac effects indicated by ECG are a low-voltage T wave, the presence of a U wave, and a prolonged Q-T interval.

      (4) Chronic exposure to low potassium damages the kidney's concentrating ability, thus producing a vasopressin-resistant diabetes insipidus.

g. **Hyperkalemia** occurs with renal failure, hemolysis, tissue necrosis, mineralocorticoid deficiency–Addison's disease, congenital adrenocortical hyperplasia, use of potassium-sparing diuretics, angiotensin converting enzyme (ACE) inhibitor therapy, overdose of K^+ supplements, or inappropriate use of salt substitutes.

   (1) Hypocalcemia, hyponatremia, acidosis, insulin deficiency, and beta-blocker therapy all exacerbate the toxicity of hyperkalemia.

   (2) The **toxic** effects are mainly cardiac. ECG changes include peaked T wave, increased P-R interval and widened QRS, depressed S-T segment, and atrioventricular or intraventricular heart block. As serum K^+ rises beyond 7.5 mEq/liter, there is grave danger of heart block, ventricular tachycardia, and ventricular fibrillation.

3. **Chloride (Cl⁻).** 1 mEq = 35.5 mg; 1 g = 28 mEq; 1 g NaCl = 18 mEq Cl⁻; plasma concentration = 99–105 mEq/liter.

   a. Cl^- is the principal anion of both intravascular fluid and gastric fluid.

   b. Abnormal losses occur with vomiting, diuretic therapy, and cystic fibrosis, and tend to lead to metabolic alkalosis.

   c. **Paradoxical aciduria** occurs in the face of Cl^- depletion with dehydration. In the absence of Cl^-, HCO_3^- is reabsorbed with Na^+. In addition, the accompanying secondary hyperaldosteronism causes the distal tubular secretion of H^+, resulting in an acid urine. This cycle of events can only be interrupted by the replacement of Cl^-.

4. **Calcium (Ca²⁺).** 1 mEq = 20 mg; 1 g = 50 mEq; plasma concentration = 9.5–10.5 mg/dl or 4.7–5.2 mEq/liter except in the newborn and premature infant.

   a. Free ionized Ca^{2+} constitutes about 47% of total serum calcium. Approximately 40% of total serum calcium is bound to serum proteins and 80 to 90% of this calcium is bound to albumin. The calcium space is approximately 25% of body weight.

   b. A change in serum albumin of 1 g/dl changes serum Ca^{2+} concentration, in the same direction, by 0.8 mg/dl.

   c. Acidosis increases ionized Ca^{2+}, whereas alkalosis decreases it.

   d. **Hypocalcemia** is most commonly seen in rickets, renal insufficiency, and the hypoalbuminemic states of liver disease or nephrosis, and in the neonate who is fed cow's milk formulas.

   Drugs that cause hypocalcemia include furosemide, glucagon, calcitonin, mithramycin, bicarbonate, and corticosteroids. **Exchange transfusion with acid citrate–preserved blood can produce hypocalcemia** (see Chap. 15, p. 457). Other conditions that produce lowered calcium are discussed in Chap. 13, p. 400.

   (1) **Symptoms** of depressed ionized Ca^{2+} include Chvostek's and Trousseau's signs, carpopedal spasm, and, occasionally, mental confusion. Neonates commonly become jittery and may have seizures with tetany of the newborn (see Chap. 6, p. 202).

   (2) The ECG shows prolongation of the Q-T interval relative to the rate.

   (3) **Treatment** of hypocalcemia includes IV and PO administration of Ca^{2+}. An IV bolus of Ca^{2+}, 10 mg/kg over 10 to 20 minutes, will transiently (for about 1 hour) raise the serum Ca^{2+} level in an emergency. Supplemental Ca^{2+}, 20 to 40 mg/kg/day IV, or oral supplements, 60 to 100 mg/kg/day, of elemental Ca^{2+} should be provided. Continuous IV administration is hazardous (cardiac arrhythmias, phlebitis, subcutaneous calcifications) and should be reserved for critical situations.

   e. **Hypercalcemia** is seen with vitamin D intoxication, sarcoidosis, cancer, immobilization, thyroid disease, Addison's disease, hypophosphatasia, hyperparathyroidism, and the milk-alkali syndrome in those taking antacids. **Symptoms** of excess Ca^{2+} include nausea, anorexia, vomiting, constipation, polyuria, dehydration, mental confusion, and eventually coma. Chronic elevation of Ca^{2+} can lead to nephrocalcinosis, extraskeletal calcification, and renal calculi.

D. Acid-base physiology

1. **General principles.** Blood pH is maintained by **blood buffering,** changes in **ventilation,** and **renal** compensatory mechanisms. Children ingest 1 to 2 mEq/kg/day (2–4 mEq/100 calories) "fixed" acid in their diet. Further acid is produced as a by-product of bone formation. Blood chemical buffers and increased elimination of carbon dioxide immediately compensate for this acid, while the kidney maintains long-term pH homeostasis.

   a. **Blood buffers** include erythrocyte hemoglobin, organic and inorganic phosphates, carbonate, and bicarbonate. About half the buffering capacity derives from bicarbonate and roughly one third from hemoglobin.

   b. **Ventilation** normally eliminates thousands of milliequivalents of carbon dioxide per day. This prevents the accumulation of the weak acid, H_2CO_3, formed when carbon dioxide remains dissolved in plasma.

   c. The **kidneys** regulate the systemic levels of HCO_3 by means of recovery of filtered HCO_3 and generation of "new" HCO_3 by the process of net acid excretion.

2. **Determination of acid-base status** requires measurement of blood pH and bicarbonate. Bicarbonate, total carbon dioxide content, and CO_2 combining power provide the same basic information. Total carbon dioxide (TCO_2) is 1 to 2 mEq/liter lower than combining power.

3. **Laboratory values.** Ideally, arterial samples are obtained for the diagnosis of significant acid-base disturbances. Normal values for arterial and venous blood are given in Table 4-2.

4. **Acid-base abnormalities.** By convention, acid-base disorders are divided by serum pH into **acidosis** or **alkalosis,** then further subdivided into the following categories (Fig. 4-1): **respiratory** versus **metabolic, acute** versus **chronic, simple** versus **mixed,** and **pure** versus **compensated.** In pure imbalances of pH, the disequilibrium results from a deviation of either PCO_2 (respiratory) or HCO_3^- (metabolic) from the norm.

   These situations prevail only for brief periods before compensatory mechanisms occur. Compensation is rarely sufficient to offset the primary disturbance completely, and the condition is usually only partially corrected, so that the patient has a compensated acid-base disorder (Table 4-3).

   a. **Respiratory acidosis** results from *retention of carbon dioxide* and a consequent *increase in H_2CO_3.* Normally, a rise in PCO_2 stimulates a ventilatory effort to eliminate the hypercapnia. In the acute phase of respiratory acidosis, pH falls rapidly as PCO_2 exceeds 50 mm Hg (see Chap. 7). When hypercapnia is sustained, renal compensation leads to an increase in plasma bicarbonate. Net acid excretion is increased. Tubular resorption of bicarbonate increases while that for chloride decreases. The kidney can raise bicarbonate to 40 mEq/liter or more to compensate for hypercapnia. Plasma bicarbonate increases by about 0.3 mEq/liter for each 1 mm increase in arterial carbon dioxide tension ($PaCO_2$). *Usually, neonates are incapable of this adaptation and will remain severely acidotic with respiratory distress syndrome.*

   b. **Respiratory alkalosis** occurs in patients who are managed with mechanical ventilators, in the early phase of salicylate intoxication, in hepatic failure or metabolic disease resulting in hyperammonemia or lactic acidosis,

Table 4-2. Normal blood values*

Blood sample	pH	PCO_2	HCO_3^-	TCO_2
Arterial	7.38–7.45	35–45 mm Hg	23–27 mEq/liter	24–28 mEq/liter
Venous	7.35–7.40	45–50 mm Hg	24–29 mEq/liter	25–30 mEq/liter

*In children less than 1 yr of age, the normal range for TCO_2 is 20–24, and pH is lower by approximately 0.05.

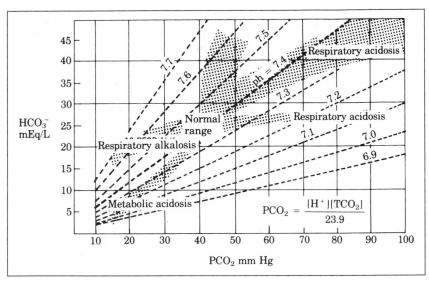

Fig. 4-1. Acid-base nomogram.

in anxious or hysterical states, and in hypermetabolic states. **Rapid correction** of metabolic acidosis can also result in respiratory alkalosis, since correction of the pH in the cerebrospinal fluid lags behind the ECF, and continuing CNS acidosis stimulates the medullary ventilatory drive.

    (1) **Acute respiratory alkalosis** can precipitate tetany (see p. 65) and causes a feeling of lightheadedness.

    (2) **Laboratory diagnosis** rests on the triad of *decreased PCO₂, elevated pH, and normal bicarbonate.*

    (3) **Hypocapnia** alkalinizes body fluids and elicits a prompt but modest reduction in plasma HCO_3^- secondary to titration of HCO_3 buffer. This is followed by a net decrease in renal acid excretion, decreased tubular HCO_3^- resorption, and enhanced tubular chloride reabsorption. Plasma bicarbonate decreases by about 0.4 to 0.5 mEq/liter for each 1 mm decrease in $PaCO_2$. Urinary loss of HCO_3 results in simultaneous loss of sodium and contraction of the ECF volume.

  c. **Metabolic acidosis** results from an *increased acid burden; renal defects* in the secretion of H⁺; and *loss of extracellular HCO₃.* In these situations bicarbonate and other blood buffers are consumed and TCO_2 falls.

    (1) The **anion gap** is an estimation of anionic substances that are not measured by the usual laboratory techniques. The anion gap is the difference between the serum cations (Na⁺) and anions (Cl⁻ and HCO_3^-).

Table 4-3. Compensation in acid-base disturbances

Acid-base disturbance	pH	HCO_3^-	PCO_2	Compensation
Metabolic acidosis	↓	↓		↓ PCO_2; acid urine
Respiratory acidosis	↓		↑	Acid urine
Metabolic alkalosis	↑	↑		↑ PCO_2; alkaline urine
Respiratory alkalosis	↑		↓	Alkaline urine

It normally is approximately 12 mEq/liter, but is somewhat higher in newborn infants. Increases in the anion gap occur when the fall in plasma bicarbonate is balanced by a rise in an anion that is not commonly measured (increased anion gap acidosis).

(2) In response to the acidemic stress, both the kidney and lung undertake corrective measures. There is a prompt increase in ventilation, and PCO_2 falls. Urinary acidification maximizes over a few days.

(3) In children, chronic metabolic acidosis most commonly can be traced to a kidney abnormality, either parenchymal disease, obstruction, or a tubular disorder, or to a metabolic disorder such as an organic acidemia. Growth failure invariably accompanies chronic acidemia.

d. Metabolic alkalosis is a disorder characterized by *elevated plasma bicarbonate* and *decreased concentrations of proton and chloride* in the ECF. Metabolic alkalosis usually occurs as part of a generalized derangement in fluid and electrolytes. Although the list of possible etiologies is long, the cause of metabolic alkalosis in the majority of affected children is *loss of acid from the gastrointestinal tract.*

(1) In acute alkalosis, K^+ moves from the ECF to the ICF to help maintain electroneutrality in the face of H^+ ion depletion. *Although serum K^+ may then be low, total body K^+ remains normal.*

(2) Paradoxical aciduria may coexist with systemic alkalosis when hypokalemia or hypovolemia is present.

e. Mixed disorders of acid-base homeostasis result from concurrent disturbances in both respiratory and renal function (Fig. 4-1). Because the shaded areas in Fig. 4-1 represent the 95% confidence bands for each disturbance (including the normal compensatory response), any combination of values of PCO_2 and HCO_3^- that falls outside these areas represents a mixed disturbance.

f. As a rule, **compensatory mechanisms** modify the acid-base disturbances as shown in Table 4-3 to the following degree:

(1) Metabolic acidosis: $PCO_2 \downarrow 1.0–1.5 \times$ fall of HCO_3^-.

(2) Metabolic alkalosis: $PCO_2 \uparrow 0.5–1.0 \times$ rise of HCO_3^-.

(3) Acute respiratory acidosis: $HCO_3^- \uparrow$ to maximum 30 mEq/liter.

(4) Chronic respiratory acidosis: $HCO_3^- \uparrow$ to 4 mEq/liter/10 mm PCO_2.

(5) Acute respiratory alkalosis: $HCO_3^- \downarrow 2.5$ mEq/liter/10 mm, $\downarrow PCO_2$ (to minimum 18 mEq/liter).

(6) Chronic respiratory alkalosis: $HCO_3^- \downarrow$ to 15 mEq/liter.

II. Maintenance of normal fluid and electrolyte balance

A. Estimation of fluid requirements

1. Rationale. *Maintenance fluid requirement* is the amount of extrinsic fluid required to balance insensible, fecal, and urinary losses. There are several methods of **estimating average** maintenance fluid requirements; **actual** maintenance requirements may vary considerably from the usual estimations because of unusual circumstances (see sec. **3** below and Table 4-4).

2. Components of maintenance fluid requirements

a. Insensible losses account for about 50% of the total fluid lost per day distributed as

(1) Respiratory = 15%.

(2) Skin (not sweat) = 30%.

(3) Feces = 5%.

b. Urine losses account for the other 50% of fluid loss.

c. Intrinsic fluid sources. Water of oxidation is water produced as a byproduct of normal metabolism; it can replace about 15% of the usual fluid losses.

3. Methods of estimating maintenance fluids

a. Surface area. Levels of renal function and body fluid requirements correlate best with body surface area (BSA). This system works well for children who **weigh more than 10 kg.** The normal water requirement is about 1,500 ml/m²/24 hr (Table 4-5).

Table 4-4. Conditions affecting normal fluid requirements

Condition	Adjustment
Increased metabolic rate	
Fever	Increase H_2O by 12%/°C
Hypermetabolic state	Increase H_2O by 25–75%
Decreased metabolic rate	
Hypothermia	Decrease H_2O by 12%/°C
Hypometabolic state	Decrease H_2O by 10–25%
Unusual insensible losses	
High environmental humidity	Decrease IWL to 0–15 ml/100 calories
Hyperventilation	Increase IWL to 50–60 ml/100 calories
Excessive sweating	Increase H_2O by 10–25 ml/100 calories

IWL = insensible water loss.

    b. Calories expended. This method computes daily water requirements from metabolic expenditure. Figure 4-2 depicts energy use as a function of weight. One allows 100 to 150 ml/24°/100 calories metabolized.

    c. Body weight. General rule is

        100 ml/kg/24° for the **first** 10 kg body weight
        50 ml/kg/24° for the **next** 10 kg body weight
        20 ml/kg/24° for each kg **above** 20 kg

    d. Changes in normal maintenance requirements are affected by several conditions, shown in Table 4-4.

  4. The fluid needs of the newborn (see Chap. 6).

B. Estimation of electrolyte requirements. Na^+, K^+, Cl^-, and HCO_3^- requirements vary significantly because of the kidney's ability to conserve them in depletion states or to excrete any excess. General guidelines to Na^+ and K^+ daily maintenance requirements calculated by three methods follow. Adjustment should be made for continuing abnormal losses (see Tables 4-7 and 4-8).

	Na+	**K+**
BSA	20–50 mEq Na^+/m^2 BSA	20–50 mEq K^+/m^2
Caloric requirement	2–4 mEq $Na^+/100$ calories	2–3 mEq $K^+/100$ calories
General method (body weight)	2–4 mEq Na^+/dl fluid	2–4 mEq K^+/dl fluid

Table 4-5. Fluid balance in children

Losses	
Respiratory and skin	775 ml/m^2/24 hr[a]
Gastrointestinal	100 ml/m^2/24 hr
Urine	875 ml/m^2/24 hr[b]
Total	1,750
Sources	
Water of oxidation	250 ml/m^2/24 hr
Net maintenance requirement	
Water	1,500 ml/m^2/24 hr

[a]Varies with size of child, e.g., 1,200 ml/m^2 in a toddler vs 700 ml/m^2 at age 8–10 yr.
[b]Based on excretion of isotonic urine, 300 mOsm/liter, and minimal solute intake, e.g., dextrose in water.

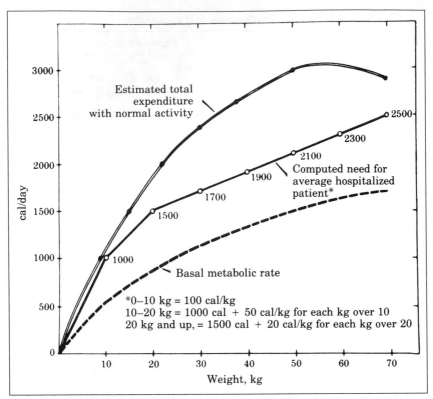

Fig. 4-2. Comparison of energy expenditure in basal and ideal state. (Reproduced with permission from WE Segar. Parenteral fluid therapy. *Curr Probl Pediatr* 3:4, 1972. Copyright © 1972 by Year Book Medical Publishers, Inc., Chicago.)

III. Assessment of abnormalities of fluid and electrolyte balance

A. General comments

1. The most useful way to consider dehydration is based on the amount of **Na⁺** and **K⁺ lost in relation to water.** Dehydration states are thus considered as isotonic (isonatremic), hypotonic (hyponatremic), and hypertonic (hypernatremic).

   a. **Hypotonic.** Na^+ <125 mEq/liter; ECF depletion with relative sparing of intracellular contents; hence, early vascular compromise.

   b. **Isotonic.** Na^+ = 130–150 mEq/liter; balanced loss of water and ions.

   c. **Hypertonic.** Na^+ >150 mEq/liter; ICF depletion; allows more chronic dehydration; the vascular space is relatively protected.

2. The best indicator of **short-term quantitative fluid loss** is change in body weight. Table 4-6 presents a rough clinical estimate of degree of dehydration.

3. **Initial assessment** of *dehydration*

   a. **History.** Urine output, weight change, infectious disease contacts, and estimate of stooling or vomiting frequency. Dietary history is important because excretion of renal solute load may aggravate dehydration by causing obligatory urinary free-water loss. *The solute stress of a given feeding is different from the formula's measured osmotic load.* Because infants cannot effectively concentrate urine much beyond 600 mOsm/kg, cow's milk causes free-water losses **three times greater** than those of human milk, while boiled skim milk imposes a fourfold free-water loss.

Table 4-6. Estimation of dehydration

	Degree of dehydration		
Clinical signs	Mild	Moderate	Severe
Weight loss (%)	5	10	15
Behavior	Normal	Irritable	Hyperirritable to lethargic
Thirst	Slight	Moderate	Intense
Mucous membrane	May be normal	Dry	Parched
Tears	Present	±	Absent
Anterior fontanel	Flat	±	Sunken
Skin turgor	Normal	±	Increased

    b. Clinical. Urine output, skin turgor, mucous membrane moisture, eye turgor, fullness of fontanel, and mental state.

    c. Laboratory. Weight, serum and urine Na^+, K^+, Cl^-, pH, TCO_2, BUN, creatinine, osmolality, glucose, and calcium; **urinalysis.**

  4. Urinalysis is particularly important. Despite a lack of *absolute* normal values for electrolyte, osmolality, and pH in the urine, there are *expected* values depending on the clinical situation. The **specific gravity** in dehydration will be well above 1.015 unless intrinsic renal disease is present. An active sediment signals underlying primary renal disease. **Alkaline urine** during dehydration or an increased urinary anion gap should raise the question of renal tubular acidosis.

  5. Water and electrolyte losses. Estimates of deficits in moderate to severe dehydration are given in Table 4-7.

B. Assessment of Na^+ and K^+ losses

  1. General. There is no practical means of assessing true K^+ loss (see p. 64). Nonetheless, one can assume in most instances that K^+ losses are equivalent to Na^+ losses.

  2. Estimations of Na^+ and K^+ deficits in a child who appears severely dehydrated and in whom the serum Na^+ is known can be made using Table 4-7.

  3. The total body Na^+ deficit ($TBNa_d^+$) is the difference between the normal total body Na^+($TBNa_n^+$) and the current (dehydrated) total body Na^+($TBNa_c^+$).

$$TBNa_d^+ = TBNa_n^+ - TBNa_c^+$$

Thus,

$$TBNa_d^+ = (TBW \times 135) - [(TBW - FL) \times Na_c^+] \ or$$

$$TBNa_d^+ = TBW(135 - Na_c^+) + FL(NA_c^+)$$

Table 4-7. Deficits in moderate to severe dehydration

		Losses			
Type of dehydration	Range of Na^+ (mEq/liter)	Water (ml/kg)	Na^+ (mEq/kg)	K^+ (mEq/kg)	$Cl^- + HCO_3^-$ (mEq/kg)
Isotonic	130–145	100–150	7–11	14–22	
Hypotonic	<125	40–80	10–14	10–14	20–28
Hypertonic	>150	120–170	2–5	2–5	4–10

Source: Modified from RW Winters. *Principles of Pediatric Fluid Therapy.* North Chicago, IL: Abbott Laboratories, 1970. P 56.

where TBW = 0.6 × normal weight, FL = the fluid loss (or equivalent of weight change), and Na_c^+ = the current serum sodium concentration (mEq/liter).

C. **Ongoing losses**
   1. **General.** *Ongoing losses are* **abnormal** losses of fluids or electrolytes, or both, that occur while the patient is under observation.
   2. **Estimation of ongoing losses**
      a. **Fluid.** Abnormal losses (nasogastric suction, surgical drainage, fistula drainage, vomitus) usually can be measured directly.
         (1) In the absence of direct measurement, **weight changes** can be used to determine fluid losses. Daily changes in weight reflect losses or gains of TBW.
         (2) Patients receiving maintenance fluids and calories should remain at a constant weight.
         (3) Patients receiving maintenance fluids, but insufficient calories, should lose about 0.5% of their weight per day.
         (4) Newborn infants should lose weight over the first 3 to 5 days of life and subsequently gain weight consistent with the usual growth curves (approximately 30 g/day for full-term infants) if given sufficient nutrition.
      b. **Electrolytes**
         (1) The electrolyte content of abnormal body fluid losses frequently can be **measured directly.** This is particularly important for **abnormal** urine losses, since the composition can vary widely.
         (2) The usual composition of body fluids is shown in Table 4-8.
         (3) The gastric Na^+ content will vary directly with the pH of gastric fluid. Above pH 2.0 (H^+ = 0.01 molar or 10 mEq/liter), the Na^+ content of the gastric fluid may be 100 mEq/liter or higher. If gastric fluid losses are large, direct measurement of electrolyte concentrations is mandatory for accurate replacement.
   3. **Strategy for replacement of ongoing losses**
      a. Ongoing losses of fluids and electrolyte are measured or calculated over fixed time periods and replaced evenly over an equivalent period of time. If there are **large** ongoing losses, these periods should be **short** (e.g., every half hour or hour). If losses are small, daily adjustment is sufficient. As a rule of thumb, monitor serum electrolyte changes after replacement volume is equal to 0.5 blood volume (approximately 25 ml/kg).
      b. **Patients without deficits at the initiation of therapy**
         (1) The therapy is designed to provide **maintenance** fluid and electrolytes and to replace the **ongoing** losses.

Table 4-8. Composition of body fluids

Source	Na^+ (mEq/liter)	K1 (mEq/liter)	Cl^- (mEq/liter)	HCO_3^- (mEq/liter)	pH	Osm (mOsm/liter)
Gastric	50	10–15	150	0	1	300
Pancreas	140	5	50–100	100	9	300
Bile	130	5	100	40	8	300
Ileostomy	130	15–20	120	25–30	8	300
Diarrhea	50	35	40	50	Alk	
Sweat	50	5	55	0		
Blood	140	4–5	100	25	7.4	285–295
Urine	0–100*	20–100*	70–100*	0	4.5–8.5	50–1,400

*Varies considerably with intake.

(2) If there are unusual urine losses or if the urine output is erratic, therapy is designed to provide **insensible** fluid losses plus urine and ongoing losses.

c. Patients who are dehydrated at the initiation of therapy (e.g., vomiting or diarrhea)

(1) The measured or estimated ongoing losses are **added to** the calculated replacement of maintenance and deficit fluid and electrolytes. Adjustments should be made **frequently.** Urine losses are ignored, since they are accounted for in the maintenance calculations.

(2) It is important **not** to recalculate the overall deficits in rehydrating a dehydrated patient with ongoing losses; this usually leads to an **underestimation** of true deficits. **Add** ongoing losses to previously estimated deficits.

IV. Correction of abnormalities of fluid and electrolyte balance

A. Acute fluid management and resuscitation

1. General concepts (see also Chap. 7)

a. Weigh the patient.

b. If shock is present, or if no urine is produced in the first half hour, give 20 to 30 ml/kg Ringer's lactate or normal saline with 5% dextrose (D5NS) or 5% albumin IV as a bolus and repeat if adequate circulation is not established.

c. After the first hour, give 10 ml/kg/hr Ringer's lactate or D5NS until shock is alleviated and actual fluid and electrolyte deficits can be accurately calculated.

d. If the patient is asymptomatic and/or dehydration is hyponatremic or isotonic, one half the fluids calculated for 24 hours should be administered in the first 8 hours. The other half should be given in the remaining 16 hours.

e. If hypertonic dehydration is present with shock, reestablish circulation and urine flow, then correct the remaining deficit **slowly and evenly** over 48 hours.

f. With **fever** add 12% of the maintenance amount per degrees centigrade (see Table 4-4).

g. In most situations, **do not add K+ to the IV solutions until after urine flow is established.**

h. In **diabetic ketoacidosis,** however, **K+ can be added** to the initial solution, since rapid correction of dehydration, acidosis, and hyperglycemia can precipitate severe hypoglycemia and hypokalemia (see Chap. 13, p. 411).

i. Adequacy of therapy is indicated by adequate urine output, normal circulation, and restoration of weight.

2. Management of dehydration states

a. Hypotonic dehydration

(1) Clinically, infants present soon after the onset of illness because **symptoms** become apparent early. For a given weight loss, the clinical signs are more marked than in isotonic or hypertonic dehydration. Thus, estimates of weight loss should follow a 3, 6, 9% rule of thumb for mild, moderate, and severe, respectively. **Vascular collapse can occur early.**

(2) General principles of treatment. Because loss is mainly ECF, replacement therapy can advance rapidly, with volume and Na+ restored by the end of 24 to 36 hours (see sec. **A.1** above).

b. Symptomatic hyponatremia. Regardless of the cause, whether Na+ loss or water excess, therapy is directed at raising the Na+ concentration **quickly,** to correct symptoms.

(1) Use *hypertonic* saline (3% = 513 mEq Na+/liter) to deliver approximately 5 mEq/kg/hr. Calculation of the approximate Na+ deficit is given in sec. **III.B.3.**

(2) Following acute correction, *the patient's acidosis may worsen.* Sodium bicarbonate (1 mEq/ml) can be mixed with the hypertonic saline to supply some of the Na^+ dose while also providing bicarbonate as the anion when severe acidosis is initially present or if acidosis persists on restoration of circulating volume.

c. The therapy of **asymptomatic hyponatremia** requires *gradual* correction. **K^+** deficit and **acidosis** both require specific therapy for correction.

d. Isotonic dehydration

(1) For a given weight loss, symptoms will be less dramatic than for hypotonic dehydration—assume a weight loss of 5, 10, or 15% for clinical estimation of mild, moderate, and severe involvement, respectively.

(2) Treatment is similar to that for hypotonic dehydration (see sec. **A.2.a.(2)** above). The solutions used are hypotonic, but since the normal kidney needs only ¼ N solution for true maintenance, these ½ N solutions provide sufficient solute even for correction of isotonic losses.

e. Hypertonic dehydration results when inappropriately high solute loads are given as replacement fluid, or when a renal concentrating defect produces a large free-water loss. Usually, sodium represents the principal excess solute.

(1) The **clinical signs of dehydration** in these infants can be deceptive.

(a) Skin turgor does not exhibit the usual tenting of advanced dehydration, but has a thick, doughy consistency. Eyeball turgor, however, is decreased as in dehydration of other causes.

(b) Other findings include a shrill cry or mewing sound, muscle weakness, tachypnea, and intense thirst in toddlers.

(c) In assessing these infants, be sure to check *serum glucose* and *calcium*, since **hyperglycemia** is present in half the patients, and **calcium deficiency** has been noted in 10%.

(d) Shock is a late manifestation. When it supervenes, one can be certain that fluid loss exceeds 10% of body weight.

(2) Treatment. The total fluid deficit must be replaced slowly over 48 hours or more, dropping serum Na^+ by 10 mEq/liter/day. Rapid correction floods the intracellular space with fluid, leading to cerebral (and sometimes pulmonary) edema. In general, *the more dilute the solution being used to correct the deficit, the slower it should be infused.*

(a) If shock is present, infuse 20 ml/kg lactated Ringer's solution, 5% albumin in lactated Ringer's solution, or 0.9% saline over 20 to 30 minutes.

(b) First hour. The goal is to reestablish satisfactory circulation and urine flow. Give 10 to 20 mg/kg Ringer's lactate to reduce the Cl^- load in favor of lactate (alkali).

(c) Over the next 4 hours, the goal is to reestablish urine output to allow steady and controlled correction of the fluid deficit and steadily reduce the serum Na^+ and serum osmolality. There is no **best** regimen.

(i) The rate of IV infusion is determined by the tonicity of the solution; that is, isotonic solutions can be infused more rapidly.

(ii) Infuse 10 mg/kg/hr of 5% dextrose in Ringer's lactate. Ringer's lactate, or a mixture of 2% dextrose and ½ N saline to which is added ¼ N bicarbonate (17 ml of 8% $NaHCO_3$/500 ml solution), depending on the degree of acidosis or hyperglycemia.

(d) The next 48 hours are utilized to replenish the fluid deficit (based on calculated deficits) together with measured ongoing losses at a steady rate.

Calculation of water deficit:

Water deficit (liters) = usual body water − current body water

Usual body water = current body water × current Osm/normal Osm

Current body water = current weight × 0.6

   (i) Children with hypernatremic dehydration, unlike adults are usually **not** significantly deficient in Na^+. **Do not try to correct the water deficit rapidly with Na^+ (normal saline or greater) solutions,** because this can lead to severe Na^+ overload and possibly to an increased serum Na^+ concentration.

   (ii) It is unwise to attempt rapid control of **hyperglycemia;** the presence of extra glucose acts as an "osmotic buffer" under whose cover the necessary ion shifts can occur as reequilibration proceeds.

   (iii) **Treatment of acute salt poisoning** (serum Na^+ ≥ 160 mEq/liter, with urine Na^+ ≥ 100 mEq/liter) requires dialysis or furosemide diuresis (1 mg/kg), replacing the urine output with a 10% dextrose in water (D/W) solution, monitoring Na^+ values q4h and repeating the administration of furosemide if urine output is not sustained.

   (e) If the serum Na^+ concentration is greater than 180 mEq/liter after circulation is reestablished, **dialysis** may be required to correct the abnormalities.

V. Monitoring fluid and electrolyte therapy
   A. The results of therapy must be assessed periodically and necessary adjustment made.
   B. The usual variables to monitor include
      1. Weight.
      2. Vital signs.
      3. Laboratory tests. Serum electrolytes, osmolality, blood sugar, calcium BUN, creatinine, and urine electrolytes and specific gravity or osmolality. Urinary electrolytes, creatinine, and the composition of abnormal losses—stool, fistulae, gastric suction—may be necessary in planning adequate correction of large and continuing losses.
      4. Total **inputs** and **outputs** of both fluids and electrolytes.
   C. A well-conceived **flowsheet** is an efficient means of monitoring and adjusting therapy.

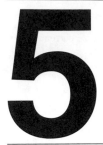

Antibiotics and Infectious Disorders

W. Charles Huskins and
Marvin B. Harper

I. Principles of antimicrobial therapy. Whenever possible, a single antimicrobial agent should be used, and the antimicrobial spectrum should be kept as narrow as possible. The use of multiple or broad-spectrum antimicrobials is associated with an increased likelihood of colonization and superinfection by drug-resistant organisms and is usually far more expensive. However, when severely ill patients or those whose defenses are impaired are suspected of being infected, they should be given broad-spectrum therapy pending the definitive results of cultures.

  A. Identification of the infecting pathogen. The most probable infecting pathogen(s) can often be determined from various host factors, the site of infection, the results of rapid diagnostic procedures, the patient's underlying illness, and local epidemiologic factors.

    1. Host factors

      a. Age. In the neonatal period the most common pathogens are *Escherichia coli*, other gram-negative enteric bacilli, group B streptococci, and staphylococci. Pneumococci and meningococci are common and serious pathogens between the ages of 2 months and 5 years. Infections caused by *Haemophilus influenzae* type b are now uncommon in areas where most children receive conjugate *H. influenzae* type (Hib) vaccines.

      b. Defects of humoral immunity (see also Chap. 16). Patients with human immunodeficiency virus (HIV) infection, congenital or acquired hypogammaglobulinemia, or defects of certain complement components, particularly C3, have an increased incidence of infections due to encapsulated pyogenic bacteria, such as pneumococci, meningococci, *H. influenzae* (type b and nontypeable strains), and *Staphylococcus aureus*.

      c. Defects in cellular immunity. The T lymphocytes and their effector cells are probably important in the defense against intracellular bacteria, *Listeria*, *Nocardia*, fungi, certain viruses, and *Pneumocystis carinii*. Human immunodeficiency virus infection is an important acquired cause of defects in cellular immunity.

      d. Granulocytopenia and granulocyte disorders (see Chap. 15, p. 452).

      e. Miscellaneous defects conferring increased risk

        (1) Patients with **splenic hypofunction** may have fulminant infections, most commonly due to the pneumococcus, meningococcus, and *H. influenzae* type b.

        (2) Patients with severe **hepatic dysfunction** have an increased frequency of bacteremias with *E. coli*, other enteric gram-negative bacilli, and occasionally the pneumococcus.

        (3) Patients with **nephrotic syndrome** have an increased incidence of infections (especially peritonitis) caused by pneumococci, gram-negative bacilli, and *H. influenzae* type b.

        (4) Primary peritonitis occurs almost exclusively in patients with ascites associated with cirrhosis or nephrosis.

    2. Site of infection. Table 5–1 lists the bacterial and fungal pathogens that cause acute infections at various sites. The list is not exhaustive. Further discussion of specific sites of infection is found in sec. **III.**

Table 5-1. Bacterial and fungal causes of acute infections in various sites

Site	Common organisms	Less common organisms	Comments
Skin (primary)	Group A streptococcus *Staphylococcus aureus*	*Haemophilus influenzae* type b Gram-negative enteric bacilli *Candida*	Face, periorbital Impaired host Paronychia, intertriginous skin, diaper dermatitis
Skin (trauma)	*S. aureus*	Group A streptococcus	Burns and surgical wounds (early)
		Pseudomonas aeruginosa	Burns (late), puncture wounds of foot
		Anaerobes	Severe trauma and abdominal wounds
		Clostridium spp	Severe trauma and abdominal wounds
		Gram negative enteric bacilli	Severe trauma and abdominal wounds
		Erysipelothrix *Pasteurella multocida*	Animal products Animal bites
Conjunctiva	*Haemophilus* species *S. aureus* Pneumococcus	Gonococcus *Chlamydia trachomatis* *P. aeruginosa*	Neonates, sexual history Neonates
Middle ear	Pneumococcus *H. influenzae* sp *Branhamella catarrhalis* Group A streptococcus	Gram-negative enteric bacilli *Mycobacterium tuberculosis*	Neonates Chronic drainage
Sinuses	*H. influenzae* (nontypable) Pneumococcus Oral anaerobes	*S. aureus* Gram-negative enteric bacilli *Pseudomonas* Group A streptococcus *Aspergillus* *Phycomycetes*	Chronic infection Impaired hosts Impaired hosts, diabetics

Table 5-1 (continued)

Site	Common organisms	Less common organisms	Comments
Cervical adenitis	Group A streptococcus S. aureus Oral anaerobes	Toxoplasma, Bartonella Nontuberculous mycobacteria M. tuberculosis	Cats Children <4 yr Contact history, abnormal chest x-ray
Mouth and pharynx	Group A streptococcus	Gonococcus Candida Oral anaerobes Corynebacterium diphtheriae Mycoplasma pneumoniae	Sexual history Antibiotic therapy, impaired host Vincent's infection Gray membrane School-aged children
Epiglottis	H. influenzae type b	C. diphtheriae Pneumococcus Group A streptococcus	Gray membrane
Lower respiratory tract	Pneumococcus M. pneumoniae	H. influenzae type b S. aureus Group A streptococcus Group B streptococcus Klebsiella and other gram-negative bacilli Oral anaerobes Bordetella pertussis M. tuberculosis C. trachomatis	Children <8 yr Influenza, impaired host, neonate Pharyngitis, large pleural effusions Respiratory distress in neonates Impaired hosts Aspiration, lung abscess Characteristic cough Exposure history Infants <12 wk
Endocardium	Viridans streptococci S. aureus Enterococcus	Staphylococcus epidermidis, diphtheroids, etc. P. aeruginosa Candida and other fungi	Prosthetic valves Addicts Large emboli

Gastrointestinal tract	*Shigella*	*Yersinia enterocolitica*	Symptoms of appendicitis
	Salmonella	*Vibrio parahaemolyticus*	Shellfish ingestion
	Campylobacter	*Vibrio cholerae*	Foreign travel
	Escherichia coli	*Aeromonas hydrophila*	Foreign travel
		Entamoeba histolytica	Waterborne
		Giardia lamblia	Foreign travel
		Clostridium difficile	Foreign travel, day care center
			Antibiotic therapy
Urinary tract	*E. coli* and other enteric gram-negative bacilli	Chronic recurrent infections	
		Enterococcus	Chronic recurrent infections
		P. aeruginosa	Adolescent and school-aged girls
		Staphylococcus saprophyticus	Bacteremia, kidney abscess
		S. aureus	
Bone	*S. aureus*	*Salmonella*	Sickle cell disease
		Pseudomonas	Foot puncture
		Streptococcus groups A and B	
		H. influenzae type b	
		M. tuberculosis	
Joints	*S. aureus*	Gram-negative bacilli	Neonates
	H. influenzae type b	Gonococcus	Neonates, sexually active adolescents
	Group A streptococcus	Pneumococcus	Prostheses
		S. epidermidis	
		M. tuberculosis	
Meninges	Pneumococcus	Enteric gram-negative bacilli	Neonates, surgery
	Meningococcus	Group B streptococcus	Neonates
	H. influenzae type b	*S. aureus*	Surgery and shunts
		S. epidermidis	Shunts
		Listeria monocytogenes	Impaired hosts, neonates
		Cryptococcus	Impaired hosts
		M. tuberculosis	

B. Choice and dosage of antimicrobial agents
   1. Antibiotic susceptibility. The recommended choice of antimicrobials for specific pathogens is outlined in Table 5–2. Dosages of specific antibiotics are listed in the formulary.
      a. Frequently, the likely pathogen(s) is (are) susceptible to several antimicrobials. A rational choice is then based on drug toxicity, pharmacologic factors relating to the patient (age, renal and hepatic function), pharmacologic factors relating to the infection (antimicrobial penetration and activity at the site of infection), and cost, especially when several antibiotics are likely to be effective against the pathogen.
      b. Agents with potentially serious side effects should be used only when they offer a definitive advantage over less toxic agents.
   2. Combinations of antimicrobial agents. Combination therapy is recommended for specific organisms or certain clinical situations. These include **endocarditis** (see p. 113) caused by enterococci or by viridans streptococci relatively resistant to penicillin, **severe *Pseudomonas* infection**, **active tuberculosis** (see p. 147), **cryptococcal** meningitis and disseminated infections caused by other yeasts, and **empiric** antibiotic therapy for severely ill patients.
      The regimen most commonly used for suspected bacterial sepsis in neonates is ampicillin and gentamicin (see Chap. 6, p. 209). For **suspected bacterial sepsis** in older infants and children, ampicillin with chloramphenicol, a third-generation cephalosporin, or ampicillin with sulbactam (if meningitis is unlikely and where high-level penicillin-resistant pneumococcus is uncommon), is acceptable. The combination of an antipseudomonal penicillin and an aminoglycoside is standard empiric coverage for immunosuppressed patients or patients with suspected nosocomial sepsis.
   3. Monitoring antimicrobial dosage. When treating a serious illness or when using an antibiotic with a narrow therapeutic-toxic ratio, antibiotic levels should be monitored. Recommended therapeutic levels of such antimicrobials are listed in the drug formulary.
      a. Peak levels should be measured 1 hour after an intramuscular dose, 30 minutes after the end of a 30-minute intravenous infusion, or immediately after a 1-hour infusion.
      b. Trough levels should be measured just before the next dose.
      c. Antibiotic levels in the serum can also be measured indirectly as bactericidal activity against the patient's pathogen (serum bactericidal level).
      d. In certain infections such as **endocarditis** and **osteomyelitis,** the level and bactericidal power of antibiotics in the patient's serum against the pathogen can be monitored during therapy. The *peak* bactericidal level should be at least 1 : 8 and the *trough* at least 1 : 2. Serum bactericidal levels are useful in monitoring compliance with and absorption of oral antibiotics.
   4. Antimicrobial activity at the site of infection
      a. Antimicrobial penetration into the CNS
         (1) Chloramphenicol, the sulfonamides, and most antituberculous agents penetrate normal meninges well.
         (2) The penicillins penetrate effectively, but only in the presence of inflamed meninges. Large doses must be given **parenterally and maintained throughout therapy.**
         (3) Some cephalosporins, including *cephalothin, cefazolin, cefaclor, cefamandole,* and *cefoxitin,* **do not penetrate the cerebrospinal fluid (CSF)** in therapeutic amounts. As a result, meningitis due to sensitive organisms may develop during parenteral treatment of bacteremic infections with cephalosporins of poor penetration.
         (4) *Cefuroxime* penetrates the meninges, but delayed sterilization of CSF in *H. influenzae* meningitis, possibly related to inadequate CSF drug level, has limited the use of cefuroxime when meningitis is suspected.
         (5) All third-generation cephalosporins have good penetration of inflamed meninges.

Table 5-2. Recommended choice of antimicrobials for specific pathogens

Organism	Drug of choice	Alternative agent
Gram-positive cocci		
Group A streptococcus	Penicillin G	Cephalosporins, erythromycin, clindamycin, vancomycin
Viridans streptococci	Penicillin G plus aminoglycoside	Vancomycin
Enterococcus	Ampicillin or penicillin G (+ aminoglycoside for endocarditis)	Vancomycin, gentamicin
Pneumococcus (penicillin sensitive)	Penicillin G	Cephalosporins, erythromycin, chloramphenicol, vancomycin
Pneumococcus (penicillin resistant)	Cephalosporin (e.g., cefotaxime or ceftriaxone) + vancomycin for life-threatening infections	Vancomycin, chloramphenicol
Staphylococcus aureus (penicillin resistant)	Semi-synthetic penicillin (e.g., oxacillin)	Cephalosporin (e.g., cephalothin, cefazolin), clindamycin, vancomycin
Staphylococcus spp (coagulase negative)	Vancomycin	
Staphylococcus spp (methicillin resistant)	Vancomycin (consider addition of rifampin and/or aminoglycoside	Trimethoprim-sulfamethoxazole (TMP/SMX)
Gram-positive bacilli		
Clostridium difficile	Oral vancomycin	Oral metronidazole
Clostridium spp	Penicillin G (+ antitoxin for tetanus)	Clindamycin, metronidazole
Listeria monocytogenes	Ampicillin ± gentamicin	TMP/SMX
Corynebacterium diphtheriae	Penicillin G + antitoxin	Erythromycin
Gram-negative cocci		
Meningococcus	Penicillin G	Cefotaxime, ceftriaxone, chloramphenicol
Gonococcus	Ceftriaxone	Cefixime, spectinomycin
Gram-negative bacilli		
Acinetobacter calcoaceticus	Imipenem	Anti-*pseudomonas* beta-lactam + amikacin, TMP/SMX
Bacteroides fragilis	Metronidazole, clindamycin	Chloramphenicol, cefoxitin, ampicillin-sulbactam
Bacteroides	Penicillin G	Clindamycin, metronidazole, ampicillin-sulbactam
Campylobacter	Erythromycin or aminoglycoside	
Citrobacter spp	An aminoglycoside	Ceftriaxone or cefotaxime, TMP/SMX
Enterobacter spp	Ceftriaxone or cefotaxime	An aminoglycoside, imipenem
Escherichia coli	An aminoglycoside	TMP/SMX, cephalosporin, aztreonam, imipenem

Table 5-2 (continued)

Organism	Drug of choice	Alternative agent
Haemophilus influenzae	Cephalosporin (e.g., cefprozil, cefotaxime, ceftriaxone)	Ampicillin-sulbactam, amoxicillin-clavulanate, TMP/SMX, chloramphenicol
Klebsiella	Ceftriaxone or cefotaxime	An aminoglycoside, TMP/SMX
Moraxella catarrhalis	Second- or third-generation cephalosporin	Ampicillin-sulbactam, amoxicillin-clavulanate, TMP/SMX
Pasteurella multocida	Penicillin G	Ampicillin, chloramphenicol, tetracycline
Proteus mirabilis	Ampicillin	Cephalexin, TMP/SMX, an aminoglycoside
Proteus (indole positive)	Ceftriaxone or cefotaxime	Imipenem, an aminoglycoside
Pseudomonas aeruginosa	Antipseudomonal beta-lactam plus aminoglycoside	Imipenem, ciprofloxacin
Salmonella spp	Ceftriaxone	Chloramphenicol, TMP/SMX, ampicillin (if sensitive)
Serratia marcescens	Ceftriaxone or cefotaxime	Imipenem, an aminoglycoside, TMP/SMX
Shigella spp	TMP/SMX	Ampicillin, chloramphenicol
Other		
Chlamydia pneumoniae *Chlamydia psittaci*	Tetracycline	Erythromycin
Rickettsia	Tetracycline	Chloramphenicol

    (6) The levels of *aminoglycoside* antibiotics in the CSF after parenteral therapy are unpredictable and are often inadequate for the therapy of gram-negative meningitis.
  b. Antimicrobial activity in the urinary tract (see p. 121). In patients with normal renal function, many antimicrobials reach much higher concentrations in urine than in serum. As a result, routine sensitivity tests based on achievable serum concentrations are not always reliable predictors of antibiotic efficacy. **Therefore, a report of antibiotic resistance should prompt a repeat urine culture** rather than a change in regimen, unless the patient's symptoms have failed to respond. An effective regimen should sterilize the urine within 12 to 24 hours.
    (1) Acidification enhances the activity of the tetracyclines, nitrofurantoin, the penicillins, and cephalosporins. **Alkalinization** markedly enhances the activity of the aminoglycosides and erythromycin, and extends the spectrum of the latter to include many gram-negative rods.
    (2) Because of ionic partitioning into acid secretions, **trimethoprim** may be particularly useful in treating recurrent urinary tract infections in females (anterior urethra) and prostatitis in males.
  c. Antimicrobial penetration into the eye. Most antibiotics have poor penetration into the aqueous and vitreous humor. For this reason, both parenteral and intraocular antibiotics are usually necessary for the treatment of endophthalmitis. Trimethoprim-sulfamethoxazole (TMP/SMZ) and chloramphenicol are the only antibiotics that penetrate the eye well when given systemically.
  5. Failure of therapy. There is variation in the rate of resolution of infections. Causes for failure of treatment should be considered when fever and signs of in-

fection are prolonged. These include inadequate antibiotic therapy, including poor compliance, complication of original infection, complications of treatment, and host factors (immune deficiency, anatomic defect, inadequate drainage, a retained foreign body).

6. **Pharmacologic considerations**
   a. **Use of antimicrobial agents in infants and young children**
      (1) In **neonates,** antimicrobial dosage must be individualized, and serum levels should be monitored, particularly when using toxic drugs. Guidelines for initial antibiotic dosage in neonates can be found in Chapter 6.
      (2) In general, dosage intervals are **longer** in younger infants than in older infants. Drug half-lives in premature infants are longer than in full-term infants. Similarly, decreases in renal function are associated with long half-lives of aminoglycoside antibiotics. Therefore, doses and intervals near the lower limits of the ranges given in Chapter 6 should be chosen in these groups.
      (3) To achieve a given blood level, older infants and children less than 10 years of age usually require higher doses of antimicrobials (based on weight) than do older children and adults.
      (4) Dosage of toxic antibiotics should be adjusted according to the age of the patient. In **gentamicin** dose recommendations rarely produce levels above the therapeutic range and levels may be subtherapeutic. A single gentamicin dosage of 60 mg/m^2 q8h produces reproducible peak levels in all age groups regardless of body habitus.
   b. **Use of antimicrobial agents in renal failure.** The routes of metabolism and excretion of antimicrobials must be considered to avoid overdosage
      (1) Antimicrobials handled mainly by the kidneys
         (a) Antimicrobials excreted primarily by renal mechanisms are best avoided in patients with severe renal failure. If their use cannot be avoided, then drug levels should be obtained, when possible, before repeat doses are administered.
         (b) Adjustment in dosage is based on estimates of renal function.
            (i) Interval extension. The standard dose of the antimicrobial is given, and the dosage interval is prolonged in direct proportion to the increase in serum creatinine concentration, as in the following equation:

            New interval = standard interval (q8h)
                 × patient's creatinine/normal creatinine

            Peak and trough levels with this method are similar to those obtained in patients with normal renal function. However, this approach can lead to relatively long periods of subtherapeutic levels before the next dose.
            (ii) Dosage adjustment. The standard dose is given (loading dose), and the standard interval is maintained. Subsequent doses (maintenance doses) are reduced in proportion to increases in the serum creatinine, as in the following equation:

            Maintenance dose = standard dose divided by patient's creatinine/normal creatinine

            Levels can be maintained within a narrower range with less chance of subtherapeutic levels. **However, this method may result in higher peak and trough levels than in** (i) **and may predispose the patient to greater toxicity.**
         (c) The serum creatinine is unreliable in acute or unstable renal disease, in severe uremia, and in intermittent dialysis. Thus, serum antibiotic levels should be measured frequently and directly to ensure therapeutic levels.

(2) Antimicrobials handled by both the kidney and extrarenal mechanisms can be used in standard doses in patients with mild or moderate renal failure (creatinine clearance > 30 ml/1.74 m² or serum creatinine < 3 mg/dl). The dosage interval should be increased if renal failure is moderate or severe. **Nitrofurantoin and all tetracyclines except doxycycline are contraindicated in severe renal failure.** In addition, sulfonamides and para-aminosalicylic acid (PAS) should be avoided in severe renal failure.

(3) **Antimicrobials handled by nonrenal mechanisms.** When these agents are used in patients with renal failure, the dosage need not be adjusted.

c. **Use of antimicrobials in hepatic failure.** Among antimicrobials metabolized by the liver, metabolic and excretory pathways differ. Therefore, specific guidelines for dosage modifications in liver failure cannot be formulated. Antimicrobials with a narrow toxic-therapeutic ratio (e.g., **nitrofurantoin**) or with a high risk of hepatotoxicity (e.g., **PAS**) are **contraindicated** in cases of severe liver failure. When possible, **clindamycin, erythromycin, chloramphenicol, tetracyclines, isoniazid (INH),** and **rifampin** should be avoided in patients with severe liver failure. If any of these agents is used, their serum levels, if possible, should be monitored.

C. **Mechanisms of antibiotic resistance** vary but usually involve enzymatic inhibition, alteration of the bacterial target, development of membrane impermeability to the antibiotic, or active pumping of the antibiotic out of the bacteria. Knowledge regarding the antibiotic resistance patterns of *local* bacterial isolates is increasingly important in managing patients.

1. **Beta-lactamases** are a family of enzymes that hydrolyze beta-lactam antibiotics. Those produced by *Enterobacter, Citrobacter, Klebsiella oxytoca*, and *Pseudomonas aeruginosa* are frequently unaffected by beta-lactamase inhibitors (e.g., clavulanate, sulbactam, tazobactam). Furthermore some beta-lactamases are chromosomally based and the emergence of resistance in patients receiving third-generation cephalosporins has been reported (most frequently with *Enterobacter*).

2. **Alteration of penicillin binding proteins (PBP).** This is the only mechanism of resistance reported among *Streptococcus pneumoniae*. Because resistance is not via beta-lactamases, antibiotics combined with beta-lactamase inhibitors offer no advantage for infections due to resistant *S. pneumoniae.*

II. **Specific antimicrobial agents.** Table 5–2 summarizes the drugs of choice for specific bacterial pathogens.

A. **Antibiotics**

1. **The penicillins** inhibit cell wall synthesis and kill growing bacteria bylysis.

a. **Penicillin**

(1) **Spectrum and indications.** Penicillin is the drug of choice for infections due to streptococci (except enterococci), *Clostridia*, oral anaerobes, spirochetes, and sensitive pneumococci and *Neisseria*. It is also used in treatment of anthrax, diphtheria, actinomycosis, leptospirosis, and rat-bite fever. Penicillin G is more active than penicillin V.

(2) **Pharmacology**

(a) **Oral preparations** are penicillin G and penicillin V (phenoxymethyl penicillin). Because penicillin G is acid labile, its absorption is **variable.** Penicillin V is well absorbed, especially when given 1 hour before meals.

(b) **Parenteral preparations** differ in their peak serum level and half-life.

(i) **Aqueous penicillin G** results in rapid attainment of high blood levels after IM or IV administration. Its rapid excretion in patients (except newborns) with normal renal function requires that it be administered frequently (usually q4h) for optimal therapy. It is prepared as a potassium or sodium salt (1.7 mEq/106 units).

(ii) **Procaine penicillin G** is absorbed slowly from IM injections and so produces relatively low but prolonged serum concentrations. It should thus be used only in infections due to highly susceptible organisms or in large dosage.

(iii) **Benzathine penicillin G** produces even lower blood levels, which last for as long as 3 to 4 weeks. It is used primarily against group A streptococci and *Treponema pallidum*, prophylactically in patients with rheumatic heart disease, and therapeutically when adherence to a program of oral penicillin is questionable.

b. **Penicillinase-resistant penicillins**

  (1) **Spectrum and indications.** These agents are resistant to hydrolysis by the beta-lactamase produced by staphylococci and are therefore the drugs of choice for penicillin-resistant staphylococcal infections. They are approximately 10 times less active than penicillin G against penicillin-sensitive organisms.

  (2) **Pharmacology.** The only clinically significant difference between preparations is in their routes of administration. Because **methicillin**, **oxacillin**, and **nafcillin** are not well absorbed after oral administration, they are used only parenterally. **Cloxacillin** and **dicloxacillin** are well absorbed orally.

c. **Ampicillin and amoxicillin**

  (1) **Spectrum and indications**

    (a) **Ampicillin** has the gram-positive spectrum of penicillin and is more active against enterococci and *Listeria*. Like penicillin, **it is inactive against penicillinase-producing staphylococci.** It is also active against many gram-negative organisms, including most *H. influenzae* strains, *Salmonella*, *Proteus mirabilis*, and some *E. coli* and *Shigella*.

    (b) The spectrum of **amoxicillin** is very similar to that of ampicillin.

  (2) **Pharmacology.** The major difference between ampicillin and amoxicillin is that the latter is better absorbed after oral administration. Amoxicillin is therefore given in lower dosage and may produce fewer gastrointestinal side effects than ampicillin. Because amoxicillin can be given q8h rather than q6h as with ampicillin, compliance may be improved. (Amoxicillin cannot be substituted for ampicillin in the therapy of *Shigella* infections.)

d. **Amoxicillin and clavulanic acid**

  (1) **Spectrum and indications.** Clavulanic acid binds irreversibly to the active site of many beta-lactamases, inactivating the enzyme. The combination of amoxicillin with clavulanic acid extends the spectrum of amoxicillin to include beta-lactamase–producing strains of *S. aureus*, *H. influenzae*, *Moraxella catarrhalis*, *E. coli*, *Proteus*, *Klebsiella pneumoniae*, and gonococci. This combination is not active against *P. aeruginosa* or many amoxicillin-resistant strains of *Enterobacter* and *Serratia*. Because of its higher cost and the side effect of diarrhea, we reserve this drug combination for second- or third-line therapy (after amoxicillin and TMP/SMZ), except for treatment of bite wounds.

  (2) **Pharmacology.** Both components are rapidly absorbed and they are excreted at similar rates in the urine. Probenecid delays renal excretion of amoxicillin but not of clavulanic acid.

e. **Ampicillin and sulbactam**

  (1) **Spectrum and indications.** Sulbactam is a penicillin-like compound that, like clavulanate, binds irreversibly to most beta-lactamases, inactivating the enzyme. When combined with ampicillin, sulbactam acts to protect the ampicillin from beta-lactamases and effectively extends the antimicrobial spectrum of ampicillin to include beta-lactamase–producing organisms, such as *H. influenzae, Moraxella catarrhalis,* many *E. coli, K. pneumoniae,* anaerobes including *Bacteroides fragilis,* and all methicillin-sensitive *S. aureus.* This combination of a well-proven and safe antibiotic (ampicillin) with a beta-lactamase inhibitor that has virtually identical pharmacokinetics and tissue penetration as ampicillin has proved to be a useful alternative to combination therapy or third-generation cephalosporins in the empiric therapy of pneumonia, cellulitis, urinary tract infection (UTI), and other community-acquired infections, especially in young children at risk for *H. influenzae.* It is not used to treat meningitis and has no activity against organisms that are resistant to ampicillin by mechanisms other than production of beta-lactamase (e.g., *Pseudomonas,* penicillin-resistant *S. pneumoniae*).

    (2) Pharmacology. Ampicillin and sulbactam have very similar pharmacokinetic profiles. Dosing is based on the ampicillin component (not to exceed 200 mg/kg/day) and administration is intravenous.

f. Carbenicillin and ticarcillin

    (1) Spectrum and indications. These agents extend the spectrum of ampicillin to include *P. aeruginosa* and some *Proteus* species. Some strains of *Enterobacter* and *Serratia* may also be sensitive. Ticarcillin is more potent than carbenicillin against *P. aeruginosa* and is therefore used in lower dosage. Both have in recent years been supplanted by newer antipseudomonal penicillins (see sec. **g** below), although oral indanyl carbenicillin remains useful as the only oral antipseudomonal antibiotic available for use in children.

    (2) Pharmacology. Oral indanyl carbenicillin attains therapeutic levels only in urine and is indicated *only* for UTIs caused by gram-negative organisms resistant to ampicillin and other oral agents.

g. Azlocillin, mezlocillin, and piperacillin

    (1) Spectrum and indications. These uride (azlocillin and mezlocillin) and piperazine (piperacillin) derivatives of ampicillin retain the activity of ampicillin to enterococci and *H. influenzae* and are more active than carbenicillin or ticarcillin against aerobic gram-negative bacilli, including *P. aeruginosa* and *Klebsiella* species. Like ticarcillin and carbenicillin, they are not active against penicillinase-producing strains of *S. aureus* or *H. influenzae.* In vitro studies demonstrate synergy with aminoglycosides against *P. aeruginosa.* Combination therapy with an aminoglycoside is advised for any serious infection. These agents have replaced ticarcillin and carbenicillin for most indications.

    (2) Pharmacology. Mezlocillin, azlocillin, and piperacillin are monosodium salts (1.8 mEq Na^+/g), whereas carbenicillin and ticarcillin are disodium salts (5 mEq Na^+/g). These drugs are administered only by the IV route.

h. Ticarcillin–clavulanic acid and piperacillin-tazobactam

    (1) Spectrum and indications. The combination of ticarcillin or piperacillin with a beta-lactamase enzyme inhibitor extends the spectrum of activity of these drugs to include beta-lactamase–producing strains of *S. aureus, H. influenzae, E. coli, Klebsiella,* and some other gram-negative bacilli. Strains of *P. aeruginosa* and gram-negative bacilli with chromosomally mediated beta-lactamases, which are resistant to ticarcillin or the piperacillin component, are still resistant to the beta-lactamase inhibitor combination. It should also be noted that the recommended dosages of piperacillin-tazobactam are not adequate for treating serious *P. aeruginosa* infections.

    (2) Pharmacology. The combination of the beta-lactam antibiotic with the beta-lactamase inhibitor does not alter the pharmacology of either drug.

2. **Cephalosporins.** The mechanism of action of the cephalosporins is similar to that of the penicillins. This class of drug has gained in popularity because of its broad-spectrum activity and relative lack of toxicity. In the discussion below, most members of each generation are discussed. However, the Children's Hospital formulary includes only cephalexin (first generation, PO), cefazolin (first, parenteral), cefoxitin (second, parenteral, used when enhanced anaerobic coverage is needed), cefprozil (second, PO), cefixime (third, PO), ceftriaxone (third, parenteral), cefotaxime (third, parenteral), and ceftazidime (third, parenteral, enhanced activity against *P. aeruginosa*). **With the exception of third-generation agents, the cephalosporins penetrate poorly into the CNS and should therefore not be used to treat meningitis or when meningitis may ensue as a complication of a bacteremic condition.**
   a. **First-generation cephalosporins**
      (1) **Spectrum and indications.** Cephalothin, and its analogues cefazolin, cephalexin, cefadroxil, cephapirin, and cephradine have similar antimicrobial spectra. They are active against gram-positive cocci, including penicillinase-producing *S. aureus*, and against gram-negative rods, including many community strains of *E. coli*, *Klebsiella*, and *P. mirabilis*. Generally, they have poor activity against enterococci or *H. influenzae*, and, despite disk sensitivity tests indicating activity against methicillin-resistant staphylococci, the cephalosporins are usually ineffective clinically against these organisms. Cephalothin and cefazolin are more resistant to staphylococcal penicillinase than other cephalosporins and are therefore the cephalosporins of choice for serious staphylococcal infections.
      (2) **Pharmacology.** Cephalothin and its analogues differ in their pharmacologic properties, especially with respect to routes of administration. Cephalothin, cefazolin, and cephapirin are available only for IM or IV administration. Cephalothin is painful when administered IM and should be given IV. Cephradine can be given parenterally or PO; cephalexin and cefadroxil are given PO only. The half-life in blood of most of these agents is very short (30–60 minutes), and parenteral therapy should therefore be given at 4-hour intervals except for cefazolin (q6–8h). Cefadroxil has an extended half-life and can be dosed once or twice a day.
   b. **Second-generation cephalosporins**
      (1) **Spectrum and indications.** Cefamandole, cefuroxime, and cefoxitin extend the spectrum of the older cephalosporins to many strains of resistant gram-negative bacteria. Cefamandole and cefuroxime are more active against *H. influenzae* type b (including ampicillin-resistant strains). Cefaclor is two to eight times more active than cephalexin against *H. influenzae* type b. However, some strains, including some beta-lactamase–producing strains, are resistant to cefaclor. Cefprozil and loracarbef each have antimicrobial activities similar to that of cefaclor but with a longer serum half-life. In general, aerobic gram-negative enteric organisms are more likely to be sensitive to gentamicin or tobramycin, anaerobes to clindamycin or ampicillin-sulbactam.
      (2) **Pharmacology.** Cefamandole, cefuroxime, and cefoxitin are given IV q6–8h. Cefprozil, loracarbef, and cefuroxime axetil can be given PO bid. Because they are excreted unchanged into the urine, the dosage should be reduced in patients with renal insufficiency. *None of the second-generation cephalosporins should be used to treat meningitis.* In general parenteral second-generation cephalosporins have been replaced by third-generation compounds for use in pediatrics.
   c. **Third-generation cephalosporins**
      (1) **Spectrum and indications.** Cefotaxime, ceftriaxone, ceftizoxime, cefixime, cefpodoxime, moxalactam, cefoperazone, and ceftazidime have broad-spectrum activity against gram-negative enteric bacteria,

many of which are resistant to the older cephalosporins and amino-glycosides. These agents are also highly active against *H. influenzae* type b (including beta-lactamase–producing strains), and *Neisseria* species. Activity against anaerobes is good but not better than that of cefoxitin. Third-generation cephalosporins generally have less activity against gram-positive cocci than do first-generation drugs, and like all cephalosporins they are inactive against enterococci and *Listeria monocytogenes*. Cefixime has no antistaphylococcal activity at all. Antipseudomonal activity is only fair except for ceftazidime. One advantage of ceftriaxone and cefixime is a long half-life, which allows q24h dosing, and makes outpatient management possible in selected cases.

(2) Pharmacology. Most third-generation drugs are excreted primarily by the kidney; ceftriaxone has both renal and hepatic excretion, and cefoperazone is excreted primarily in bile. Ceftriaxone and cefixime have a serum half-life of 4 to 6 hours, allowing q12–24h dosing. All others have a 1- to 2-hour half-life and q6–8h dosing. Cerebrospinal fluid penetration is good through inflamed meninges. Ceftizoxime has not been adequately evaluated for safety in infants less than 6 months of age.

3. **Aminoglycosides** inhibit protein synthesis.
   a. **Spectrum and indications.** The aminoglycosides are effective against a broad range of enteric gram-negative bacilli and *S. aureus*, but the various analogues differ in their antimicrobial spectra. Aminoglycosides are valuable and proven antibiotics; however, they have a narrow therapeutic index and careful attention must be given to proper dosing and drug level monitoring. Despite the recent popularity of cephalosporins, aminoglycosides remain a mainstay of antimicrobial therapy in the neonate and young infant as well as in hospitalized children.
      (1) They are not effective against streptococci, pneumococci, anaerobes, and spirochetes.
      (2) Many gram-negative bacilli, especially in hospitals, have become resistant to **streptomycin** and **kanamycin**. In addition, neither agent is active against *P. aeruginosa*. **Streptomycin** is now used only as an antituberculosis agent.
      (3) Gentamicin is active against most gram-negative rods, including *P. aeruginosa*, and is the aminoglycoside of choice for the empiric treatment of gram-negative infections, in which resistant gram-negative bacilli are common.
      (4) Tobramycin is more active than gentamicin against *P. aeruginosa* (2–4 times).
      (5) Amikacin is active against many enteric gram-negative bacilli that are resistant to gentamicin. Unless such organisms are common, this agent should be reserved for infections that have proved resistant to the other aminoglycosides or for settings in which gentamicin-resistant organisms are common.
      (6) Netilmicin is an aminoglycoside with antibacterial activity similar to that of tobramycin. Netilmicin may be associated with less ototoxicity than other aminoglycosides, but it has not gained wide use in pediatrics.
   b. **Pharmacology**
      (1) The aminoglycosides are poorly absorbed from the GI tract. However, they can reach toxic levels after oral administration in patients with a damaged intestine or with renal failure.
      (2) Because the aminoglycosides have a narrow toxic-therapeutic ratio, dosage must be adjusted to obtain safe, effective serum levels.
      (3) Aminoglycoside levels should be **monitored** to minimize the risk of ototoxicity and nephrotoxicity. We routinely monitor pre- and post-dose levels every 2 to 3 days in critically ill patients and in all patients

who are receiving prolonged courses of therapy. However, in otherwise healthy children with normal renal function who are started on standard-dose aminoglycoside therapy empirically with the intention of stopping therapy within 48 to 72 hours (a usual time for culture results to become available), measuring levels is of limited use. **If therapy is continued beyond 48 to 72 hours, levels should be monitored.** Aminoglycoside-related ototoxicity and nephrotoxicity are most likely to occur with prolonged administration or improper dosing.

(4) Aminoglycosides are excreted almost entirely by the kidneys. The dosage must be adjusted when there is even a minor degree of renal impairment.

c. Side effects

(1) Nephrotoxicity due to renal tubular damage is enhanced by the concurrent use of cephalothin or vancomycin and diuretics (especially when sodium depletion occurs) and by preexisting renal disease. It is usually reversible. **The serum creatinine should be monitored in all patients receiving aminoglycoside therapy.**

(2) Ototoxicity (both vestibular and auditory) is enhanced by preexisting ear disease, concurrent administration of diuretics, and preexisting renal disease. It may be irreversible unless recognized early.

(3) Neuromuscular blockade with respiratory paralysis has been described, usually after peritoneal irrigation with high concentrations of aminoglycoside or in association with botulism.

4. Newer antibiotics: carbapenems, monobactams, and quinolones

a. Imipenem-cilistatin. Imipenem, a carbapenem, has the widest spectrum of any lactam antibiotic yet released and is available only in combination with cilistatin, an enzyme inhibitor that is important in achieving effective concentrations. Activity includes nearly all gram-positive organisms, including enterococci but excluding methicillin-resistant staphylococci. It is highly active against most Enterobacteriaceae species and anaerobes, including *B. fragilis.* Although highly active, it is not usually used as monotherapy against *Pseudomonas* because resistance can develop while a patient is undergoing therapy. Its use in pediatrics is currently limited to very specific infections with organisms resistant to other antibiotics. **In the treatment of meningitis, imipenem-cilastin use has been associated with a high rate of seizures.**

b. Aztreonam. This first monobactam antibiotic has no significant gram-positive or anaerobic activity, but is highly active against most Enterobacteriaceae and *P. aeruginosa.* Although combination therapy will often be needed, aztreonam has the potential to replace aminoglycosides in many gram-negative infections.

c. Ciprofloxacin. As synthetic agents based on the structure of naladixic acid, quinolones are highly active against gram-negative bacteria in addition to many gram-positive organisms. Quinolones are well absorbed after oral administration. Their use in pediatrics is limited because they have been shown to damage cartilage in growing animals. Limited data do not show evidence of similar toxicity in children; however, the data are insufficient currently to recommend use of quinolones for children except in special circumstances.

5. The **macrolide antibiotics** erythromycin, clarithromycin, and azithromycin inhibit bacterial protein synthesis by binding to ribosomes.

a. Spectrum and indications. Erythromycin, clarithromycin, and azithromycin are bacteriostatic at low concentrations against *Mycoplasma pneumoniae,* spirochetes, and most gram-positive organisms. They can be used as alternative drugs in penicillin-allergic patients with group A streptococcal and pneumococcal infections. Erythromycin and clarithromycin are only moderately active against *H. influenzae.* Macrolides are the drugs of choice for *Legionella* and *M. pneumoniae* infections, pertussis, the diphtheria carrier state, *Campylobacter* infections, and chlamydia pneumonia. Clarithromycin and azithromycin have the advantage of bid and once-daily dosing, respectively; they cause fewer gastrointestinal symptoms and are therefore much better tolerated than erythromycin. Clarithromycin is being utilized (often in combination with other antibiotics) for the treatment of atypical mycobacterial infections. Azithromycin in a single 1-g oral dose will cure chlamydia genital infections.

   b. **Pharmacology.** Erythromycin base is acid labile and poorly absorbed. Erythromycin estolate is well absorbed, even in the presence of food, but must be hydrolyzed to the active base by the liver. A variety of parenteral preparations are also available. Active erythromycin is excreted in low concentrations in urine and in higher concentrations in bile. Clarithromycin and particularly azithromycin do not achieve high serum concentrations but retain adequate and prolonged in situ and intracellular concentrations.

6. **Clindamycin** inhibits bacterial protein synthesis.

   a. **Spectrum and indications**

      (1) Clindamycin has a spectrum similar to that of erythromycin, except that it is inactive against *M. pneumoniae, Neisseria gonorrhoeae, Neisseria meningitidis,* and *H. influenzae.* It is quite active against nonenterococcal gram-positive organisms and most anaerobes.

      (2) Clindamycin is often used for serious anaerobic infections due to *B. fragilis* and is popular as part of the "triples" regimen with ampicillin and gentamicin to provide empiric coverage for perforated appendix or other forms of peritonitis. It is an alternative to penicillin for infections due to group A streptococci and pneumococci, and to penicillinase-resistant penicillins for staphylococcal infections. However, resistance to clindamycin may emerge during therapy, and staphylococcal endocarditis may relapse after clindamycin treatment.

   b. **Pharmacology.** Absorption is not decreased by the presence of food. Clindamycin is metabolized by the liver.

   c. **Side effects.** Gastrointestinal side effects (nausea, vomiting, abdominal cramps, diarrhea) are common. **Pseudomembranous colitis,** which is also associated with many other antibiotics, can develop and become severe if treatment is continued.

7. **The tetracyclines** inhibit bacterial protein synthesis and are not used commonly in early childhood because of their side effects.

   a. **Spectrum and indications**

      (1) The tetracyclines have broad-spectrum bacteriostatic activity against gram-positive organisms, enteric gram-negative bacilli, anaerobes, *Mycoplasma,* spirochetes, and rickettsiae. *Serratia, Proteus,* and *P. aeruginosa* are almost always resistant.

      (2) Tetracyclines are the drugs of choice for brucellosis, cholera, Q fever, relapsing fever, Rocky Mountain spotted fever (in children older than 8 years), psittacosis, lymphogranuloma venereum, and nonspecific urethritis. They are second-line drugs for *Mycoplasma* pneumonia, tularemia, gonorrhea, syphilis, melioidosis, and granuloma inguinale.

   b. **Pharmacology.** The absorption of tetracycline is impaired by concurrent food intake and the presence of divalent cations (calcium, iron). The serum half-life is relatively short (6 hours). Doxycycline and minocycline are absorbed more completely than tetracycline, and have a longer half-life (14–20 hours). Most tetracyclines are excreted mainly by the kidney, but also reach high concentrations in bile. **Doxycycline,** which is eliminated mainly by nonrenal mechanisms, **is the only tetracycline that can be safely used in renal failure.**

   c. **Side effects.** Tetracyclines may produce **permanent yellow discoloration of the deciduous teeth** (when given during the second and third trimester of pregnancy and the first 3 months of life) and of permanent teeth (when given to children 3 months–8 years of age). Tetracyclines should therefore be avoided during these periods. Other side effects include upper and lower **GI symptoms,** candidal superinfection, and dose-related **hepatitis.**

8. **Vancomycin** inhibits bacterial cell wall synthesis.
   a. **Spectrum and indications.** Vancomycin is bactericidal for most gram-positive organisms but is only bacteriostatic for enterococci. It is active against staphylococci, beta-hemolytic streptococci, viridans streptococci, pneumococci, *Corynebacterium*, and *Clostridium*.
      (1) Vancomycin is useful in the treatment of serious infection caused by methicillin-resistant staphylococci.
      (2) Vancomycin and gentamicin combined are the treatment of choice for enterococcal endocarditis in patients with allergy to penicillin.
      (3) Oral vancomycin is effective treatment for staphylococcal entero-colitis and antibiotic-induced colitis associated with enterotoxin-producing *Clostridium*.
   b. **Pharmacology.** Vancomycin is not absorbed after oral administration. After parenteral administration it enters tissues well, but diffuses poorly across inflamed meninges. It is excreted primarily by the kidneys, and dosage must be adjusted in renal failure and serum levels must be followed. **It is not eliminated by hemodialysis.** To avoid a histamine-like reaction (red man syndrome), vancomycin is infused over at least 30 minutes and can be preceded by antihistamine administration if necessary.

9. **The sulfonamides** block the synthesis of dihydrofolic acid from para-aminobenzoic acid in bacterial cells.
   a. **Spectrum and indications**
      (1) Sulfonamides have a broad bacteriostatic spectrum, including most gram-positive cocci (but not enterococci); gram-positive bacilli; most gram-negative organisms, including *H. influenzae, Chlamydia, Actinomyces*, and *Nocardia;* and protozoa (malaria, *Toxoplasma*, and *Pneumocystis*).
      (2) The **major indications** for sulfonamides include uncomplicated UTI, *Nocardia* infections, and, together with other drugs, toxoplasmosis and *P. carinii* pneumonia.
      (3) Erythromycin with a sulfonamide is a second-line regimen for otitis media. Trimethoprim combined with sulfamethoxazole is an important drug in pediatrics and is discussed below.
      (4) Sulfonamides provide effective rheumatic fever prophylaxis but cannot be relied on for the treatment of group A streptococcal infections.
      (5) Sulfonamides compete with bilirubin for albumin-binding sites, thereby increasing the risk of **kernicterus** in neonates. **They are contraindicated in pregnancy near term and in jaundiced infants or infants at risk of developing severe jaundice** (e.g., ABO incompatibility).
   b. Pharmacology (e.g., sulfisoxazole). Most sulfonamides are well absorbed orally. They are metabolized by the liver, and both active drug and metabolites are excreted primarily by the kidney. Products of tissue necrosis inhibit the action of sulfonamides. Therefore, these agents should not be used for severe suppurative infections.

10. **Trimethoprim-sulfamethoxazole.** Both drugs inhibit folic acid synthesis.
    a. **Spectrum and indications**
       (1) The antimicrobial spectrum includes most gram-positive cocci, *H. influenzae, M. catarrhalis* and *P. carinii*, and many enteric gram-negative bacilli.
       (2) The **major indications** include treatment and prophylaxis of otitis media, UTIs, and *P. carinii* pneumonia. It is a very effective and inexpensive drug in the treatment of acute otitis media, especially after amoxicillin failure, and is useful in the treatment of shigellosis, *Salmonella* infections, and infections caused by susceptible gram-negative bacilli.

(3) As a well-tolerated antibiotic with near complete bioavailability after oral administration, TMP/SMZ is useful for oral outpatient continuation therapy of many infections due to susceptible organisms. Serum concentrations after oral administration are equivalent to levels obtained with parenteral dosing.

b. Pharmacology. The dosage should be decreased in patients with severe renal dysfunction. Intravenous usage for *P. carinii* is discussed on p. 110.

c. Side effects

(1) Rash, nausea, vomiting, and thrombocytopenia are the most common side effects. Hematologic suppression due to weak inhibition of folic acid metabolism may be reversible with folinic acid. **The drug should be used with caution in patients with preexisting hematologic disease, in patients receiving immunosuppressive therapy, or in patients who are dehydrated.**

(2) Mild, reversible renal impairment may occur.

11. Nitrofurantoin may inhibit bacterial carbohydrate metabolism.

a. Spectrum and indications

(1) Nitrofurantoin is active against most gram-positive cocci (including enterococci) and gram-negative urinary pathogens. Sensitive organisms usually do not become resistant during therapy.

(2) The only indications for nitrofurantoin are the treatment and prophylaxis of UTIs.

b. Pharmacology. The drug reaches therapeutically effective levels only in the urine, which is its major route of excretion.

12. Metronidazole is reduced by enzymes in anaerobic bacteria. The reduction products disrupt DNA and inhibit nucleic acid synthesis.

a. Spectrum and indications

(1) Most aerobic organisms are resistant, but metronidazole is bactericidal for almost all anaerobic organisms, including *B. fragilis* and *Clostridium.*

(2) Metronidazole is probably the drug of choice only for endocarditis due to *B. fragilis* (because of its bactericidal activity) and for *B. fragilis* infections that are resistant to other drugs. It is equally effective as oral vancomycin in treatment of *Clostridium difficile* pseudomembranous colitis. Metronidazole is also useful in the treatment of trichomoniasis, amebiasis, and giardiasis.

b. Pharmacology

(1) Metronidazole is well absorbed from the GI tract and enters into all tissues, including the CSF. Serum concentrations after oral dosage are similar to those achieved with equal IV doses.

(2) The drug is largely metabolized in the liver and excreted by the kidney. No alteration in dosage is necessary for renal insufficiency; however, the dosage in patients with hepatic disease should be decreased and serum levels monitored.

13. Rifamycins (rifampin and rifabutin) are bactericidal because they inhibit DNA-dependent RNA polymerase at the beta-subunit preventing chain initiation. Bacteria rapidly develop resistance through mutations; therefore, rifamycins should not be used as monotherapy (except as meningitis prophylaxis with rifampin, or *Mycobacterium avium-intracellulare* (MAI) prophylaxis in selected HIV-infected patients with rifabutin).

a. Spectrum and indications

(1) Rifampin is extremely active against staphylococci, *N. meningitidis, N. gonorrhoeae, H. influenzae,* and *Legionella.* A common use of rifampin has been in meningitis prophylaxis because of its efficacy in eradicating nasopharyngeal colonization with *N. meningitidis, and H. influenzae.*

(2) Rifampin and rifabutin have good activity against most species of mycobacteria. They are commonly used in antimycobacterial prophylaxis and treatment.

b. Pharmacology
   (1) Rifampin and rifabutin are well absorbed from the GI tract and enter into all tissues, including the CSF.
   (2) They are largely metabolized in the liver.
c. Side effects
   (1) Orange discoloration of the urine is common and staining of soft contact lenses can occur.
   (2) Hepatotoxicity especially in combination with other medications.
   (3) The serum concentrations of many other medications with hepatic clearance are reduced; these include oral contraceptives, digoxin, warfarin, and glucocorticoids.
   (4) Rifabutin can cause uveitis.

III. Treatment of infectious diseases by site
  A. Ocular infections
    1. Preseptal cellulitis. The preseptal space consists of elastic connective tissue. A layer of dense connective tissue separates this space from the orbit, face, and forehead.
     a. Etiology
      (1) If the infection arises after an insect bite, local trauma, or an infection of the eyelid, *S aureus* or group A streptococci are the most common causes.
      (2) If the patient has no history or evidence of cutaneous inoculation, sinusitis—particularly ethmoid sinusitis—is a common associated finding. Organisms that cause sinusitis, including *Sp. pneumoniae*, nontypeable *H. influenzae*, *M. catarrhalis*, and anaerobes, are the most common etiologies.
      (3) *Haemophilis influenzae* type b is now a rarity.
     b. Evaluation. It is critical to distinguish **preseptal cellulitis** from **orbital cellulitis.**
      (1) Examination should focus on determining the
       (a) Location of the infection.
       (b) Source of the infection (cutaneous inoculation, infection of eyelid, or sinusitis).
      (2) If orbital infection is suspected, a **CT scan or MRI** of the orbit and sinuses is necessary.
      (3) Blood culture should be performed.
      (4) Lumbar puncture may be indicated.
      (5) Sinus x-rays are indicated if sinusitis is suspected.
     c. The **diagnosis** is established clinically by the presence of warmth, erythema, induration, and tenderness of the eyelids and surrounding tissues of the preseptal space. Fever may or may not be present. An exaggerated inflammatory reaction due to an insect bite may be difficult to distinguish from infection.
     d. Therapy. Given the present rarity of *H. influenzae* type b infection in the United States, **outpatient** management of children with mild infection may be considered *if orbital cellulitis is excluded* and close follow-up is assured. **Indications for inpatient management and parenteral antimicrobial therapy** include cases in which the distinction between preseptal or orbital cellulitis is not clear, the infection is moderate or severe, the child is toxic or unable to tolerate oral therapy, or close follow-up cannot be assured.
      (1) Antibiotic therapy
       (a) If cutaneous inoculation is the likely cause, antistaphylococcal therapy is indicated. Oxacillin or cefazolin is appropriate for intravenous therapy; cephalexin, dicloxacillin, or erythromycin is appropriate for oral therapy.
       (b) If sinusitis is present or cutaneous inoculation is not a likely cause, therapy should be directed toward organisms that

cause sinusitis (see sec. **a** above) as well as *S. aureus* and group A streptococci. Appropriate intravenous agents are cefuroxime or ampicillin-sulbactam as single agents or combination therapy with oxacillin and a third-generation cephalosporin or chloramphenicol. Appropriate oral agents are cefuroxime, cefprozil, or ampicillin-clavulanate.

- **(c)** Uncomplicated cases that respond to parenteral therapy can be switched to an appropriate oral agent to finish the course of treatment.
- **(d)** Duration of therapy is 7 to 10 days. If sinusitis is present the duration of treatment should be 2 to 3 weeks.

(2) Warm compresses provide symptomatic relief.

2. Orbital cellulitis

- **a. Etiology.** *Staphylococcus aureus*, group A streptococci, and organisms that cause sinusitis, such as *S. pneumoniae* or nontypeable *H. influenzae*, *M. catarrhalis*, and anaerobes, are the most common etiologies. Orbital cellulitis in an immunocompromised child may be caused by an invasive fungal infection of the sinuses and orbit.
- **b. Evaluation**
  - **(1)** A detailed **examination** is necessary to evaluate for evidence of decreased visual acuity, limitation of extraocular movements, chemosis, proptosis, and congestion of the blood vessels of the fundus.
  - **(2)** An **ophthalmologist should be consulted** if orbital involvement is suspected.
  - **(3)** A **CT scan or MRI** of the orbit and sinuses should be performed.
  - **(4)** **Blood culture** should be performed.
- **c.** The **diagnosis** is suggested clinically by swelling of the eyelid and surrounding tissues accompanied by eye pain, decreased visual acuity, limitation of extraocular movement, chemosis, and/or proptosis. A definitive diagnosis is made by a CT scan or MRI. Cavernous sinus thrombosis and infection involving the meninges or brain parenchyma are rare complications.
- **d. Therapy**
  - **(1) Hospitalization and immediate consultation with an ophthalmologist** are required.
  - **(2) Drainage** is necessary in some cases.
  - **(3) Parenteral antibiotics** should be given in high doses. Treatment should include an antistaphylococcal agent, such as oxacillin, and a second- or third-generation cephalosporin, such as cefuroxime, cefotaxime, or ceftriaxone. Clindamycin as a single agent is an alternative in penicillin-allergic patients.

3. Trachoma is uncommon in the US, but is one of the leading causes of blindness in parts of the world where the infection is endemic. It begins as chronic follicular conjunctivitis with mucopurulent discharge, progresses with exacerbations and remissions of inflammation and neovascularization of the cornea, and can lead to extensive scarring and blindness.

- **a. Etiology.** Trachoma is caused by specific serovars of *Chlamydia trachomatis*, which are spread by direct and indirect contact between children.
- **b. Evaluation.** Examination is usually sufficient in areas of the world where the disease is endemic.
- **c.** The **diagnosis** is usually made clinically.
- **d. Therapy.** Treatment is difficult and requires a long course of therapy.
  - **(1) Topical therapy.** Erythromycin, tetracycline, sulfacetamide ointment two times a day for 2 months or twice a day for the first 5 days of the month for 6 months.
  - **(2) Oral therapy.** Erythromycin or doxycycline for 40 days.

B. Oral infections

1. Stomatitis

a. **Etiology.** Herpes simplex virus (HSV) is a common cause year round. Herpangina caused by enteroviruses (coxsackievirus and echoviruses) is more common in the summer. Varicella causes stomatitis but occurs in the setting of systemic illness. There are a variety of other causes of stomatitis of undetermined etiology.

b. **Evaluation**

(1) **Examination** should focus on the presence and location of ulcers and the involvement of the gingiva and lips. Lesions on other areas of the body should be sought.

(2) In severe or recurrent cases, indirect **immunofluorescence tests or viral culture** will determine if HSV is the causative agent. Enteroviruses can be isolated from viral cultures, but this is rarely helpful clinically.

c. The **diagnosis** is based on clinical findings. **Herpes simplex virus gingivostomatitis** typically involves the anterior portion of the oral cavity. **Herpangina** usually involves the posterior portion of the oral cavity and the pharynx. **Other conditions** include varicella, Kawasaki's disease, FAPA (fever, aphthous ulcers, and adenopathy) syndrome, Stevens-Johnson syndrome, aphthous stomatitis, Behçet's disease, and stomatitis-mucositis in the immunocompromised child. Noma is a rare, severe gangrenous stomatitis seen in the malnourished or debilitated child.

d. **Therapy**

(1) **Supportive care** is usually sufficient. Children with severe stomatitis may require intravenous hydration if they are unable to tolerate oral hydration.

(2) Data on the efficacy of **oral acyclovir** for HSV gingivostomatitis in normal children are not available. Treatment may reduce symptoms but is likely to be of marginal benefit in mild or uncomplicated cases. Severe or prolonged cases may benefit from oral acyclovir. Parenteral acyclovir can be used to treat children with severe stomatitis who are unable to tolerate oral medication.

(3) **Parenteral acyclovir** is indicated for treatment of hospitalized immunocompromised children (5–7mg/kg/day or 750 mg/m^2/day divided q8h).

e. **Suppressive therapy**

(1) Data on the efficacy of suppressive acyclovir for recurrent oral HSV stomatitis in normal children are not available. Children who have frequent recurrences of HSV stomatitis may benefit from a period of suppressive acyclovir (10 mg/kg/day divided bid).

(2) Recurrent HSV stomatitis in immunocompromised children is a common problem. These children often benefit from suppressive acyclovir (10 mg/kg/day divided bid).

2. **Oral candidiasis (oral moniliasis, thrush)** is a common infection of neonates and young infants and may occur in conjunction with candidal diaper rash. It is commonly seen during or after systemic antimicrobial treatment. Severe oral candidiasis in an infant or disease in an older child, especially when it is recurrent or does not respond well to therapy, may be an indicator of an underlying immunodeficiency.

a. **Etiology.** *Candida albicans* is the most common pathogen, but other species can cause disease.

b. **Evaluation**

(1) **Examination** of the mucosal membranes is sufficient. Milk, food, or coating on the tongue may be confused with plaques.

(2) **Gram's stain and potassium hydroxide (KOH) prep** are helpful but not necessary if the clinical findings are characteristic.

(3) **Cultures** are generally not useful except when the diagnosis is in question.

(4) Tests of immune function are *not* necessary in otherwise healthy children if disease is not severe or recurrent.

(5) Although older children may complain of mouth pain, the infection is usually asymptomatic in infants.

(6) Fever or other signs of systemic infection should prompt evaluation for another focus of infection.

c. The **diagnosis** is made clinically by the finding of white plaques that do not brush away easily on a base of inflamed mucosa. Plaques are usually on the buccal mucosa but may involve the gingiva and pharynx. The demonstration of yeast and pseudohyphae in scrapings of mucosal lesions is diagnostic. Oral candidiasis is a common finding in immunocompromised children and is commonly seen with candidal esophagitis.

d. **Therapy**

(1) Spontaneous resolution is common, especially if antimicrobial therapy is discontinued.

(2) Acute infection is usually treated.

(a) Topical agents are effective for most cases.

(i) Nystatin suspension (100,000 units) qid for 7 to 14 days is the most commonly used treatment for infants.

(ii) Gentian violet is effective but causes staining.

(iii) Clotrimazole troches tid or qid can be used in older children.

(b) Systemic therapy

(i) Oral fluconazole (2–6 mg/kg qd) for 14 days has replaced ketoconazole for treatment of difficult cases.

(ii) Parenteral therapy is used for severe cases often accompanied by candidal esophagitis: amphotericin, 0.25–0.50 mg/kg qd, and fluconazole, 6 mg/kg qd.

(3) Suppressive therapy is commonly used in immunocompromised children with recurrent oral candidiasis or esophagitis, or both.

(a) Nystatin suspension bid is often effective.

(b) Clotrimazole troches bid can be used by older children.

(c) Oral fluconazole (2–4 mg/kg qd) has replaced ketoconazole for chronic suppression because of better tolerance, although elevation of hepatic transaminases can also be seen with fluconazole.

C. Ear, upper respiratory tract, and neck infections

1. Otitis externa. Children with congenital or acquired narrowing of the external auditory canal are predisposed to this infection.

a. **Etiology.** *Staphylococcus aureus* is the most common cause. *Pseudomonas aeruginosa* and other gram negative bacteria are associated with swimming, chronic draining otitis media, and immunocompromised children. Fungi are an uncommon cause.

b. **Evaluation**

(1) Examination typically reveals partial or complete occlusion of the external auditory canal by drainage or edematous tissues. Marked pain on chewing or manipulation of the tragus is a characteristic sign. In small children, the presence of a foreign body should be excluded.

(2) Examination by an otorhinolaryngologist may be necessary in moderate to severe cases to rule out a foreign body and to insert a wick to facilitate drainage and use of topical agents. Removal of debris and purulent drainage is helpful, if possible.

(3) A culture taken by an otorhinolaryngologist who can first remove debris and drainage from the canal and directly swab infected areas may be more helpful in guiding antimicrobial therapy.

(4) In severe cases, a **CT scan or MRI** may help define the extent of the infection and identify areas that require surgical drainage.

c. The **diagnosis** is established clinically by the constellation of ear pain, seropurulent drainage, induration of the tissues of the external canal and periauricular area, and tenderness of the tragus during manipulation.

d. **Therapy**

(1) Local therapy will help reduce swelling, treat infection, and provide analgesia. In mild cases, the following should be administered topically.

(a) A solution of 1% acetic acid may be sufficient.

(b) Cortisporin (polymyxin, neomycin, and hydrocortisone) tid or qid is useful for its antimicrobial and anti-inflammatory properties.

(c) Topical antibiotics, such as topical colistin, gentamicin, or clindamycin tid, are also effective.

(d) Treatment should continue for 1 to 2 weeks, depending on the severity.

(2) Systemic therapy is necessary in moderate and severe infections with significant surrounding inflammation.

(a) **Oral therapy** with an antistaphylococcal agent, such as cephalexin, is sufficient in all but the most severe cases.

(b) **Parenteral therapy**, which is reserved for severe cases or immunocompromised children, should include a combination of an antistaphylococcal agent, such as oxacillin, and an antipseudomonal agent, such as tobramycin or ceftazidime.

2. Otitis media. Eustachian tube dysfunction causes inadequate ventilation of the middle ear, resulting in a negative middle ear pressure. Persistent negative pressure produces a sterile transudate within the middle ear. Concurrent or subsequent contamination of the middle ear with infected nasopharyngeal contents occurs by aspiration and insufflation during crying and nose blowing.

a. Acute otitis media

(1) Etiology

(a) *Streptococcus pneumoniae*, nontypable *H. influenzae*, *M. catarrhalis*, and group A streptococci are the most common causative organisms; *S. aureus* and enteric gram-negative bacilli (in neonates) are less frequent causes.

(b) Viruses and *M. pneumoniae* have been isolated from middle-ear fluid; their significance is uncertain.

(c) Of *Haemophilus* isolates, the nontypeable *H. influenzae* (nonencapsulated) species comprise the majority of middle ear isolates, are not associated with invasive infection, and are responsible for a small but significant proportion of infections in older children and adults. *Haemophilus influenzae* type b is uncommon.

(2) Evaluation

(a) **Pneumotoscopy** is required to make the diagnosis.

(b) **Tympanometry** may be helpful in difficult cases.

(c) **Tympanocentesis.** Middle ear aspiration should be performed on children who are seriously ill, have a poor response to antibiotics, or have a complication of acute otitis media. It is also useful in newborns and immunocompromised children. Diagnostic tympanocentesis should be performed under semisterile conditions with the aid of an operating microscope or otoscope with operating head; a spinal needle is inserted through the anteroinferior segment of the tympanic membrane.

(3) Diagnosis. A bulging, opacified, discolored eardrum through which the landmarks are poorly visualized, together with decreased mobility of the drum, defines acute otitis media.

(4) Treatment

(a) Oral antimicrobial agents are prescribed for all patients, generally for 10 days. Amoxicillin is the first drug of choice as it is safe and inexpensive. Recurrent otitis shortly after amoxicillin therapy or amoxicillin failure is reason to use alternative antibiotics. In some areas with high levels of beta-lactamase–producing *H. influenzae* or *M. catarrhalis*, alternative antibiotics might be given initially. We generally use TMP/SMZ as a second-line drug, as it is inexpensive, well tolerated, and likely to treat infection caused by beta-lactamase–producing pathogens. Erythromycin-sulfisoxazole can also be effective. Direct comparisons of alternative antibiotics are limited but suggest that amoxicillin-clavulanate is superior to cefaclor as a third-line agent. Amoxicillin-clavulanate, cefprozil, cefaclor, cefixime, cefpodoxime, locarbacef, and clarithromycin cost three to five times as much as amoxicillin or TMP/SMZ. We do not advocate use of cefaclor given the potential for a serum sickness reaction and because alternative agents are available.

    (i) Penicillin-resistant *S. pneumoniae*, which are increasing in frequency in many areas, are a more difficult problem. These organisms are often resistant to one or more of the alternative agents, including TMP/SMZ, erythromycin, the cephalosporins, and ampicillin-clavulanate. Of the oral agents, clindamycin has the most reliable in vitro activity against penicillin-resistant *S. pneumoniae*.

(b) Analgesics (acetaminophen, codeine) may be indicated.

(c) Antihistamines and decongestants are not indicated in otitis media, except to relieve coryza symptoms.

(d) The patient should be reevaluated within 30 days after starting therapy to determine whether effusion persists. If complete resolution has occurred, the patient is discharged. Periodic monitoring is required for patients with repeated episodes of otitis media. If effusion persists after 4 weeks, treatment is the same as that for chronic otitis media.

(e) Repeated episodes of otitis media with clearing of middle ear effusion between attacks can be managed by the use of prophylactic antibiotics including TMP/SMZ (4 mg and 20 mg, respectively/kg/day) or sulfisoxazole (50 mg/kg/day) in a single daily dose.

3. Streptococcal pharyngitis (tonsillitis)

  a. Etiology. Group A beta-hemolytic streptococci cause virtually all streptococcal pharyngitis, with rare outbreaks of group C and G.

  b. Evaluation

    (1) A **history** in the patient or family of recent streptococcal pharyngitis, scarlet fever, rheumatic fever, or penicillin allergy should be noted.

    (2) **Examination** is helpful in deciding on further evaluation. The presence of exudative pharyngitis, tender cervical adenopathy, and fever increases the likelihood of streptococcal versus viral pharyngitis. Conversely, the presence of cough and nasal congestion decreases this likelihood. In infants, streptococcal infection is more likely to present as persistent nasopharyngeal discharge with fever and excoriation of the nares.

    (3) A properly obtained specimen is critical for either a rapid streptococcal antigen test or a throat culture and must be performed by vigorously swabbing both tonsillar areas and the posterior pharynx. If done properly, this usually induces a gag reflex.

    (4) **Rapid streptococcal antigen tests** have replaced throat culture in many areas and, if performed properly, are highly specific (i.e., a positive test is highly correlated with isolation of group A streptococci in culture). However, these tests are generally not as sensitive as a properly collected and processed throat culture, especially when small numbers of group A streptococci are present.

    (5) Short of serologic confirmation, **throat culture** remains the gold standard for identification of streptococcal pharyngitis. Some clinics obtain a specimen for rapid streptococcal antigen test and throat culture at the same time and process the throat culture only if the rapid strep test is negative.

c. The **diagnosis** is supported by a positive throat culture or rapid antigen detection and confirmed by a rising antistreptolysin O titer (500 Todd units as an absolute value on a single specimen, or a 2-tube rise in serial specimens analyzed simultaneously).

d. **Therapy**

(1) **Antibiotic therapy** is necessary to prevent sequelae, such as rheumatic fever.

(a) **Intramuscular penicillin (benzathine)** ensures treatment for a sufficient length of time. Children should be given a single injection of 600,000 to 1,200,000 units. The larger dose is preferable for children over 60 lb.

(b) **Oral therapy** is dependent on the cooperation of the patient and the parents. For prevention of acute rheumatic fever, therapy must be continued for the *entire* 10 days, even though the temperature returns to normal and the patient is asymptomatic.

(i) Penicillin, 125 mg (children) or 250 mg (older children and adolescents) tid–qid.

(ii) For patients with documented penicillin allergy, oral erythromycin, 40 mg/kg/day in four divided doses, or clindamycin, 10 to 20 mg/kg/day in four divided doses for 10 days, is recommended. Cephalosporins are also effective. Sulfonamides, while effective in the prophylaxis of streptococcal infection, are ineffective in their treatment.

(2) Bed rest is not necessary. After 24 hours of antibiotic therapy, children are no longer contagious and can return to school.

(3) Follow-up cultures are not necessary unless the child remains symptomatic or other family members become infected.

(4) Throat cultures are indicated for symptomatic family members but are not necessary for others unless recurrent streptococcal pharyngitis occurs in the family. Such recurrences may necessitate empiric antibiotic treatment of the entire family.

4. **Abscesses** involving the peritonsillar, retropharyngeal, or parapharyngeal spaces may complicate infections in and around the oropharynx.

a. **Peritonsillar abscesses** commonly occur in children over 10 years of age.

(1) **Etiology.** Group A streptococci and oral anaerobes are the causative agents.

(2) **Evaluation**

(a) The soft palate and uvula may be swollen and displaced toward the unaffected side.

(b) The patient complains of severe throat pain and may speak with a muffled, "hot-potato" voice.

(c) Trismus is present due to spasm of the internal pterygoid muscle, and drooling occurs due to dysphagia.

(3) **Diagnosis.** Surgical drainage of the abscess usually yields the organism.

(4) **Therapy**

(a) **Surgical drainage** is the cornerstone of effective therapy and should be performed under general anesthesia using a cuffed endotracheal tube to minimize the chances of aspiration or mediastinitis, or both.

(b) After effective surgical drainage, **the antibiotic treatment** of choice is a 10-day course of penicillin, initially IV until acute manifestations have subsided and then continued PO.

b. **Retropharyngeal or parapharyngeal abscesses** commonly occur in children younger than 3 years.

(1) **Etiology.** Group A streptococci, *S. aureus*, and oral anaerobes. The possibility of an embedded foreign body should never be overlooked.

(2) Evaluation. History includes sore throat, fever, dysphagia, odynophagia, and voice change. Abscesses in these locations should be suspected with displacement of structures or a mass in the posterior pharynx. A lateral neck x-ray or CT scan may be necessary to evaluate the thickness of the retropharyngeal tissues.

(3) Diagnosis. Culture of aspirated surgical drainage may yield the organisms.

(4) Therapy

    (a) Surgical drainage is the mainstay of treatment.

    (b) Because of the high incidence of mixed infections at these sites, a penicillinase-resistant penicillin should be given in addition to penicillin G. Alternatively, ampicillin-sulbactam can be used.

    (c) Clindamycin is an alternative drug for the penicillin-allergic patient.

5. Cervical adenitis. Lymph nodes often enlarge in response to localized or systemic infection. Marked enlargement (≥3 cm) associated with tenderness and erythema indicates progressive infection within the node.

  a. The **etiology** varies with the location of the infected neck glands and the acuity of the process.

    (1) Tonsillar nodes (at the angle of the jaw) are likely to be infected by organisms from the pharynx, such as group A streptococci, *S. aureus*, and mouth anaerobes.

    (2) Submandibular node infection follows oral or facial disease. Unilateral, "cold" submandibular nodes that are chronic and unresponsive to antibiotic treatment suggest infection with atypical (nontuberculous) mycobacteria.

    (3) Posterior cervical node infection suggests an adjacent skin infection.

    (4) Bilateral cervical node enlargement of marked degree indicates Epstein-Barr virus or cytomegalovirus infection, toxoplasmosis, secondary syphilis, a phenytoin reaction, or infiltrative node disease.

    (5) *Bartonella henselae* (the cat-scratch agent) can cause unilateral cervical or preauricular adenitis, but more commonly results in axillary adenitis.

    (6) Recurrent episodes of adenitis should raise the suspicion of chronic granulomatous disease or immunoglobulin (IG) deficiency.

  b. Evaluation

    (1) The **history** should investigate the presence of other symptoms (pharyngitis, neck stiffness, dysphagia), significant exposures (cats, tuberculosis, tick bites), and prior episodes.

    (2) Examination of the area should define the nodes involved as well as associated findings of fever, warmth, induration, tenderness, and fluctuance. Torticollis is a relatively common finding.

    (3) If fever is present, a **complete blood count and differential** is necessary.

    (4) A **blood culture** should be obtained although the yield is low.

    (5) A **throat culture or rapid streptococcal antigen test** is useful in determining if group A streptococcus is a likely pathogen.

    (6) A **tuberculin skin test with control** should be placed. A positive tuberculin skin test mandates a chest x-ray.

    (7) Other laboratory tests should be ordered only as indicated: ASLO titer, Monospot, antibody titers for Epstein-Barr virus and *Toxoplasma gondii*, urine for cytomegalovirus rapid diagnosis and/or culture, and a rapid plasma reagin (RPR).

    (8) Ultrasound or CT scan are useful when it is difficult to determine whether suppuration is sufficient to warrant drainage.

    (9) Needle aspiration of the node offers a simple, safe means of diagnosis. Gram's and acid-fast stains of aspirates may provide immediately helpful information. Aspirates should be cultured for aerobes, anaerobes, and mycobacteria.

c. The **diagnosis** is made by the clinical findings and evaluation described above.

d. Therapy

(1) Surgical drainage or excisional biopsy is appropriate for infected nodes that are fluctuant ("pointing") or refractory to broad-spectrum antibiotic therapy. The therapy of choice for atypical mycobacterial adenitis is excisional biopsy. In some cases, biopsy is necessary to rule out malignancy.

(2) Antibiotic therapy. Unless stains of the node aspirate suggest another organism, a penicillinase-resistant penicillin or first-generation cephalosporin should be given as *initial therapy*, because the most likely organisms are *S. aureus* or group A streptococci. Oral anaerobes can be isolated from some nodes but other pathogens, such as *H. influenzae* type b, are seen only rarely.

(a) Streptococcal adenitis. When group A streptococcus is isolated, penicillin G, either IM or IV in severe cases, is given until the fever and localized inflammation have subsided. This response should occur within 2 to 3 days, after which a 10-day course of oral penicillin (penicillin G, 50,000 units/kg/day, or penicillin V, 50 mg/kg/day) can be completed. Hot compresses and antipyretics also are prescribed.

(b) Staphylococcal adenitis. Because the organism is often penicillin resistant, one of the penicillinase-resistant semisynthetic penicillins or a first-generation cephalosporin is given. Severity of the illness determines whether the IV route and hospitalization are necessary. The duration of treatment is determined by the patient's response, but a 10- to 14-day course is usually sufficient.

(i) Recommended *parenteral* preparation is nafcillin, oxacillin, or methicillin, 100 to 200 mg/kg/day q4h, or cefazolin, 80 mg/kg/day q8h.

(ii) Recommended *oral* preparation is dicloxacillin, 25 mg/kg/day qid, or cephalexin, 25 to 50 mg/kg/day qid.

(c) Tuberculous adenitis. Antituberculous drugs are given (see p. 147).

(d) Nontuberculous mycobacterial adenitis. Although the natural history of this disease is variable, the adenopathy will often resolve spontaneously. When increasing adenopathy or related symptoms indicate the need for more aggressive management, complete surgical excision of the involved nodes is recommended and is often curative. Antituberculous therapy should be given postoperatively until culture reports demonstrate that *M. tuberculosis* is not present. Clarithromycin and rifampin can be used for complicated cases where surgical excision is impossible or incomplete.

(e) *Bartonella henselae* **(the cat-scratch agent) adenitis.** Most cases resolve spontaneously. There is no known effective treatment.

6. Epiglottitis (see Chap. 7, p. 225).

D. Lower respiratory tract infections

1. Croup (see Chap. 7, p. 226).

2. Bacterial tracheitis (see Chap. 7, p. 228).

3. Bronchiolitis and bronchitis (see Chap. 7, p. 231).

4. Pertussis

a. Etiology. The etiologic agent is *Bordetella pertussis*, a fastidious, gram negative pleomorphic bacillus. A syndrome similar to pertussis may be caused by a closely related bacteria, *Bordetella parapertussis* and *Bordetella bronchiseptica* and some adenoviruses (type 11).

b. Evaluation

(1) A **history** of a disease characterized by mild upper respiratory symptoms (catarrhal stage) that progresses to paroxysms of cough (paroxysmal stage), particularly when the cough lasts longer than 2 weeks, is strongly suggestive. An inspiratory whoop is characteristic but is not often heard in young infants. Posttussive vomiting is common. Cyanosis with coughing episodes is of concern, especially in young infants.

(2) **Nasopharyngeal culture** should be obtained whenever the disease is suspected. Positive cultures may be obtained in the catarrhal or early paroxysmal phases. False-negative cultures are common later in the disease course or when the patient has been treated with antimicrobials. The culture should be obtained using a Dacron or calcium alginate swab and inoculated onto special media (Regan-Lowe or Bordet-Gengou) at the bedside.

(3) **Direct immunofluorescent assay** (DFA) of nasopharyngeal secretions has variable sensitivity and specificity.

(4) **Serologic tests** are available for a number of specific *B. pertussis* antigens.

(5) **Complete blood count** will usually reveal an absolute lymphocytosis.

(6) **Chest x-ray** should be performed to rule out an accompanying pneumonia and other etiologies.

(7) Complications of pertussis include secondary bacterial pneumonia, seizures, and encephalopathy.

c. The **diagnosis** is confirmed by a positive culture. Serologic tests also confirm the diagnosis if there is a marked rise in titer between sera drawn at presentation and during convalescence; a single high titer is also diagnostic. The presence of a marked absolute lymphocytosis ($>20,000/mm^3$) suggests the diagnosis, but lesser degrees of lymphocytosis are often seen in pertussis as well as in *Chlamydia* and viral respiratory infections. A history of cough in a person known to have been exposed to pertussis or during a documented outbreak is sufficient for the diagnosis when culture is not possible or feasible.

d. **Therapy**

(1) **Supportive care** includes avoidance of factors that provoke paroxysms of coughing, humidified oxygen if necessary, adequate hydration, and suctioning and positioning to assist in the removal of secretions. Infants less than 6 months old and other children with severe disease should be hospitalized.

(2) **Antimicrobial therapy**

(a) All patients and their close contacts should be given antibiotics to reduce the potential for transmitting the infection to others. Erythromycin, 40 to 50 mg/kg/day divided qid, eliminates the organism from the nasopharynx in 3 to 5 days, but should be continued for 14 days. TMP/SMZ (8–10 mg/kg/day TMP component) or clarithromycin, 15 mg/kg/day divided bid, can be substituted for patients who cannot tolerate erythromycin, but their efficacy has not been proved.

(b) Therapy that is begun in the catarrhal phase may shorten the course of the disease, but if therapy does not begin until the paroxysmal phase it is unlikely to have an effect on the course of the disease.

(c) Secondary bacterial pneumonia should be treated with antimicrobial therapy (see below).

e. **Prevention.** See Table 5–3 for post exposure prophylaxis measures.

5. **Pneumonia**

a. **Etiology**

(1) **Neonates.** Gram-positive cocci, particularly group B streptococcus and occasionally *S. aureus*, and gram-negative enteric bacilli cause most neonatal bacterial pneumonias.

(2) **Children 1 month to 5 years of age**

(a) Respiratory viruses cause the majority of pediatric pneumonias.

Table 5-3. Postexposure prophylaxis regimens for children and adolescents

Disease	Indication	Regimen
Botulism	Ingestion of food known to contain botulinum toxin	Administration of botulinum antitoxin is not routinely recommended due to the potential for hypersensitivity reactions. Contact the state health department or the CDC.
Diphtheria	Contacts, regardless of vaccination status[a]	Contacts should be cultured and observed for 7 days. Erythromycin, 40–50 mg/kg/d, maximum 2.0 g/d, for 7 days or benzathine penicillin G, 600,000 units for children < 30 kg and 1,200,000 units for children ≥ 30 kg IM, should be administered after the culture is obtained. If compliance with the oral regimen cannot be assured, the IM regimen should be used.
		Repeat cultures should be obtained after prophylaxis is complete in persons with positive initial cultures. If the primary vaccination series is complete (>3 doses of diphtheria toxoid), note the following:
		If a vaccine dose has been given in the past 5 yr, no booster dose is needed.
		If no vaccine dose has been given within the past 5 yr, give a booster dose.
		If the primary vaccination series is not complete or the vaccination status is unknown, give an age-appropriate dose of vaccine and complete the primary vaccination series.
Chlamydial genital infection	Sexual contacts	Treat as indicated after evaluation (see p. 129).[b] If the last contact was within 30 days of a symptomatic index case or within 60 days of an asymptomatic index case, treat as infected.
Gonorrhea	Sexual contacts	Treat as indicated after evaluation (see p. 127).[b]
Hepatitis A	Household and sexual contacts	Immune globulin (IG), 0.02 ml/kg IM[b]
	Contacts (enrollees and staff) in child care and household contacts of child care enrollees	Recommendations vary according to the age of enrolled children, whether the children are toilet trained, the number of cases in enrolled children, staff and household contacts, and the elapsed time since the index case.[c] Contact the state health department or the CDC.
	Contacts in institutions for custodial care	IG, 0.02 ml/kg IM
	Contacts in schools and health care facilities	IG is generally not indicated, but can be considered in some situations or during outbreaks.

Table 5-3 (continued)

Disease	Indication	Regimen
Hepatitis B	Infants < 12 mo of age with acutely infected primary caregiver	If the vaccination series is complete, no prophylaxis. If the vaccination series has not started or is not complete, give hepatitis B immune globulin (HBIG), 0.5 ml IM, and hepatitis B vaccine (HBV); complete the vaccination series.
	Household contacts of person with acute infection[d]	Therapy is not immediately indicated; wait to determine if person becomes hepatitis B surface antigen (HBsAg) carrier. An alternative approach is to begin the vaccination series if not already complete.
	Household contacts of HBsAg carrier[d]	If the vaccination series is complete, no prophylaxis. If the vaccination series has not started or is not complete, give HBV; complete the vaccination series.
	Sexual contacts of person with acute infection	If the vaccination series is complete, no prophylaxis.[b] If the vaccination series has not started or is not complete, give HBIG, 0.06 ml/kg IM, and HBV; complete the vaccination series.[b]
	Sexual contacts of HBsAg carrier	If the vaccination series is complete, no prophylaxis.[b] If the vaccination series has not started or is not complete, give HBV; complete the vaccination series.[b]
	Percutaneous or permucosal contact with blood or infectious body fluids[e] from person with acute infection or HBsAg carrier	If the vaccination series is complete, no prophylaxis. An alternative approach if the vaccination series is complete is to check the hepatitis B surface antibody (HBsAb) level. If the level is adequate[f], no prophylaxis. If the level is inadequate, give HBIG, 0.06 ml/kg IM, and HBV. If the vaccination series has not started or is not complete, give HBIG, 0.06 ml/kg IM, and HBV; complete the vaccination series.
Human immunodeficiency virus (HIV)	Sexual contacts	No prophylaxis with established effectiveness is available; an individualized approach should be followed involving counseling and follow-up serologic testing.[b]
Infection/acquired immunodeficiency syndrome (AIDS)	Percutaneous or permucosal contact with blood or infectious body fluids[e]	No prophylaxis with established effectiveness is available; an individualized approach should be followed involving counseling, follow-up serologic testing, and, possibly, the use of antiretroviral agents.[g]

Table 5-3 (continued)

Invasive bacterial disease

Neisseria meningitidis	Contacts in households, child care, school, and health-care facilities[h]	Rifampin is the recommended agent. Infants < 2 mo of age: 10–20 mg/kg/d PO divided bid for 2 d. All others: 20 mg/kg/d, 600 mg/d maximum, PO divided bid for 2 d. Ceftriaxone can be used when rifampin is contraindicated. Children < 12 yr: 125 mg IM once. Persons ≥ 12 yr: 250 mg IM once. Ciprofloxacin, 500 mg PO once, has been shown to be effective in adults. Prophylaxis should be given as soon as possible, especially for household contacts. In outbreaks due to types A, C, Y, and W-135, vaccination may be helpful. Contact the state health department or the CDC.
Haemophilus influenzae type b disease	Contacts in households with at least one unvaccinated or incompletely vaccinated[i] contact < 48 mo of age[h]	Rifampin is the only agent with established efficacy. Infants < 2 mo of age: 10–20 mg/kg/d PO divided bid for 4 d. All others: 20 mg/kg/d, 600 mg/d maximum, PO divided bid for 4 d. All members of the household should receive prophylaxis. Index cases should receive rifampin as dosed above at the conclusion of their treatment course.
	Contacts in child care[h]	When 1 case has occurred: If all contacts are ≥ 2 yr of age, rifampin prophylaxis is not necessary. If contacts include unvaccinated or incompletely vaccinated children[i] < 2 yr of age and if contact time is ≥ 25 hr/wk, rifampin prophylaxis as described for household contacts should be considered. When 2 cases have occurred within 60 d and unvaccinated or incompletely vaccinated children[i] attend, rifampin prophylaxis as described for household contacts should be given. Unvaccinated or incompletely vaccinated children[i] should be given a dose of conjugate vaccine and their immunization status should be brought up to date. All enrollees and staff should receive prophylaxis as soon as possible.
Streptococcus pneumoniae	Household contacts, child care, and school contacts[h]	Prophylaxis is not generally recommended but may be useful in some situations, such as an outbreak of penicillin-resistant invasive pneumococcal infection.

Table 5-3 (continued)

Disease	Indication	Regimen
Measles	Household contacts who are not immune[j]	IG, 0.25 ml/kg IM once
	Contacts 6 mo–1 yr of age[k,l]	Measles vaccine or measles-mumps-rubella (MMR) vaccine as soon as possible and within 72 hr. IG, 0.25 ml/kg IM once as soon as possible if > 72 hr since exposure has elapsed and within 6 d.
	Contacts who are not immune[j,k] Immunocompromised children[k]	Measles vaccine or MMR vaccine as soon as possible and within 72 hr IG, 0.5 ml/kg, maximum 15 ml, IM once[m]
Mumps	Contacts who are not immune[n]	Mumps vaccine has not been demonstrated to be effective in preventing or modifying infection after exposure, but can be administered to nonimmune persons to provide protection against subsequent exposures.
Parvovirus (erythema infectiosum, fifth disease)	Contacts who are not immune[o]	IG has not been demonstrated to be effective in preventing or modifying infection after exposure, but may be considered in some situations.
Pertussis	Household contacts regardless of vaccination status	Erythromycin, 40–50 mg/kg/d PO divided qid for 14 days. If erythromycin is not tolerated, clarithromycin, 15 mg/kg/d PO divided bid, or trimethoprim-sulfamethoxazole, 10 mg/kg/d (trimethoprim component) PO divided bid for 14 d, can be used, although their efficacy is not established. Unvaccinated or incompletely vaccinated (<4 doses of diphtheria-tetanus-pertussis [DTP] or diphtheria-tetanus-acellular pertussis [DTaP]) children < 7 yr of age, should be given a dose of vaccine and the vaccine series completed. Children who have received 4 doses of vaccine should receive a booster dose unless the last dose was given <3 yr ago or they are > 6 yr of age.
Rabies	Bites, scratches, or exposures to saliva or other infectious material on mucous membranes or nonintact skin from potentially or confirmed rabid animal (see p. 143)	Cleanse the wound with soap and water. Rabies immune globulin (RIG), 20 IU/kg infiltrated in the wound (½ the dose) and IM (the remainder). Human diploid cell rabies vaccine (HDCV) or rabies vaccine, absorbed (RVA), 1 ml IM, should be given at a different site, with subsequent doses on days 3, 7, 14, and 28.

Table 5-3 (continued)

Rubella	Contacts who are not immune[k,n]	Rubella vaccine has not been demonstrated to be effective in preventing or modifying infection after exposure but can be administered to nonimmune persons to provide protection against subsequent exposures. Routine use of IG in susceptible women early in pregnancy is not recommended. If termination of pregnancy is not an option, IG, 0.55 ml/kg, should be considered but does not necessarily prevent infection of the mother or the fetus.
Syphilis (acquired)	Sexual contacts	Treat as indicated after evaluation (see p. 125)[b] Contacts within the past 3 mo who are seronegative may have early acquired syphilis and should be treated as infected.
Tuberculosis	Household contacts ≥ 4 yr of age	Examine and apply a tuberculin and control skin test. If skin test is positive, evaluate and treat as indicated (see p. 147). If skin test is negative and not anergic, retest in 12 wk. If skin repeat test is positive, evaluate and treat as indicated. If skin test is negative without anergy and exposure has ended (contact is no longer present or is known to have responded to therapy), no treatment is necessary.
	Household contacts < 4 yr of age or immunocompromised children	Examine and apply a tuberculin and control skin test; perform chest x-ray and other tests as indicated (see p. 147). If skin test is positive or there is evidence of infection, treat as indicated. If skin test is negative and there is no evidence of infection, treat with isoniazid (INH), 10–15 mg/kg qd, and retest in 12 wk. If repeat skin test positive or evidence of infection, evaluate and treat as indicated (see p. 147). If skin test is negative without anergy, there is no evidence of infection, and exposure has ended (contact is no longer present or is known to have responded to therapy), prophylaxis can be discontinued. If skin test is negative but anergic, treat for 9–12 mo.
Tetanus	Clean wounds	If tetanus immunization is incomplete (< 3 previous doses of toxoid) and/or > 10 yr have elapsed since the last dose, give 0.5 ml (DT, DTP, or DTaP in children < 7 yr old, Td in children 7 yr and older) IM once.
	Contaminated wounds[p]	If tetanus immunization is incomplete (<3 previous doses of toxoid) and/or > 5 yr have elapsed since the last dose, give vaccine as described above and administer human tetanus immunoglobulin (TIG), 250–500 units IM in a separate injection site.
Varicella	Immunocompromised children with a negative history for varicella[q,r]	Varicella zoster immunoglobulin (VZIG), one vial (125 units) for each 10 kg weight IM once as soon as possible and within 96 hr of exposure.[m,s]

Table 5-3 (continued)

[a] The definition of a contact is difficult to define absolutely, and clinical judgment is necessary. Close, person-to-person contact should generally be regarded as sufficient to warrant prophylaxis, although the duration of contact is also important. Brief, face-to-face encounters are not necessarily significant; on the other hand, contact that occurs over extended periods, such as contact between persons living in the same household, is almost always significant. Contact between infected persons and their primary caregivers or medical or dental professionals is usually more intense and may be significant depending on the individual circumstances.

[b] Sexual contacts should be examined, tested, and treated for other sexually transmitted diseases. Testing for HIV infection should be offered in conjunction with appropriate counseling, including counseling regarding the prevention of sexually transmitted diseases.

[c] See the 1994 Red Book. The Report of the Committee on Infectious Diseases, American Academy of Pediatrics. Pp 223–224.

[d] If percutaneous or permucosal contact with blood or infectious body fluids of person with acute infection or HBsAg carrier, see recommendations below.

[e] Infectious body fluids include visibly bloody body fluids of any kind, amniotic fluid, pericardial fluid, peritoneal fluid, pleural fluid, synovial fluid, cerebrospinal fluid, semen, and vaginal or cervical secretions.

[f] An adequate HBsAb level is ≥ 10 mIU.

[g] If antiretroviral agents are to be used, they should be started as soon as possible after exposure, preferably within a few hours.

[h] Contacts should be carefully observed. Exposed individuals in whom a febrile illness develops should receive a prompt medical evaluation.

[i] Complete vaccination is defined as at least 1 dose of conjugate vaccine at ≥12 mo. If the household contains an immunocompromised child, prophylaxis should be administered regardless of the age or vaccination status of that child.

[j] Immunity consists of documentation of physician-diagnosed measles, serologic evidence of immunity to measles, or documentation of receipt of 2 doses of measles vaccine on or after 12 mo of age.

[k] Transmission is via the airborne route; consequently, contact does not require person-to-person contact. Infants ≤ 5 mo of age usually have partial or complete immunity as a result of passively acquired maternal antibody. However, infants in this age group should be considered for prophylaxis if their mother has no history of measles or has not been vaccinated or if the infant was significantly premature (<32 wk gestation).

[m] Children receiving monthly high-dose IV immunoglobulin (IVIG, 100–400 mg/kg/dose) are likely to be protected and do not require prophylaxis if the last dose of IVIG was given in the 3 wk before exposure.

[n] Immunity consists of documentation of physician-diagnosed disease, serologic evidence of immunity, or documentation of receipt of a dose of measles vaccine on or after 12 mo of age.

[o] Immunity consists of documentation of physician-diagnosed disease or serologic evidence of immunity.

[p] Examples are wounds contaminated with dirt, feces, soil, and saliva; puncture wounds; avulsions; and wounds that result from missiles, crushing, burns, and frostbite.

[q] Prophylaxis should be considered in some immunocompromised children regardless of the prior history of infection, such as severely immunocompromised children with HIV infection, children with congenital severe combined immunodeficiency, or children who have recently undergone bone marrow transplantation.

[r] In general, children receiving short courses of corticosteroids for asthma treatment are not regarded as immunocompromised. Management of these children should take into account the likelihood of exposure, the time frame of the administration of steroids in relation to the development of varicella, and the dose and duration of treatment with corticosteroids.

[s] Monitor closely for signs of infection. Acyclovir should be administered if evidence of infection develops, but prophylactic use of acyclovir is not recommended since its efficacy has not been adequately studied and may result in an alteration of the incubation time or immune response.

Source: Adapted from recommendations included in the 1994 Red Book. The Report of the Committee on Infectious Diseases, American Academy of Pediatrics.

(b) *Chlamydia trachomatis* causes an afebrile pneumonia in infants under 16 weeks of age.

(c) The major bacterial pathogens in this age group are *S. pneumoniae* and *H. influenzae* type b. *M. catarrhalis*, group A streptococci, and *S. aureus* are occasional pathogens.

(3) Children 5 years of age and older

(a) *Streptococcus pneumoniae* is the major cause of bacterial pneumonia in this age group.

(b) *Mycoplasma pneumoniae* is a common cause of pneumonia in school-aged children, adolescents, and young adults.

(c) *Chlamydia pneumoniae* is a common etiology in adolescents and college students.

(4) Immunocompromised hosts are subject to pneumonia caused by any organism. In addition to the pathogens described above, *Pneumocystis carinii*, cytomegalovirus, gram-negative bacteria, and fungi are common causes of pneumonia in these patients.

(5) Anaerobic bacteria, especially penicillin-sensitive oral anaerobes, can cause pneumonia and lung abscess in patients who aspirate.

(6) In any age group, *S. aureus*, group A streptococcus, and *S. pneumoniae* can cause bacterial pneumonia *after* a viral respiratory infection.

(7) Tuberculosis should always be considered as a possible cause of infectious pneumonia, especially in the child who responds slowly or not at all to antibiotic therapy.

(8) A variety of other agents, such as *Francisella tularensis*, *Legionella*, *Chlamydia psittaci*, and *Coxiella burnetii* (Q fever), are rare causes of pneumonia in children.

b. Evaluation

(1) Chest x-ray (posteroanterior and lateral).

(2) Tuberculin skin test by intradermal purified protein derivative with a *Candida* control.

(3) Sputum or deep tracheal aspirate for Gram's stain and culture is helpful when a good-quality specimen (a specimen not contaminated with oral secretions) can be obtained. Cultures for bacteria from the nasopharynx should be interpreted with great caution.

(4) Fluorescent antibody techniques for rapid diagnosis of certain viruses (e.g., respiratory syncytial virus) are now more widely available. **Cultures for respiratory viruses** are useful in cases with severe pneumonia or pneumonia in immunocompromised children.

(5) Blood culture(s) may be positive in children with bacterial pneumonia and thus reveal the etiologic agent.

(6) Leukocyte and differential counts are occasionally helpful, but are not specific enough to reliably distinguish bacterial pneumonia from other causes.

(7) A **diagnostic thoracentesis** if pleural fluid is present.

(8) Serologic titers (acute and convalescent) are not very satisfactory for most pathogens, but for *Mycoplasma* (cold agglutinin titer > 1 : 64, or complement fixation titers), group A streptococcus (antistreptolysin O titer), *Chlamydia*, *Legionella*, and *Rickettsia* (Q fever), they may be the most useful means to make a presumptive diagnosis.

(9) Rapid diagnostic techniques for bacterial antigens in body fluids.

(10) Bronchoscopy with bronchoalveolar lavage and protected brush biopsy or open lung biopsy is necessary to establish the etiologic diagnosis to guide antimicrobial therapy in critically ill or immunocompromised children.

c. The **diagnosis** is usually established by the chest x-ray and physical signs of consolidation. The following clinical features may assist in etiologic diagnosis:

(1) A history of conjunctivitis is present in 50% of *Chlamydia trachomatis*, eosinophilia is common, and the chest x-ray shows hyperinflation and diffuse interstitial or patchy infiltrates.

(2) Pneumococci commonly cause lobar or segmental consolidation, but bronchopneumonia is not infrequent. *Haemophilus influenzae* type b can mimic pneumonia caused by a number of organisms and is not infrequently associated with extrapulmonary infection.

(3) Group A streptococci can cause a rapidly progressive bilateral pneumonia, often accompanied by pleural effusion and bacteremia.

(4) *Staphylococcus aureus* is suggested by rapidly evolving respiratory distress, empyema, and the characteristic radiologic features of rapid progression, lobular ectasia, and pneumatoceles in a child less than 3 years old. Even in an extremely ill child, however, the initial x-ray film may demonstrate only faint local mottling.

d. Therapy (see also p. 232)

    (1) Symptomatic care should include oxygen if necessary, maintenance of adequate hydration, high humidity (such as the use of a humidifier in the home), bronchodilators if bronchospasm is present, and suctioning of children with an ineffectual cough.

    (2) Antimicrobial therapy

      (a) Children who are mildly ill with features suggestive of viral disease can be managed without antibiotics, provided they can be followed closely.

      (b) Therapy should be directed toward the most likely pathogens.

        (i) Neonates should receive parenteral treatment with a penicillinase-resistant penicillin and an aminoglycoside or third-generation cephalosporin.

        (ii) The hospitalized child should be treated with a second- or third-generation cephalosporin or ampicillin-sulbactam. If an *S. aureus* pneumonia is suspected, a penicillinase-resistant penicillin (oxacillin, 200 mg/kg/day q4h) should be used in combination with a second- or third-generation cephalosporin. Clindamycin is an alternative for patients with a history of allergy to beta-lactam antibiotics. Ampicillin-sulbactam or clindamycin should be used when an aspiration pneumonia is suspected. Ampicillin alone can be used when infection with *S. pneumoniae* is strongly suspected and is much cheaper than any of the above regimens.

        (iii) The nonhospitalized child should be given an antibiotic such as amoxicillin that is effective against both *S. pneumoniae* and *H. influenzae* type b. TMP/SMZ, ampicillin-clavulanate, and an oral second-generation cephalosporin (cefuroxime, cefprozil) are alternatives and also provide staphylococcal and ampicillin-resistant *H. influenzae* coverage.

        (iv) If *Mycoplasma*, *Chlamydia*, or *Legionella* is suspected, treatment should include erythromycin (30–50 mg/kg/day in 4 daily doses for 10 days). Clarithromycin, 15 mg/kg/day divided bid, is a more expensive alternative but has fewer gastrointestinal side effects. Tetracycline can be used in children 9 years of age or older.

        (v) If *P. carinii* pneumonia (PCP) is suspected, the treatment is TMP/SMZ (TMP, 20 mg/kg/day) in four divided doses IV or PO for 21 days. Pentamidine isethionate, 4 mg/kg IV qd as a single dose for 21 days, is an alternative for patients with hypersensitivity reactions to TMP/SMZ. Corticosteroids (prednisone, 2 mg/kg/day initially and as a tapering dose over 21 days) should strongly be considered as adjunctive therapy in any child with PCP that requires oxygen therapy.

        (vi) Suspected pulmonary tuberculosis should receive prompt treatment (see p. 147).

    (c) Identification of the pathogen or failure to respond to these regimens necessitates reevaluation of the choice of antibiotics.

    (d) The **duration** of antimicrobial therapy is based on the individual patient's clinical response, but, in general, staphylococcal pneumonia requires 3 weeks of parenteral therapy followed by 1 to 3 weeks of oral therapy. *Haemophilus influenzae* and streptococcal pneumonia usually respond to 1 to 2 weeks of therapy, and uncomplicated pneumococcal pneumonia will resolve with only 7 days of therapy.

  (3) **Indications for hospitalization** include the following: significant hypoxia, respiratory distress or toxicity, cyanosis, age under 6 months, empyema or significant pleural effusion, possible staphylococcal pneumonia, and inadequate home care.

  (4) **Drainage** of an associated empyema, by repeated aspiration or insertion of a chest tube, may be necessary.

  (5) **Postural drainage** and **physiotherapy** may be helpful, particularly with underlying bronchiectasis.

  (6) **Follow-up** of the ambulatory patient should be on a day-to-day basis until definite clinical improvement has occurred.

  (7) **Radiologic resolution** may lag behind clinical improvement, but persistence of radiologic abnormalities without improvement for more than 4 to 6 weeks should alert the physician to possible underlying pulmonary disease (e.g., tuberculosis, foreign body, cystic fibrosis).

E. Cardiovascular system

  1. Acute rheumatic fever

    a. Etiology. Acute rheumatic fever (ARF) is a sequela of pharyngeal infection with a group A streptococcus, but the exact pathogenesis is still unknown.

    b. Evaluation

      (1) The **history** should emphasize antecedent infections, fever, arthralgia, previous episodes of ARF, and a family history of ARF.

      (2) **Physical examination** should look for evidence of arthritis, rashes, subcutaneous nodules, murmurs, and neurologic abnormalities.

      (3) **Laboratory studies** should include erythrocyte sedimentation rate (ESR) or C-reactive protein, CBC, ECG, chest x-ray, streptococcal antibodies (antistreptolysin O, anti-deoxyribonuclease[DNase] B, anti-NADase, antihyaluronidase), and throat culture.

    c. Diagnosis

      (1) No single laboratory test, symptom, or sign is pathognomonic, although several combinations are suggestive of ARF.

      (2) According to the **revised Jones criteria**, ARF is likely in the presence of one major and two minor criteria or two major criteria plus evidence of a preceding streptococcal infection. **Chorea** alone may be sufficient for a diagnosis.

        (a) Major criteria

          (i) Carditis. The valvular endocardium, myocardium, and pericardium are typically involved together in a pancarditis. The murmur of mitral insufficiency (apical systolic murmur transmitted to the axilla) is the most common manifestation of valvular involvement. The murmur of *aortic insufficiency* (diastolic murmur at the left sternal border) is also present in some patients. An echocardiographic finding of mitral insufficiency without an audible murmur is **not** sufficient for the diagnosis of carditis.

          (ii) Migratory polyarthritis. The arthritis of ARF is characteristically migratory and particularly affects the knees, ankles, elbows, and wrists. It rarely affects the spine or the small joints of the hands and feet.

  (iii) **Subcutaneous nodules** are found on the extensor surfaces of the joints and usually occur only in children with chronic rheumatic heart disease or severe, untreated carditis of several weeks' duration.

  (iv) **Erythema marginatum** is an uncommon finding in ARF and is not specific to the disease.

  (v) **Chorea** occurs long after the preceding streptococcal infection. Emotional instability is a common associated finding.

  (b) **Minor criteria**

  (i) **Fever.** Rarely above 40°C (104°F); associated with shaking chills.

  (ii) **Arthralgias.** Joint pain without objective findings.

  (iii) **Prolonged P-R interval on the ECG** (not in and of itself diagnostic of carditis).

  (iv) **Increased ESR, C-reactive protein, leukocytosis.**

  (v) **Previous history of ARF or rheumatic heart disease.**

  (c) **Previous evidence of a streptococcal infection** includes a positive rapid streptococcal antigen test or throat culture, elevated levels of antibodies to streptococcal antigens, or a history of scarlet fever.

 d. **Treatment**

  (1) **Antibiotics.** Treatment with penicillin or another antibiotic with activity against streptococci is indicated in order to eradicate any streptococci.

  (2) **Anti-inflammatory agents**

  (a) **Aspirin** is indicated for arthritis without carditis and possibly for children with mild cardiac involvement. The dosage of acetylsalicylic acid is 100 mg/kg/day in four to six divided doses for 3 to 4 weeks. The optimal serum level is about 20 to 25 mg/day. Although salicylates undoubtedly give symptomatic relief, there is no proof that they alter the course of the myocardial damage.

  (b) **Corticosteroids** have been controversial in the therapy of ARF since their introduction.

  (i) Corticosteroids are almost mandatory in patients with severe carditis and congestive heart failure (CHF). Prednisone, 2 mg/kg/day for 4 to 6 weeks, is given, with tapering over the next 2 weeks. Corticosteroids reduce inflammation promptly, but there is no conclusive evidence that they prevent residual valvular damage.

  (ii) In patients with carditis without cardiomegaly or CHF, the use of corticosteroids instead of salicylates remains controversial and more a matter of personal preference.

  (3) **Anticongestive measures,** including digitalis, should be used in patients with ARF in the same fashion as in other patients with CHF, despite possible increased sensitivity of the inflamed myocardium.

  (4) **Bed rest** is accepted during the acute phase when CHF is present. In the absence of objective data of CHF, we think it is prudent to keep children on limited activity until the ESR returns to normal.

  (5) Children with **chorea** should be moved to a quiet environment and should be protected against self-inflicted injury due to uncontrollable movements. Drug treatment with phenobarbital, chlorpromazine, diazepam, and haloperidol has been tried, with varying success.

 e. **Prevention of recurrences of ARF**

  (1) All children with documented ARF with or without carditis—and all those with rheumatic heart disease—should receive prophylaxis against recurrences of ARF.

  (2) Any of the following approaches is acceptable, provided compliance is assured. If severe residual heart disease is present or the patient is unreliable, the first alternative is preferable.

(a) Benzathine penicillin, 1.2 million units every 3 to 4 weeks (some data indicate that every 3 weeks is more effective).

(b) Penicillin G or V, 200,000–250,000 U PO qd-bid

(c) Sulfadiazine, 0.5 mg per day for those weighing under 30 kg; 1 gm per day for those weighing over 30 kg

(d) Erythromycin, 250 mg PO bid, in patients sensitive to both sulfonamides and penicillin

2. **Infective endocarditis.** In children, congenital heart disease is present in most cases of bacterial endocarditis. Predisposing lesions include tetralogy of Fallot, ventricular septal defect, patent ductus arteriosus, aortic stenosis, transposition of the great vessels, and coarctation. Endocarditis in children with rheumatic heart disease (RHD) is uncommon in the United States, but may be seen in areas where RHD is prevalent. Endocarditis may also be seen in the setting of damage to the tricuspid valve caused by intravascular catheters. A prior event leading to bacteremia (e.g., dental manipulation or infection) or prior cardiac surgery is frequently, although not always, implicated as a precipitating factor.

   a. Etiology

   (1) Alpha-hemolytic streptococcus is the most common etiology.

   (2) *Staphylococcus aureus* is the second most common etiology and can occur in children without underlying structural heart disease. It is the most common etiology in intravenous drug users.

   (3) *Enterococcus, S. pneumoniae,* group A streptococci, *Haemophilus* species, other fastidious organisms, anaerobes, gram-negative bacilli, and fungi are rare causes.

   (4) In the first several months after cardiac surgery, *S. aureus, Staphylococcus epidermidis, Enterococcus,* and gram-negative bacteria are the most common causes.

   (5) *Staphylococcus epidermidis* is a common etiology in children with prosthetic valves.

   b. Evaluation

   (1) The **history** should focus on fever (particularly its duration, height, and time of onset), malaise, and symptoms of embolism to the eyes, skin, brain, or kidneys.

   (2) **Physical examination** should emphasize auscultation for new or changing murmurs; cutaneous manifestations, such as petechiae, splinter hemorrhages, Osler's nodes, and Janeway lesions; splenomegaly; and, if indicated, needle marks from illicit drug use.

   (3) **Blood cultures.** Properly obtained and incubated blood cultures are critical for diagnosis and treatment since therapy will be guided by the specific organism isolated and by susceptibility testing.

   (a) In a child who is not critically ill, three to six separate blood cultures should be obtained over a 48-hour period from different sites before therapy is started.

   (b) In the seriously ill child who requires immediate therapy, three sets of blood cultures should be obtained.

   (c) Because bacteremia is continuous in endocarditis, there is no advantage to culturing only with temperature spikes or to drawing blood for culture from arteries rather than veins.

   (d) Blood cultures should be incubated for 4 weeks to enable detection of fastidious organisms.

   (e) Isolates should be saved for bactericidal testing.

   (4) **Laboratory studies** should include a CBC, ESR, and urinalysis.

   (5) A **chest x-ray** should be performed to look for cardiac enlargement.

   (6) A baseline **electrocardiogram** should be obtained.

   (7) **Echocardiographic evaluation** is helpful if a vegetation is visualized, but a negative study does not rule out the diagnosis.

   c. The **diagnosis** is established by one or more positive blood cultures in association with a compatible clinical picture. The bacteremia is typically low grade and continuous; consequently, the majority (85–90%) of blood cultures are positive. The development of a new regurgitant murmur and extracardiac findings indicating systemic emboli or vasculitis are highly suggestive of the diagnosis. Splenomegaly is common. While non-specific, characteristic laboratory abnormalities, such as anemia, leukocytosis with a shift to the left, elevated ESR, microscopic hematuria, and hyperglobulinemia, support the diagnosis. When the blood cultures are negative, a presumptive diagnosis is based on the typical clinical syndrome. The previous distinction between acute and subacute endocarditis has been discarded; classification based on the specific organism causing the infection is preferred.

d. Therapy

(1) Antibiotics

(a) If the diagnosis is clinically evident, initiation of antibiotics should begin while the results of the blood cultures are still pending.

(b) Empiric therapy

(i) If viridans streptococci or enterococci are suspected, therapy with penicillin or ampicillin plus gentamicin should be initiated.

(ii) If *S. aureus* is suspected, a penicillinase-resistant penicillin or vancomycin plus gentamicin should be initiated immediately.

(iii) In postoperative cases or in children with prosthetic valves, vancomycin and gentamicin should be initiated.

(c) For viridans streptococci and *Streptococcus bovis* that is susceptible to penicillin (minimum inhibitory concentration [MIC] ≤ 0.1 µg/ml):

(i) Aqueous crystalline penicillin G, 150,000–200,000 units/kg/day (maximum 20 million units/day) IV continuously or divided q4h for 4 weeks.

(ii) Aqueous crystalline penicillin G (dose as above) for 2 to 4 weeks, plus gentamicin, 2.0 to 2.5 mg/kg (maximum 80 mg) IV or IM q8h, or streptomycin, 15 mg/kg (maximum 500 mg) IM q12h for the first 2 weeks of therapy.

(iii) Cephalothin, 100 to 150 mg/kg/day (maximum 12 g/day) IV divided q4–6h, or cefazolin, 80 to 100 mg/kg/day (maximum 3 g/day) IV divided q8h, can be used in patients with manifestations of penicillin allergy other than immediate hypersensitivity.

(iv) Vancomycin, 40 mg/kg/day (maximum 2 g/day unless serum levels indicate higher dosing) IV divided q6–12h for 4 weeks, can be used in patients with a history of immediate hypersensitivity to beta-lactam antimicrobials.

(d) For staphylococci that are susceptible to methicillin and in the absence of prosthetic material:

(i) Nafcillin or oxacillin, 150 to 200 mg/kg/day (maximum 12 million units/day) IV continuously or divided q4–6h for 4 to 6 weeks with the optional addition of gentamicin (as dosed above) for the first 3 to 5 days of therapy.

(ii) Cefalothin or cefazolin (as dosed above) for 4 to 6 weeks with the optional addition of gentamicin (as dosed above) for the first 3 to 5 days of therapy can be used in patients with manifestations of penicillin allergy other than immediate hypersensitivity.

(iii) Vancomycin (as dosed above) for 4 to 6 weeks can be used in patients with a history of immediate hypersensitivity to beta-lactam antimicrobials.

(e) **Serum bactericidal tests** are helpful in guiding therapy in difficult cases. A serum bactericidal level of 1 : 8 or greater at the time of peak antibiotic concentration is desirable. We do not routinely use bactericidal testing in uncomplicated cases of endocarditis caused by viridans streptococci that are fully sensitive to penicillin.

(2) **Monitoring**

(a) **Blood cultures** during antibiotic treatment should be obtained to document clearing of the bacteremia, particularly for difficult-to-treat organisms. Repeat blood cultures after therapy is complete are a traditional part of follow-up.

(b) **Daily physical examinations** for new or changing murmurs and evidence of embolization are necessary in the acute period. Once a clinical response has been achieved, these examinations can be spaced out.

(c) **Fever** may persist for 5 to 7 days despite adequate antibiotic therapy.

(d) **ESR** should be checked at weekly intervals.

(3) **Surgical replacement** of the infected valve, when indicated, may be lifesaving. The indications for surgery in endocarditis include congestive heart failure refractory to medical therapy, more than one major embolic episode, worsening valve function, ineffective therapy (as in fungal endocarditis), mycotic aneurysm, and most cases of prosthetic valve endocarditis.

e. **Prevention of endocarditis.** Prophylactic antibiotic regimens are outlined in Table 5–4. The choice of regimen should be individualized according to both the risk of the underlying heart disease and the risk of the procedure. The regimens that require parenteral administration of potentially toxic antibiotics should be reserved for high-risk situations.

(1) Patients with prosthetic heart valves or grafts are at highest risk; patients with rheumatic heart disease are also at high risk. Patients with congenital heart diseases, such as ventricular septal defect, atrial septal defect, patent ductus arteriosus, and the "click-murmur" syndrome, are at lower risk.

(2) High-risk procedures are dental manipulations, especially surgery and tooth extractions in patients with poor oral hygiene, and manipulations of the infected genitourinary tract, especially when enterococci are present. Procedures such as bronchoscopy, endoscopy, proctosigmoidoscopy, barium enemas, and liver biopsies may be associated with bacteremia but have a lower risk.

3. **Myocarditis** (see Chap. 10, p. 316).

4. **Pericarditis** (see Chap. 10, p. 317).

F. **Gastrointestinal and abdominal infections**

1. **Bacterial and protozoal causes of diarrhea**

a. **Etiology.** This section discusses diarrhea caused by bacteria and protozoa that are common in the US. Amebiasis is discussed in 2 below.

(1) **Bacterial agents** common in the US are *Salmonella enteritidis*, *Shigella sonnei*, and, in some areas, *Campylobacter fetus* subspecies *jejuni*. *Escherichia coli* 0157:H7, the prototype of enterohemorrhagic *E. coli* (EHEC), has been associated with an increasing number of outbreaks and sporadic cases throughout the US. Other agents include *Yersinia enterocolitica*, *Aeromonas hydrophila*, and *Vibrio parahaemolyticus* (which causes shellfish poisoning). Diarrhea caused by enterotoxigenic *E. coli* (ETEC) and enteropathogenic *E. coli* (EPEC) is uncommon in the US.

(2) **Protozoal agents** common in the US are *Giardia lamblia* and *Cryptosporidium parvum*. Infection with these organisms is common in young children and in older children and in adults who care for young

Table 5-4. Prevention of bacterial endocarditis for children and adolescents

Conditions	Procedure	Regimen
Prosthetic heart valves, including bioprosthetic and hemograph valves Previous bacterial endocarditis Most congenital cardiac malformations (but not uncomplicated secundum atrial septal defect) Rheumatic and other acquired valvular dysfunction, even after surgery Hypertrophic cardiomyopathy Mitral valve prolapse with valvular regurgitation	Dental, oral, and upper respiratory procedures[a]	Standard regimen[b]: Amoxicillin, 50 mg/kg, 3.0 g maximum, PO 1 hr before the procedure; then half the dose PO 6 hr after the initial dose *For amoxicillin–penicillin–allergic patients:* Erythromycin ethylsuccinate 20 mg/kg, 800 mg maximum, or erythromycin stearate, 20 mg/kg, 1.0 g maximum, PO 2 hr before the procedure; then half the dose PO 6 hr after the initial dose Clindamycin, 10 mg/kg, 300 mg maximum, PO 1 hr before the procedure; then half the dose PO 6 hr after the initial dose Alternative regimen for patients unable to take oral medications[b]: Ampicillin, 50 mg/kg, 2.0 g maximum, IV or IM 30 min before the procedure; then half the dose IV or IM or 25 mg/kg, 1.5 g maximum, PO 6 hr after the initial dose *For amoxicillin–penicillin–allergic patients:* Clindamycin, 10 mg/kg, 300 mg maximum, IV 30 min before the procedure; then half the dose IV or 5 mg/kg, 150 mg maximum, PO 6 hr after the initial dose Alternative regimen for patients considered at high risk[b,c]: Ampicillin, 50 mg/kg, 2.0 g maximum, IV or IM plus gentamicin, 2.0 mg/kg in children and 1.5 mg/kg in older children and adolescents, 80 mg maximum, IV or IM 30 min before the procedure; then amoxicillin, 25 mg/kg, 1.5 g maximum, PO 6 hr after the initial dose or repeat the parenteral regimen 8 hr after the initial dose *For amoxicillin–penicillin–allergic patients:* Vancomycin 20 mg/kg, 1.0 g maximum, IV over 1 hr starting 1 hr before the procedure; no repeat dose is necessary

| Same as above | Gastrointestinal and genitourinary procedures[d] | Standard regimen[b]:
Ampicillin, 50 mg/kg, 2.0 g maximum, IV or IM plus gentamicin, 2.0 mg/kg in children and 1.5 mg/kg in older children and adolescents, 80 mg maximum, IV or IM 30 min before the procedure; then amoxicillin, 25 mg/kg, 1.5 g maximum, PO 6 hr after the initial dose or repeat the parenteral regimen 8 hr after the initial dose

For amoxicillin-penicillin–allergic patients:
Vancomycin, 20 mg/kg, 1.0 g maximum, IV over 1 hr, plus gentamicin, 2.0 mg/kg in children and 1.5 mg/kg in older children and adolescents, 80 mg maximum, IV or IM 1 hr before the procedure; this regimen can be repeated 8 hr after the initial dose

Alternative regimen for patients considered at low risk[b,c]:
Amoxicillin, 50 mg/kg, 3.0 g maximum, PO 1 hr before the procedure; then half the dose PO 6 hr after the initial dose |

[a]Includes dental procedures known to induce gingival or mucosal bleeding, including professional cleaning; tonsillectomy or adenoidectomy, or both; surgical procedures involving the respiratory mucosa; bronchoscopy with rigid bronchoscope; and incision and drainage of infected tissue. See the reference below for procedures for which prophylaxis is not recommended.

[b]If an infection is present, therapy should be directed against the most likely pathogen.

[c]Individuals with prosthetic heart valves, a previous history of endocarditis, or surgically constructed systemic pulmonary shunts or conduits are at high risk for development of endocarditis. Because of the logistical and financial barriers of parenteral administration and because oral regimens are effective in these patients, the standard (oral) regimens are recommended. However, some physicians may wish to administer parenteral agents.

[d]Includes surgical procedures involving the intestinal tract, sclerotherapy for esophageal varices, esophageal dilatation, gallbladder surgery, cystoscopy, urethral dilatation, urethral catheterization or urinary tract surgery if urinary tract infection is present, prostatic surgery, incision and drainage of infected tissue, vaginal hysterectomy, and vaginal delivery in the presence of infection. See the reference below for procedures for which prophylaxis is not recommended.

Source: Adapted from AS Dajani, AL Bisno, KJ Chung, et al. Prevention of bacterial endocarditis. Recommendations of the American Heart Association. *JAMA* 265:1686–1688, 1990.

children. Waterborne outbreaks have been described. *Entamoeba histolytica* is discussed in a separate section (see p. 120).

(3) Antibiotic-associated colitis (pseudomembranous colitis) is caused by *C. difficile* toxin, produced as the organism overgrows the residual gut flora of antibiotic-treated patients.

(4) Traveler's diarrhea, a self-limited disease that lasts for several days, is usually caused by ETEC, although *Shigella* and *Salmonella*, other bacteria, viruses, and *G. lamblia* have been implicated. *Vibrio cholerae* infection is very uncommon in travelers, but should be considered in children with watery diarrhea shortly after they return from endemic areas.

(5) Food poisoning can be caused by several bacteria (usually toxin producing), including staphylococci, *Clostridium perfringens*, *Clostridium botulinum* (botulism), *V. parahaemolyticus*, and *Bacillus cereus*. Diarrhea is an associated symptom with food poisoning, but other symptoms, such as vomiting and hypotonia (botulism), are usually more prominent.

b. Evaluation

(1) The **history** should include an assessment of potential epidemiologic exposures; the character, frequency, and duration of the abnormal stools; associated symptoms such as abdominal pain and tenesmus; and the patient's state of hydration.

(2) Examination should include assessment of hydration status, toxicity, and abdominal tenderness.

(3) A **stool guaiac test** should be performed to detect occult blood.

(4) Microscopic examination for fecal leukocytes should be performed.

(5) Stool cultures are indicated in the presence of significant numbers of fecal leukocytes, bloody stools, toxicity, severe diarrhea, chronic disease or impaired host defenses, diarrhea in neonates and young infants (<3 months of age), and epidemic diarrhea. Stool cultures handled routinely will identify *Salmonella* and *Shigella*. If *Campylobacter*, *Yersinia*, or *Vibrio* is suspected, the laboratory should be alerted.

(6) Stool examination for ova and parasites should be performed if *Giardia* or *Cryptosporidium* is suspected. An enzyme-linked immunosorbent assay (ELISA) for *Giardia* antigen performed on stool is more sensitive than traditional stool examination.

(7) An **assay for *C. difficile toxin*** should be performed in patients with significant diarrhea during or after antimicrobial treatment.

(8) Special isolation and latex agglutination tests can be performed to identify *E. coli* **0157:H7;** however, the microbiology laboratory must be alerted to perform these tests.

(9) Blood cultures should be obtained in hospitalized patients with fever and diarrhea.

(10) Toxin-producing *E. coli* (ETEC) is reliably identified only by special assay for enterotoxin.

c. Diagnosis

(1) The presence of fever, abdominal pain, bloody stool, and fecal leukocytes strongly suggests an **inflammatory diarrhea.** Lack of fever or systemic toxicity and watery stools with no blood or fecal leukocytes suggest a **secretory diarrhea.**

(2) Traveler's diarrhea is a nonspecific definitional diagnosis and generally refers only to a mild to moderate secretory diarrhea in a traveling child. Children with fever, abdominal tenderness, or systemic illness should be investigated thoroughly to determine the specific cause.

(3) Antibiotic-associated diarrhea is another definitional diagnosis. If diarrhea is significant, tests should be done to determine whether *C. difficile* toxin is responsible.

(4) In **food poisoning** the contaminating organism can be inferred from the incubation period (time from ingestion to onset of symptoms)— for *S. aureus*, 3 to 6 hours, but as early as 30 minutes; for *C. perfringens*, 1 to 25 hours, usually 8 to 12 hours; and for *Salmonella*, 12 to 18 hours, up to 72 hours—or from careful epidemiologic history and the physical signs as with botulism.

d. Therapy. Rehydration and correction of electrolyte disturbances represent the first priority of management (see Chap. 4).

e. Antimicrobial therapy

(1) *Salmonella enteritidis.* Because antibiotics may prolong the carrier state, most patients with *Salmonella* in the stool are not treated. **Indications for treatment** are infection in infants less than 3 months of age, immunodeficiency, hemoglobinopathy, chronic inflammatory bowel disease, severe toxicity, and enteritis with bacteremia if fever and toxicity persist by the time the positive blood culture is obtained. Antibiotic choice should be directed by local resistance patterns and susceptibility testing on the specific isolate. Options include

  (a) Oral therapy

    (i) Amoxicillin can be used if the isolate is susceptible.

    (ii) TMP/SMZ is our choice for empiric therapy.

    (iii) Cefixime is an alternative.

    (iv) Ciprofloxacin can be used for multiply resistant organisms.

  (b) Parenteral therapy

    (i) Ampicillin can be used if the isolate is susceptible.

    (ii) Cefotaxime or ceftriaxone is our first choice for empiric therapy.

    (iii) Chloramphenicol is an alternative.

    (iv) Ciprofloxacin can be used for multiply resistant organisms.

(2) *Shigella sonnei*

  (a) Amoxicillin can be used if the isolate is susceptible, but this is uncommon.

  (b) TMP/SMZ is our choice for empiric therapy.

  (c) Cefixime is an alternative.

  (d) Ciprofloxacin can be used for multiply resistant organisms

  (e) Antidiarrheal drugs should be avoided.

(3) *Campylobacter* can be treated with erythromycin (40 mg/kg/day PO q6h for 5–7 days) if symptoms have not resolved by the time the culture result is available.

(4) *Yersinia* can be treated with TMP/SMZ (10 mg TMP/kg/day PO q6h for 5–7 days) if symptoms have not resolved by the time the culture result is available.

(5) Treatment of diarrhea caused by *E. coli* 0157:H7 is controversial. Additional data are needed before recommendations can be given.

(6) *Giardia.* Options are

  (a) No treatment; many cases will resolve spontaneously.

  (b) Furazolidone (5 mg/kg/day in divided doses qid for 7–10 days) is available in suspension.

  (c) Metronidazole (15 mg/kg/day in divided doses tid for 5–10 days, maximum 750 mg/day) is effective.

  (d) Quinacrine (6–9 mg/kg/day in divided doses tid for 5–7 days, maximum 300 mg/day) is the most effective but tastes bitter and has more side effects.

  (e) Treatment failures can be treated again with the same medication.

(7) *Cryptosporidium.* Most cases recover spontaneously. No therapy has been conclusively established as effective.

(8) Traveler's diarrhea

  (a) Most cases resolve spontaneously. TMP/SMZ can be used empirically and usually decreases the duration of symptoms.

    (b) *Vibrio cholerae* infection should be treated to reduce the duration of symptoms and infectivity. Options are

      (i) Tetracycline (50 mg/kg/day, maximum 2 g/day, divided qid for 3 days).

      (ii) Doxycycline (6 mg/kg, maximum 300 mg, for one dose).

      (iii) TMP/SMZ (10 mg TMP/kg/day divided bid for 3 days).

      (iv) Furazolidone (5–8 mg/kg/day divided tid for 3 days).

    (c) Preventing infection by drinking only boiled or carbonated water or other processed beverages and avoiding unpeeled fruits, salads and ice is the best approach.

    (d) We do not advocate prevention using pharmacologic agents.

  (9) Antibiotic-associated colitis (pseudomembranous colitis)

    (a) Withdrawal of the implicated antibiotic is sufficient in most mild cases.

    (b) When the presence of *C. difficile* toxin in the stool has been confirmed, there are two options:

      (i) Oral metronidazole (35 mg/kg/day in four divided doses) is cheap and is usually effective.

      (ii) Oral vancomycin (40 mg/kg/day in 4 divided doses) is expensive and is believed by some experts to be more effective. We use this agent in severe or relapsed cases.

    (c) Therapy should be continued for 7 to 10 days

    (d) Follow-up stool tests for the toxin are necessary only if symptoms persist.

    (e) Relapses are common and require retreatment.

  (10) Food poisoning is treated symptomatically with fluid replacement and antiemetics.

2. Amebiasis

  a. Etiology. Amebiasis is worldwide in distribution, and the human is the only known host. Sporadic localized epidemics occur in the United States, and the disease is endemic in many institutionalized populations.

  b. Evaluation and diagnosis

    (1) Intestinal amebiasis

      (a) Intestinal amebiasis varies in presentation from the asymptomatic carrier state (by far the most common) to fulminant colonic disease.

        (i) Mild colonic infection is characterized by alternating diarrhea and constipation.

        (ii) Amebic dysentery presents most frequently as subacute illness. Mild tenderness, bloody diarrhea, low-grade fever, weakness, and malaise are characteristic. The tempo of the illness may clinically distinguish it from more acute, bacillary dysentery. Abdominal tenderness is common, particularly over the sigmoid and cecal areas; appendicitis is sometimes erroneously diagnosed.

      (b) Confirmation in acute cases is obtained by **demonstrating motile amebic trophozoites in fresh stool, or cysts in the carrier state.** Proctoscopy may be useful if multiple stool samples are negative.

      (c) Erythrocytes are plentiful and leukocytes are minimal in the stool, which is helpful in distinguishing between amebic and bacillary dysentery.

      (d) Eosinophilia is **not** found.

    (2) Extraintestinal amebiasis most commonly affects the liver.

      (a) Disease may occur without the signs or symptoms of intestinal infection. Fever, chills, or enlarged tender liver, elevated right diaphragm, minimal liver function abnormalities, and the finding of a filling defect on liver scan are highly suggestive. Of all amebic abscesses, 95% are single and situated in the upper part of the right lobe of the liver.

- **(b) Serologic tests** for invasive amebiasis (indirect hemagglutination, counter immunoelectrophoresis, complement fixation) are extremely accurate.
- **(c) Percutaneous liver aspiration** is recommended in large abscesses only. Aspirated material may show amebas. However, their absence does not rule out hepatic infection because organisms tend to be located at the margins of the abscess.
- **(d)** A therapeutic trial is an accepted diagnostic measure **in a severely ill patient.**

- **c. Therapy.** All stages of amebiasis are treated.
  - **(1) Asymptomatic carrier state**
    - **(a)** Diiodohydroxyquin, 30 to 40 mg/kg/day in divided doses tid for 20 days (maximum 2 g/day), or
    - **(b)** Diloxanide furoate, 20 mg/kg/day in divided doses tid for 10 days (maximum 1.5 g/day).
  - **(2) Intestinal infection**
    - **(a)** Metronidazole, 35 to 50 mg/kg/day in divided doses tid for 10 days (maximum 2.25 g/day).
    - **(b)** As a second choice, paromomycin, 25 to 30 mg/kg/day in divided doses tid for 5 to 10 days, can be used alone.
    - **(c)** In severe cases, use metronidazole, 35 to 50 mg/kg/day in divided doses tid for 10 days (maximum 2.25 g/day), **and** diiodohydroxyquin as above. For alternative therapy, use dehydroemetine hydrochloride, 1.0 to 1.5 mg/kg/day intramuscularly for 5 days (maximum 90 mg/day), **and** diiodohydroxyquin as above.
  - **(3) Hepatic infection**
    - **(a)** Metronidazole, as in sec. **(2)**, and
    - **(b)** Diiodohydroxyquin, as in sec. **(1)**, or
    - **(c)** Dehydroemetine, as in sec. **(2)**, followed by
    - **(d)** Chloroquine phosphate, 10 mg base/kg/day for 21 days (maximum 300 mg base/day), **and**
    - **(e)** Diiodohydroxyquin, as in sec. **(1)**.
  - **(4)** In addition to specific amebicidal therapy, **supportive care** is important in invasive amebiasis.
  - **(5) Follow-up stool examinations** should be done at 1- and 2-month intervals to ensure that a cure has been achieved.

3. **Hepatitis** can be caused by a wide range of viruses, most commonly hepatitis A, hepatitis B, or hepatitis C (which accounts for most of what was formerly called non-A, non-B hepatitis). Hepatitis delta virus causes hepatitis only in conjunction with hepatitis B virus infection and is not common in the US. Hepatitis E virus is transmitted enterically and has not been reported in the US although cases have occurred in travelers. Other viruses that can cause hepatitis include Epstein-Barr virus, cytomegalovirus, and coxsackieviruses A and B. There is no specific therapy for hepatitis A, B, C, delta, or E. See Table 5–3 for postexposure prophylaxis.

G. Genitourinary infections

1. **Urinary tract infections**
   - **a. Etiology**
     - **(1)** First infections are most commonly caused by *E. coli.*
     - **(2)** Other pathogens include *Proteus, Klebsiella, Pseudomonas, Streptococcus faecalis, S. saprophyticus,* and *S. aureus.*
     - **(3)** *Candida* species cause infections in hospitalized patients.
   - **b. Evaluation**
     - **(1)** History includes dysuria, frequency, urgency, and flank pain. Previously toilet-trained small children may be enuretics. Fever may suggest pyelonephritis.

(2) Physical examination should include blood pressure measurement, a search for congenital malformations, and a careful examination of the abdomen, genitalia, and perineum.

(3) Laboratory studies

    (a) Urine microscopy can provide an accurate provisional diagnosis of UTI if used to quantitate the concentration of bacteria in a fresh, clean sample: One or more bacteria per oil field in gram-stained, uncentrifuged urine are equivalent to 10^5 colonies/ml. The presence of numerous bacteria per high-power field in the centrifuged urine sediment does not necessarily indicate infection.

    (b) Urinalysis is a critical component of the evaluation.

        (i) Pyuria is not specific for bacterial infection but is usually present in UTI.

        (ii) Microscopic hematuria is common.

        (iii) Proteinuria and gross hematuria are *uncommon* with UTI.

        (iv) White blood cell casts may be present in pyelonephritis.

    (c) Urine culture provides proof of infection, **provided the specimen is collected properly and interpreted appropriately.** A negative culture is helpful in ruling out infection.

        (i) Infected urine will generally contain more than 10^5 colonies/ml (except in some neonates, in whom $>10^4$ colonies may indicate infection).

        (ii) Repetition of cultures increases diagnostic precision in all age groups. A single, midstream, clean-catch specimen will accurately predict the presence of UTI 80% of the time; two consecutive positive cultures increase the accuracy to 95%.

        (iii) Diagnostic precision is greatest with urine obtained by **suprapubic bladder aspiration**, for which any growth of bacteria should be considered significant, or **sterile catheterization**, for which more than 10^4 colonies/ml are significant. In skilled hands, both procedures are safe. While cultures of urine specimens obtained by collection of urine in an externally placed bag may be helpful if they are negative, they are contaminated so often that they are nearly useless in directing management. **Cultures obtained in this manner should not be used for any infant who will be started on antibiotic therapy before culture results are available.**

        (iv) Contaminated cultures usually contain several species in concentrations less than 10^5 colonies/ml, but they may contain more than 10^5 colonies/ml of a single species.

        (v) Urine specimens should be processed promptly or refrigerated at $4°C$ and cultured right away to avoid growth of contaminants.

    (d) A **blood culture** should be obtained in patients with pyelonephritis and in neonates or young infants with UTI.

    (e) Serum electrolytes, BUN, and creatinine should be checked in all patients experiencing their first UTI.

    (f) A **renal ultrasound** is indicated when pyelonephritis is suspected.

c. The **diagnosis** is based on the results of the urine culture, urinalysis, and clinical findings. **Asymptomatic bacteriuria** is most common in preschool and school-aged girls. **Cystitis** is associated with suprapubic pain, dysuria, frequency, urgency, and enuresis. **Pyelonephritis** is suggested by high fever, toxicity, flank pain, and costovertebral angle tenderness and is commonly associated with ureteral reflux. However, clear differentiation between cystitis and pyelonephritis may be difficult, especially in young children. The presence of white cell casts in the urine sediment is diagnostic.

d. Therapy

  (1) Oral therapy

   (a) Uncomplicated UTIs and mild cases of pyelonephritis in older children often respond to oral therapy.

   (b) An oral agent should be chosen on the basis of susceptibility results.

   (c) Commonly used agents include sulfisoxazole (120–150 mg/kg/day PO qid), amoxicillin (25 mg/kg/day PO tid), TMP/SMZ (8 mg/kg/day TMP PO bid), cefixime (8 mg/kg/day PO qd), and nitrofurantoin (5 mg/kg/day PO qid).

   (d) Candidal UTIs usually respond to fluconazole (2–6 mg/kg/day PO qd).

   (e) Duration of therapy is 10 days.

  (2) Parenteral therapy

   (a) Infants less than 6 months old, children with moderate or severe pyelonephritis, children with a prior history of pyelonephritis, and children with compromised renal function should be treated initially with parenteral antimicrobial agents.

   (b) Ampicillin (100–200 mg/kg/day q6h IV) is effective against many urinary tract pathogens, but is generally combined with sulbactam or an aminoglycoside for initial therapy of suspected pyelonephritis. Alternatively, aztreonam, a second- or third-generation cephalosporin, or parenteral TMP/SMZ can be used.

   (c) Clinical improvement should be evident within 48 to 72 hours. Failure to respond should increase suspicion of an underlying anatomic abnormality or abscess.

   (d) Once the patient is afebrile, therapy can be switched to oral antibiotics.

   (e) Duration of therapy is usually 10 to 14 days, but severe cases of pyelonephritis may require longer (3 weeks) therapy.

  (3) Adequate **hydration** of the patient is important.

  (4) Continuous bladder drainage by an indwelling catheter should be done only when absolutely necessary and discontinued at the earliest possible time; a closed drainage system is mandatory.

e. Follow-up of a UTI should be carefully organized because infection tends to recur, often in asymptomatic form. Recurrence is most likely during the first 6 to 12 months after an infection.

  (1) After therapy is discontinued, a **follow-up urine culture** is indicated 1 week later to document resolution. Additional cultures are not necessary in uncomplicated cystitis without evidence of reflux. If reflux is present, follow-up cultures should be performed. We suggest that they be performed every month during the subsequent 3 months, every 3 months during the next 6 months, and then twice a year.

  (2) A **voiding cystourethrogram (VCUG)** should be obtained in boys of all ages and in girls less than 5 years of age to investigate the possibility of vesicoureteral reflux. The test should be performed when acute symptoms have resolved but does not need to be delayed for a long time. We usually perform the test 5 to 14 days after presentation.

  (3) A **renal ultrasound** is indicated in children with vesicoureteral reflux, children with documented or suspected urologic malformations, or when pyelonephritis is present.

  (4) Among patients with **significant vesicoureteral reflux,** recurrent infection is prevented by prophylactic antibiotic therapy, which is continued until reflux resolves or is repaired. TMP/SMZ (4 mg TMP/kg/day PO in one dose) or nitrofurantoin (2 mg/kg/day in one dose) can be used.

(5) Some normal girls experience **multiple recurrences** of UTI. They should be carefully assessed for correctable contributing factors. When infections are frequent, socially distressing, or associated with renal scarring, prophylactic antibiotic therapy is often prescribed for 6 to 12 months. TMP/SMZ (2 mg TMP/kg/day PO in one dose) or nitrofurantoin (2 mg/kg/day in one dose) can be used.

2. Vulvovaginitis in prepubertal girls (see Chap. 14, p. 418).

3. Vaginal infections (non-sexually transmitted) in postpubertal girls (see Chap. 14, p. 421).

4. Sexually transmitted diseases (STDs). (see also Chap. 14). In evaluating a child or adolescent with a possible STD, a specific diagnosis should be established whenever possible because of the requirements for reporting these infections and to facilitate partner notification and treatment. Remember that more than one infection may be present in a single individual. The ideal is to diagnose and treat each infection, but in some cases empiric treatment for common coexisting infections (i.e., gonorrhea and chlamydial infection) is the most practical approach. Because coexisting syphilis and HIV infection may be asymptomatic, testing for these infections should be offered to all patients with an STD, regardless of the circumstances or source of the infection. Abstinence from sexual activity during treatment until the period of contagiousness is past must be emphasized. Counseling regarding the risks of STDs and effective methods for prevention should be provided. **The diagnosis of an STD in a prepubertal child should prompt an investigation into the probability of child abuse.**

a. Genital herpes

(1) Etiology. Usually involves HSV type 2; HSV type 1 occurs less frequently.

(2) Evaluation

(a) Examination for painful vesicular or ulcerative lesions on the genitals.

(b) Tzanck preparation of vesicle base scrapings (not vesicular fluid) to look for multinucleated giant cells.

(c) Immunofluorescent antibody (IFA) stain of vesicle base scrapings.

(d) Viral culture of a vesicle swab.

(3) The **diagnosis** can often be made clinically, but a Tzanck preparation, an IFA stain, or viral culture is easy to perform and establish a definitive diagnosis.

(4) Therapy

(a) First clinical episode. Oral acyclovir shortens both duration of symptoms and shedding of virus in primary genital herpes infections, but does not affect the risk or severity of subsequent recurrent genital lesions.

(i) Genital lesions are treated with acyclovir, 200 mg PO five times a day for 7 to 10 days or until clinical resolution.

(ii) Proctitis is treated with acyclovir, 400 mg PO five times a day for 7 to 10 days or until clinical resolution.

(iii) Topical therapy is less effective.

(b) Recurrent genital lesions

(i) Daily suppressive therapy can reduce the frequency of recurrences by 75% or more in persons with frequent recurrences (6 or more times per year). However, lesions may develop at the pretherapy recurrence rate after suppression is discontinued. Suppressive therapy does not eliminate symptomatic or asymptomatic shedding or the potential for transmission. The safety and efficacy of daily suppressive therapy for as long as 5 years has been documented and the development of viral resistance to acyclovir has not been a significant problem. After a year suppression should be stopped to allow assessment of the frequency of recurrences. The recommended dose for an adult is 400 mg acyclovir PO bid. An alternative regimen is 200 mg PO three to five times a day with use of the minimum dose that provides symptomatic relief.

(ii) Initiation of acyclovir at the first sign of recurrence may be helpful for some persons, but is usually of limited benefit and is not generally recommended.

b. Chancroid

(1) Etiology. *Haemophilus ducreyi* is the causative agent.

(2) Evaluation

(a) Examination for painful vesicular or ulcerative lesions on the genitals and inguinal adenopathy.

(b) Culture of the ulcer requires special media that are not generally available.

(3) The **diagnosis** can be made definitively if a painful ulcer and suppurative inguinal adenopathy are present or by culture. If significant adenopathy is not a prominent finding, a probable diagnosis can be made if herpes simplex and syphilis are excluded as etiologies.

(4) Therapy. Treatment should result in prompt improvement of symptoms and resolution of the ulcer. Adenopathy may respond more slowly. Recommended treatment regimens include

(a) Azithromycin, 1 g PO as a single dose.

(b) Ceftriaxone, 250 mg IM as a single dose.

(c) Erythromycin base, 500 mg PO qid for 7 days.

c. Syphilis. This section discusses *acquired* syphilis. Congenital syphilis is discussed in Chapter 6, p. 205.

(1) Etiology. The infecting organism is *Treponema pallidum.*

(2) Evaluation

(a) Clinical findings

(i) In **primary infection**, an ulcer or chancre is seen at the site of infection.

(ii) Latent infection is the asymptomatic period after the spontaneous resolution of primary infection.

(iii) In **secondary infection**, fever, a polymorphic rash classically involving the palms and soles, mucocutaneous lesions, lymphadenopathy, splenomegaly, and arthritis are common.

(iv) In **tertiary infection**, cardiac, neurologic, ophthalmologic, auditory, or gummatous lesions of the bone, skin, or other organs are seen.

(b) Dark-field examination or direct immunofluorescent antibody stains of exudate from lesions or tissue are the most specific tests if they are available. This material is infectious and should be handled with care.

(c) Serologic tests

(i) Nontreponemal tests are used as screening tests for infection since they are inexpensive, easily performed, and sensitive. They may be falsely negative in early primary, latent, or late congenital syphilis and falsely positive in other infectious and inflammatory processes. They also correlate with disease activity and so are useful in monitoring response to therapy. Commonly used tests include RPR, automated reagin test (ART); and VDRL slide test.

(ii) Treponemal tests provide definitive evidence of infection when screening tests are positive. After infection, these tests remain positive for life and so are not helpful in assessing reinfection or monitoring the response to therapy. They may be falsely positive in persons with other spirochetal diseases, including Lyme disease, leptospirosis, rat-bite fever, yaws, and pinta. Two commonly used tests include the fluorescent treponemal antibody absorption test (FTA-ABS) and the microhemagglutinin test for antibody to *T. pallidum* (MHA-TP).

(d) **Examination of the CSF** is necessary in persons with neurologic or ophthalmologic symptoms, other manifestations of tertiary syphilis, treatment failure, HIV infection, or serum nontreponemal titers of 1 : 32 or greater (unless the duration of infection is known to be less than 1 year), and for whom nonpenicillin therapy will be prescribed (unless the duration of infection is known to be less than 1 year).

   (i) The **CSF leukocyte count and protein** are usually elevated in neurosyphilis.

   (ii) A **CSF VDRL** should be obtained when neurosyphilis is suspected.

(e) **Slit lamp examination** is done in persons with symptoms or signs of ophthalmologic involvement.

(3) A definitive **diagnosis** is established by a positive dark-field or immunofluorescent stain examination. A presumptive diagnosis is established by clinical findings and positive serologic testing.

(a) **Primary syphilis** consists of a chancre at the site of inoculation. During this stage, serologic tests may be negative, but become reactive during the following 1 to 4 weeks.

(b) **Latent syphilis** is the term for the asymptomatic period following primary infection. Persons infected in the preceding year are defined as having early latent syphilis; persons with a duration of infection longer than a year are defined as having late latent infection.

(c) **Secondary syphilis** is characterized by fever, malaise, rash, condyloma lata, lymphadenopathy, splenomegaly, and arthritis.

(d) **Tertiary syphilis** is characterized by aortitis, neurosyphilis, or gummatous lesions. A reactive CSF VDRL is diagnostic for neurosyphilis.

(4) **Therapy.** Extensive experience with penicillin G has shown it to be an effective agent for treatment of syphilis. Skin testing and desensitization should be considered for persons with a history of penicillin allergy. The optimal dose, duration, and preparation of penicillin used for therapy of the various stages of syphilis have been determined primarily by clinical experience. Treatment failures can occur with any regimen; consequently, response to therapy must be closely monitored. A fourfold increase in nontreponemal test titers should be considered as a treatment failure or reinfection. Failure of the nontreponemal test to decline fourfold by 3 months suggests treatment failure. Follow-up examination of CSF is necessary in persons with neurosyphilis.

(a) **Primary and secondary syphilis**

   (i) In adolescents and adults, benzathine penicillin G, 2.4 million units IM as a single dose.

   (ii) In children, benzathine penicillin G, 50,000 units/kg IM, up to the adult dose, as a single dose.

   (iii) For penicillin-allergic persons, doxycycline, 100 mg PO bid for 14 days, or tetracycline, 500 mg PO qid for 14 days.

(b) **Early latent syphilis**. Treatment is as described for primary and secondary syphilis.

(c) **Late latent syphilis or latent syphilis of unknown duration**

   (i) In adolescents and adults, benzathine penicillin G, 7.2 million units total administered as three doses of 2.4 million units IM each at 1-week intervals.

   (ii) In children, benzathine penicillin G, 150,000 units/kg total, up to the adult dose, administered as three doses of 50,000 units/kg IM each at 1-week intervals

(iii) For penicillin-allergic persons, doxycycline, 100 mg PO bid for 14 days, or tetracycline, 500 mg PO qid for 14 days, if the duration of infections is known to be less than one year; otherwise treatment should be extended to 28 days.

(d) **Tertiary syphilis (excluding neurosyphilis).** Treatment is as described for latent syphilis.

(e) **Neurosyphilis**

(i) In adolescents and adults, aqueous crystalline pencillin G, 12 to 24 million units/day administered as 2 to 4 million units IV q4h for 10 to 14 days, or procaine penicillin, 2.4 million units IM once a day plus probenecid, 500 mg PO qid for 10 to 14 days.

(ii) Some experts administer a dose of benzathine penicillin at the conclusion of therapy to provide a similar duration of therapy to that of latent syphilis.

(iii) For penicillin-allergic persons, treatment regimens are not well established. Desensitization should be considered.

(f) **Syphilis in HIV-infected persons.** In general, treatment is the same as for non–HIV-infected persons. However, HIV-infected persons are at increased risk for neurologic involvement and treatment failure. Close follow-up for HIV-infected persons is particularly important.

(g) The **Jarisch-Herxheimer reaction** may occur in the first 24 hours after therapy for any stage of syphilis. The reaction consists of fever, headache, myalgia, arthralgias, and other symptoms.

(5) **Prevention.** See Table 5–3 for postexposure prophylaxis measures.

d. **Gonorrhea**

(1) **Etiology.** The infecting organism is *N. gonorrhoeae*.

(2) **Evaluation**

(a) **Clinical findings**

(i) Infection in males is almost always symptomatic and is characterized by mucopurulent penile discharge and dysuria.

(ii) In adolescent or adult females, uncomplicated infection is usually asymptomatic, although mucopurulent cervical or vaginal discharge or vaginal bleeding, or both, may be seen. Symptoms or signs of pelvic inflammatory disease are seen as a complication of infection in females (see p. 129).

(iii) In prepubertal girls, infection may present as purulent vulvovaginitis.

(iv) Disseminated disease in either sex is manifested by fever, petechial or pustular acral skin lesions, asymmetrical arthralgias, tenosynovitis, or septic arthritis.

(v) Conjunctivitis, hepatitis, endocarditis, and meningitis are rarely seen.

(b) **Specimens**

(i) In **males**, urethral specimens can be obtained by "stripping" the penis.

(ii) In **females**, pelvic examination should be performed to evaluate cervical and adnexal tenderness and to obtain a specimen from the cervix. Specimens should be collected during routine examination of high-risk women in order to identify asymptomatic infection.

(iii) In prepubertal girls, vaginal discharge is an adequate specimen.

(iv) The rectum and pharynx should be cultured in both males and females.

(c) **Gram stain** should be performed to document the number of white blood cells (≥ 5 WBCs per high-power field are seen in urethritis and cervicitis) and to look for gram-negative intracellular diplococci.

(d) Culture

  (i) Specimens should be inoculated onto prewarmed Thayer-Martin media and placed in a high carbon dioxide $_2$ atmosphere (e.g., candlejar) or in a special packet with a CO_2-generating pellet.

  (ii) Transport medium should be used when direct cultures are not practical.

(e) Blood culture should be performed in suspected disseminated infection.

(f) Examination of synovial fluid is useful in cases with frank arthritis. Test should include

  (i) Culture as described above.

  (ii) Cell count and differential.

  (iii) Glucose.

(3) The **diagnosis** of gonorrhea is made by the demonstration of gram-negative intracellular diplococci on Gram's stain of appropriately obtained specimens or by isolation of the organism in culture. Disseminated disease is diagnosed by clinical findings; isolation of the organism from clinical specimens establishes a definitive diagnosis.

(4) Therapy

  (a) Uncomplicated infection in adolescents or adults. Any of the regimens listed below is effective for genital and anal infection. Pharyngeal infection should be treated with ceftriaxone or ciprofloxacin.

  (i) Ceftriaxone, 125 mg IM as a single dose, or

  (ii) Cefixime, 400 mg PO as a single dose, or

  (iii) Ciprofloxacin 500mg PO as a single dose, or

  (iv) Ofloxacin, 400 mg PO as a single dose, plus

  (v) A regimen effective against possible infection with *C. trachomatis*, such as doxycycline, 100 mg PO bid for 7 days.

  (vi) Alternative treatment regimens using other injectable or oral cephalosporins, other quinolones, and spectinomycin are available but are either not as effective or not studied as extensively.

  (b) Uncomplicated infection in prepubertal children. Any of the regimens listed below is effective for genital and anal infection. Pharyngeal infection should be treated with ceftriaxone or ciprofloxacin.

  (i) Ceftriaxone, 125 mg IM as a single dose, plus

  (ii) A regimen effective against possible infection with *C. trachomatis*, such as erythromycin, 40 mg/kg/day PO divided bid for 7 days.

  (c) Conjunctivitis (nonneonatal). A single dose of ceftriaxone, 1 g IM, is effective.

  (d) Disseminated infection

  (i) In adolescents, ceftriaxone, 1 g IV or IM once a day, or cefotaxime, 1 g IV q8h, or ceftizoxime, 1 g IV q8h for 7 days, plus a regimen effective against possible infection with *C. trachomatis* as described above.

  (ii) In children, ceftriaxone, 50 mg/kg IV or IM once a day, or cefotaxime, 1 g IV q8h, or ceftizoxime, 1 g IV q8h for 7 days, plus a regimen effective against possible infection with *C. trachomatis* as described above.

  (e) Meningitis and endocarditis

  (i) In adolescents, ceftriaxone, 1 to 2g IV bid for 10 to 14 days for meningitis and for 4 weeks for endocarditis

(ii) In children, ceftriaxone, 50 mg/kg IV once or twice a day for 10 to 14 days for meningitis and for 4 weeks for endocarditis

(f) Follow-up. Test of cure cultures are not necessary in uncomplicated cases. Infection after treatment is usually due to reinfection rather than treatment failure.

(5) Prevention. See Table 5-3 for postexposure prophylaxis measures.

e. **Chlamydia genital infection**

(1) Etiology. The infecting organism is usually *C. trachomatis.*

(2) Evaluation

  (a) Clinical findings

    (i) Infection in **males** is characterized by mucopurulent penile discharge and dysuria but may be asymptomatic.

    (ii) In adolescent or adult **females,** uncomplicated infection is usually asymptomatic. Symptoms or signs of pelvic inflammatory disease are seen as a complication of infection in females (see p. 130).

    (iii) In prepubertal females, infection may present as vaginitis.

  (b) Specimens should be obtained as described for gonorrhea. (see sec. **d** below).

  (c) A **Gram's stain and culture** should be performed to exclude gonorrhea.

  (d) Tests for *C. trachomatis* (see also Chap. 14, p. 418)

    (i) Culture (most reliable).

    (ii) Direct immunofluorescence test looking for basophilic, intracytoplasmic inclusion bodies.

    (iii) Indirect immunofluorescence antibody test.

    (iv) ELISA.

    (v) DNA probe.

(3) The **diagnosis** is dependent on clinical manifestations and laboratory results.

(4) Therapy

  (a) In **adolescents** and **adults,** a number of effective regimens are available. Clinical experience is greatest with doxycycline. Azithromycin offers the benefit of single-dose therapy. Erythromycin and sulfisoxazole are less effective.

    (i) Doxycycline, 100 mg PO bid for 7 days.

    (ii) Azithromycin, 1 g PO as a single dose.

    (iii) Ofloxacin, 300 mg PO bid for 7 days.

    (iv) Erythromycin base, 500 mg PO qid for 7 days or erythromycin ethylsuccinate, 800 mg PO qid for 7 days.

    (v) Sulfisoxazole, 500 mg PO qid.

  (b) In **children,** treatment regimens are generally limited to erythromycin. Since the effectiveness of erythromycin is approximately 80%, a second dose may be necessary.

    (i) In children less than 45kg, 50 mg/kg/day PO divided qid for 10 to 14 days.

    (ii) In children 45 kg or greater but less than 8 years of age, erythromycin base, 500 mg PO qid, or erythromycin ethylsuccinate, 800 mg PO qid for 7 days.

    (iii) In children 8 years or older, adult treatment regimens of doxycycline.

  (c) Follow-up. Test of cure cultures are not necessary in uncomplicated cases unless symptoms persist or reinfection is likely.

(5) Prevention. See Table 5-3 for postexposure prophylaxis measures.

f. **Pelvic inflammatory disease (PID).** PID comprises a group of infections of the upper female genital tract, including endometritis, salpingitis, tuboovarian abscess, and pelvic peritonitis.

  (1) Etiology. *Neisseria gonorrhoeae* and *C. trachomatis* are responsible for the majority of cases. However, other flora of the female genital tract can cause PID, including gram-positive and gram-negative anaerobes, gram-negative enteric rods, *Gardnerella vaginalis*, group B streptococci, *Mycoplasma hominis*, and *Actinomyces israelii*.

(2) Evaluation

    (a) A **history** of acute lower abdominal pain with vaginal discharge, fever, and chills suggests the diagnosis. Symptoms may be mild. The menstrual period is often a precipitating factor.

    (b) **Pelvic examination** findings include cervical motion or adnexal tenderness, and sometimes a mass.

    (c) **Specimens for Gram's stain, culture, and tests for *C. trachomatis*** should be obtained as described above.

    (d) **Other laboratory tests**
        (i) A peripheral **WBC** should be obtained.
        (ii) An **ESR** should be obtained.

    (e) **Ultrasound** can help delineate the location and extent of infection.

    (f) **Laparoscopy** is useful in obtaining a more accurate assessment of the involvement of the fallopian tubes and ovaries and to obtain cultures.

    (g) If surgical drainage is required, **intraoperative cultures** should be obtained.

(3) Diagnosis. Minimal criteria are the presence of lower abdominal pain, cervical motion tenderness, and adnexal tenderness. Additional criteria that improve the specificity of a clinical diagnosis include fever, abnormal cervical or vaginal discharge, elevated ESR or C-reactive protein, and laboratory documentation of infection with *N. gonorrhoeae* or *C. trachomatis*. Ultrasound, laparoscopy, and endometrial biopsy are helpful in establishing a definitive diagnosis.

(4) Therapy. Empiric therapy should not be delayed awaiting additional evaluation or culture results.

    (a) Absolute **indications for admission** to the hospital include toxicity, uncertain diagnosis, suspected pelvic abscess, signs of peritonitis, pregnancy, inability to take oral medications, failure of response to outpatient therapy, and poor follow-up arrangements. Because of the long-term complications associated with poor compliance, many experts recommend hospitalization for all cases.

    (b) A variety of regimens have proved effective for reducing symptoms; however, the efficacy of treatment regimens in eradicating infection in the fallopian tubes or in reducing long-term consequences, such as infertility, have not been determined.

    (c) **Inpatient therapy** must be individualized, and surgical drainage may be necessary. Some regimens for PID follow.

        (i) Cefoxitin, 2.0 g IV q6h, or cefotetan, 2 g IV q12h, plus doxycycline, 100 mg IV or PO bid. Continue for at least 48 hours after the patient's condition improves. Then continue doxycycline, 100 mg PO bid, to complete 10 to 14 days total therapy.

        (ii) Clindamycin, 900 mg IV q6h, plus gentamicin, 2 mg/kg IV or IM as the first dose and followed by 1.5 mg/kg q8h, plus doxycycline, 100 mg IV bid. Continue IV drugs at least 48 hours after the patient's condition improves. Then continue doxycycline, 100 mg PO bid, to complete 10 to 14 days total therapy. Therapy may be completed with oral clindamycin to provide improved anaerobic coverage in cases of tuboovarian abscess, but the efficacy of this agent against *C. trachomatis* is not well established.

        (iii) Ampicillin-sulbactam plus doxycycline and ofloxacin administered IV has been effective, but has not been studied extensively.

(iv) Sufficient evidence is not present for use of a single agent for inpatient treatment.

(d) Outpatient therapy

(i) Cefoxitin, 2 g IM, accompanied by probenecid, 1 g PO as a single dose, or ceftriaxone 250 mg IM, plus doxycycline, 100 mg PO bid for 10 to 14 days.

(ii) Ofloxacin, 400 mg PO bid for 14 days, plus either clindamycin, 450 mg PO qid, or metronidazole, 500 mg PO bid for 14 days.

(e) Follow-up

(i) Patients should be reevaluated in 2 to 3 days; those who do not respond favorably should be hospitalized.

(ii) Microbiologic reevaluation 7 to 10 days after completing therapy should be performed. The need for additional microbiologic evaluation in not established, but practitioners should reassess the potential for reinfection frequently.

(5) Prevention. See Table 5–3 for postexposure prophylaxis measures.

g. Epididymitis

(1) Etiology. *Neisseria gonorrhoeae* and *C. trachomatis* account for the majority of sexually transmitted causes of epididymitis. *Escherichia coli* can cause infection after anal intercourse.

(2) Evaluation

(a) A **history** of unilateral testicular pain and tenderness is characteristic. Urethritis is common.

(b) Specimens for Gram's stain, routine culture and culture for *N. gonorrheae*, and tests for *C. trachomatis* should be obtained as described above.

(c) Ultrasound can help distinguish epididymitis from testicular torsion.

(3) A clinical **diagnosis** can be established by the clinical features. A specific diagnosis can be established by identification of the etiologic agent.

(4) Therapy

(a) Bed rest and scrotal elevation may offer symptomatic relief.

(b) Treatment usually results in prompt improvement.

(i) Ceftriaxone,250 mg IM as a single dose, plus doxycycline, 100 mg PO bid for 10 days.

(ii) Azithromycin and ofloxacin may be effective but have not been studied extensively.

(c) Follow-up

(i) Patients should be reevaluated in 48 to 72 hours; those who do not respond favorably should be hospitalized.

(ii) Microbiologic reevaluation 7 to 10 days after completing therapy should be performed. The need for additional microbiologic evaluation is not established, but practitioners should reassess the potential for reinfection frequently.

(5) Prevention. See Table 5–3 for postexposure prophylaxis measures.

h. Genital and anal warts

(1) Etiology. Several types of human papilloma virus (HPV) (especially types 6 and 1) cause exophytic warts. Other types of HPV can lead to warts but can also cause subclinical infection. Human papilloma virus infection is strongly associated with genital dysplasia and carcinoma.

(2) Evaluation

(a) Examination will identify exophytic warts (condylomata acuminata).

(b) Application of acetic acid on a suspicious lesion results in whitening of the lesion, but false-positive results are common.

(c) Papanicolaou (Pap) smear is helpful but does not correlate well with detection of HPV DNA in cervical cells.

    (d) Histologic examination of a specimen obtained by colposcopy or biopsy is the most specific test.

    (e) Tests that detect HPV DNA are available.

  (3) The **diagnosis** is established by examination in symptomatic cases. Histologic examination or tests for HPV DNA establish a definitive diagnosis.

  (4) Therapy

    (a) The **goal of treatment** is directed toward improvement of cosmetic appearance. Spontaneous resolution is not uncommon. Treatment does not affect the potential for subsequent carcinoma.

    (b) Treatments of all types are associated with a high rate of recurrence. The anatomic site, size, and number of the warts and the expense, convenience, comfort, and adverse effects should be considered in choosing a specific regimen. (see also Chap. 14).

      (i) Cryotherapy with liquid nitrogen or cryoprobe is relatively inexpensive and does not result in scarring if performed correctly. Special equipment is necessary. Pain is a common side effect in the immediate posttreatment period.

      (ii) Trichloroacetic acid (TCA) 25–85% can be applied just to the lesion and does not need to be washed off. Aloe vera gel or normal saline can be applied immediately afterward to help alleviate the burning sensation. TCA should be applied weekly.

      (iii) Podofilox 0.5% applied in cycles to genital warts bid for 3 days followed by 4 days of no therapy can be used for self-therapy.

      (iv) Podophyllin 10–25% applied weekly can be used for external vaginal and urethral meatus warts and washed off several hours later. It should not be used for anal warts. Dosing guidelines need to be followed to avoid systemic toxicity.

      (v) Electrodesiccation or electrocautery requires local anesthesia.

      (vi) Carbon dioxide laser treatment is useful when lesions are extensive or other therapies have failed.

    (c) Subclinical infections are generally not treated.

    (d) Follow-up

      (i) Follow-up is necessary until patients are no longer symptomatic.

      (ii) Women should receive Pap smear annually regardless of a history of genital warts.

  i. Vaginitis in children (see chap. 14).

  j. Vaginitis in adolescents (see chap. 14).

H. Skin and soft tissue infections

  1. Superficial fungal infections of the skin, hair, and nails. See Chap. 17, p. 480

  2. Nonbullous impetigo

    a. Etiology. Caused primarily by streptococci and sometimes secondarily infected by *S. aureus*. Glomerulonephritis can result from impetigo caused by **streptococci M, type 49 or 55.**

    b. Evaluation.

      (1) Gram's stain is rarely helpful due to frequent secondary infection.

      (2) Laboratory evaluation is usually not required. If glomerulonephritis or nephritogenic strains are suspected, throat and skin cultures should be done on close contacts.

    c. Diagnosis

      (1) Subjective findings. The patient may have a history of antecedent minor trauma, insect bites, or exposure to other infected children.

The lesions are usually relatively asymptomatic, but occasionally pruritus is a prominent feature.

(2) Objective findings. Multiple lesions, most numerous on the face and extremities, are characterized by a thick, adherent, yellowish-brown crust. Involved areas spread centrifugally and coalesce into large, irregularly shaped lesions with no tendency for central clearing. Regional lymphadenopathy is common.

d. Treatment

(1) Minimal disease. Local cool water soaks can be used to remove crusts. The area is washed with povidone-iodine (Betadine) or chlorhexidine gluconate (Hibiclens), and a topical antibiotic (mupirocin, bacitracin, or erythromycin gluceptate [Ilotycin]) is applied two to three times a day. However, if the lesions do not resolve quickly with topical care, systemic antibiotic therapy is indicated.

(2) Moderate or extensive disease. Topical mupirocin, cephalexin, dicloxacillin, or erythromycin usually is effective therapy. Although impetigo is often caused by penicillin-sensitive organisms and frequently responds to penicillin, the presence of *S. aureus* is common enough to justify therapy with an agent that is also active against this organism.

3. Bullous impetigo, scalded skin syndrome, and staphylococcal scarlet fever represent a spectrum of dermatologic manifestations of staphylococcal infection resulting from release of soluble toxins by *S. aureus*.

a. Etiology. The infecting organism is *S. aureus* (usually bacteriophage group II).

b. Evaluation

(1) Cultures of the skin, nose, throat, and blood should be made (exceptions include children with only localized bullous impetigo and older children who are afebrile and nontoxic).

(2) Gram's stain of the denuded skin or bullous fluid, or both, will differentiate direct staphylococcal skin invasion from the more common toxin-mediated skin changes. The fluid aspirated from intact bullae will be sterile in scalded skin syndrome, but may contain *S. aureus* in bullous impetigo.

c. The **diagnosis** is established by the clinical picture in association with recovery of *S. aureus* from the patient. Nikolsky's sign (gentle rubbing of the skin results in sloughing of the epidermis) is usually indicative of the scalded skin syndrome; its absence does not exclude the diagnosis.

d. Therapy

(1) A 7- to 10-day course of a penicillinase-resistant penicillin or first-generation cephalosporin generally is sufficient. Except in mild bullous impetigo, the antibiotic is usually given parenterally (e.g., oxacillin, 100–200 mg/kg/day divided q4h IV, or cefazolin, 150 mg/kg/day divided q8h IV).

(2) After a good clinical response has been achieved, therapy can be completed with oral dicloxacillin or cephalexin.

(3) Contact precautions are indicated until the lesions have resolved.

(4) Corticosteroids have not been demonstrated to be beneficial.

(5) In patients with extensive skin losses, hydration and maintenance of normal body temperature are important. Avoid unnecessary skin trauma (e.g., adhesive from tape).

4. Infestations (see Chap. 17, p. 484).

5. Cellulitis

a. Etiology

(1) *Staphylococcus aureus* and group A streptococci are the primary pathogens.

(2) *Haemophilus influenzae* type b is now a rarity in the US.

(3) Group B streptococcal infection can occur in neonates and infants in the first few months of age.

(4) Gram-negative bacteria (*P. aeruginosa*) should be considered in immunocompromised children.

b. Evaluation

(1) A **blood culture** and antigen detection studies (e.g., latex agglutination) should be done in patients with severe cellulitis, fever, generalized toxicity, or impaired host defenses.

(2) **Needle aspiration** of the advancing border of an active lesion should be carried out for Gram's stain and culture.

c. The **diagnosis** is usually established by the characteristic warm, erythematous, tender, and indurated skin.

(1) Group A streptococcal cellulitis (erysipelas) is suggested by advancing, well-demarcated, heaped-up borders; facial involvement may assume a butterfly distribution.

(2) *Pseudomonas aeruginosa* cellulitis (ecthyma gangrenosum) is suggested by an ulcer or an eschar in an immunocompromised host.

(3) *Haemophilus influenzae* type B is suggested by a purple discoloration of the skin. Most patients with *H. influenzae* type b cellulitis are bacteremic, and additional sites of infection should be considered (e.g., septic arthritis or meningitis).

d. Therapy

(1) Application of local heat (e.g., warm compresses) 10 to 20 minutes qid or more provides symptomatic relief.

(2) The affected area should be immobilized and elevated.

(3) Suppurative foci of infection should be incised and drained.

(4) **Antibiotic therapy.** Localized cellulitis without fever can be treated with oral antibiotics. However, if evidence of systemic toxicity is present, parenteral antibiotics should be given until sustained clinical improvement has occurred. It is important to note that the cellulitis, with advancing erythema, does not halt immediately once effective therapy has been given. It is common for the cellulitis to appear to spread over the first 24 to 36 hours after the start of effective therapy. Clinical judgment and evidence of toxicity should be considered before antibiotics are changed.

(a) **Empiric therapy** includes a penicillinase-resistant penicillin, a first-generation cephalosporin, clindamycin, cefuroxime, or ampicillin-sulbactam.

(b) **Streptococcal disease or erysipelas** usually responds to benzathine penicillin G, 0.6 to 1.2 MU IM in one dose, or oral penicillin V, 125 to 150 mg qid. More severely ill patients may initially require IV penicillin, 100,000 units/kg/day q4h. Treatment should be continued for 7 to 10 days.

(c) **Staphylococcal cellulitis** is usually treated with a penicillinase-resistant penicillin or cephalosporin (nafcillin or oxacillin, 100–200 mg/kg/day IV q4h, or cefazolin, 150 mg/kg/day IV q8h) for severe infections or with oral dicloxacillin or cephalexin for milder infections.

(d) *Haemophilus influenzae* cellulitis, in view of the high incidence of positive blood cultures in this disease, is treated parenterally with ampicillin-sulbactam; cefuroxime, cefotaxime, ceftriaxone, or choramphenicol can be used pending ampicillin sensitivity testing.

(e) For therapy in immunocompromised patients, an antibiotic that is effective against gram-negative enteric organisms and *Pseudomonas* should be included.

I. Bone and joint infections

1. Septic arthritis

a. Etiology

(1) *Staphylococcus aureus* is the most common etiology, either due to hematogenous seeding of the joint or penetrating injuries.

(2) Group B streptococci represent an important etiology in infants a few months of age but may also be seen later in the first year of life.

(3) Group A streptococci can cause involvement of multiple joints.

(4) *Haemophilus influenzae* type b was a common etiology in young children in the prevaccination era but is now a rarity.

(5) *Neisseria gonorrhoeae* can cause suppurative arthritis, sterile inflammatory arthritis, and tenosynovitis (see **G.4.d**).

(6) Gram-negative enteric bacteria, pneumococci, and *N. meningitidis* are less commonly involved.

(7) Tuberculous arthritis is uncommon.

(8) Lyme disease may mimic septic arthritis.

b. Evaluation

(1) Careful **examination** of the joints for range of motion, warmth, erythema, and effusion is necessary. Joint infection, particularly hip involvement, may be overlooked in the infant who is not ambulating, the young child who cannot verbalize joint pain, and the toxic, prostrate child with bacteremia. Repeated examination of the hips and all other joints is an important aspect of the management of febrile or bacteremic patients, or both. Delayed diagnosis can result in extensive damage to growth cartilages.

(2) **X-rays** should be obtained of the joint(s) for evidence of effusion and of adjacent bones for evidence of osteomyelitis.

(3) **Ultrasound** examination is very sensitive in detecting the presence of an effusion in the hip joint.

(4) At least one **blood culture** should be obtained.

(5) A CBC and an ESR should be obtained initially; these laboratory markers of inflammation will be used in follow-up.

(6) **Arthrocentesis.** Analysis of the joint fluid includes Gram's stain, culture (including plating on prewarmed chocolate agar if *H. influenzae* or *Neisseria* is suspected), WBC and differential, total protein, and joint-blood glucose ratio.

c. Diagnosis. Isolation of pathogenic bacteria in a culture of the joint fluid establishes the diagnosis. In the absence of a positive joint fluid culture, the diagnosis can also be made by a combination of characteristic clinical findings, presence of a high WBC count with a polymorphonucleocyte predominance in the joint fluid, and blood culture results. Joint or blood cultures, or both, are positive in most but not all patients with septic arthritis. Osteomyelitis of the adjacent bone may also be present in neonates and in children with septic arthritis of the hip.

d. Therapy

(1) **Drainage.** Prompt aspiration of the affected joint is both diagnostic and therapeutic. Adequate drainage is critical to the prevention of sequelae. Whether open surgical drainage, arthroscopy with irrigation, or repeated needle aspiration is chosen depends on the **joint involved** (the hip and shoulder require surgical drainage; the knee is particularly amenable to arthroscopic irrigation), **age** (infants and young children may require surgical drainage), **viscosity** of the synovial exudate, the offending **pathogen** (staphylococcal disease usually necessitates surgical drainage, whereas meningococcal or gonococcal arthritis may require only needle aspiration), and the **response** of the patient to antibiotics.

(2) **Antibiotics**

(a) **Parenteral therapy**

(i) Empiric therapy should be begun with an intravenous antistaphylococcal antibiotic, such as oxacillin or cefazolin.

(ii) For children in whom infection with *H. influenzae* is a possibility, empiric therapy should include coverage for this organism in addition to *S. aureus*. In this situation, appropriate agents include cefuroxime or ampicillin-sulbactam, a combination of oxacillin and chloramphenicol,or a second- or third-generation cephalosporin.

(iii) Neonates should have adequate coverage for *S. aureus*, group B streptococci, and gram-negative bacteria. Oxacillin and gentamicin or a third-generation cephalosporin are appropriate.

(iv) In children with underlying diseases or immunodeficient children, coverage for gram-negative organisms is necessary. Oxacillin and gentamicin or a third-generation cephalosporin are appropriate.

(v) Since systemically administered antibiotics diffuse well into synovial fluid, additional local instillation is unnecessary.

(vi) Once the pathogen is identified, therapy may require modification to provide the most effective drug with the least toxicity.

(b) **Oral therapy**

(i) After an initial period of IV antibiotic therapy, when the clinical condition has stabilized, we finish therapy with oral antibiotics.

(ii) Care must be taken to choose an oral drug based on in vitro sensitivities and pharmacokinetics that is tolerated at two to three times the normal oral dose. Commonly used oral agents for *S. aureus* septic arthritis are dicloxacillin (80–100 mg/kg/day divided qid) and cephalexin (100 mg/kg/day divided qid).

(iii) Compliance with the oral therapy regimen must be ensured.

(c) The **duration of antibiotic therapy** is usually a total of 2 to 3 weeks.

(d) **Serum bactericidal levels** are useful to monitor absorption of oral antibiotics and to assess compliance. However, they are often logistically difficult to obtain and measure. Serum should be obtained 1 to 2 hours after oral dosing and should have a titer of 1 : 8 or better. Dosing can be adjusted or probenecid added to the regimen (for penicillins and cephalosporins) to achieve desired serum levels.

(3) **Response to therapy** should be assessed by follow-up examinations and an ESR at periodic intervals.

(4) **Other therapeutic measures** include early immobilization of the joint and physical therapy when the inflammation subsides.

2. **Acute osteomyelitis.** Most osteomyelitis in children is caused by hematogenous seeding of the cancellous bone present in the metaphysis of the long bones. Osteomyelitis due to penetrating injuries, extension from a contiguous site of infection, or in postoperative wounds is considerably less common. Infection of nontubular bones, such as the pelvic bones, the vertebral bodies, the bones of the thorax, the small cuboidal bones of the hand and foot, and the skull, account for about 10% of cases in children.

a. **Etiology**

(1) *Staphylococcus aureus* is the organism responsible in 75 to 80% of cases.

(2) Other organisms include group A streptococci, pneumococci, and *H. influenzae*. Special associations include *Salmonella* in sickle cell anemia, gram-negative enteric pathogens and group B streptococci in neonates and young infants, and *P. aeruginosa* following a penetrating injury of the foot or in drug addicts. Mycobacteria are rare causes.

b. **Evaluation**

(1) As with septic arthritis, a careful **examination** is necessary to avoid overlooking the site of infection. Bony tenderness is common but not universal.

(2) X-rays should be obtained, although evidence of osteomyelitis may not be seen until the second week.

(3) At least one **blood culture** should be obtained.

(4) A **CBC** and a **ESR** should be obtained initially; as laboratory markers of inflammation, these tests will help gauge improvement.

(5) A **bone scan** is helpful to identify osteomyelitis early in the course of the infection.

(6) MRI is very sensitive and is particularly useful in cases in which the location of the infection is difficult to assess by clinical findings and other radiographic studies (i.e., pelvic osteomyelitis).

(7) In the presence of localized bony tenderness or a positive bone scan, **needle aspiration or open biopsy of the bone** for Gram's stain and culture is indicated.

c. The **diagnosis** is based on a combination of clinical findings, radiographic studies, and the results of needle aspiration, bone biopsy, and/or blood culture.

d. Therapy. The approach to therapy is similar to that used in septic arthritis (see p. 135).

(1) Drainage. Surgical intervention is necessary to drain collections of pus in the bone, below the periosteum, and in the adjacent soft tissues. Necrotic bone (sequestra) should be debrided.

(2) Antibiotics. The approach to empiric therapy while awaiting culture results is similar to that for septic arthritis.

(a) Parenteral therapy

(i) Empiric therapy is similar to that used for septic arthritis (see p. 135).

(ii) Children with sickle cell anemia require appropriate coverage for both *S. aureus* and *Salmonella*. Ampicillin-sulbactam, cefuroxime, or oxacillin and chloramphenicol or a second- or third-generation cephalosporin provide both.

(iii) In children with penetrating injuries of the foot, coverage for *S. aureus* is appropriate acutely. When the infection is chronic, coverage for *P. aeruginosa*, such, as piperacillin or ceftazidime plus an aminoglycoside is used.

(iv) Once the pathogen is identified, therapy may require modification to provide the most effective drug with the least toxicity.

(b) Oral therapy is the same as for septic arthritis (see p. 136). However, the **duration of antibiotic therapy** is usually a total of 4 to 6 weeks.

(3) Serum bactericidal levels are useful to monitor absorption of oral antibiotics and to assess compliance. However, they are often logistically difficult to obtain and measure.

(4) Response to therapy should be assessed by follow-up examinations, x-rays, and an ESR at periodic intervals.

J. Nervous system infections

1. Meningitis. This section discusses common bacterial, mycobacterial, and fungal causes of meningitis. For a discussion of **neonatal meningitis,** see Chap. 6, p. 210.

a. Etiology

(1) Hematogenous seeding of the meninges is responsible for most episodes of meningitis.

(a) *Neisseria meningitidis* and *S. pneumoniae* account for most cases of acute bacterial meningitis in children over 2 months of age.

(b) Group B streptococci, gram-negative bacteria, and *Listeria* are the most common causes in neonates.

(c) *Haemophilus influenzae* type b, previously the most common etiologic agent in children less than 2 years of age, is now a rarity in the United States.

(d) Mycobacterium tuberculosis is most common in young children, but can affect children of any age.

(e) Infrequently involved bacteria are group A streptococci, *S. aureus*, and gram-negative enteric bacteria.

(f) *Cryptococcus neoformans* and *L. monocytogenes* cause meningitis in immunocompromised patients.

(g) Fungi, such as *Histoplasma, Coccidioides, Paracoccidiodes*, and *Blastomycoses*, are rare causes in children. *Candida, Aspergillus*, and *Mucor* may occur in immunocompromised or hospitalized children.

(h) Syphilis is a rare cause of meningitis in children.

(i) Other causes include Lyme disease, *Brucella* species, *Leptospira iterrogans*, and a variety of parasitic agents.

(2) **Direct inoculation** of the CSF occurs in children with penetrating injuries, tears in the meninges with CSF leak into the sinuses or ear canal, and spinal dysraphism, and in children undergoing neurosurgical procedures or with CSF shunts.

(a) *Streptococcus pneumoniae* cause most episodes of meningitis in association with CSF leaks.

(b) Skin flora are the most common etiology, including *S. aureus, S. epidermidis*, diphtheroids, *Proprionibacterium acnes* and, less commonly, gram-negative bacteria.

(3) **Extension of infection from a contiguous focus**, such as parameningeal infection (sinusitis, mastoiditis, subdural empyema, epidural abscess), can also cause meningitis.

b. **Evaluation**

(1) **Presenting symptoms and signs**

(a) In infants, presently signs and symptoms are nonspecific and include a high-pitched cry, irritability, anorexia, vomiting, lethargy, and/or a full fontanel. Fever is not always present. Close attention must be paid to alterations in consciousness in order to make an early diagnosis.

(b) In children and adolescents, headache, photophobia, stiff neck, vomiting, and an altered level of consciousness are common symptoms.

(c) **Meningismus** is uncommon in infants and toddlers but is a more reliable indicator in children over the age of 2 years. Kernig's sign (inability to extend the knee >135 degrees when the hip is flexed at 90 degrees) and Brudzinski's sign (flexion of the neck with the patient supine causes involuntary flexion of the hips and knees and pain in the small of the back) are useful indicators.

(d) **Convulsions** may be an early manifestation of meningitis. Convulsions associated with fever are generally an indication for CSF examination in children under 2 years unless a diagnosis of a simple febrile seizure is made, the patient has a history of epilepsy, or meningismus is absent in a child over 2.

(e) **Focal neurologic deficits** can occur from vasculitis or thrombosis of blood vessels, particularly meningeal vessels, or direct invasion of the brain parenchyma.

(f) **Papilledema** is an uncommon presenting sign unless the case is very advanced.

(g) Patients with evidence of bacteremia should be carefully assessed for meningitis.

(2) **Examination of the CSF**

(a) **Papilledema suggests increased intracranial pressure and is a relative contraindication to lumbar puncture (LP).** A neurosurgical consultation should be considered before proceeding.

  (b) A **lumbar puncture or a shunt tap** should be performed as soon
as the diagnosis is suspected. The following test sshould be performed.

   (i) Gram's stain

   (ii) Culture for bacteria and, if *Cryptococcus* is suspected, fungal culture.

   (iii) Latex agglutination tests to detect capsular polysaccharide antigens. These tests vary in their sensitivity: *H. influenzae* type b and group B streptococci are the most sensitive; *N. meningitidis* and *S. pneumoniae* are less sensitive.

   (iv) Cell count and differential.

   (v) Total protein and glucose. A blood glucose level should
be obtained for comparison with the CSF glucose, preferably before the lumbar puncture is performed.

   (vi) Cryptococcal antigen test if *Cryptococcus* is suspected.

   (vii) Acid-fast stain and mycobacterial culture if tuberculous
meningitis is suspected.

  (3) Other laboratory tests

   (a) Blood culture.

   (b) Other cultures as indicated (e.g., stool, urine, joint, abscess,
middle ear).

   (c) Serum electrolytes, BUN, creatinine.

   (d) Urine electrolytes and serum and urine osmolarity should be
checked if SIADH (syndrome of increased antidiuretic hormone)
is suspected.

   (e) Tuberculin test and chest x-ray if tuberculous meningitis is
suspected.

   (f) A serum **RPR and a CSF VDRL** should be obtained if syphilis is
suspected.

   (g) Serologic tests for Lyme disease, brucellosis, and leptospirosis
should be performed if the patient has a suggestive epidemiologic history.

  (4) A **CT scan or MRI** is necessary in some cases to assess the possibility
of a brain abscess or other parameningeal focus or an infarct.

  (5) An **electroencephalogram** is indicated if seizures are a prominent
aspect of the case.

 c. The **diagnosis** can be established only by examination of the spinal fluid.
In bacterial meningitis the CSF is characteristically cloudy and under increased pressure, usually with more than 100 WBC/mm³, predominantly
neutrophils; elevated total protein; low glucose (<½ of the blood glucose
concentration); and organisms seen in the CSF Gram's stain. However,
some of these findings are often absent, and any of these abnormalities
must be viewed with suspicion, particularly the presence of any neutrophils. The CSF culture is necessary and/or other tests described above
are necessary to determine the etiology. A variety of noninfectious
processes, including Kawasaki's disease, Mollaret's meningitis, intracranial
epidermoid cysts, and a number of inflammatory processes, can cause
meningitis.

 d. Therapy. Intravenous antibiotic therapy should be initiated immediately
after bacteriology specimens have been obtained. The initial choice of antibiotics usually is based on the gram-stained smear of CSF and on the patient's age.

  (1) Antibiotic therapy

   (a) Empiric therapy

    (i) Infants less than 2 months old (see Chap. 6).

    (ii) Children over 2 months of age. Because of the increas-
ing incidence of penicillin- and cephalosporin-resistant *S.
pneumoniae*, we now begin therapy with **vancomycin,** 60

mg/kg/day, **and either cefotaxime** (200 mg/kg/day q6h) **or ceftriaxone** (75–100 mg/kg/day q12–24h) until culture results and susceptibility tests are available. In areas where resistant *S. pneumoniae* are rare or absent, either ampicillin (300–400 mg/kg/day q6h) and chloramphenicol (100 mg/kg/day q6h) or cefotaxime (200 mg/kg/day q6h) or ceftriaxone (75–100 mg/kg/day q12–24h) are equally acceptable for empiric therapy.

(iii) Ampicillin (300 mg/kg/day divided q4–6h) should be used empirically if *L. monocytogenes* is suspected.

(iv) Because it may take weeks before mycobacterium tuberculosis is identified in culture, therapy for tuberculous meningitis must be initiated empirically if the diagnosis is suspected (see p. 149).

(v) Amphotericin (test dose, then 1.0 mg/kg/day) should be initiated if cryptococcal meningitis or another fungal etiology is suspected.

(b) Directed therapy. Once the organism is identified and susceptibility tests are available, directed therapy should be given.

(i) Treatment of **penicillin-sensitive *S. pneumoniae*** or *N. meningitidis* is accomplished with high-dose penicillin (200,000–250,000 units/kg/day divided q4h) or ampicillin (300 mg/kg/day divided q4–6h).

(ii) Treatment of resistant *S. pneumoniae* is potentially complicated. The regimen should be based on the susceptibility results of the specific isolate. Consultation with an infectious disease specialist is recommended.

(iii) Treatment of *H. influenzae* type b can be completed with ampicillin (300 mg/kg/day divided q4–6h) if the isolate is susceptible. Chloramphenicol is an option if the isolate is susceptible; otherwise cefotaxime or ceftriaxone is adequate.

(iv) *Listeria* meningitis should be treated with ampicillin (300 mg/kg/day divided q4–6h) with gentamicin for the first 5 to 7 days.

(v) The treatment of gram-negative meningitis usually involves use of two agents, such as a third-generation cephalosporin and an aminoglycoside. The regimen should be based on the susceptibility results of the specific isolate. Consultation with an infectious disease specialist is recommended.

(vi) Treatment of other causes of bacterial meningitis should be based on the susceptibility results of the specific isolate. Consultation with an infectious disease specialist is recommended.

(vii) Treatment of tuberculous meningitis is discussed on p. 147.

(viii) Treatment of neurosyphilis in children and adolescents is discussed on p. 127. Treatment of neonatal neurosyphilis is discussed in Chap. 6.

(ix) Treatment of Lyme disease is discussed on p. 146.

(x) Leptospirosis should be treated with high-dose parenteral penicillin.

(xi) Treatment of meningitis caused by brucellosis must be prolonged; relapses are common if the duration of therapy is inadequate. Agents used include tetracyclines, TMP/SMZ, and gentamicin. Consultation with an infectious disease specialist is recommended.

(xii) Treatment of fungal meningitis is difficult and relapses are common. While amphotericin is the principal drug used, new antifungal agents, such as fluconazole, penetrate into the CNS and are useful in some situations, such as cryptococcal meningitis. The regimen should be based on the specific isolate and clinical considerations. Consultation with an infectious disease specialist is recommended.

(c) The **duration of therapy** depends on the patient's clinical course, but antibiotics should generally be administered for 5 to 7 days for meningococcus, 7 to 10 days for *H. influenzae* type b, and 10 to 14 days for pneumococcal meningitis.

(d) **Parenteral therapy should be used in most situations.** In cases of meningitis caused by a chloramphenicol-sensitive organism, a portion of therapy can be completed with oral chloramphenicol if the child is able to take oral medication, adequate serum levels are demonstrated on oral therapy, and compliance is assured.

(2) **Other aspects of management**

(a) **Dexamethasone.** Dexamethasone has been conclusively shown to be effective only in reducing the incidence of sensorineural hearing loss after *H. influenzae* type b meningitis. The regimen is 0.6 mg/kg/day given q6h IV for the first 4 days of therapy.

(b) **Blood pressure, perfusion, and hydration**

(i) **Maintenance of blood pressure and cerebral perfusion pressure** is of primary importance.

(ii) Most patients who present with meningitis have been ill and febrile for 12 to 24 hours before diagnosis, and they are typically dehydrated on admission. **Rehydration** to restore a euvolemic state should precede any fluid restriction.

(iii) The **SIADH** commonly occurs in bacterial meningitis, usually within the first 72 hours of therapy. After rehydration has been accomplished and if blood pressure and perfusion are adequate, fluids should be restricted to three-fourths maintenance until it is documented that SIADH is absent.

(c) **Frequent observation** of vital signs, daily neurologic examinations, measurement of head circumference, and transillumination of the head (if the fontanel is open) should be performed.

(d) A **repeat lumbar puncture** or shunt tap should be performed after 24 to 48 hours of therapy only in patients whose disease is severe, who respond poorly to treatment, or who are infected with antimicrobial-resistant or difficult-to-treat (gram-negative bacteria) organisms. Cultures and stains are usually negative after 24 to 48 hours if treatment is effective.

(e) **Fever during therapy** most commonly results from phlebitis, drugs, nosocomial infection, subdural effusion (which may occur in up to 50% of infants and children during the acute illness, usually without producing symptoms or fever), or coexisting viral infection. Unless an obvious cause is found, **prolonged (>7 days) or secondary fever during therapy should prompt a repeat CSF examination** and a search for localized infection in the subdural space, bones, joints, pericardium, or pleural spaces.

(f) A **CT scan** is useful to document subdural effusions, but we do not routinely perform scans on all patients. A CT scan should be obtained in all cases of gram-negative meningitis, especially in neonates, because abscesses are a common complication.

(g) Selected children with uncomplicated cases of bacterial meningitis can finish therapy with oral chloramphenicol (same dose as IV; check levels) or ceftriaxone, 50 to 75 mg/kg q24h, given IM once a day. We do not routinely repeat a lumbar puncture or observe patients in the hospital after completion of therapy.

e. **Prevention.** See Table 5–3 for postexposure prophylaxis measures.

2. Brain abscess. Normal brain tissue is resistant to bacterial infection. However, ischemic brain injury (e.g., cyanotic heart disease), parameningeal infection (sinusitis, mastoiditis, skull osteomyelitis), and skull trauma increase the risk of brain abscess.

  a. Etiology

    (1) Causative bacteria are usually derived from the upper airway or mouth. Mixtures of aerobes (streptococci, *S. aureus*, diphtheroids, *Haemophilus*) and anaerobes (*Peptococcus, Bacteroides*) are common.

    (2) Gram-negative bacteria are uncommon causes in children. An exception is gram-negative meningitis in neonates, which is frequently complicated by formation of brain abscesses.

    (3) Other agents, such as *Nocardia, Actinomyces*, and fungi, are occasionally responsible, usually in immunocompromised patients.

  b. Evaluation. Brain abscess must be considered in patients with evidence of a rapidly progressive intracranial mass.

    (1) The **history** should focus on possible predisposing causes. Headache and seizures are common. Fever is seldom prominent.

    (2) **Examination** should focus on detection of foci of extracranial infection and assessment of neurologic deficits and elevated intracranial pressure (ICP).

    (3) A **CT scan with contrast or an MRI** is necessary.

    (4) **Needle aspiration** of the abscess is useful in order to establish an etiologic diagnosis. Aspirated fluid should be submitted for complete microbiologic examination, including Gram's stain, aerobic and anaerobic culture, fungal stain, fungal culture, AFB stain, and mycobacterial culture.

    (5) **Laboratory examination**

      (a) One or more **blood cultures** should be obtained from all patients.

      (b) A **CBC and differential** should be performed, although leukocytosis may or may not be present.

      (c) **CSF examination should be avoided in patients with increased ICP.** It seldom adds to the evaluation (CSF changes are neither universally present nor pathognomonic for brain abscess).

    (6) An **EEG** is necessary if the patient has a history of seizures.

  c. The **diagnosis** is made by visualization of a ring-enhancing intracranial mass, usually with surrounding inflammatory edema, on a contrast CT scan or MRI. Even small abscesses can be localized by skilled personnel and generally make an arteriogram unnecessary. In some cases a definitive diagnosis can only be made by needle aspiration or excisional biopsy.

  d. Therapy

    (1) Although surgical drainage may be necessary in cases with life-threatening increased intracranial pressure, many cases can be managed medically with antibiotic therapy. Ideally, therapy should be preceded by a **needle aspiration** of the abscess to obtain a specimen for microbiologic examination.

    (2) **Careful monitoring** by neurologic examination and CT scan is necessary to assess the efficacy of empiric therapy in this setting.

    (3) **Antibiotic therapy**

      (a) **Empiric therapy** should always include a regimen of two or more parenterally administered agents and be directed toward the likely causative agent(s). Several options exist.

        (i) Penicillin (300,000 units/kg/day divided q4h) and chloramphenicol (100 mg/kg/day divided q6h).

        (ii) Oxacillin (200–300 mg/kg/day divided q4h) plus chloramphenicol or a third-generation cephalosporin (cefotaxime,

200 mg/kg/day divided q6h, or ceftriaxone, 100 mg/kg/day divided q12h, or ceftazidime, 200 mg/kg/day divided q8h).

(iii) Vancomycin (45–60 mg/kg/day divided q8–12h) should be substituted for oxacillin in the regimen described in sec. **(ii)** if methicillin-resistant *S. aureus* or *S. epidermidis* are suspected.

(iv) If the regimen in sec. **(ii)** using a third-generation cephalosporin is chosen, metronidazole (35–50 mg/kg/day divided q8h) can be added to provide better anaerobic coverage.

- **(b) Directed therapy** should be based on the susceptibility results of the specific isolate. Consultation with an infectious disease specialist is recommended.
- **(4) Fluid management** should be as described in the section on meningitis (see sec. **1.d.2** above).
- **(5) Hyperosmotic agents,** such as mannitol, and **dexamethasone** may also help to reduce cerebral edema (see Chap. 7).
- **(6) Follow-up CT scans** are used to monitor resolution of the abscess and to help determine the duration of antibiotic therapy.
- **(7) Parameningeal foci of infection responsible for brain abscess may also require surgical intervention** (sinusitis, mastoiditis).

IV. Special infectious disease topics
A. Bites
1. Animal bites
- **a. Etiology.** Potential pathogens include *S. aureus,* anaerobic and microaerophilic streptococci, other anaerobic cocci, *Clostridium* species (including *C. tetani*), *Pasteurella multocida, Streptobacillus moniliformis,* and *Spirillum minus* (the latter two cause the two types of rat-bite fever).
- **b. Evaluation** includes an assessment of the patient's immunity to tetanus as well as the extent of the wound. A bacterial complication of an animal bite is suggested by the finding of cellulitis.
- **c. Therapy**
  - **(1)** Cleansing, irrigation, local antisepsis, and surgical care of the bite, including debridement if necessary, should be performed.
  - **(2)** Antimicrobial prophylaxis is used when the bite is on the face or hands and when a puncture wound (e.g., cat bite) is present. Antimicrobial treatment is indicated if evidence of cellulitis is present. Ampicillin-clavulanate is useful for oral therapy; ampicillin-sulbactam or the combination of penicillin and oxacillin is useful for parenteral administration.
  - **(3)** The need for prophylactic measures for rabies and tetanus (see Table 5–3) should be considered.
2. Rabies prophylaxis. The recommendations are based on those of the Centers for Disease Control (CDC) (*MMWR* RR-33:1–19, 1991).
- **a. Evaluation.** Capture and evaluation of the biting animal, whenever possible, is critical. Healthy domestic animals are observed for signs of rabies for 10 days in confinement. Domestic animals with signs of rabies and all wild animals should be killed and immunofluorescent antibody testing for rabies antigen performed on brain tissue. Viral culture can be performed, but takes considerably longer. The decision to administer rabies prophylaxis should be made with the assistance of the local public health department, which should have information regarding the risk of rabies in particular areas and animals. The following factors should be considered:
  - **(1) Species of biting animal.** Carnivorous wild animals (especially skunks, raccoons, foxes, coyotes, and bobcats) and bats are more likely to be infective than are other animals. Postexposure prophylaxis should be initiated after the bite of one of these animals unless the animal is tested and shown not to be rabid or the geographic area

is known to be free of rabies. Rabies in domestic dogs and cats is uncommon in most of the US, but depends on local epidemiology. Livestock, rodents, and lagomorphs are rarely infected.

   (2) Vaccination status of the biting animal. An adult animal immunized properly with one or more doses of rabies vaccine has only a minimal chance of having rabies and transmitting the virus.

   (3) Circumstances of the biting incident. An unprovoked attack is more likely to indicate that the animal is rabid than is a provoked attack. Bites sustained during attempts to feed or handle an apparently healthy animal should generally be regarded as provoked.

   (4) Type of exposure. The likelihood that rabies infection will result from a bite varies with its extent and location. A nonbite exposure (scratches, abrasions, open wounds, or mucous membrane contamination with saliva or other potentially infectious material from a rabid animal) may rarely result in rabies virus transmission. Casual contact, such as petting a rabid animal without sustaining a bite, may not be an indication for prophylaxis.

   b. Postexposure prophylaxis. See Table 5–3.

3. **Human bites,** especially those that occur on the palmar surface of the hand, can result in extensive, rapidly developing infection.

   a. Etiology. Infections are usually polymicrobial and may include staphylococci, gram-negative anaerobes and spirochetes from the mouth, and aerobic streptococci. Hepatitis B can be transmitted if the biter is a hepatitis B virus carrier, although the risk is small. HIV has not been demonstrated to be transmitted or acquired by a human bite.

   b. Evaluation. The principles of management are similar to those for management of animal bites, but irrigation, debridement, and provision for drainage assume much greater importance. Because of the potential for anaerobic infection, these wounds are usually not sutured. Testing the "biter" for hepatitis B infection should be considered in some situations but is not routine.

   c. Therapy

   (1) Wound care is the same as described for animal bites.

   (2) Antimicrobial prophylaxis is indicated for all human bites due to the high risk of infection. Appropriate antimicrobial agents are the same as those described for animal bites.

   (3) The need for prophylactic measures for tetanus should be considered (see Table 5–3).

   (4) Hepatitis B immune globulin and hepatitis B vaccine should be administered if the biter is a hepatitis B virus carrier.

B. Toxic shock syndromes. Staphylococcal toxic shock syndrome (STSS) is a multisystem illness that was initially identified in menstruating women, but can also occur in children who have foci of staphylococcal infection. **Group A streptococcal toxic shock syndrome (GASTSS)** is a multisystem illness that occurs in association with localized group A streptococcal (GAS) infections. Most often GASTSS occurs in children as a complication of superinfected varicella lesions.

1. **Etiology.** STSS is caused by one or more extracellular toxins produced by *S. aureus*. It is most often associated with infections caused by strains of *S. aureus* that produce TSS toxin-1 (TSST-1). GASTSS is caused by one or more extracellular toxins produced by GAS. Pyrogenic exotoxin a and b (the same toxins associated with scarlet fever) have been implicated in GASTSS. These toxins may act as super antigens, similar to TSST-1, activating a cascade of immunologic phenomena.

2. **Evaluation**

   a. A careful history and physical examination are critical since the diagnosis is based on clinical criteria.

   b. A careful search for foreign bodies and foci of localized infection should be performed.

    c. Laboratory evaluation should include a complete blood count and differential, liver function tests, BUN, creatinine, creatinine phosphokinase (CPK), and urinalysis.

    d. Cultures of the blood, vagina, nasopharynx, anus, pharynx, and any wound or skin lesions should be obtained in suspected cases.

    e. Evaluation should rule out a number of other conditions that may mimic toxic shock syndrome, including Kawasaki's disease, scarlet fever, Rocky Mountain spotted fever, measles, leptospirosis, and other febrile mucocutaneous diseases.

3. The **diagnosis** of STSS and GASTSS is based on clinical criteria.

    a. STSS

        (1) The clinical criteria established by the CDC (*MMWR* 39 [RR-13]:38–39, 1990)] for STSS are based on the presence of four of the following five signs.

            (a) Fever of 38.9°C (102.0°F) or greater.

            (b) Presence of a diffuse macular erythroderma.

            (c) Desquamation 1 to 2 weeks after onset of the illness, particularly on the palms, soles, fingers, and toes.

            (d) Hypotension.

            (e) Involvement of three or more of the following organ systems:

                (i) Gastrointestinal (vomiting or diarrhea at the onset of illness).

                (ii) Muscular (severe myalgia or serum CPK level ≥ 2 times the upper limit for age).

                (iii) Mucous membrane (vaginal, oropharyngeal, or conjunctival hyperemia).

                (iv) Renal (BUN or serum creatinine ≥ 2 times the upper limit for age or ≥ 5 white blood cells per high-power field in the absence of a UTI).

                (v) Hepatic (transaminases or total bilirubin ≥ 2 times the upper limit for age).

                (vi) Hematologic (platelets $\leq 100 \times 10^9$/liter).

                (vii) CNS (disorientation or alterations in consciousness without focal neurologic signs when fever and hypotension are absent).

        (2) In addition, the following conditions must be fulfilled:

            (a) Negative blood, throat, or CSF cultures (except in the uncommon cases in which *S. aureus* bacteremia is present).

            (b) Negative serologic tests for Rocky Mountain spotted fever, leptospirosis, and measles.

        (3) Isolation of *S. aureus* from a mucosal site or from a localized infection lends support to the diagnosis. However, *S. aureus* can be isolated from the nares or vagina in 30% of healthy individuals and 30% of these strains can be demonstrated to produce TSST-1. Consequently, isolation of a TSST-1 strain is only presumptive evidence of STSS.

    b. Criteria for the **diagnosis** of GASTSS were established by the Working Group on Severe Streptococcal Infections (*JAMA* 269:390–391, 1993). A definite case is defined as fulfilling criteria in secs. **(1)(a), (2)(a),** and **(2)(b)** below. A probable case is defined as fulfilling criteria in secs. **(1)(b), (2)(a),** and **(2)(b)** below.

        (1) Isolation of GAS

            (a) From a normally sterile site (e.g., blood CSF, pleural or peritoneal fluid, tissue biopsy, surgical wound, etc.).

            (b) From a nonsterile site (e.g., throat, sputum, vagina, superficial skin lesion, etc.).

        (2) Clinical signs

            (a) Hypotension (systolic blood pressure of ≤ 90 mm Hg for adults; <5th percentile by age for children <16 years of age), and

            (b) Two or more of the following findings.

      (i) Renal impairment (creatinine ≥ 2 times the upper limit for age).

      (ii) Coagulopathy (platelets ≤ 100 x 10^9/liter or disseminated intravascular coagulation).

      (iii) Liver involvement (transaminases or bilirubin ≥ 2 times the upper limit for age).

      (iv) Adult respiratory distress syndrome (ARDS).

      (v) Generalized erythematous macular rash that may desquamate or soft tissue necrosis, including necrotizing fasciitis, myositis, or gangrene.

4. Therapy

  a. Volume replacement and pressor support may be required to maintain adequate blood pressure and perfusion.

  b. For STSS, penicillinase-resistant penicillin therapy should be given parenterally (e.g., oxacillin, 200 mg/kg/day IV in divided doses q4h). For GASTSS, parenteral penicillin therapy should be given (e.g., penicillin G, 200,000–400,000 units/kg/day divided q4h).

  c. Foreign bodies should be removed (tampons, contraceptive sponges, wound drains and packing).

  d. Foci of local infection should be explored and drained.

  e. Supportive care for respiratory failure, electrolyte abnormalities, renal failure, coagulopathy, and thrombocytopenia should be provided.

  f. Corticosteroid therapy and intravenous immune globulin have been reported to be helpful, but have not been studied in well-designed clinical trials.

  g. Menstruating patients should be advised about the possible recurrence of STSS if tampons are used during subsequent menstrual periods.

C. Lyme disease

  1. Etiology. *Borrelia burgdorferi* is the tick-borne spirochete that causes Lyme borreliosis (Lyme disease). Humans are usually infected after prolonged (> 24 hour) attachment of an infected tick of the *Ixodes ricinus* complex. *Ixodes dammini* (deer tick) is the most common member of this tick group in the northeastern US.

  2. Evaluation

    a. Clinical manifestations are dependent on the stage of the disease: stage 1 (early localized), stage 2 (early disseminated), and stage 3 (late persistent phase).

      (1) Erythema chronicum migrans (ECM), the characteristic rash seen in early Lyme infection, occurs in about 60 to 80% of cases. The lesion characteristically begins as a red macule, which expands to form an annular erythema with central clearing. Lesions vary in size but usually expand to greater than 5 cm in diameter if untreated. Additional skin findings are often noted days to weeks after initial infection and may resemble the primary ECM lesion or present as malar, urticarial, or diffuse erythematous rash.

      (2) Arthritis along with **arthralgia** and **myalgia,** often brief and recurrent, are common findings of the second stage of Lyme disease. Chronic arthritis reflects the persistent infection of the third stage.

      (3) Seventh cranial nerve (Bell's) palsy is common a few weeks to months after infection, reflecting the early disseminated stage. **Meningitis** may present as classic summertime "aseptic" meningitis in the second stage of disease or as a chronic condition in the third stage. Less commonly, **peripheral neuropathies** are found in both the second and third clinical stages. Chronic neurologic involvement, including **encephalomyelitis, ataxia, and polyradiculitis,** is a manifestation of late-stage Lyme disease and may occur years after initial infection.

      (4) Carditis has been found in 4 to 8% of children within several weeks of infection. Atrioventricular blocks of varying types have been reported. Less commonly, pericarditis and myocarditis occur. Cardiac manifestations are usually brief.

(5) **Acrodermatitis chronica atrophicans**, a chronic localized sclero-derma-like rash, can occur years after the primary infection and represents persistent disease.

b. **Serology**. Serologic testing for evidence of infection by *B. burgdorferi* infection is useful, but there is considerable interlaboratory variation in results.

(1) ELISA is performed for immunoglobulin G (IgG) and immunoglobulin M (IgM).

(2) Western blot is performed for sera positive by ELISA and detects antibody to specific antigens.

3. **Diagnosis**. Lyme disease is primarily a clinical diagnosis. If ECM is present, serologic confirmation is unnecessary. Serology is useful when clinical findings are consistent with those seen in Lyme disease and confirmation of infection by *B. burgdorferi* is necessary. Immunoglobulin G and IgM ELISA titers need to be interpreted with reference to the clinical stage of disease suspected. As antibody is first detectable after 2 to 4 weeks of illness, children may be antibody negative at the time ECM is present and early treatment may ablate the expected antibody response. Children with stage 1 or 2 symptoms may have only IgM antibodies; alternatively, a child with more than 2 to 3 months of "early" symptoms or with symptoms of persistent infection may have negative IgM titers and positive IgG titers. Positive serologic tests in the absence of clinical findings consistent with past infection should not be viewed as an indication for therapy.

4. **Therapy**. The choice and length of therapy is dependent on the stage of disease, clinical findings, and response to therapy.

a. **Early infection (ECM), isolated seventh cranial nerve (Bell's) palsy, mild arthritis, and mild carditis**

(1) Amoxicillin, 25 to 50 mg/kg/day (maximum 2 g day) divided tid for 14 to 30 days, is the preferred agent.

(2) Penicillin V, 25 to 50 mg/kg/day (maximum 2 g day) divided tid for 14 to 30 days, is an alternative.

(3) Doxycycline, 100 mg bid for 14 to 30 days, can be used for children 9 years of age and older.

(4) Cefuroxime and erythromycin can be used in penicillin-allergic children.

(5) Retreatment is sometimes necessary.

b. **Persistent arthritis, CNS disease, severe carditis, or failure of oral therapy**

(1) Ceftriaxone, 75 to 100 mg/kg/day (maximum 2 g) given as a single IV or IM dose for 14 to 21 days, is the preferred agent.

(2) Penicillin G, 300,000 units/kg/day (maximum 20 million units/day) IV in six divided doses daily for 14 to 21 days is an alternative.

D. **Tuberculosis**

1. **Etiology**. *Mycobacterium tuberculosis* is the etiologic agent. Rarely, *Mycobacterium bovis* is the etiologic agent in nonpulmonary TB.

2. **Evaluation**

a. **Tuberculin skin test.** The tuberculin skin test is the best means of identifying infected children.

(1) The skin test (Mantoux test) should be performed using 5 tuberculin units of purified protein derivative (PPD) injected intradermally.

(2) Multiple puncture tests should not be used because of higher rates of false-positive and false-negative results.

(3) The skin test interpretation depends on several factors. A positive reaction is defined as

(a) 15 mm for children 4 years of age or older without any risk factors.

(b) 10 mm for children at risk of disseminated disease, such as children less than 4 years of age, children with underlying medical conditions, and children with increased environmental exposure.

(c) 5 mm for children in close contact with persons known or suspected to have tuberculosis, children suspected of having tuberculosis on the basis of a chest x-ray or clinical findings, and HIV-infected or immunocompromised children.

(4) A positive skin test usually develops 3 to 6 weeks (at most 3 months) after exposure and remains positive for life even with treatment.

(5) Prior vaccination with bacillus Calmette-Guérin (BCG) is not a contraindication to skin testing and does not affect the interpretation of the test.

(6) Nontuberculous (atypical) mycobacteria may cause cross-reaction with intermediate-strength PPD, but the reaction is usually less than 10 mm unless infection is recent.

(7) A negative skin test does not exclude *M. tuberculosis* infection or disease, as approximately 10% of immunocompetent children with tuberculosis have negative skin tests.

b. Clinical manifestations of childhood tuberculosis include

(1) Persistent cough, pulmonary infiltrates, atelectasis, pleural effusion, and/or enlarged hilar nodes.

(2) Occult fever, failure to thrive, weight loss, and anemia or hepatosplenomegaly.

(3) Lymphadenopathy.

(4) Aseptic meningitis.

(5) Chronic draining otitis media.

(6) Aseptic pyuria.

(7) Monoarticular arthritis, dactylitis, back pain, or bony tenderness.

c. Clinical specimens

(1) Types of clinical specimens

(a) Sputum is an excellent specimen if the child is capable of producing it.

(b) Specimens obtained by **bronchoalveolar lavage** are useful, but are not as sensitive as gastric aspirates.

(c) Gastric aspirates obtained in the morning immediately on the patient's awakening are the most sensitive specimens in young children. Three gastric aspirates on successive mornings should be obtained.

(d) A first-voided morning **urine specimen** is helpful when renal infection is suspected.

(e) Other useful specimens, if available, include cerebrospinal fluid, liver biopsies, bone marrow biopsies, pleural biopsies, lymph node aspirates or biopsies, and bone biopsies.

(2) Mycobacterial culture should be obtained in all suspected cases to confirm the diagnosis as well as determine drug susceptibilities.

(3) Acid-fast bacilli (AFB) stain should be performed on all specimens to allow rapid identification of mycobacteria, although *M. tuberculosis* cannot be distinguished from nontuberculous (atypical) mycobacteria.

(4) Polymerase chain reaction (PCR) and DNA probes are available in some settings and are promising though not yet routine methods for the identification of *M. tuberculosis*.

d. A **chest x-ray** should be obtained in all children with suspected tuberculosis.

e. Cerebrospinal fluid (CSF) examination, including culture and acid-fast stain, is necessary in all children with suspected tuberculous meningitis and in all infants under 6 months with suspected tuberculosis regardless of the site of infection.

f. Liver function tests are useful if miliary tuberculosis is suspected.

g. In proven cases of tuberculosis, **skin tests and chest x-rays of family members and contacts** are indicated.

3. The **diagnosis** of asymptomatic skin test conversion is based on the presence of a new positive skin test, the absence of symptoms, a negative chest x-ray, and negative AFB and mycobacterial culture results from sputum or gastric aspirates, or both. The presumptive diagnosis of tuberculosis is based on the presence of characteristic symptoms and a positive skin test or identification of acid-fast organisms in clinical specimens. A definitive diagnosis is made by the isolation of the *M. tuberculosis* in culture.

4. Therapy is complicated by the need for several medications and long courses of treatment and the increased incidence of multiple-drug–resistant *M. tuberculosis*. All children with tuberculosis should be tested for HIV infection.

a. Asymptomatic PPD skin test converter

(1) When the index infection is caused by INH-susceptible strains or when INH resistance is unlikely, INH, 10 to 15 mg/kg (maximum of 300 mg) PO qd for 9 months.

(2) When infection is caused by INH-resistant, rifampin-susceptible strains, rifampin, 10 to 20mg/kg PO qd for 9 months.

(3) When infection is likely to be caused by resistant strains but susceptibility results are not available, INH and rifampin (doses as above) for 9 months.

(4) Optimal therapy for infection caused by strains with documented INH and rifampin resistance is not known.

b. Pulmonary tuberculosis (including hilar adenopathy and pleural effusion)

(1) Six-month (standard) regimens

(a) Isoniazid, 10 to 15mg/kg (maximum 300 mg) PO qd, plus rifampin, 10 to 20mg/kg (maximum 600 mg) PO qd, plus pyrazinamide, 20 to 40 mg/kg (maximum 2 g) PO qd, for 2 months followed by INH and rifampin qd for 4 months.

(b) Isoniazid plus rifampin plus pyrazinamide (doses as in above) for 2 months followed by INH, 20 to 30 mg/kg (maximum 900 mg) PO, and rifampin, 10 to 20 mg/kg (maximum 600 mg) PO twice a week for 4 months.

(c) If drug resistance is possible, ethambutol 15 mg/kg (maximum 2.5 g) PO qd or 50 mg/kg (maximum 2.5 g) PO twice a week, or streptomycin, 20 to 40 mg/kg (maximum 1 g) IM qd, should be added until susceptibility results are known.

(2) Nine-month (alternative) regimens

(a) Isoniazid plus rifampin qd (doses as in sec. **(1)(a)** above) for 9 months.

(b) INH plus rifampin qd (doses as in sec. **(1)(a)** above) for 1 month followed by INH and rifampin twice a week (doses as in sec. **(1)(b)** above) for 8 months.

(c) Regimens using two agents should not be used if drug resistance is suspected.

c. Extrapulmonary tuberculosis (including adenitis, but not meningitis, miliary disease, and bone/joint disease) can be treated as pulmonary tuberculosis.

d. Tuberculous meningitis, miliary tuberculosis, and bone/joint tuberculosis

(1) Isoniazid, 10 to 15 mg/kg (maximum 300 mg) PO qd, plus rifampin, 10 to 20 mg/kg (maximum 600 mg) PO qd, plus pyrazinamide, 20 to 40 mg/kg (maximum 2 g) PO qd, plus streptomycin, 20 to 40 mg/kg (maximum 1 g) IM qd for 2 months, followed by INH and rifampin qd for 10 months.

(2) Isoniazid plus rifampin plus pyrazinamide plus streptomycin qd (doses as above) for 2 months followed by INH and rifampin twice a week (doses as in sec. **(1)(b)** above) for 10 months.

(3) Pyrazinamide is particularly important in tuberculous meningitis because it achieves better CSF concentrations than ethambutol or streptomycin.

(4) If streptomycin resistance is common, capreomycin, 15 to 30 mg/kg (maximum 1 g) IM qd, or kanamycin, 15 to 30 mg/kg (maximum 1 g) IM qd can be used in place of streptomycin until susceptibility results are known.

e. Drug-resistant *M. tuberculosis*

    (1) Resistance is most common in

        (a) Foreign-born persons from high-risk areas, such as Asia, Africa, and Latin America.

        (b) New York City and several other cities where drug-resistant tuberculosis is common.

        (c) Homeless persons.

        (d) Persons who have previously received treatment for tuberculosis.

        (e) Children whose adult source case is in one of the above groups.

    (2) Treatment should always include at least two bactericidal drugs to which the organism is susceptible. Bactericidal drugs include INH, rifampin, streptomycin, pyrazinamide, and high-dose ethambutol.

    (3) Other agents that may be useful include capreomycin, ciprofloxacin, cycloserine, ethionamide, kanamycin, and ofloxacin.

    (4) Treatment duration should be 12 to 18 months.

    (5) Consultation with an expert who has experience in treating drug-resistant tuberculosis in children should be obtained.

f. Pyridoxine, 25 to 50mg once a day, can be used in children with inadequate nutrition.

g. Corticosteroids given in conjunction with antimicrobial therapy may lessen the inflammatory complications of tuberculous pericarditis and pleuritis. They may also be indicated when large hilar lymph nodes are obstructing the passage of air and when severe respiratory distress complicates diffuse pulmonary tuberculosis. Dexamethasone should be administered in tuberculous meningitis since use of this agent lowers mortality and long-term neurologic morbidity.

h. Directly observed therapy (DOT). A major cause of treatment failure and the development of multiple drug resistance is nonadherence to the treatment regimen. DOT is one method of ensuring adherence and should be considered as an option in all cases of tuberculosis.

i. Follow-up

    (1) Although general recommendations for treatment durations are listed above, the length of treatment in an individual patient should be determined by the clinical and chest x-ray response, follow-up sputum smear and culture results (if possible), and susceptibility test results from the patient or the index case. In most situations, monthly clinical evaluations for the first 3 months and every 1 to 3 months thereafter are sufficient.

    (2) Hilar adenopathy may persist for several years. A normal x-ray is not a requirement to terminate treatment if other parameters are consistent with successful treatment.

    (3) Isoniazad treatment commonly causes a transient asymptomatic elevation of liver enzymes during the first 3 months of therapy. Routine laboratory testing for hepatotoxicity is unnecessary in uncomplicated cases but is required in severe cases, when high doses of INH are used, when initial therapy is administered for an extended time, in the presence of liver or biliary disease, during pregnancy and the first 6 weeks postpartum, or in the presence of overt hepatotoxicity.

    (4) Interruptions in therapy require that the duration of treatment be extended.

5. Prevention. See Table 5–3 for postexposure prophylaxis measures.

E. Rocky Mountain spotted fever

1. Etiology. *Rickettsia rickettsii,* a member of the spotted fever group of rickettsiae, is the causative agent. The organism is transmitted primarily by the dog tick, *Dermacentor variabilis,* in the eastern US, by the wood tick, *Dermacentor andersoni,* in the western US, and by the Lone Star tick, *Amblyomma americanum,* in the central US. Transmission is highest in seasons of peak tick activity, usually the spring and summer.

2. Evaluation

   a. Clinical findings

      (1) Fever is virtually always present.

      (2) Headache, myalgia, nausea, and vomiting are also common presenting symptoms.

      (3) A characteristic **rash** is usually present after several days of illness, although in some cases the rash may develop late or not at all. The rash is usually erythematous and maculopapular but becomes petechial. It generally begins on the extremities, often on the wrists and ankles, and spreads to the trunk.

      (4) Abdominal pain may be present.

      (5) CNS, cardiac, pulmonary, gastrointestinal, and renal involvement; disseminated intravascular coagulation; and shock may be present in severe cases.

   b. Laboratory tests should include

      (1) A CBC.

      (2) BUN and creatinine.

      (3) Liver function tests.

   c. Serologic testing. A variety of serologic tests are available. The immunofluorescent antibody and indirect hemagglutination tests are the most sensitive and specific. Acute and convalescent sera should be tested. The Weil-Felix serologic reaction becomes positive 10 to 14 days into the illness but is not very sensitive or specific.

   d. Immunofluorescent staining of a skin biopsy specimen from the site of the rash is very specific, but is not widely available.

   e. Culture is not attempted because it is technically difficult and hazardous for laboratory workers.

3. The **diagnosis** must be based on clinical and epidemiologic features because no widely available microbiologic test is positive early in the course of the disease. A fourfold rise in titer between acute and convalescent sera provides a retrospective, definitive diagnosis.

4. Therapy

   a. Early treatment is essential. Delay in diagnosis can lead to death.

   b. Chloramphenicol, tetracycline, and doxycycline are comparable in efficacy, although tetracycline is considered the drug of choice by some.

   c. Therapy is continued until the patient is afebrile for 2 to 3 days; a usual course is 6 to 10 days.

F. Human immunodeficiency virus (HIV) infection and acquired immunodeficiency syndrome (AIDS)

1. Etiology. Human immunodeficiency virus is a human retrovirus that has a tropism for cells with CD4 receptors, particularly CD4 (T-helper) lymphocytes. There are two types of HIV, HIV-1 and HIV-2. Almost all of the HIV infection occurring in the US is caused by HIV-1. The course of HIV infection is variable, but eventually the progressive destruction of CD4 lymphocytes results in AIDS.

2. Evaluation and diagnosis

   a. Risk factors for HIV infection should be evaluated, although their absence does not rule out the diagnosis.

      (1) Maternal HIV infection. Transmission of HIV from infected women to their offspring accounts for the vast majority of pediatric HIV infection in the US. The rate of transmission in the US is approximately 20%. HIV can be transmitted in utero, in the perinatal period (presumably due to exposure to blood or genital secretions during the birth process), and postnatally by breast feeding. Women at risk for HIV infection include those who use intravenous drugs, those who are the sexual partners of HIV-infected men or intravenous drug users, female commercial sex workers, and women who have received transfusions of blood products (see below). However, many infected women will not have acknowledged risk factors.

(2) **Receipt of blood products.** This risk was greatest for persons receiving blood products between 1979 and 1985. Most hemophiliacs treated with factor VIII concentrate before 1985 are infected with HIV. Since 1985, blood has been screened for antibody against HIV, which has drastically reduced, but not eliminated, the risk. HIV infection has not been demonstrated to occur after gamma globulin infusion.

(3) **Sexual activity.** HIV infection among sexually active adolescents has increased dramatically in recent years. A history of other sexually transmitted diseases increases the risk of HIV infection.

(4) **Intravenous drug use.** The incidence of HIV infection among intravenous drug users is very high in many areas of the US.

(5) **Percutaneous exposure to HIV-infected blood or other body fluids**. The risk of HIV infection after a percutaneous exposure to HIV-infected blood is estimated at 0.3%.

b. **Tests for HIV infection**

(1) **Serologic testing** is the preferred method for screening children over the age of 15 months. The presence of antibody against HIV in these children, if repeated, is definitive evidence of HIV infection. Children younger than 15 months, particularly those younger than 9 months of age, may harbor maternally derived antibodies to HIV. A positive test in these children indicates maternal HIV infection but is not definitive evidence of HIV infection in the child.

  (a) **ELISA** is a very sensitive and specific test for a variety of antibodies produced against HIV antigens; however, false-positives can occur.

  (b) A **Western blot** should be performed on any sera positive by ELISA. This test provides definitive proof of the presence of antibodies against HIV antigens.

(2) **Tests to detect the presence of HIV** are particularly useful in the evaluation for infection in young infants. A child born to an HIV-infected mother should have two of these tests (preferably HIV culture or PCR) performed in the first 6 months of life (preferably 1 month apart during the period between 1 and 3 months of age). A positive test should be repeated for confirmation.

  (a) Culture of HIV from peripheral blood mononuclear cells provides definitive evidence of infection at any age. This test is generally available only in research centers. A positive culture at birth indicates in utero infection. However, cultures performed at birth are negative in 50 to 75% of children who are ultimately found to be HIV infected, presumably because the virus was transmitted in the perinatal period and is not yet present in detectable amounts. Culture is positive in fewer than 90% of infected children by 3 months of age.

  (b) **Polymerase chain reaction** is similar to culture of HIV in terms of its sensitivity and specificity, but may offer faster turnaround time. It is generally available only in research centers.

  (c) **Immune complex dissociated p24 antigen** (p24 is a component of the viral capsid) is a less sensitive test than culture or PCR, but is cheaper, may have faster turnaround time, and is more readily available.

c. **Clinical features**

(1) **Age at presentation**. The age at onset of symptoms is extremely variable. Nonetheless, symptoms can often be recognized in the first year

of life in vertically infected children. The majority, but not all, of vertically infected children will be symptomatic by 2 years of age.

    (2) Clinical features in symptomatic HIV-infected children are

        (a) Poor weight gain or weight loss.

        (b) Developmental delay.

        (c) Generalized lymphadenopathy.

        (d) Hepatosplenomegaly.

        (e) Persistent or recurrent oral candidiasis.

        (f) Persistent or recurrent otitis media.

        (g) Persistent or recurrent diarrhea.

        (h) Persistent or recurrent parotitis.

        (i) Hepatitis.

        (j) Autoimmune anemia or thrombocytopenia.

        (k) Nephropathy.

        (l) Cardiomyopathy.

    (3) AIDS-defining illnesses for HIV-infected persons of all ages are

        (a) Opportunistic infections, such as *P. carinii* pneumonia; *Candida* infection of the esophagus, trachea, bronchi, or lungs; chronic or progressive cytomegalovirus (CMV) infection; chronic or disseminated HSV infection; disseminated *Mycobacterium avium* complex infection; disseminated or extrapulmonary tuberculosis; chronic intestinal cryptosporidiosis or isosporiasis; disseminated or CNS cryptococcal infection; disseminated or extrapulmonary histoplasmosis or coccidioidomycosis; and CNS toxoplasmosis.

        (b) HIV encephalopathy.

        (c) Wasting syndrome.

        (d) Progressive multifocal leukoencephalopathy.

        (e) Lymphoma (uncommon in children).

        (f) Kaposi's sarcoma (very rare in children).

    (4) Additional AIDS-defining illnesses in children less than 13 years of age are

        (a) Recurrent, serious bacterial infections (bacteremia, sinusitis, and pneumonia are the most common).

        (b) Lymphoid interstitial pneumonitis.

    (5) Additional AIDS-defining illnesses in adolescents 13 years of age and older are

        (a) Pulmonary tuberculosis.

        (b) Recurrent pneumonia.

        (c) Recurrent *Salmonella* bacteremia.

        (d) Invasive cervical cancer.

        (e) Total CD4 lymphocyte count (TCD4) less than 200 cells/μl or percentage of CD4 lymphocytes (CD4%) less than 14%.

  d. Lymphocyte subset studies, including determination of the percentage of CD4 lymphocytes (CD4%) and the total CD4 lymphocyte count (TCD4), are useful in following the course of the disease, estimating the degree of immunosuppression, and serving as an indicator for the need to initiate antiretroviral therapy and prophylaxis for specific opportunistic infections. The frequency of monitoring CD4% and TCD4 is dictated by the stage of disease, but is generally performed every 3 months, except when counts are already extremely low.

  e. Complete blood counts are necessary to calculate the TCD4, to monitor blood counts, and to monitor for toxicity from antiretroviral therapy (especially zidovudine [AZT]).

  f. Liver function tests are necessary to monitor for anicteric hepatitis and toxicity from therapy.

  g. Quantitative immunoglobulin assays will usually reveal hypergammaglobulinemia but are useful in identifying the occasional child with hypogammaglobulinemia who may benefit from intravenous immunoglobulin (IVIG; see p. 156).

h. A **chest x-ray** should be obtained as a baseline for future comparison and during any significant respiratory illness.

i. Children with documented CMV infection should be monitored with regular **ophthalmologic examinations** to screen for retinitis since they may not report significant visual disturbances.

j. We obtain yearly cardiologic evaluations, including an **ECG and echocardiography for qualitative and quantitative assessment of cardiac function**, as subclinical but significant diminution in cardiac function can occur. **Holter monitor evaluations** are obtained as indicated.

k. **Tuberculin skin tests** and two control skin tests (i.e., *Candida*, tetanus, mumps) should be monitored on a yearly basis.

3. Therapy

a. **Antiretroviral therapy.** The indications for antiretroviral therapy and optimal treatment regimens as well as strategies for managing disease progression and adverse effects of therapy are evolving constantly. Consultation with or referral to an expert in the treatment of pediatric HIV infection is recommended. Other sources of information include the National Pediatric HIV Resource Center (800-362-0071) and guidelines and updates published periodically in the *Pediatric Infectious Diseases Journal*.

(1) **Initiation of therapy.** There is a general belief that early initiation of therapy is helpful in limiting ongoing viral replication, although the benefits and consequences (development of viral resistance, adverse effects of therapy) are not clear and a matter of considerable controversy. A decision to initiate therapy should take into account the circumstances of the individual case and the wishes of the caregivers. The following are general indications for initiation of antiretroviral therapy.

(a) Development of AIDS.

(b) Significant symptomatology related to HIV or associated conditions (see p. 153).

(c) TCD4 count

(i) Less than 1,750 for children 0 to 1 year of age.

(ii) Less than 1,000 for children 1 to 2 years of age.

(iii) Less than 750 for children 2 to 5 years of age.

(iv) Less than 500 for children greater than 5 years of age.

(2) **Agents and regimens.** In the past, antiretroviral treatment in children was generally initiated with a single agent, usually zidovudine (ZDV, 90–180 mg/m^2/dose PO qid) or didanosine (ddI, 100 mg/m^2/dose PO bid). Of these two agents, ddI is now the preferred agent for monotherapy. Combination therapy may be more effective in reducing HIV replication, although its effect on clinical outcomes and the frequency and nature of adverse reactions have not yet been completely described. Other agents available for use in combination regimens (but not yet approved for use in children) include nucleoside analogues (zalcitabine [ddC], 0.005–0.01 mg/kg/dose PO tid; lamivudine [3TC], 4 mg/kg/dose PO bid; stavudine [d4T], 1 mg/kg/dose PO bid) and protease inhibitors (saquinavir, ritonavir, and indinavir). Combination regimens in use at the time of this writing in children are ZDV plus ddI and ZDV plus 3TC.

(3) **Monitoring.** The effect of therapy on clinical and laboratory parameters should be monitored at regular intervals. Measurement of the total count and percentage of CD4 lymphocytes should be performed at 3-month intervals. Measurements of viral load are being used increasingly to gauge the effect of antiretroviral therapy. The occurrence of adverse effects with these agents should be monitored closely (see manufacturer's recommendations). If disease progression occurs, consideration should be given to switching to another agent or adding another agent.

b. Immunizations (see also Chap. 16, p. 471 and Chap. 3, p. 27)

(1) Hepatitis B vaccine, diphtheria-tetanus-pertussis (DTP) vaccine, and H. influenzae b-conjugate vaccine should be administered following the routine vaccination schedule.

(2) Inactivated polio vaccine (IPV) should be used instead of oral polio vaccine (OPV) in all HIV-infected children.

(3) The **measles-mumps-rubella (MMR) vaccine** administered at 12 months of age is recommended for both symptomatic and asymptomatic HIV-infected children because of the potential severity of measles in these children and because serious consequences from administration of this live virus vaccine have not been observed.

(4) Varicella vaccine is currently not recommended.

(5) Influenza vaccine should be administered every year.

(6) Pneumococcal vaccine at 2 years of age and again at 3 to 4 years of age is potentially beneficial to children who are capable of responding to the antigens.

(7) Live vaccines other than MMR (e.g., yellow fever vaccine) should be avoided unless the potential benefits greatly exceed the potential adverse effects of administration of these vaccines to an immunocompromised host.

c. Prophylactic therapy

(1) Varicella-zoster immune globulin (VZIG) should be administered to susceptible children after exposure to varicella.

(2) Immune globulin should be administered to susceptible children after exposure to measles.

(3) PCP prophylaxis. Although the TCD4 and the CD4% are useful markers to predict the risk of PCP, they are not sufficiently reliable in the first 12 months of life and especially in the first 6 months, the period of life with the highest incidence of PCP.

 (a) Initiation of prophylaxis. Prophylaxis should be initiated according to the following guidelines.

  (i) All infants 4 weeks to 12 months of age born to HIV-infected mothers regardless of the TCD4 or CD4%, unless clinical findings and laboratory tests indicate that HIV infection is very unlikely.

  (ii) Children 1 to 2 years with a TCD4 less than 750/µl.

  (iii) Children 2 to 6 years of age with a TCD4 less than 500/µl.

  (iv) Children 6 to 12 years with a TCD4 less than 200 cells/µl or CD4% less than 15%.

  (v) All children with a previous episode of PCP regardless of their TCD4 or CD4%.

 (b) Agents

  (i) Trimethoprim-sulfamethoxazole, trimethoprim component 8 mg/kg/day or 150 mg/m²/day, given either three times a week or daily PO in one or two divided doses, is the preferred agent.

  (ii) Dapsone, 2 mg/kg PO as a single daily dose, is an alternative agent for children who do not tolerate TMP/SMZ.

  (iii) Intravenous pentamidine, 4 mg/kg IV given every 2 to 4 weeks, is an alternative for children who cannot tolerate TMP, SMZ or dapsone.

  (iv) Aerosolized pentamidine is an alternative for children old enough to cooperate with its administration.

(4) Prophylaxis against *M. avium* complex infection should be initiated when the TCD4 is less than 50 cells/µL. Rifabutin, 6 mg/kg as a single daily dose, is the preferred agent. A blood culture for mycobacteria should be obtained first to rule out preexisting infection. Children should be monitored for drug interactions and toxicity (i.e., gastrointestinal symptoms and painful but reversible uveitis). Clarithromycin,

15 mg/day PO divided bid is a potential alternative; however, there is insufficient experience to recommend this agent at the present time.

(5) **Intravenous gamma globulin** reduces the frequency of serious bacterial infections (pneumococcal bacteremia and sinopulmonary infections) in some children. It is particularly helpful in reducing the likelihood of pneumococcal bacteremia. Some centers use IVIG for all or at least a majority of the HIV-infected children they follow. However, because not all children benefit from this therapy and because of its expense and the need for monthly intravenous infusions, we generally reserve monthly IVIG therapy for children who have had at least one serious bacterial infection or an episode of bacteremia or those who are hypogammaglobulinemic.

d. **Treatment of specific infections**

(1) Bacterial infections are particularly common and typically involve encapsulated bacteria, such as *S. pneumoniae*. See sec. **III** for recommendations for the treatment of infections at specific sites (pp. 93.*ff.*).

(2) *Pneumocystis carinii* pneumonia is treated with either TMP/SMZ or pentamidine (see p. 110).

(3) **Thrush and *Candida* esophagitis** is treated with intravenous amphotericin or fluconazole or oral nystatin, clotrimazole, or fluconazole (see p. 96).

(4) **Herpes simplex infection** is treated with intravenous or oral acyclovir (see Table 5-5).

(5) **Varicella and herpes zoster** are treated with intravenous or oral acyclovir (see Table 5-5).

(6) **Cytomegalovirus (CMV)** infection is treated with intravenous ganciclovir (see Table 5-5).

(7) **Measles** can be very severe in HIV-infected patients and may warrant treatment with ribavirin and vitamin A (see Table 5-5).

(8) **Parvovirus** can cause chronic anemia, which may improve with treatment with IVIG.

(9) **Diarrhea** is common in HIV-infected patients. Treatment is generally the same as for non–HIV-infected patients, although *Salmonella* infection usually warrants treatment.

(10) **Disseminated *M. avium* infection.** Treatment involves use of multiple agents (usually ≥4) because multiple drug resistance is common. Regimens must be individualized; clarithromycin, rifampin or rifabutin, ethambutol, ciprofloxacin, amikacin, cefoxitin, and clofazime are among the agents most commonly used. Consultation with an expert in treatment of this infection is recommended.

(11) **Tuberculosis.** Manifestations may be unusual and can include extrapulmonary disease. Performing adequate tests to isolate and complete susceptibility testing of isolates of *M. tuberculosis* causing infection is particularly critical in HIV-infected children. Most cases respond well to therapy, but optimal doses and durations have not been defined. Initial therapy should involve at least two agents that are likely to have bactericidal activity. Generally, this requires three drugs; a fourth agent should be added if extrapulmonary disease or drug resistance is suspected. Treatment duration may need to be extended.

(12) **Syphilis** (see p. 126).

(13) **Toxoplasmosis**. Toxoplasmosis, including CNS toxoplasmosis, is unusual in pediatric patients.

e. In addition to medical management, appropriate nursing care and social support are critical to effective care both in the hospital and at home.

f. As the disease is ultimately fatal, appropriate judgment must be used when considering use of life support systems.

G. **Viral infections.** Table 5–5 reviews therapy for some specific viral infections. Also, see Table 5–3, p. 103 for recommendations for postexposure prophylaxis.

H. Fungal infections
1. **Candidiasis.** Infections caused by *Candida* are discussed elsewhere: thrush (see p. 95), *Candida* skin infection (see Chap. 17, p. 479), and *Candida* vaginitis (see Chap. 14, p. 420).
2. **Cryptococcosis**
   a. **Etiology.** The causative organism is *C. neoformans.*
   b. **Evaluation.** Symptoms are often vague. Meningoencephalitis is the most frequently recognized form of infection, with headache, nausea, and vomiting as common presenting symptoms. Infections of lungs, heart, skin, bones, and joints also occur.
   c. **Diagnosis.** The presence of cryptococcal antigen in the CSF, serum, or urine or a "positive" CSF India ink smear strongly suggests the diagnosis. The diagnosis is established by the growth of cryptococci from a normally sterile site (e.g., CSF, blood, lung tissue). India ink results should be confirmed with an antigen test.
   d. **Therapy**
      (1) **Cryptococcal meningitis**
         (a) Treatment should include a combination of amphotericin B, 0.3 mg/kg/day, and 5-fluorocytosine, 150 mg/kg/day PO divided q6h for at least 6 weeks. Patients with severe marrow impairment in whom further marrow suppression from 5-fluorocytosine may develop, can be treated with amphotericin B alone (0.5 mg/kg/day) for 10 weeks. Fluconazole is the drug of choice for patients who require maintenance therapy and may be an alternative for primary treatment of cryptococcal meningitis as well.
         (b) **Monitoring** with weekly examination of the CSF by culture, India ink smear, and cryptococcal antigen concentration is neces-

Table 5-5. Therapy for specific viral infections

Viral infection	Treatment
Herpes simplex virus	
Acute oral/genital	Treatment is not usually prescribed, but may reduce disease severity and duration, acyclovir 5 mg/kg/dose (maximum 400 mg) PO tid
Recurrent oral/genital	Chronic suppressive therapy can be used for frequent or severe episodes, acyclovir 5 mg/kg/dose (maximum 400 mg) PO tid
Oral/disseminated, immunocompromised host	Acyclovir 750 mg/m^2/day IV divided q8h; foscarnet 120 mg/kg/day IV divided q8h for infection caused by resistant virus
Neonatal	See Chap. 6, p. 204
Encephalitis	Acyclovir 1500 mg/m^2/day IV divided q8h
Keratoconjunctivitis	Trifluridine 1% solution one drop q2h; in neonates, systemic therapy should also be used
Varicella zoster virus	
Varicella, immunocompetent host	Acyclovir 20 mg/kg PO quid for 5 days reduces disease severity and duration if begun within 24 hours of onset
Varicella, immunocompromised host	Acyclovir 1500 mg/m^2/day IV divided q8h
Herpes zoster, immunocompetent host	Treatment is not usually prescribed; acyclovir 20 mg/kg PO qid in severe cases
Herpes zoster, immunocompromised host, not severe	Acyclovir 20 mg/kg PO qid; if progresses, use IV therapy (see below)
Herpes zoster, immunocompromised host, severe	Acyclovir 1500 mg/m^2/day IV divided q8h

Table 5-5 (continued)

Viral infection	Treatment
Cytomegalovirus	
Acute disease, immunocompetent host	No treatment is indicated
Acute disease, immuno-compromised host	Ganciclovir 10 mg/kg/day IV divided q12h; foscarnet 180 mg/kg/day IV divided q8h for infection that does not respond to ganciclovir
Suppressive therapy, immuno-compromised host	Ganciclovir 5 mg/kg IV qd 5 days per week, or foscarnet 90 mg/kg/day IV
Epstein-Barr virus	Prednisone 1–2 mg/kg/day PO for 5–7 days for airway compromise or marked splenomegaly
Measles virus	
Children 6–24 mo hospitalized with measles and children >6 mo with immunodeficiencies, ophthalmologic evidence of vitamin A deficiency, impaired intestinal absorption, moderate to severe malnutrition, or living in or recent immigration from areas where mortality from measles is >1%	Vitamin A 100,000 IU PO once for children 6–12 mo 200,000 IU PO once for children >12 mo Additional doses should be given the next day and at 4 weeks for children with ophthalmologic evidence of vitamin A deficiency Intravenous ribavirin 20–35 mg/kg/day for 7 days may be useful in cases of severe measles, but has not been approved for this indication by the FDA
Parvovirus	
Immunocompetent hosts	No treatment indicated
Immunocompromised hosts with chronic anemia	High dose immune globulin (400 mg/kg/day IV for 5 days)
Respiratory syncytial virus	See Chapter 7, p. 231
Human immunodeficiency virus	See p. 154

sary until cultures become sterile and at the conclusion of therapy. Microscopy should show a decrease in the number of organisms, and antigen testing should demonstrate at least a fourfold decrease in level during treatment.

(c) **Suppressive therapy** with fluconazole is necessary in HIV-infected patients to prevent relapse.

3. **Histoplasmosis**
   a. **Etiology.** The causative organism is *Histoplasma capsulatum*.
   b. **Evaluation and diagnosis.** Clinical manifestations may be severe in the infant or immunocompromised patient with fever, cough, adenopathy, pneumonitis, hepatosplenomegaly, and pancytopenia. Acute pulmonary histoplasmosis presents with fever, headache, cough, chest pain, and pulmonary infiltrates. Chronic pulmonary histoplasmosis can mimic tuberculosis. Skin testing with the histoplasmin skin test indicates current or past infection. Serum and urine can be tested for the presence of antigen. Acute and convalescent sera can be tested for specific IgG titer rise. Tissue, bone marrow, blood, and sputum can be cultured, stained, or tested by DNA probe as well.
   c. **Therapy**
      (1) Uncomplicated acute pulmonary histoplasmosis requires no treatment.
      (2) Itraconazole is now the drug of choice for treatment and prophylaxis of adults but pediatric experience is limited.
      (3) Amphotericin B remains the drug of choice for life-threatening disease, dosed at 0.5 to 1.0 mg/kg/day for 6 weeks or more.
4. **Blastomycosis**

   a. Etiology. The causative organism is *Blastomyces dermatitidis.*
   b. Evaluation and diagnosis. Children most commonly have pulmonary disease though cutaneous and disseminated disease also occurs. Symptoms vary widely and diagnosis depends on microscopic wet-mount evaluation of fresh specimens, growth in culture, or the use of specific DNA probes.
   c. Therapy. Itraconazole is now the treatment of choice for adults with nonmeningeal, non–life-threatening infections. More severe infections are treated with amphotericin B.
 5. Aspergillosis
   a. Etiology. A variety of *Aspergillus* species are pathogenic in humans, the most common being *A. fumigatus.*
   b. Evaluation and diagnosis should include
      (1) Careful examination for sinusitis, necrotic nasal lesions, pneumonia, pleuritic pain, and necrotizing skin lesions.
      (2) X-ray or CT scans of the sinuses and chest.
      (3) Direct microscopic examination and culture of sputum and biopsy specimens from suspected sites. Early diagnosis is essential, and biopsies should be performed promptly.
   c. The **therapy** for invasive aspergillosis is amphotericin B, 1.0 to 1.5 mg/kg/day (for a total dosage of 30–35 mg/kg over a period of 6 weeks or longer) and aggressive surgical debridement of lesions when feasible. The addition of flucytosine or rifampin should be considered. Itraconazole has been successfully used to cure *Aspergillus* infections in patients who are unable to tolerate amphotericin B therapy as well as to replace amphotericin B after the initial phase of treatment.
 I. Toxoplasmosis
 1. Etiology. *Toxoplasma gondii,* an obligate intracellular parasite, is responsible for this infection. Congenital transmission has been clearly established. Postnatally acquired infection is thought to occur via ingestion of improperly cooked meat and exposure to cat feces. Transmission from asymptomatic donors via blood product transfusion and organ donation has occurred
 2. Evaluation and diagnosis
   a. Infection is largely asymptomatic. Serologic evidence of prior infection is demonstrated in 25 to 40 percent of the population of the US. Several symptomatic forms are recognized.
      (1) Congenital infection (see Chap. 6, p. 204).
      (2) Acquired infection shows clinical variations ranging from a mild virus-like illness with lymphadenopathy to chorioretinitis without systemic illness. Fatal, usually focal, disease (pneumonia and encephalitis), which is nearly always reactivation disease, can occur in the compromised host.
   b. Demonstration of **rising antibody titers** by complement fixation (CF), hemagglutination (HA), indirect fluorescent antibody tests (IFA), and the Sabin-Feldman dye test establishes the diagnosis. Newborn infections can be diagnosed by demonstration of IgM (by capture enzyme-linked immunosorbent assay [ELIA]) or IgA *Toxoplasma* antibodies or the persistence of high titers of CF, HA, or IFA IgG antibodies beyond 4 months of age. Maternal *Toxoplasma* IgG is usually undetectable in the infant by 6 to 12 months of age.
   c. Rarely, in special circumstances, the diagnosis may be established by the demonstration of organisms in tissue sections or smears of body fluids. To determine if an infection is recent, however, rising serologic titers are still required.
 3. Therapy
   a. Congenital infection (see Chap. 6, p. 204).
   b. Acquired infection. Treatment depends on the clinical severity of the illness. Dosage for pyrimethamine is 1 mg/kg/day for the initial few weeks, then change to qod. Dosage for sulfadiazine should be increased to 100 to 200 mg/kg/day (maximum 6 g/day). Duration of therapy is 3 to 4 weeks. Folinic acid should also be given to prevent hematologic toxicity.

c. Reactivitation disease in immunocompromised host. Pyrimethamine and sulfadiazine in the above suggested doses are the initial recommended therapy. Obtain an infectious disease consultation if alternative therapies are necessary.

J. Malaria

1. **Etiology.** Malaria, among the most lethal of worldwide human infections, is transmitted by the bite of an *Anopheles* mosquito infected with *Plasmodium*. Four species of *Plasmodium* infect humans: *P. falciparum*, *P. vivax*, *P. ovale*, and *P. malariae*. *Plasmodium falciparum* is the most lethal of the four and also presents the problem of drug resistance.

2. **Evaluation and diagnosis**

   a. The most important factor when considering the diagnosis of malaria is the patient's immune status with respect to malaria. *Plasmodium falciparum* malaria in a nonimmune patient is a much more rapidly fatal disease.

   b. The common clinical manifestations of acute malaria infection are fever, rigors, malaise, headaches, myalgias, and arthralgias. **Splenomegaly** is the most consistent physical finding. In children, GI complaints, including loss of appetite, vomiting, or diarrhea, may predominate particularly in nonimmunes. In infants, pallor or jaundice is also seen.

   c. Fever in a nonimmune individual with *P. falciparum* is rarely periodic. The fever pattern may become periodic *after* infection is well established (patients from endemic areas): q48h in *P. vivax* and *P. ovale* infections, q72h in *P. malariae* infections, and q36–48h in *P. falciparum* malaria. Typically, the patient appears well between fever paroxysms.

   d. **It is exceedingly important in a nonimmune individual to distinguish between relapsing malaria** *(vivax and ovale)* **and falciparum malaria.** Documented malarial infections in nonimmune individuals should be treated as falciparum malaria. Mixed infections do occur, and one should be aware of this possibility. Textbooks of parasitology should be consulted to aid in species differentiation.

   e. The complications of *P. falciparum* infection include cerebral malaria (presenting as coma, delirium, and convulsions), massive hemolysis, disseminated intravascular coagulation, renal failure, pulmonary edema, and cardiovascular collapse.

   f. A history of residence or travel in an endemic area is almost always elicited.

   g. **The diagnosis rests on the demonstration of malaria parasites in the peripheral blood.**

   h. Nonimmune individuals are usually symptomatic with very low parasitemias. Therefore, a single negative blood smear **does not rule out malaria.** Serial smears over 48 to 72 hours should be done if no other source of fever or symptoms can be identified.

3. **Therapy.** The choice of antimalarial drugs depends on the infecting species and the geographic area of acquisition of infection.

   a. In **relapsing malaria,** therapy must be directed against both the erythrocytic and exoerythrocytic parasites to prevent relapse. There is no resistance to chloroquine, but relapse may occur if this agent is used alone.

   b. *Plasmodium falciparum* infections in nonimmune individuals, even when the level of parasitemia is low, should be treated immediately. The patient should be observed in the hospital until clinical improvement or a decrease in parasitemia is noted. *Plasmodium falciparum* infections in individuals from indigenous areas can be treated on an outpatient basis, based on clinical symptoms with follow-up blood smears at 7 and 28 days. Malaria, other than that caused by *P. falciparum*, can be treated on an outpatient basis.

   c. In addition to vigorous antimalarial therapy, the complications of falciparum malaria require intensive supportive measures. Transfusions with packed RBCs are given in severe hemolytic anemia. Mannitol can be used in renal failure, and dialysis may be necessary. Careful attention to fluid and electrolyte balance is essential. Anticonvulsants are often required in cerebral malaria.

d. **Recommended treatment regimens.** Given the rapidly evolving problem of drug resistance in falciparum malaria, the CDC maintains a 24-hour-a-day service for treatment and prophylaxis recommendations: 404–639–1610. This information is also available on the World Wide Web: http://www.cdc.gov.

  (1) Relapsing malaria
    (a) Chloroquine phosphate, 10 mg base/kg (16.6 mg/kg salt, maximum 600 mg base), followed by 5 mg/kg 6 hours later (maximum 300 mg), then 5 mg/kg/day (maximum 300 mg) for 2 days, and
    (b) Primaquine, 0.3 mg/kg/day for 14 days (maximum 15 mg base/day). **All patients at risk for glucose 6-phosphate dehydrogenase deficiency should be screened before therapy with primaquine.**

  (2) Falciparum malaria
    (a) Nonchloroquine-resistant area
      (i) Chloroquine phosphate, as in sec. **(1)(a)** above, or if parenteral therapy is required then either quinidine gluconate, 10 mg/kg over 1 to 2 hours, then 0.02 mg/kg/min until oral therapy can begin, or quinine dihydrochloride, 25 mg/kg/day (maximum 1,800 mg/day) divided tid given in normal saline over 2 to 4 hours until oral therapy can begin. Whenever parenteral therapy with quinidine gluconate or quinine dihydrochloride is used, ECG and blood pressure monitoring are recommended.
    (b) Chloroquine-resistant area
      (i) Quinine sulfate, 25 mg/kg/day in divided doses tid for 3 days (maximum 2 g/day), and
      (ii) Pyrimethamine-sulfadoxine (Fansidar): less than 1 year, a single dose of a ¼ tablet; 1 to 3 years, single dose of ½ tablet; 4 to 8 years, single dose of 1 tablet; 9 to 14 years, single dose of 2 tablets; and more than 14 years, single dose of 3 tablets, or
      (iii) Tetracycline (5 mg/kg/dose qid for 7 days, maximum 250 mg/dose) or clindamycin (20–40 mg/kg/day divided tid for 3 days) can be substituted for pyrimethamine-sulfadoxine if necessary.
      (iv) Mefloquine hydrochloride at 25 mg/kg (maximum 1,250 mg) can be used as alternative therapy. However, there is little experience with its use in small children, and it should not be used in pregnant women or in patients who are using beta blockers.
      (v) If the patient is critically ill and unable to take medication PO, use quinidine gluconate as in sec. above.
    (c) Multiply resistant areas. Should standard therapy fail in areas with multiply resistant strains of *P. falciparum*, the combination of quinine (as above) and tetracycline (5 mg/kg qid for 7 days) is recommended.
    (d) Response to therapy is evidenced by dramatic clinical improvement. Repeated blood smears show disappearance of parasitemia. **Pyrimethamine and primaquine are contraindicated in pregnancy.**

4. **Prevention.** Barrier protection from mosquitoes should be practiced whenever possible, especially between dusk and dawn. Persons traveling through or residing in malarious areas should receive prophylactic suppressive therapy as follows.
  a. **Chloroquine-sensitive area**

Table 5-6. Helminthic infections

Helminth	Clinical Features	Treatment
Roundworms		
Pinworms (*Enterobius vermicularis*)	Perianal pruritus	Mebendazole, 100 mg once; repeat in 2 wk Pyrantel pamoate, 10–20 mg/kg once; repeat
Ascaris (*A. lumbricoides*)	Vague abdominal distress; cough and pneumonia during lung migration	Pyrantel pamoate, 11 mg/kg in 1 dose, or Mebendazole, 100 mg for 3 d, or Piperazine citrate, 75 mg/kg/d for 2 d
Hookworm (*Necator* spp and *Ancyclostoma* spp)	Vague abdominal distress; anemia in severe infections	Mebendazole, 100 mg bid for 3 d Pyrantel pamoate, 11 mg/kg (maximum 1 g)/day for 3 days Albendazole, 400 mg once
Whipworm (*Trichuris trichiura*)	Rarely symptomatic; occasional colitis	Mebendazole, 100 mg bid for 3 days, or Albendazole, 400 mg once
Strongyloides (*S. stercoralis*)	Urticarial eruptions, abdominal pain, diarrhea; marked eosiniphilia	Thiabendazole, 25 mg/kg bid for 2 days (maximum 3 g/day)
Visceral larva migrans (*Toxocara canis* and *cati*)	Fever, hepatosplenomegaly; cough or wheezing; rarely identified in stool; marked eosinophilia	No therapy in mild cases Severe cases and ocular involvement: Diethylcarbamazine, 6 mg/kg/d divided tid for 7–10 d, or Albendazole, 400 mg bid for 3–5 d Corticosteroids and/or antihistamines may be helpful
Trichinosis (*Trichinella spiralis*)	History of ingestion of undercooked pork; fever, periorbital edema, headache, conjunctivitis, severe muscle pain	Mebendazole, 200–400 mg tid for 3 days, followed by 400–500 mg tid for 10 days Corticosteroids may help severe symptoms

Tapeworms (cestodes)		
Beef and pork tapeworms (*Taenia saginata* and *solium*)	Most patients are asymptomatic	Praziquantel, 10–20 mg once, or Niclosamide: 11–34 kg, 1 g in 1 dose; 34–50 kg, 1.5 g in 1 dose; >50 kg, 2 g in 1 dose
Cysticercosis (*T. solium*)	Systemic infection involving muscle, subcutaneous tissue, eye, and brain Symptoms occur with death of the cysticerci	Albendazole, 15 mg/kg/day in 3 doses for 28 days, or Praziquantel, 50 mg/kg/day in 3 doses for 15 day Dexamethasone is usually given concurrently
Fish tapeworm	Most are asymptomatic Vitamin B_{12} deficiency may occur	Same as for beef and pork tapeworm
Hydatid disease	Most are asymptomatic Liver and lung are primary sites	Surgical removal in some cases; contents should not be spilled Albendazole, 10 mg/kg/day for several months may be of benefit
Schistosoma	Serum sickness–like illness 4–8 wk after exposure; occult bloody diarrhea, hepatomegaly, portal hypertension, bladder fibrosis, pulmonary hypertension, CNS granulomas	*S. haematobium* or *mansoni*: praziquantel, two 20-mg/kg doses, 12 hr apart *S. japonicum* or *mekongi*: praziquantel, 20 mg/kg q8h for 3 doses

(1) Chloroquine phosphate, 5 mg base/kg (8.3 mg salt/kg; maximum 300 mg base) once a week, to be started 1 week before travel and continued for 4 weeks after the last exposure.

(2) To prevent relapsing malaria, a 14-day course of primaquine should be taken concurrently with the final 2 weeks of chloroquine therapy.

b. Chloroquine-resistant area

(1) For children 15 kg or greater, weekly mefloquine can be used for prophylaxis (15–19 kg, ¼ tablet; 20–30 kg, ½ tablet; 31–45 kg, ¾ tablet) to be started 1 week before travel and continued for 4 weeks after the last exposure. Mefloquine should not be given to travelers with epilepsy, a psychiatric disorder, cardiac conduction problems, or in the first trimester of pregnancy.

(2) For children who cannot take mefloquine and are 8 years of age or older, doxycycline (2 mg/kg/day; maximum 100 mg/day) can be used beginning the day before they enter the malarial area and continued for 4 weeks after they leave.

(3) For smaller and younger children, recommendations are more complex and should be done in consultation with a Traveler's Clinic or the CDC.

K. Helminthic infections. Table 5–6 outlines clinical features and therapy for specific infections.

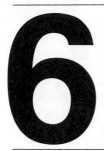

Management of the Sick Newborn*

Anne R. Hansen and
Charles F. Simmons

I. **Anticipation of high-risk delivery.** The majority of pregnancies result in the delivery of a healthy newborn. However, it is essential to identify maternal, fetal, perinatal, and neonatal conditions that increase the risk of neonatal illness. If possible, infants earlier than 32 weeks' gestation and those with known anomalies should be delivered in a hospital with an intensive care nursery. Intensive perinatal management (tocolytics, steroids, and fetal monitoring) can often optimize neonatal outcome.

A. **General antenatal assessment.** Factors associated with high-risk pregnancy are listed in Table 6-1. When assessing a high-risk pregnancy, it is most important to obtain information regarding gestational age, maturity of specific organ systems, fetal size and rate of growth, and fetal-placental health.

1. **Gestational age.** Accurate obstetric dating should supersede postnatal estimates unless there is a major discrepancy (>2 wk). Obstetric dating is a composite estimate based on the following information.

   a. **Date of the last menstrual period.**

   b. **Date of first reported fetal activity.** "Quickening" is first felt at approximately 16 to 20 weeks.

   c. **Date of first recorded fetal heart sounds,** approximately 10 to 12 weeks by ultrasonic Doppler and about 20 weeks by fetoscope.

   d. **Pregnancy tests.** Quantitative assessment of beta–human chorionic gonadotropin (beta-HCG).

   e. **Uterine size** is an accurate predictor in the absence of multiple gestations and structural abnormalities.

   f. **Early ultrasonographic findings.**

   g. **Dated fertility procedures** provide the exact gestational age.

2. **Maturity of specific organ systems.** Pulmonary maturation can be predicted from measurement of amniotic fluid phospholipids (see p. 178).

3. **Real-time ultrasonography** can identify structural malformations, fetal position, multiple gestations, abnormalities of fetal growth, ascites and hydrops, and other conditions revealed through amniocentesis or fetal blood and tissue sampling

4. **Fetal size and rate of growth** can be determined from uterine size and by ultrasonographic estimates of biparietal diameter, femur length, and abdominal circumference.

5. **Fetal well-being.** Fetuses at risk for intrapartum asphyxia require the pediatrician to be prepared for newborn resuscitation. Tests of fetal well-being include

   a. **Nonstress monitoring.** Assesses reflex acceleration of fetal heart rate, and is reliable from 32 weeks' gestation.

      (1) Reactive: reassuring.

      (2) Nonreactive: concerning, repeat. If nonreactive again, proceed to sec. **b** or **c** below.

   b. **Oxytocin challenge test** assesses fetal reserve during uterine contractions.

*For a more comprehensive discussion of newborn management, consult JP Cloherty, AR Stark (eds). *Manual of Neonatal Care* (3rd ed). Boston: Little, Brown, 1991.

Table 6-1. Perinatal risk factors associated with an increased risk to the newborn

Condition	Risk to newborn
Maternal condition	
Maternal age > 35	Chromosomal abnormalities, SGA
Maternal age < 16	Prematurity
Poverty	Prematurity, infection, SGA
Infertility, assisted reproductive technology	SGA, congenital anomalies, increased prenatal mortality
Smoking	SGA, increased perinatal mortality
Drug or alcohol abuse	SGA, fetal alcohol syndrome, withdrawal syndrome, sudden infant death
Anemia	SGA, asphyxia, stillbirth
Diabetes	Stillbirth, hyaline membrane disease, congenital anomalies
Heart or lung disease	SGA, stillbirth, prematurity
Hypertension, chronic or preeclampsia	SGA, asphyxia, stillbirth, prematurity
Isoimmunization (platelets)	Stillbirth, bleeding
Isoimmunization (red cell antigens)	Stillbirth, anemia, jaundice
Renal disease	SGA, stillbirth
Thrombocytopenia	Stillbirth, bleeding
Thyroid disease	Goiter, hypothyroidism, hyperthyroidism
TORCH infections	See TORCH infections, sec. **VIII.A.1**
Polyhydramnios	Anomalies (anencephaly, GI obstruction, renal disease, goiter)
Uterine malformation, uterine trauma, incompetent cervix	Prematurity
Preeclampsia	SGA
Low urinary estriols	SGA, stillbirth, anencephaly
Bleeding in early pregnancy	Prematurity, stillbirth
Bleeding in third trimester	Anemia, prematurity, stillbirth
Premature rupture of membranes, fever, infection	Infection, prematurity
Past history of infant with jaundice, respiratory distress syndrome, or anomalies	Increased risk of recurrence in neonate
Maternal medications, corticosteroids, antimetabolites, antithyroid medications, reserpine, salicylates, etc.	See individual package inserts; see also JP Cloherty, AR Stark (eds). *Manual of Neonatal Care.* Boston: Little, Brown, 1991
Fetal conditions	
Multiple birth	Prematurity, twin transfusion syndrome, asphyxia, SGA
Poor fetal growth	Asphyxia, stillbirth, congenital anomalies
Abnormal fetal position	Trauma, hemorrhage, deformities
Abnormality of fetal heart rate or rhythm	Asphyxia, heart failure, heart block
Acidosis	Asphyxia, respiratory distress syndrome
Condition of labor or delivery	
Premature labor	Respiratory distress, asphyxia
Labor occurring 2 wk or more after term	Stillbirth, asphyxia, meconium aspiration
Long labor	Asphyxia, stillbirth
Meconium-stained amniotic fluid	Asphyxia, meconium aspiration syndrome, stillbirth
Prolapsed cord	Asphyxia
Maternal hypotension	Asphyxia, stillbirth
Rapid labor	Trauma
Analgesia and anesthesia	Respiratory depression, hypotension

Table 6-1 (continued)

Condition	Risk to newborn
Neonatal condition	
Low Apgar score	Intracranial hemorrhage, respiratory distress, anoxic-ischemic encephalopathy
Foul smell of baby, amniotic fluid, or membranes	Infection
Placental anomalies	
Small placenta	SGA
Large placenta	Hydrops, heart failure
Torn placenta	Blood loss
Vasa previa	Blood loss

SGA = small for gestational age; TORCH = toxoplasmosis, rubella, cytomegalic inclusion disease, and herpes simplex.

    c. Ultrasound biophysical profile (BPP)
       (1) Ten-point scale, similar to Apgar score.
       (2) Two points each for fetal breathing, tone, activity, heart rate (non-stress test), and amniotic fluid volume.
       (3) Interpretation: 3 or less—intervene; 4 to 7—retest/suspect; 8 or greater—reassuring.
    d. Intrapartum fetal heart rate monitoring.
    e. Fetal scalp pH. Concerning if less than 7.25.
    f. Percutaneous umbilical blood sampling to assess fetal acid-base status (see below).
  B. Identified fetal risks. High-risk pregnancies should be referred to a perinatal center for evaluation.
    1. Maternal medical problems. Women with serious preexisting or acquired medical conditions, such as preeclampsia, should be evaluated for delivery at a tertiary care center.
    2. Maternal infection
      a. Routine screening: rubella, hepatitis B (hepatitis B surface antigen [HBsAg]), and syphilis exposure (rapid plasma reagin [RPR]).
      b. Additional screening: group B streptococcus genitourinary colonization, tuberculosis.
    3. Genetics. Fetuses may demonstrate an abnormal karotype or inherited Mendelian disorder.
    4. Anomalies identified by prenatal ultrasound.
  C. Intrapartum tests of fetal well-being
    1. Fetal heart rate monitoring
      a. Baseline rate
        (1) Normal: 120 to 160 beats per minute.
        (2) Bradycardia: fetal congenital heart malformation, maternal systemic lupus erythematosus (SLE) with fetal heart block.
        (3) Tachycardia: maternal fever, chorioamnionitis, fetal tachyarrhythmia +/- fetal congestive heart failure (CHF).
      b. Beat-to-beat variability
        (1) Normal: 5 to 10 beats per minute.
        (2) Reduced: fetal CNS depression due to hypoxia, fetal sleep, fetal immaturity, maternal narcotic or sedative exposure.
      c. Decelerations
        (1) Early (type I): coincident with onset of uterine contractions, secondary to head compression; normal.
        (2) Late (type II): start after onset of uterine contractions, suggest fetal hypoxia.

(3) Variable (type III): no consistent temporal relationship to contractions. May suggest umbilical cord compression but is often normal. Concerning when associated with other abnormalities of fetal monitoring.

II. Care of the newborn in the delivery room

A. Preparation

1. A thorough knowledge of the maternal and fetal history is essential (see sec. **I**).
2. The factors associated with increased risk to the newborn are listed in Table 6-1. Two clinicians experienced in the resuscitation of the newborn should be present at the delivery of a high-risk infant. One clinician must be skilled in intubation.
3. Before the delivery of a high-risk infant, the pediatric clinicians should discuss the expected condition and prognosis of the infant with the parent.
4. **Equipment** should be located and tested before delivery
   a. Preheated radiant warmer bed, prewarmed blankets.
   b. Cord-cutting materials and clamp.
   c. **Suction** with manometer. Suction should be set to 80 to 100 cm H_2O.
   d. Infant suction bulb.
   e. **Oxygen** source with flowmeter and an **anesthesia bag** or self-inflating bag with a reservoir capable of delivering 100% oxygen, an adjustable valve or "pop-off" control, and an in-line manometer for observing airway pressure. Oxygen should flow at 5 to 8 liters per minute and valve position should be tested.
   f. Infant **face masks** large enough to cover the mouth and nose without covering the eyes.
   g. **Infant stethoscope.**
   h. **Laryngoscope** with size 0 and 1 **blades**, fresh batteries, and bulbs.
   i. Uniform-diameter **endotracheal tubes** with 2.5-, 3.0-, and 3.5-mm internal diameters (at least two of each). Stylets should be used with caution because of the risk of airway trauma.
   j. **Feeding tube** (No. 8 French [F]), 20-ml syringe, and adhesive tape for gastric decompression.
   k. **Drugs. Epinephrine,** 1 : 10,000; **NaHCO₃,** 0.5 mEq/ml (4.2%); **naloxone** (Narcan), 0.4 or 1.0 mg/ml; saline; and albumin (5%). *The use of NaHCO₃ during neonatal resuscitation should be reserved for those infants with metabolic acidosis and effective ventilation.*
   l. **Umbilical catheterization tray** with 3.5F and 5F catheters, three-way stopcock, and 10- and 20-ml syringes.
   m. A prewarmed transport **Isolette** with portable oxygen supply.
   n. Caps, masks, goggles or face shield, gloves, and gown should be worn routinely as universal precautions.

B. Immediately after delivery (Fig. 6-1)

1. **General procedures**
   a. Place the infant on a warming table.
   b. Dry the infant and remove wet linen.
   c. Position the infant with the neck slightly extended.
   d. If effective respirations do not begin, *stimulate* the infant briefly by vigorously rubbing the back or flicking/slapping the soles.
   e. **Evaluate the infant's respirations.**
      (1) If respirations are spontaneous and effective, evaluate heart rate.
      (2) If infant is apneic, or respirations are ineffective, proceed with positive pressure ventilation (PPV) (see **3** below).
   f. **Evaluate the heart rate**
      (1) If heart rate is greater than 100, check skin color.
      (2) If heart rate is less than 100, proceed with PPV (see **3** below).
   g. **Evaluate skin color**
      (1) If no central cyanosis is present, observe.
      (2) If central cyanosis is present, administer free-flow oxygen at 5 to 8 liters per minute, with tubing held steadily 1 cm from nares or with

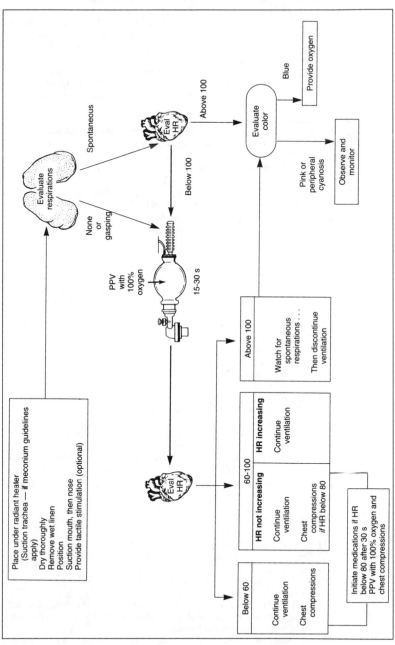

Fig. 6-1. Overview of resuscitation in the delivery room. (Reproduced with permission from RS Bloom, C Cropley, and the AHA/AAP Neonatal Resuscitation Program Steering Committee. *Textbook of Neonatal Resuscitation*, 1987, 1990, 1994. Copyright American Heart Association.)

firmly applied oxygen mask. Slowly withdraw and observe carefully for recurrence of cyanosis.

  h. All infants should have a brief examination for anomalies.

2. Meconium at delivery

  a. If thick meconium is present, the obstetrician should suction the oropharynx before the shoulders are delivered. When received from the obstetrician, intubate and suction the trachea before triggering the first breath by drying and stimulating the infant.

  b. If thick meconium is not present, bulb suction the mouth first, then the nose. **Gastric aspiration and deep suctioning in the first 5 minutes of life can produce bradycardia and should not be done routinely.**

  c. Continue as in **1** above.

3. Resuscitative procedures

  a. If infant is apneic or cyanotic, or respirations are ineffective, positive pressure ventilation should be administered with 100% oxygen. Ventilate at a rate of 40 to 60 breaths per minute.

   (1) The following initial pressures are recommended.

     (a) First breath: 30 to 40 cm H_2O.

     (b) Succeeding breaths: 15 to 20 cm H_2O is often adequate.

     (c) Pulmonary disease: 20 to 40 cm H_2O may be required.

   (2) If there is inadequate chest movement with PPV:

     (a) Reapply mask to face (adequate seal).

     (b) Reposition the head (adequate airway).

     (c) Suction secretions, if present (adequate airway).

     (d) Ventilate with the infant's mouth slightly open (for blocked airway).

     (e) Increase pressure to 20 to 40 cm H_2O (adequate pressure).

   (3) After 15 to 30 seconds, the heart rate, (HR) should be rechecked.

     (a) If the heart rate is greater than 100 and spontaneous respirations are observed, apply free-flow oxygen and then withdraw as above.

     (b) If the heart rate is 60 to 100 and increasing, continue PPV, then recheck after another 15 to 30 seconds.

     (c) If the heart rate is less than 100 and not increasing, PPV is continued. Start chest compressions if HR is less than 80 and not increasing.

  b. An orogastric catheter should be inserted and left in place if bag-and-mask ventilation is required for more than 2 minutes. The length of the inserted catheter should be equal to the distance from the bridge of the nose to the earlobe to the xiphoid. A 20-ml syringe is used to remove the gastric contents. The catheter is taped to the infant's cheek.

  c. Chest compressions, if necessary, should be performed by depressing the lower third of the sternum (below a line between the nipples and above the xiphoid) with two thumbs (with the hands encircling the torso) or the index and middle fingers. The sternum should be depressed ½ to ¾ in. at a rate of 120 times per minute.

  d. Endotracheal intubation is necessary in the following situations (see sec. **III.A.2**).

   (1) Prolonged positive pressure ventilation is required.

   (2) Bag-and-mask ventilation is ineffective.

   (3) Tracheal suctioning is required.

   (4) Diaphragmatic hernia is suspected (see also sec. **XIII.D.3**).

  e. Medications (Table 6-2 and Fig. 6-2).

   (1) Epinephrine is indicated if the heart rate is zero or remains below 80 despite adequate ventilation (with 100% oxygen) and chest compressions for a minimum of 30 seconds.

   (2) Naloxone is indicated if the infant exhibits respiratory depression and has a history of maternal narcotic exposure.

   (3) Common sites of drug administration

     (a) Epinephrine and naloxone diluted in 1 to 2 ml normal saline

Table 6-2. Medications for neonatal resuscitation

Medication	Concentration to administer	Preparation	Dosage/route	Rate/precautions
Epinephrine	1 : 10 000	1 ml	0.01–0.03 mg/kg 0.1–0.3 mg/kg IV or ET	Give rapidly Can dilute with normal saline to 1–2 ml if giving ET
Volume expanders	Whole blood 5% albumin-saline Normal saline Ringer's lactate	40 ml	10 ml/kg IV	Give over 5–10 min Give by syringe or IV drip
Sodium bicarbonate	0.5 mEq/ml (4.2% solution)	20 ml *or* Two 10-ml prefilled syringes	2 mEq/kg IV only (4 ml/kg)	Give slowly, over at least 2 min Give only if infant is being effectively ventilated
Naloxone hydrochloride	0.4 mg/ml	1 ml	0.1 mg/kg (0.25 ml/kg) IV, ET, IM, SQ	Give rapidly
	1.0 mg/ml	1 ml	0.1 mg/kg (0.1 ml/kg) IV, ET, IM, SQ	IV, ET preferred IM, SQ acceptable

ET = endotracheal.
Source: RS Bloom, C Cropley, and the AHA/AHP Neonatal Resuscitation Program Steering Committee. *Textbook of Neonatal Resuscitation*, 1987, 1990, 1994. Copyright American Heart Association.

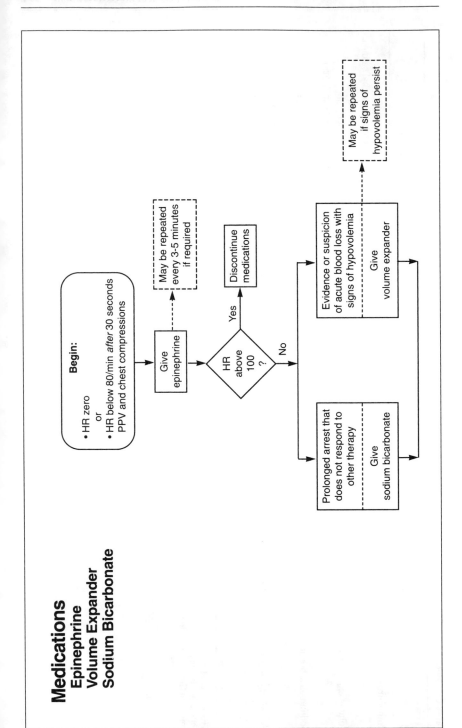

Medications
Epinephrine
Volume Expander
Sodium Bicarbonate

Begin:

- HR zero
  or
- HR below 80/min *after* 30 seconds
  PPV and chest compressions

Give
epinephrine

May be repeated
every 3-5 minutes
if required

HR
above
100
?

Yes → Discontinue
medications

No

Prolonged arrest that
does not respond to
other therapy

Give
sodium bicarbonate

Evidence or suspicion
of acute blood loss with
signs of hypovolemia

Give
volume expander

May be repeated
if signs of
hypovolemia persist

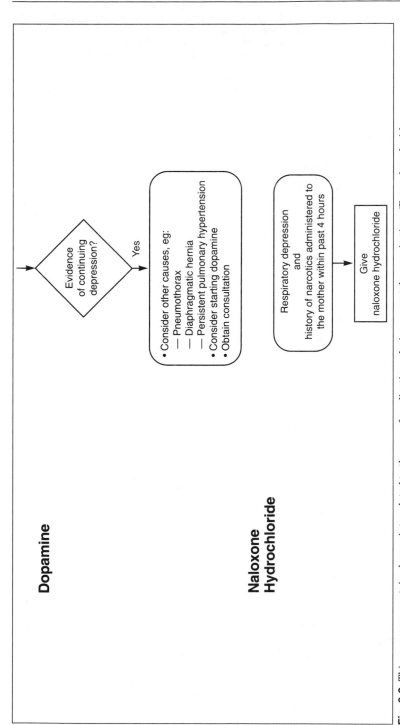

Fig. 6-2. This summary contains key points related to the use of medications during neonatal resuscitation. (Reproduced with permission from RS Bloom, C Cropley, and the AHA/AAP Neonatal Resuscitation Program Steering Committee. *Textbook of Neonatal Resuscitation*, 1987, 1990, 1994. Copyright American Heart Association.)

can be administered by endotracheal instillation until vascular access is available.

  (b) An **umbilical venous catheter** can be inserted into the vein of the umbilical stump until the tip of the saline-flush catheter is just below the skin level and free flow of blood is present.

  f. Inform the parents of assessment and plan when feasible. If the infant appears well, encourage the parents to hold the infant when appropriate.

  g. **Apgar scores** are assigned to describe the infant's condition at 1 and 5 minutes, and every 5 minutes until the score is greater than 7 (Table 6-3).

III. Intensive care of the sick newborn
  A. Management of the airway and respiration
    1. Establish patency of the airway. The infant can usually be adequately ventilated by bag and mask until preparations are made for intubation.
    2. Intubation in the delivery room
      a. Equipment. In the delivery room or in an emergency, *oral* intubation is quickest and easiest. *Nasotracheal* placement may be more stable for long-term use. Endotracheal tube size (internal diameter in mm) can be determined using the table below, or can be calculated as follows:

$$\text{ETT size} = \frac{\text{postconceptional age in weeks}}{10}$$

Infant weight (g)	Tube size	Laryngoscope blade
<1,000	2.5	0
1,000–2,000	3.0	0
>2,000	3.5	0–1

      b. Method
        (1) Suction the stomach and oropharynx.
        (2) If the intubation is elective, attach a cardiac monitor and an oximeter or transcutaneous oxygen tension (PO_2) monitor.
        (3) Determine the proper tube length before intubation. For orotracheal intubation, a mnemonic is "1–2–3 kg, 7–8-9 cm, tip to lip." For nasotracheal intubation, add 2 to 3 cm.
        (4) The baby should be ventilated with a bag and mask just before intubation.
        (5) The infant's head should be placed in a neutral position, *avoiding excessive extension or flexion of the neck.* Hold the laryngoscope between the thumb and first finger of the left hand. Use the second and third fingers to hold the chin and stabilize the head. Open the mouth with the right hand. Push down on the larynx with the fifth finger of the left hand (or have an assistant do it) and keep the infant's head straight. Pass the laryngoscope into the right side of the mouth and then swing it to the midline, pushing the tongue out of the way.
        (6) Hold the endotracheal tube with the right hand and insert it directly between the vocal cords to about 2 cm below the glottis. Most commercial tubes are marked with a circumferential ring, which should

Table 6-3. Apgar score*

Sign	0	1	2
Heart rate	Absent	Slow, <100 beats/min	>100 beats/min
Respiratory effort	Absent	Weak cry, hypoventilation	Crying lustily
Muscle tone	Limp	Some flexion of extremities	Well flexed
Reflex irritability	No response	Some motion	Crying
Color	Blue, pale	Pink body, blue extremities	Entirely pink

*Score infant at 1 and 5 min of age.

come to rest at the vocal cords. During nasotracheal intubation, Magill forceps are usually necessary to guide the tube between the cords. If the fifth finger is pressing on the trachea, the tube can be felt as it slips into place. *A stylet should be used only if necessary, to stiffen the endotracheal tube.* Resistance can indicate incorrect positioning of the infant or anatomic abnormality of the upper airway.

(7) During the procedure, one person should continually observe the infant and monitor the heart rate. **The infant should not be allowed to become hypoxic or bradycardic during intubation.** If bradycardia occurs, if there is doubt about successful tube placement, or if intubation has not been accomplished within 20 seconds, stop the procedure and ventilate the infant with a bag and mask.

(8) Check the tube position by auscultation to ensure equal aeration of both lungs. If air entry is poor over the left chest, pull back the tube until aeration improves. Auscultate the area over the stomach to evaluate the possibility of an esophageal intubation.

(9) If air entry remains asymmetric despite tube repositioning, evaluate the infant for possible pneumothorax by auscultation, transillumination, or portable chest x-ray. If chest movement is poor, the tube is in a good position, no pneumothorax is present, and adequate ventilatory pressure is being used, consider anatomic or developmental abnormalities (e.g., diaphragmatic hernia, hypoplastic lungs, severe lung immaturity) with poor lung compliance.

(10) Tape the tube securely and obtain an x-ray to check its position.

3. **Ventilation**
   a. **Continuous positive airway pressure (CPAP)** is indicated for
      (1) Hyaline membrane disease (HMD), when an inspired oxygen concentration (FiO_2) greater than 0.4 to 0.6 is required to maintain an arterial oxygen tension (PaO_2) of 50 to 70 mm Hg, or when there is significant clinical worsening during the first day of life. Application of CPAP early in the course of HMD can decrease the time spent in high oxygen concentrations, reduces alveolar collapse, and avoids the need for mechanical ventilation.
      (2) Apnea that is unresponsive to other forms of therapy (see p. 184).
      (3) Postextubation management for babies with reduced respiratory reserve.
   b. **Intermittent positive pressure ventilation (IPPV)** is indicated for
      (1) HMD, when the PaO_2 is less than 60 mm Hg at an FiO_2 of 0.4 to 0.6 on adequate CPAP. **Surfactant** administration is often warranted in these circumstances (see p. 179).
      (2) Respiratory failure: **carbon dioxide tension (PCO_2) is greater than 60 to 70 mm Hg;** pH is less than 7.20.
      (3) Apnea unresponsive to CPAP.
   c. The actual levels of PaO_2 and arterial carbon dioxide tension ($PaCO_2$) selected for intervention depend on the disease course.
      (1) For hyaline membrane disease, ventilation is adjusted to maintain PaO_2 = 50–70 mm Hg, $PaCO_2$ = 45–55 mm Hg, and pH = 7.28–7.35.
      (2) Patients with persistent pulmonary hypertension may require a respiratory alkalosis with systemic alkalosis (see p. 183).
      (3) Patients with exclusively alveolar disease should be ventilated normally.

B. **Shock in the delivery room.** Blood pressure in healthy newborns varies by birth weight. Emergency packed red cells, 5% albumin, or normal saline may be required for volume expansion in cases of acute perinatal hemorrhage.

C. **Other emergency procedures**
   1. **Blood gas sampling**
      a. Capillary (arterialized) blood obtained from a warmed heel in a heparinized Natelson tube, by heel stick.

    b. Direct puncture of the radial or posterior tibial artery. Avoid brachial and femoral arterial punctures.

    c. If the infant's condition is unstable, cannulation of the umbilical, radial, posterior tibial, or dorsalis pedis arteries may be necessary.

    d. Catheters in the temporal artery are relatively contraindicated.

2. Umbilical artery catheters. Indwelling arterial catheters increase the risk of life-threatening infection and thromboembolism.

    a. Indications

        (1) Patients with a high risk of death from their primary disease (e.g., extreme prematurity, birth weight < 1,000 g, HMD, persistent pulmonary hypertension, severe aspiration pneumonia, shock).

        (2) Patients who require frequent arterial blood sampling.

        (3) Alternatives to invasive arterial monitoring include use of transcutaneous PO_2 monitoring and pulse oximetry.

    b. Methods

        (1) Use sterile procedure (gloves, gown, mask, and cap).

        (2) Measure shoulder to umbilical distance before draping patient, in order to calculate appropriate catheter insertion length. Estimate the insertion depth by referring to Fig. 6-3 or by using one of the following formulas (for high lines).

            (a) Shoulder-umbilical cord distance + 2 cm.

            (b) (3 × birth weight in kg) + 9 cm.

        (3) Carefully wash the cord and surrounding area with povidone-iodine (Betadine) and then alcohol. Excessive iodine exposure can induce either transient hypothyroidism or hyperthyroidism. Drape the infant's abdomen with sterile towels.

        (4) Cut the cord 1.0 cm from the skin. Tie the base with a cord tie.

        (5) Identify the two umbilical arteries. Gently insert one, then two tips of a pair of iris forceps into the lumen of one artery. Slowly allow the forceps to expand and dilate the artery.

        (6) Insert a saline-filled catheter (5 Fr for infants who weigh over 1,250 g and 3.5F for infants who weigh under 1,250 g) the precalculated distance into the artery.

        (7) Obtain a radiograph after placement of all umbilical catheters. The tip should be either at or below the level of L3–L4 or just above the diaphragm (T6-T10).

        (8) Secure the properly positioned catheter with a suture and adhesive tape.

        (9) Infuse a solution containing 0.5 to 1.0 units heparin/ml infusate to minimize thrombosis.

        (10) Remove arterial catheters as soon as possible.

3. Peripheral arterial catheters can be placed as an alternative to an umbilical aterial catheter (see Chap. 7).

4. Umbilical vein catheters

    a. Indications. Umbilical vein catheters are used for emergency access to the circulation, for exchange transfusion, and for central venous access in very sick or very small (<750 g) infants.

    b. Methods

        (1) Prepare as for umbilical artery (UA) catheterization.

        (2) Identify the vein, remove visible clots, and dilate with a pair of iris forceps.

        (3) Insert a saline-filled 5F catheter. If the infant weighs less than 1,250 g, a 3.5F catheter may be necessary. A multiholed catheter is used for exchange transfusions, and a single-holed catheter for long-term placement. Estimate insertion depth and confirm position by x-ray before hypertonic infusions are begun by referring to Fig. 6-4, or by using one of the following formulas.

            (a) Two thirds of shoulder-umbilical cord distance.

            (b) (½ UA line calculation) − 1 cm (see **2.b.(2)** above).

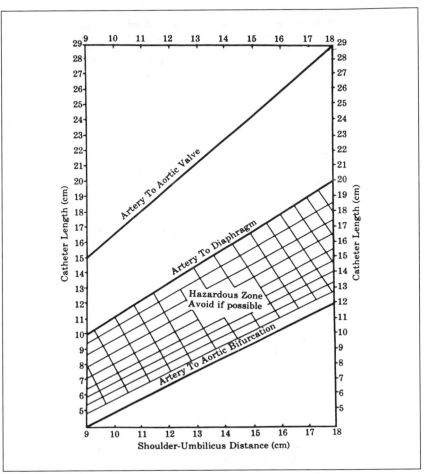

Fig. 6-3. Shoulder-umbilical distance measured above lateral end of clavicle to umbilicus versus length of umbilical artery catheter needed to reach designated level. (From PM Dunn. *Arch Dis Child* 41:69, 1966.) Alternative calculation by weight is: Catheter length (in cm) = 3(birth weight in kg) + 9. (From H Shukla. *Am J Dis Child* 140:786, 1986. Copyright 1986, American Medical Association.)

> **(4)** For exchange transfusion, insert the catheter until free blood flow is achieved (usually 5–7 cm). Keep the catheter and surrounding area sterile during placement and transfusion. Following exchange, place a purse-string silk suture around the vein before removing the catheter. For subsequent exchanges, the cord should be soaked with warm saline until it is soft. The suture will assist in identification of the vein and reinsertion of the catheter.

IV. Respiratory diseases

A. Hyaline membrane disease (HMD)

1. **Etiology.** Absence or deficiency of surfactant, a complex phospholipid and protein mixture that normally lines alveoli and decreases surface tension. The risk of HMD is increased with prematurity and factors that impair lung maturation and surfactant production.

2. Prenatal evaluation
  a. Reliable amniotic fluid indices of fetal lung development include the lecithin-sphingomyelin (L/S) ratio, disaturated phosphatidylcholine (DSPC) concentration, and fetal lung maturity (FLM) test. The predictive value of an assessment of fetal lung maturity depends on the gestational age of the fetus (prior probability) and value of the L/S, SPC, or FLM.
    (1) An L/S ratio that exceeds 2.0 predicts less than a 5% risk of HMD in fetuses of 28 to 32 weeks' gestation.
    (2) The L/S ratio must be greater than 3.5 : 1 or the DSPC greater than or equal to 1,000 to predict pulmonary maturity in infants of diabetic mothers. The predictive value of the FLM in diabetic women has not been established
    (3) The risk is less than 1% if the DSPC is greater than or equal to 500 µg/dl.
  b. Maternal corticosteroid therapy. If an infant of less than 34 weeks' gestation with evidence of pulmonary immaturity (L/S < 2 : 1) must be delivered, pulmonary maturity can be accelerated by treatment with maternal glucocorticoids.
    (1) Betamethasone or **dexamethasone,** administered over 48 hours.
    (2) Reassessment of fetal lung maturity indices will guide subsequent glucocorticoid therapy if the infant remains undelivered for more than 7 days and the risk of premature delivery remains high.
3. Postnatal evaluation must rule out sepsis, pneumonia, transient tachypnea of the newborn, pneumothorax, and congenital heart disease.
  a. Physical examination. Signs of HMD in the premature infant include grunting respirations, flaring, retractions, tachypnea, and hypoxia in room air, with onset of signs shortly after birth.
  b. Laboratory
    (1) Chest radiograph.
    (2) An arterial blood gas (ABG) should be obtained and oximeter or transcutaneous PO_2 monitoring should be initiated.
    (3) Hypoxemic infants should be evaluated for congenital heart disease (see sec. **V,** p. 185).
    (4) Blood culture.
    (5) Complete blood count, including a platelet count.
4. Diagnosis is confirmed by the chest radiograph. The radiographic appearance of HMD includes low lung volumes and a generalized haziness or a reticulogranular "ground glass" pattern with air bronchograms.
5. Treatment
  a. Temperature must be carefully regulated, especially in the low-birthweight infant.
  b. Oxygen
    (1) Dosage. The lowest concentration of oxygen to maintain the PaO_2 at about 55 to 65 mm Hg should be administered. Oxygen should be properly warmed and humidified, and the humidity chamber changed daily to minimize bacterial growth. Oxygen should be administered via oxygen-air blenders with precise control over the concentration of administered oxygen, and **checked at least every hour.** If an infant requires intermittent assisted ventilation with an anesthesia bag, the oxygen concentration administered via the bag should be similar to that usually required by the infant. Blood gases should be obtained 15 to 20 minutes after a change in respiratory therapy and regularly while receiving oxygen. The use of a transcutaneous PO_2 ($TcPO_2$) monitor or pulse oximeter allows the continuous assessment of the infant's oxygenation and decreases the need for frequent blood gas monitoring.
    (2) Oxygen toxicity. Prolonged PaO_2 over 100 mm Hg may contribute to retinopathy of prematurity in infants less than 1,500 g.

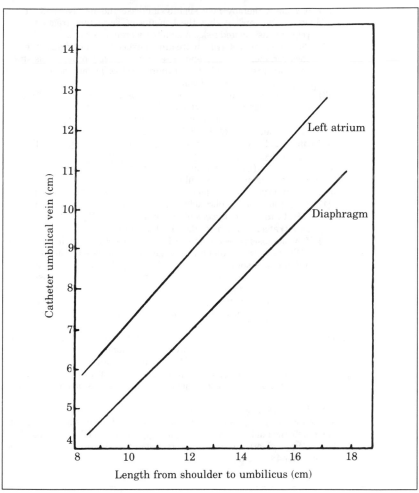

Fig. 6-4. Length from shoulder to umbilicus versus length of umbilical vein catheter. (From PM Dunn. *Arch Dis Child* 41:69, 1966.) Alternative calculation by weight is: Catheter length (in cm) = ½(UA catheter length) + 1 (see legend Fig. 6-3). (From H Shukla. *Am J Dis Child* 140:786, 1986. Copyright 1986, American Medical Association.)

Administration of high concentrations of oxygen can also be toxic to the lungs of all newborns.

- **(3) Delivery of oxygen.** If the infant's oxygen requirement exceeds that which can be delivered by hood (PaO$_2$ < 50 mm Hg despite FiO$_2$ > 0.6), or if hypercapnia (PaCO$_2$ > 60 mm Hg) or apnea uncontrolled by other therapies is present, CPAP or mechanical ventilation is indicated (see sec. III.A.3).
- **c. Surfactant replacement therapy.** Early administration of exogenous surfactant to premature infants with surfactant deficiency can significantly reduce the severity of HMD, decrease the incidence of pneumothorax, and improve survival rates.

(1) Surfactant therapy may slightly increase the relative risk of pulmonary hemorrhage but the benefits of surfactant treatment outweigh the associated risks. Absolute risk remains small.

(2) The benefit of prophylactic treatment exceeds that of rescue therapy. However, increased risk and expense accompany prophylaxis strategies since respiratory distress syndrome (RDS) would never have developed in many treated babies.

(3) Currently, there are two Food and Drug Administration (FDA)–approved preparations of surfactant in the United States.

  (a) Survanta, 4 cc/kg via endotracheal tube (ETT) q6h × 4.

  (b) Exosurf, 5 cc/kg via ETT q12h × 2–4.

d. Fluid and electrolyte balance should be maintained (see p. 213). Relative dehydration decreases the incidence and severity of HMD, bronchopulmonary dysplasia (BPD), and patent ductus arteriosus (PDA).

e. Severe **metabolic acidosis** should be corrected with bicarbonate infusion if the patient is ventilating adequately to excrete excess carbon dioxide.

  (1) In profound metabolic acidosis (pH < 7.10), infuse a solution of $NaHCO_3$ to correct the calculated base deficit (mEq = 0.3 × kg × base deficit) at a rate no faster than 1 mEq/kg/min.

  (2) If the acidosis is less severe (pH 7.10), correct by slow infusion of an $NaHCO_3$-dextrose solution to replace the calculated deficit over several hours. A solution of 15 mEq $NaHCO_3$/dl in 5 or 10% dextrose in water (D/W) will provide adequate treatment of the acidosis while avoiding the use of hyperosmolar solutions, which have been associated with intraventricular hemorrhage in the premature neonate. Infusion of sodium bicarbonate obligates a sodium load and can expand extracellular fluid volume.

f. Follow **blood pressure** and cardiac output carefully (Fig. 6-5). If the infant is hypovolemic, support intravascular volume with infusions of normal saline, 5% albumin, or packed RBC as appropriate.

g. Maintain adequate **oxygen-carrying capacity** by transfusion of packed RBCs. Monitor blood glucose frequently during transfusions to avoid hypoglycemia.

h. Antibiotic coverage (ampicillin and an aminoglycoside) should be considered after appropriate cultures have been obtained, since pneumonia can mimic the clinical and radiographic appearance of HMD. If clinical and laboratory evaluation of infection are negative, antibiotics can be discontinued after 48 to 72 hours.

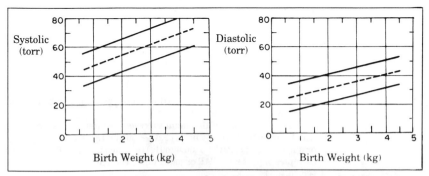

Fig. 6-5. Linear regressions (*broken lines*) and 95% confidence limits (*solid lines*) of systolic (*left*) and diastolic (*right*) aortic blood pressures on birth weight in 61 healthy newborn infants during the first 12 hours after birth. (From HT Versmold et al. *Pediatrics* 67:607, 1981. Copyright 1981, American Academy of Pediatrics.)

  i. Hypocalcemia and hyperbilirubinemia should be corrected as described on p. 203 and p. 192.
  j. Appropriate nutrition should be provided. Feedings can often be started by the third or fourth day in mild illnesses. In more severe illnesses, however, this may not be possible, and IV hyperalimentation should be given to provide additional carbohydrate, lipid, and protein (see Chap. 11).
  k. The risk of **complications of prematurity,** such as intraventricular hemorrhage, PDA, pneumothorax, nosocomial infection, bronchopulmonary dysplasia, retinopathy of prematurity, and hearing loss, increase with severity of respiratory illness.
B. Perinatal meconium aspiration can obstruct newborn airways, impair gas exchange, increase pulmonary vascular resistance, and result in severe respiratory distress and hypoxemia.
  1. Etiology. Passage of meconium in utero and subsequent aspiration; can result from hypoxic and ischemic stress.
  2. Evaluation and diagnosis
    a. History. Severity of disease is related to the thickness of the meconium, amount aspirated, and presence of persistent pulmonary hypertension or sequelae of neonatal depression.
    b. Physical examination. Respiratory distress can be mild to severe.
    c. Laboratory
      (1) ABG. Systemic hypoxemia is more prominent than respiratory acidosis.
      (2) Chest radiographs can demonstrate coarse, irregular, pulmonary alveolar densities. Also, 10 to 20% of infants will have associated pneumothorax or pneumomediastinum.
      (3) A CBC and blood culture are indicated because meconium aspiration increases the risk of bacterial pneumonia.
  3. Therapy
    a. Prevention
      (1) Prevention of passage of meconium in utero. Tests of fetal well-being can be done in pregnancies at risk for uteroplacental insufficiency, including postterm (> 42 weeks) pregnancies.
      (2) Prevention of meconium aspiration
        (a) Thick, particulate, or "pea-soup" meconium (see p. 170).
        (b) Immediately after birth, the infant should be passed to a warming table. A clinician should intubate and suction the trachea under direct laryngoscopy with a 3.0- to 3.5-mm endotracheal tube. Wall suction (set at 100 mm H_2O) should be used. Intubation and suction should be performed until the meconium has been cleared. One or two intubations are usually sufficient.
        (c) Oxygen by mask should be administered as soon as the trachea has been cleared.
        (d) The airway should be cleared and ventilation initiated before significant bradycardia occurs.
        (e) It is not necessary to suction the trachea of infants born through thin meconium who have effective respirations at the time of delivery. Risk of intubation exceeds the benefit of suctioning in this circumstance.
      (3) Respiratory physiotherapy and **oropharyngeal suction** should be provided to assist pulmonary toilet.
      (4) Hypoxia should be treated with supplemental oxygen. Severe metabolic acidosis should be corrected with a bicarbonate infusion (see sec. **A.5.e** above). Careful monitoring of blood gases is essential, and the placement of an indwelling arterial catheter for blood sampling may be required. Treatment of persistent hypoxia (PaO_2 < 50 mm Hg) or severe hypercapnia ($PaCO_2$ > 60 mm Hg) requires intubation and mechanical ventilation (see pp. 174–5).

(5) Maintenance fluid and electrolytes should be provided.

(6) If a radiographic infiltrate is evident, broad-spectrum antibiotics should be administered after blood cultures have been obtained.

(7) Hypoxia and acidosis can contribute to **persistent pulmonary hypertension** with resultant hypoxemia due to right-to-left shunting of blood via the patent ductus arteriosus or foramen ovale, or both.

C. Air leak

    1. Etiology: results from dissection of air into the pulmonary parenchyma outside the alveolar and bronchial tree.

    2. Evaluation and diagnosis

        a. History. Increased risk of pneumothorax occurs in infants with HMD or pneumonia, infants who have required resuscitation, or infants with meconium aspiration syndrome.

        b. Physical examination

            (1) Clinical signs of **pneumothorax** develop rapidly and include moderate to severe respiratory distress, cyanosis, reduced breath sounds, chest asymmetry, a shift of the apical beat away from the side of pneumothorax, and a decline in blood pressure and perfusion.

            (2) Pneumomediastinum can cause distant heart sounds and may be a harbinger of other air leak. It is most reliably diagnosed by chest radiograph.

            (3) Pneumopericardium causes immediate deterioration in blood pressure, heart rate, and arterial oxygen saturation and can be lethal if not diagnosed and treated quickly. It should be considered in the presence of pneumomediastinum and pneumothorax.

            (4) Pneumoperitoneum. Air can dissect into the abdomen through the posterior mediastinum. Rarely a cause of significant respiratory compromise, a perforated abdominal viscus must be excluded. Accurate diagnosis requires evaluation of clinical condition and radiographic imaging of the abdomen.

        c. Diagnosis

            (1) Anteroposterior and cross-table lateral **chest radiographs.**

            (2) A fiberoptic transilluminator; the room must be sufficiently dark for effective transillumination.

    3. Treatment

        a. Pneumothorax

            (1) Observation. Infants without respiratory distress, underlying pulmonary disease, or the need for positive pressure ventilation can be managed with conservative therapy. This consists of close observation, frequent small feedings to minimize crying, and a follow-up x-ray. Extrapulmonary air usually resolves in 24 to 48 hours. The use of 100% oxygen (for <24 hr), while effective in speeding the resolution of pneumothorax, **is not recommended** in premature infants because of the danger of retinopathy of prematurity.

            (2) Needle aspiration is a useful therapeutic and/or diagnostic procedure in the critically ill infant with respiratory or hemodynamic compromise possibly due to pneumothorax.

                (a) Place the infant in a supine position.

                (b) Attach a 23- or 25-gauge "butterfly" or a 20 to 22-gauge angiocath needle to a 20-cc syringe via a three-way stopcock.

                (c) Insert the needle through the second intercostal space in the midclavicular line. Walk the needle over the rib to minimize the chance of bleeding from the intercostal artery. Avoid the nipple.

                (d) Apply continuous suction with the syringe as the needle is inserted. A rapid flow of air will occur when the pleural air space is entered.

                (e) If air continues to leak, a chest tube must be inserted. Because the needle can puncture the lung parenchyma (with a small chance of bronchopleural fistula), remove as soon as possible.

(3) Chest tube placement. Continued air leak in infants with significant pulmonary disease or positive pressure airway support, or both, should be treated with **chest tube** placement and suction for evacuation of extrapleural air. This should be performed or supervised by an experienced practitioner.

(4) Persistent pneumothorax may require selective bronchus intubation or catheter occlusion to stabilize pulmonary gas exchange.

(5) High-frequency ventilation can provide effective support of gas exchange and reduce the degree of pleural gas accumulation.

b. Pneumomediastinum requires no specific therapy.

c. Pneumopericardium

(1) Symptomatic pneumopericardium should be treated by immediate drainage of pericardial air.

(a) Following sterile preparation, insert a 20-gauge needle or catheter connected via a three-way stopcock to a 10 to 20-cc syringe in the subxiphoid region, directed superiorly toward the posterior left shoulder. With suction on the syringe, advance the needle until air appears.

(b) When the air stops flowing, withdraw the needle.

(2) Often, a single aspiration results in clinical improvement. Recurrent symptomatic pneumopericardium, which should be aspirated, will occur in 25 to 40% of patients.

(3) Refractory pneumopericardium will require placement of a 16-gauge Intracath or a surgically placed catheter.

D. Neonatal persistent pulmonary hypertension (PPHN) is a syndrome of suprasystemic pulmonary vascular resistance that induces systemic hypoxemia as a result of right-to-left shunting at the ductus arteriosus or foramen ovale, or both.

1. Etiology

a. PPHN is a multifactorial syndrome that results from failure of postnatal decline of pulmonary vascular resistance, sometimes accompanied by hypertrophy and distal extension of pulmonary artery smooth muscle and constriction of the pulmonary vascular bed.

b. The failure of transitional circulation can be associated with

(1) Aspiration syndromes (meconium, blood, amniotic fluid).

(2) Pneumonia, sepsis (especially in term infants).

(3) Diaphragmatic hernia and pulmonary hypoplasia.

(4) Rarely, alveolar-capillary dysplasia.

2. Evaluation and diagnosis

a. With shunting, preductal oxygen saturation is greater than postductal by 3 to 4%.

b. Echocardiogram confirms right to left shunting at the atrial or ductal level.

3. Treatment

a. Minimize pulmonary vasoconstriction

(1) Avoid pulmonary hypoxia by increasing FiO_2 to achieve a PaO_2 of 60 to 80 (or higher in severe cases).

(2) Induce systemic alkalemia via metabolic alkalosis (bicarbonate therapy) or respiratory alkalosis (hyperventilation), or both, to raise pH to 7.45 to 7.50.

(3) A proven selective pulmonary vasodilator does not exist, although clinical trials of nitric oxide are in progress.

b. Maintain cardiac output and oxygen-carrying capacity

(1) Maintain preload and intravascular volume with normal saline, albumin, packed red blood cells (PRBCs), or fresh frozen plasma (FFP) as appropriate.

(2) Provide inotropic and chronotropic support with dopamine or dobutamine, or both. These agents will increase cardiac output and reduce discrepancy in systemic and pulmonary vascular resistance.

    c. Alternative therapy

       (1) High-frequency ventilation is indicated in selected infants with PPHN who remain hypoxemic despite conventional mechanical ventilation. Ventilated infants with air leak disease may benefit from high-frequency ventilation.

       (2) Infants in whom conventional management fails may benefit from rescue therapy with extracorporeal membrane oxygenation (ECMO).

E. Apnea can precipitate bradycardia, cyanosis, pallor, hypotonia, or metabolic acidosis. Most premature infants under 30 weeks' gestational age have occasional apneic spells. Apnea generally begins at 1 to 2 days of age and may recur until the infant is about 35 weeks' gestational age, or longer in infants born at less than 28 weeks' gestational age.

    Prolonged apnea is defined as cessation of spontaneous respirations beyond 15 seconds in a full-term infant and more than 20 seconds in preterm infants. **Bradycardia** and **cyanosis** usually occur after 20 seconds of apnea, although they may occur more rapidly in the small premature infant. After 30 to 40 seconds, **pallor** and **hypotonia** are seen, and the infant may be unresponsive to tactile stimulation.

    Periodic breathing is defined as pauses in breathing of 3 seconds or longer, interrupted by respirations for less than 20 seconds. This respiratory pattern is normal in preterm infants.

    1. Etiology

       a. Hypoxemia or diaphragmatic fatigue can result from respiratory disease (HMD, pneumonia), anemia, hypovolemia, and congenital heart disease.

       b. Respiratory center depression can result from hypoglycemia, electrolyte abnormalities (including hypocalcemia), sepsis, drugs, or intracranial disorders.

       c. Apnea associated with abnormal or hyperactive reflexes can be induced by suction or stimulation of the pharynx, fluid in the airway or pharynx from feeding, or gastroesophageal reflux.

       d. Airway obstruction and apnea can result from neck flexion, pressure on the lower rim of a face mask, submental pressure, or supine position.

       e. Temperature. The presence of a skin-core temperature gradient decreases the incidence of apnea. Infants in Isolettes servocontrolled to maintain skin temperatures at 36.8°C (98.2°F) have more frequent spells than do those maintained at 36.0°C (96.8°F). Sudden increases in incubator temperature increase the frequency of apneic spells.

       f. Apnea of prematurity results from decreased carbon dioxide sensitivity or decreased afferent stimulation from peripheral receptors, or both.

    2. Evaluation and diagnosis

       a. All infants less than 34 weeks' gestational age or weighing under 1,800 g should be placed on heart rate monitors for at least 5 to 7 days. Because impedance apnea monitors may not detect apnea due to airway obstruction, the heart rate should be simultaneously monitored.

       b. When a monitor alarm sounds, the clinician should *evaluate the infant, not the monitor.* Check for bradycardia, cyanosis, and airway obstruction.

       c. A first apneic spell, apnea in the first 24 hours, or in infants greater than 34 weeks' gestational age should be evaluated for etiologies in addition to apnea of prematurity.

    3. Treatment

       a. Anesthesia bag and mask should be available near every infant who is being monitored for apnea. Use an oxygen concentration similar to that which the infant has been breathing, to minimize hypoxia or hyperoxia. Equipment for intubation and full resuscitation should be available.

       b. Infants with apnea episodes that do not immediately self-resolve, or respond to gentle shaking, should be ventilated with bag and mask.

       c. Infants with repeated, prolonged spells, that is, more than two to three per hour or spells that require frequent bagging, necessitate further interventions. Staged interventions should include the following:

(1) The environmental temperature can be decreased to the low end of the neutral thermal environment range. Placing a heat shield around a small premature infant may prevent swings in temperature.

(2) Stimuli that can trigger apnea should be avoided. These may include suctioning, nipple feeding, and cold or warm stimulation of the trigeminal area of the face.

(3) Aminophylline (2.0–8.0 mg/kg/day IV/PO) in divided doses q4–12h should be started if the preceding measures fail.

    (a) If the neonate has severe apneic spells and more rapid action is desired, a loading dose of aminophylline, 7 to 8 mg/kg IV/PO, can be given. The maintenance doses can be given after 6 hours.

    (b) Serum aminophylline concentrations should be obtained during therapy, and the dosage should be adjusted to maintain the concentration in the range of 4 to 15 mg/ml. The dosage should be reduced if tachycardia or GI toxicity (vomiting) becomes evident.

    (c) The maximum response may take up to 4 days.

(4) Caffeine citrate, a related xanthine stimulant, is an alternative medication. As with theophylline, the acute and long-term toxicity of caffeine in newborn infants is not well established, although the therapeutic range is broader and therefore the medicine is probably safer. A suggested **dosage schedule** for caffeine citrate is a loading dose of 10 to 20 mg/kg PO or IV, followed by a maintenance dose of 5 to 10 mg/kg/day in a single dose. When serum concentrations are monitored, optimal levels are 5 to 20 µg/ml.

(5) Small increases in FiO_2 may reduce the frequency of apneic spells. Continuous monitoring of arterial oxygenation is necessary to minimize the **risk of retinopathy of prematurity** in very-low-birth-weight (VLBW) infants.

(6) Administration of CPAP (3–5 cm H_2O) can reduce apnea frequency or severity, or both.

(7) Apnea associated with severe anemia may respond to a packed RBC transfusion by increasing the oxygen-carrying capacity of the blood.

(8) If all these interventions fail, **mechanical ventilation** may be required until the infant achieves respiratory maturity.

(9) Most neonates with apnea of prematurity attain maturity of respiratory control by the time they are otherwise ready for discharge from the hospital. If infants are free of apnea for 5 to 7 days while being monitored in the hospital, their medication can be stopped. If they remain free of apnea off medication for 5 to 7 days while being monitored in the hospital, and are 34 to 35 weeks' gestational age, they can be discharged home, with only standard baseline risk of adverse events.

(10) If there is any concern about the recurrence of apnea, a **pneumogram** to assess breathing patterns, obstructive apnea, and bradycardia may be useful. The use of the pneumogram to predict the future risk of apnea is controversial. If there is a documented need for medication (abnormal pneumogram or clinical apnea off medication), a pneumogram can objectively document the response of the infant to the medication. Infants on medication, with no evidence of apnea by pneumogram, can be discharged home, without a monitor, as long as they remain on the successful treatment regimen.

(11) Reassessment of apnea frequency as the patient's serum theophylline or caffeine concentration declines can guide subsequent need for medication. This assessment can occur while monitored either at home or in the hospital.

(12) Home monitoring may be required for infants with persistent apnea despite optimized medication regimens.

V. Cardiac disease in the newborn. Severe congenital heart disease affects approximately 1 in 400 infants. Because many benign murmurs occur in the neonatal period, asymptomatic infants in stable condition can be followed clinically. Symptomatic infants will often present with either congestive failure, cyanosis, or an arrhythmia. (see also Chap. 10).

A. Congestive heart failure (CHF)

1. **Etiology.** CHF results from elevated ventricular end-diastolic pressures.
   a. Patent ductus arteriosus is the most common cause of CHF in the premature infant.
   b. Large ventricular septal defect (VSD).
   c. Endocardial cushion defect.
   d. Left-sided obstructive lesions (hypoplastic left heart syndrome, interrupted aortic arch, coarctation of the aorta).
   e. Functional cardiac failure can result from cardiomyopathies (asphyxial, diabetic, or viral), peripheral arteriovenous fistulae, and prolonged paroxysmal tachycardias.

2. **Evaluation**
   a. Common signs of heart failure in the newborn include poor feeding, tachycardia, tachypnea, diaphoresis, hepatomegaly, and cardiomegaly. Murmurs, S3 and S4, may be present.
   b. Pre- and postductal ABGs, chest x-rays, four-extremity blood pressures, and an ECG are the basic tools of diagnosis.

3. **Diagnosis**
   a. **PDA.** A significant left-to-right shunt through a PDA is often manifested by a hyperdynamic precordium, systolic or continuous murmur, and accentuated palmar pulse (Table 6-4). The diagnosis of a PDA can be confirmed and the amount of the left-to-right shunt quantitated by two-dimensional echocardiography.
   b. The diagnosis of other acyanotic cardiac lesions that can result in CHF are given in Table 6-4.

4. **Treatment**
   a. An ill infant suspected of having serious cardiac disease should be transferred immediately to a regional neonatal intensive care unit.
   b. Restrict sodium and administer diuretics to achieve a negative sodium balance. This will decrease extracellular fluid (ECF) and lower ventricular filling pressures.
   c. Reduce workload by providing gavage rather than oral feedings. Maintain a neutral thermal environment.
   d. Maintain oxygen delivery
      (1) Maintain the hematocrit at over 40% (use packed RBCs, 5 ml/kg, given over 2–4 hr and repeated as necessary), and
      (2) Provide FiO_2 to maintain PaO_2 at 60 to 80 mm Hg. Mechanical ventilation may be required to assure adequate gas exchange.
   e. **Cardiotonic drugs** are the cornerstone of CHF treatment.
      (1) For specific recommendations regarding **digoxin** and **diuretics,** see Chapter 10.
      (2) **Dopamine** (2.5–20 µg/kg/min) and dobutamine (5–20 µg/kg/min) are used in the newborn for inotropic support.
   f. **CHF** associated with a hemodynamically significant PDA warrants a trial of indomethacin therapy to medically close the PDA.

B. Cyanosis

1. **Etiology**
   a. Cardiac: transposition of the great arteries, critical pulmonary stenosis or atresia, tetralogy of Fallot, tricuspid atresia, total anomalous pulmonary venous return, Ebstein's anomaly, hypoplastic left heart, and truncus arteriosus. (Table 6-5).
   b. Noncardiac: persistent pulmonary hypertension, hemoglobinopathy, or pulmonary etiologies, for example, HMD, meconium aspiration pneumonia, hypoplastic lungs, or pneumothorax.

2. **Evaluation** of the cyanotic infant includes ECG, radiograph, right radial (i.e., preductal) and postductal ABGs in room air and 100% oxygen, and an echocardiogram. A cardiologist should be consulted promptly.

Table 6-4. Acyanotic cardiac lesions that can result in congestive heart failure

Diagnosis	Physical findings	Onset of heart murmur	Onset of CHF	ECG findings	CXR findings	Associated pathology
Severe AS	SEM and SEC	Birth onward	3 d onward	Usually LVH; RVH if hypoplastic LV	CE with PV congestion	EFE, MS, or MR
Severe coarctation	Decreased femoral pulses; differential cyanosis	Variable	First month	Usually RVH	CE with PV congestion	Bicuspid AoV, VSD, AS, AR
IAA	Decreased femoral pulses; differential cyanosis	Variable	4 d onward	Usually RVH	CE with PV congestion	VSD, PDA, complex CHD, DiGeorge's syndrome
VSD	SRM; MDR	2–3 d onward	Usually 3–6 wk	RVH or BVH	CE with ↑ PBF	Prematurity; chromosomal anomalies
CAVC	SRM	Birth onward	Usually 3–6 wk	Superior axis with CCWL, RVH, or BVH	CE with ↑ PBF	Down syndrome; heterotaxy
PDA	Continuous murmur; bounding pulses; hyperdynamic precordium	2–3 d onward	First wk onward	RVH normal for age	CE with ↑ PBF	Prematurity

Table 6-4 (continued)

Diagnosis	Physical findings	Onset of heart murmur	Onset of CHF	ECG findings	CXR findings	Associated pathology
Transient myocardial ischemia	Transient SRM; quiet precordium	Birth	Birth	NSSTTWA	CE with PV congestion	Perinatal asphyxia
Myocarditis	Other signs of infection (e.g., seizures)	Variable	Birth onward	NSSTTWA; arrhythmia (20%)	CE with PV congestion	Perinatal infection
EFE	Muffled heart sounds; gallop rhythm	Variable	Usually in first 6 mo	RVH in newborns; LVH in infants	CE with PV congestion	
Pompe's disease (acid maltase deficiency)	Hypotonia and weak cry; protruding tongue	Variable	Usually within 2 mo	LAD with LVH; deep Q waves; PR < 0.09 sec	CE	

CHF = congestive heart failure; ECG = electrocardiogram; CXR = chest x-ray; AS = aortic stenosis; SEM = systolic ejection murmur; SEC = systolic ejection click; LVH = left ventricular hypertrophy; RVH = right ventricular hypertrophy; LV = left ventricle; CE = cardiac enlargement; PV = pulmonary venous; EFE = endocardial fibroelastosis; MS = mitral stenosis; MR = mitral regurgitation; AoV = aortic valve; VSD = ventricular septal defect; AR = aortic regurgitation; IAA = interrupted aortic arch; PDA = patent ductus arteriosus; CHD = congenital heart disease; SRM = systolic regurgitant murmur; MDR = middiastolic murmur; BVH = biventricular hypertrophy; PBF = pulmonary blood flow; CAVC = common atrioventricular canal defect; CCWL = counterclockwise vector loop; NSSTTWA = nonspecific ST-T wave abnormalities; LAD = left axis deviation.
Source: JP Cloherty, AR Stark (eds). *Manual of Neonatal Care* (3rd ed). Boston, Little, Brown, 1991. Pp 258–259.

Table 6-5. Cyanotic congenital heart disease presenting with PaO$_2$ less than 50 mm Hg

Diagnosis	Heart murmur	ECG findings	CXR findings
D-TGA with IVS	None	RVH normal for age	No CE with ↑ PBF
TAPVR with PV obstruction	None	RVH	PV congestion
Ebstein's anomaly	± TR murmur	RAE, RBBB, WPW	Massive CE; normal or ↓ PBF
Tricuspid atresia with PS or PA	± PS murmur	Superior axis, LVH	No CE with ↓ PBF
PA with IVS	± TR murmur, ± continuous murmur	LVH, QRS axis 0–90 degrees	± CE with ↓ PBF
Severe PS	PS murmur	RVH, QRS axis 0–90 degrees	± CE with ↓ PBF
Severe TOF	PS murmur	RVH	No CE with ↓ PBF
TOF with PA	± Continuous murmur	RVH	No CE with ↓ PBF

ECG = electrocardiogram; CXR = chest x-ray; D-TGA = D-transposition of the great arteries; IVS = intact ventricular septum; RVH = right ventricular hypertrophy; CE = cardiac enlargement; PBF = pulmonary blood flow; TAPVR = total anomalous pulmonary venous return; PV = pulmonary venous; TR = tricuspid regurgitation; LVH = left ventricular hypertrophy; RAE = right atrial enlargement; RBBB = right bundle branch block; WPW = Wolff-Parkinson-White syndrome; PS = pulmonary stenosis; PA = pulmonary atresia; TOF = tetralogy of Fallot; ↑ = increased; ↓ = decreased; ± = present or absent.
Source: Adapted from MD Freed. Congenital Cardiac Malformations. In ME Avery, HW Taeusch (eds). *Schaffer's Diseases of the Newborn* (5th ed). Philadelphia: Saunders, 1984. Reprinted from JP Cloherty, AR Stark (eds). *Manual of Neonatal Care* (3rd ed). Boston: Little, Brown, 1991. P 262.

   3. Diagnosis
      a. In 100% oxygen, a PaO$_2$ over 150 significantly reduces the probability of significant cyanotic heart disease, though a PaO$_2$ of 250 to 300 is most reassuring.
      b. Early measurement of PaO$_2$ in 100% oxygen in a child with developing pulmonary disease is important. Many infants with HMD may have a PaO$_2$ greater than 100 mm Hg in 100% oxygen early in their disease, but not by day 2 or 3.
   4. Treatment
      a. Cyanotic congenital heart disease is a **medical emergency.**
      b. Prostaglandin E$_1$ (PGE$_1$) may be required to maintain patency of the ductus arteriosus until definitive surgical therapy can be instituted.
  C. Rhythm disturbances (see also Chap. 10, pp. 324 *ff.*)
   1. Bradycardia
      a. Etiology
         (1) Sinus bradycardia
            (a) Elevated intracranial pressure.
            (b) Hypertension.
            (c) Hyperkalemia.
            (d) Hypothyroidism.
            (e) Congenital heart disease.
            (f) Maternal medications (e.g., beta blockers).
         (2) Congenital heart associated with maternal collagen vascular disease (e.g., systemic lupus erythematosus).
         (3) Benign low resting heart rate (90–100 beats/min)
            (a) Term infants with neonatal encephalopathy secondary to birth depression.

   (b) Postmature infants.

 b. Evaluation and diagnosis

  (1) When fetal heart rate monitoring indicates a persistent fetal bradycardia, a cardiologic consultation should be arranged before delivery. The timely distinction between fetal distress and fetal bradycardia due to congenital heart block must be quickly defined by clinical context and ultrasonography.

  (2) Electrocardiography confirms the diagnosis.

 c. Treatment. The goal of treatment is to maintain an appropriate cardiac output.

  (1) Treat the underlying cause if possible. Asymptomatic bradycardia should be observed for at least 72 hours without intervention.

  (2) In infants with a heart rate under 50, respiratory distress, cyanosis, and CHF frequently develop. Treatment can begin with a chronotropic agent such as isoproterenol to acutely raise the heart rate. If symptomatic bradycardia persists when medication is begun or withdrawn, insertion of a pacemaker may be necessary.

2. Tachycardia is more common than bradycardia in the newborn period.

 a. Supraventricular tachycardia (SVT)

  (1) Etiology

   (a) Wolff-Parkinson-White syndrome.

   (b) Structural congenital heart disease.

   (c) Idiopathic.

  (2) Evaluation and diagnosis

   (a) Electrocardiogram. In 1 : 1 atrioventricular conduction, SVT results in a heart rate of 200 to 300 beats per minute. P waves are rarely seen, and the QRS interval may be normal or prolonged.

   (b) Prolonged SVT in utero can cause CHF, with the possibility of fetal hydrops or stillbirth. Frequent assessment by ultrasound guides obstetric management.

  (3) Therapy

   (a) In utero: maternal digoxin therapy.

   (b) Treatment after delivery aims to convert the infant to sinus rhythm. Infants who are in stable condition at delivery can usually tolerate up to 24 hours of tachycardia without CHF.

    (i) Vagal stimulation: ice to the malar area, suctioning, abdominal pressure.

    (ii) Adenosine therapy can convert neonatal SVT. The starting dose is 50 µg/kg by rapid (1–2 sec) IV push through the most proximally located IV line. The half-life of adenosine is less than 10 seconds. Therefore, the dose can be repeated q2min, doubling it to a maximum of 250 µg/kg.

   (c) Intraesophageal pacing by a pediatric cardiologist to convert SVT to normal sinus rhythm.

   (d) Maintenance therapy with digoxin should be considered in the infant with recurrent SVT.

   (e) Cardioversion may be necessary in infants with refractory SVT (see Chap. 10).

 b. Ventricular tachycardia must be distinguished as hemodynamically stable or unstable.

  (1) Etiology

   (a) Congenital cardiac malformation, accessory conduction system, hamartoma (e.g., in tuberous sclerosis), aneurysm, Ebstein's anomaly.

   (b) Congenital long Q-T syndrome.

   (c) Maternal drug ingestion (e.g., cocaine).

   (d) Severe metabolic abnormalities.

  (2) Treatment

(a) Hemodynamically unstable: The infant may require immediate cardioversion.

(b) Long-term treatment may require antiarrhythmic medications, specific ablation, or cardiac surgery.

VI. Hematologic problems (see also Chap. 15, pp. 436*ff.*)

A. Jaundice

1. Etiology

a. **Physiologic hyperbilirubinemia** in full-term infants appears on or after the third day of life and resolves before 10 days.

(1) **Unconjugated hyperbilirubinemia:** total serum bilirubin less than 12 mg/dl; direct fraction less than 15% of the total.

(2) Caused by a combination of increased bilirubin production, and impaired hepatic uptake, conjugation, and excretion of bilirubin.

(3) The immature liver of the premature infant further decreases bilirubin metabolism and leads to higher peak serum bilirubin concentrations.

(4) Breast-fed infants exhibit higher peak serum bilirubin values and slower resolution than do formula-fed infants.

b. **Nonphysiologic jaundice** results from abnormal bilirubin production, metabolism, or excretion. It should be suspected in the very-low-birthweight infant, in the presence of clinical jaundice in the first 36 hours of life, when serum bilirubin concentration increases by more than 5 mg/dl/day, when the total bilirubin is over 15 mg/dl in a formula-fed full-term infant or over 17 mg/dl in a breast-fed term infant, or if clinical jaundice persists beyond 8 days in a full-term infant or beyond 2 weeks in a premature infant.

(1) **Indirect hyperbilirubinemia:** direct bilirubin less than 15% of the total bilirubin. Causes of indirect hyperbilirubinemia:

(a) *Excess bilirubin production* due to

(i) Immune hemolysis secondary to maternal-fetal blood group incompatibility.

(ii) Hereditary hemolytic anemia, red cell membrane defects, enzyme defects, hemoglobinopathies.

(iii) Acquired hemolytic anemia: infection, disseminated intravascular coagulation (DIC).

(iv) Extravasation of blood.

(v) Polycythemia.

(vi) Swallowed maternal or fetal blood.

(vii) Increased enterohepatic circulation of bilirubin seen in pyloric stenosis, delayed emptying of the intestine, and after bowel surgery.

(b) *Decreased clearance of bilirubin* due to

(i) Inborn errors of metabolism, including familial nonhemolytic jaundice types I and II (Crigler-Najjar syndrome), Gilbert syndrome, Dubin-Johnson syndrome, Rotor syndrome, galactosemia, tyrosinosis, and hypermethioninemia.

(ii) Prematurity.

(iii) Hypothyroidism and hypopituitarism.

(iv) Infants of diabetic mothers.

(v) Reduced hepatic perfusion.

(2) **Direct hyperbilirubinemia:** direct bilirubin greater than 15% of the total bilirubin. Causes:

(a) Bacterial sepsis.

(b) Intrauterine viral infections.

(c) Neonatal hepatitis.

(d) Intrahepatic and extrahepatic biliary atresia.

(e) Biliary tract obstruction (by a choledochal cyst, an abdominal mass, or annular pancreas).

(f) Inherited disorders: trisomy 18, galactosemia, tyrosinemia, Rotor syndrome, Dubin-Johnson syndrome, hypermethioninemia, alpha-1-antitrypsin deficiency, cystic fibrosis.

(g) Posthemolytic disease of the newborn syndrome (inspissated bile syndrome).

(h) Hypopituitarism, hypothyroidism.

(i) Prolonged administration of total parenteral nutrition.

2. **Evaluation and diagnosis**
   a. **Physical examination.** Clinical jaundice appears at serum bilirubin levels greater than 6 mg/dl.
   b. **Laboratory tests**
      (1) Direct and indirect bilirubin, the blood types of mother and infant
         (a) A full-term infant whose bilirubin is over 5 mg/dl within the first 24 hours of life, over 10 mg/dl within the first 48 hours, or over 13 mg/dl after 72 hours requires investigation.
         (b) Premature or sick infants should have regular serum bilirubin measurements until values have peaked and begin to decline. Infants known to be at high risk of hyperbilirubinemia, such as infants born to Rh-sensitized mothers, should have cord blood bilirubin concentrations measured.
      (2) Direct Coombs' test and, if positive, identification of the antibody if it is positive, a hematocrit, a blood smear for red cell morphologic study, and a reticulocyte count.
      (3) In persistent jaundice or direct hyperbilirubinemia, tests of liver function and thyroid function, tests for viral or bacterial infection, and tests for galactosemia may be indicated.
      (4) Additional hematologic tests include glucose 6-phosphate dehydrogenase (G6PD), hemoglobin electrophoresis, and RBC enzymes.
      (5) **Kernicterus** is a central nervous system pathologic state associated with elevated serum bilirubin concentrations. Susceptibility to kernicterus is increased by factors that decrease albumin binding (hypoalbuminemia, elevated free fatty acids, lipid infusion or sepsis with catecholamine-stimulated lipolysis, acidosis, hypoglycemia, sulfonamides, organic anions) and factors that increase diffusion of free bilirubin into the brain (increased concentration of bilirubin and/or increased duration of exposure to elevated levels of bilirubin; anoxic-ischemic encephalopathy).

3. **Treatment**
   a. The goal of treatment is to avoid kernicterus or sublethal bilirubin encephalopathy.
      (1) In *full-term infants*, kernicterus is unlikely to occur if indirect bilirubin concentrations are kept under 20 mg/dl, provided there are no factors disturbing the blood-brain barrier or interfering with the binding of bilirubin to albumin. **A bilirubin concentration less than 25 mg/dl in a well full-term infant without hemolytic disease is unlikely to be toxic.**
      (2) Kernicterus has been described at autopsy in *premature* infants whose bilirubin levels never exceeded 10 mg/dl. Bilirubin encephalopathy in low-birth-weight infants may be promoted by alterations in the blood-brain barrier caused by anoxia, ischemia, or hyperosmolarity.
   b. General treatment guidelines for term infants (*Pediatrics* 1994, 94:565) are summarized in Table 6-6.
      (1) Establish that the baby has adequate fluid intake and correct any state of dehydration. In breast-fed infants, supplement the diet if indicated.
      (2) Correct hypotension, hypoxia, hypothermia, and hypoglycemia. Avoid drugs administered to mother or newborn that may interfere with the binding of bilirubin to albumin (e.g., sulfonamides, moxalactam, aspirin, rapid infusions of ampicillin, long-chain free fatty acids).

Table 6-6. Management of hyperbilirubinemia in the healthy term newborn

	TSB level (mg/dl)			
Age (hr)	Consider phototherapy[a]	Phototherapy	Exchange transfusion if intensive phototherapy fails[b]	Exchange transfusion and intensive phototherapy
≤24c	—	—	—	—
25–48	≥12	≥15	≥20	≥25
49–72	≥15	≥18	≥25	≥30
>72	≥17	≥20	≥25	≥30

TSB = total serum bilirubin.
[a]Phototherapy indicated at the discretion of the clinician.
[b]Intensive phototherapy should produce a decline of TSB of 1–2 mg/dl within 4–6 hr, and the TSB level should continue to fall and remain below the threshold level for exchange transfusion. If this does not occur, it is considered a failure of phototherapy.
[c]Term infants who are clinically jaundiced at ≤24 hr old are not considered healthy and require further evaluation.
Source: Modified from American Academy of Pediatrics. Practice parameter: Management of hyperbilirubinemia in the healthy term newborn. Pediatrics 1994;94:558–565.

c. Phototherapy
   (1) Indications
      (a) Phototherapy should be instituted if there is a risk that unconjugated bilirubin will rise to levels that might saturate albumin-binding sites or result in the need for an exchange transfusion.
      (b) Early phototherapy (< 24 hours of age) may be indicated in special circumstances (i.e., in immature VLBW infants and in severely bruised premature infants). In hemolytic disease, phototherapy is used as an adjunct to exchange transfusion.
      (c) Effectiveness. The amount of skin exposed to radiant energy per cm^2 and the wavelength spectrum of light determine the effectiveness of phototherapy. Blue light (wavelength 450–500 nm) is more effective in lowering bilirubin, but cool white light provides better visualization of cyanosis in the infant. Fiberoptic blankets provide a convenient way to increase exposure to radiant energy.
   (2) Technique of phototherapy
      (a) Shield the infant's eyes, avoiding nasal obstruction.
      (b) Properly ground all electrical outlets.
      (c) Use a Plexiglas shield to protect the infant from ultraviolet light.
      (d) Placing lights over, beside, and under the baby will increase the exposure. The underside of the baby can be exposed to phototherapy by a phototherapy blanket.
      (e) Monitor the temperature q2h to prevent hypo- or hyperthermia.
      (f) Weigh the infant frequently to guide fluid requirements.
      (g) Monitor serum bilirubin frequently, as the clinical assessment of jaundice becomes less sensitive in infants under phototherapy.
      (h) Change the lamps every 2,000 hours or every 3 months.
   (3) Side effects include
      (a) Increased insensible water loss, which may require a 10 to 20% increase in fluid intake.
      (b) Transient exanthemas, usually on exposed areas of skin.
      (c) Diarrhea.

(d) Bronze baby syndrome, a rare complication usually seen in infants with direct hyperbilirubinemia who are treated with phototherapy. **Phototherapy should therefore be used with caution in infants with liver disease or obstructive jaundice.**

(e) No significant long-term toxicity has been described.

d. Exchange transfusion

(1) Indications

(a) Exchange transfusion should be instituted to correct severe anemia or if the rate of rise or absolute serum bilirubin concentration predicts a significant risk of bilirubin encephalopathy (see sec. **A.2** above; Table 6-6). The level of bilirubin at which exchange transfusion is recommended for low-birth-weight infants is controversial. There are no studies that permit recommendations for the treatment of low-birth-weight infants with bilirubins under 20 mg/dl. Current recommendations from the American Academy of Pediatrics (*Guidelines for Perinatal Care*, 1992) state:

> Some pediatricians use guidelines that recommend aggressive treatment of jaundice in low-birth-weight neonates, initiating phototherapy early and performing exchange transfusions in certain neonates with very low bilirubin concentrations (<10 mg/dl). However, this approach will not prevent kernicterus consistently. Some pediatricians prefer to adopt a less aggressive therapeutic stance and allow serum bilirubin concentrations in low-birth-weight neonates to approach 15–20 mg/dl (257-342 µmol/liter) before considering exchange transfusions. At present, both of these approaches to treatment should be considered reasonable. In either case, the finding of low bilirubin kernicterus at autopsy in certain low-birthweight neonates cannot necessarily be interpreted as a therapeutic failure or equivalent to bilirubin encephalopathy. Like retinopathy of prematurity, kernicterus is a condition that cannot be prevented in certain neonates, given the current state of knowledge.

(b) Serum bilirubin concentration rising more rapidly than 0.5 µg/dl/hr despite phototherapy.

(c) Early exchange transfusion is often indicated in the presence of hydrops, in a known sensitized infant, or in an infant with splenomegaly or anemia due to hemolytic disease.

(d) The indications for immediate (at birth) exchange transfusion are hydrops or severe anemia. When the delivery of hydropic fetus is expected avoid delays by alerting blood bank personnel.

(e) A cord hemoglobin of less than 11 µg/dl and a cord indirect bilirubin greater than 4.5 mg/dl are usually indications for exchange transfusion. However, the rate of rise of the indirect serum bilirubin is the best indication. A bilirubin rise of over 1.0 mg/dl/hr or a rise of 0.5 mg/dl/hr with a hemoglobin concentration between 11 and 13 g/dl despite phototherapy usually signifies a need for exchange transfusion.

(f) Late exchange transfusion in hemolytic disease is recommended if serum bilirubin in full-term infants exceeds 20 mg/dl or the rate of rise predicts that it will go over 20 mg/dl.

(2) Blood preparations for exchange transfusions (see p. 454)

(a) Fresh (< 24-hr old) **whole blood** should be used in sick infants. Use of blood that is less than 72 hours old will minimize problems with hyperkalemia and acidosis.

(b) **Irradiated blood** is preferred for all exchange transfusions to minimize risk of graft-versus-host disease.

(c) **Viral** for the AIDS virus, in addition to hepatitis B, hepatitis C, and syphilis. Ideally, all neonatal blood products should be tested for cytomegalovirus (CMV). PRBCs should be frozen and washed, or white cell filtered.

(d) **Citrate-phosphate-dextrose (CPD) blood** has the *advantage* that it can be used up to 72 hours after drawing and that there is no rise in nonesterified free fatty acids in recipients. The *disadvantages* are low pH (6.9–7.0), hypernatremia, hyperglycemia that can cause rebound hypoglycemia in hyperinsulinemic infants with erythroblastosis, and a tendency to reduce ionized calcium and magnesium. Measurement of whole blood electrolytes and pH helps to assess the safety of blood that is more than 48 hours old.

(e) Heparinized blood is used less frequently in exchange transfusions because of associated risks of hypoglycemia and elevated serum free fatty acids.

(f) Fresh (< 24-hr old) CPD blood should be used in hydropic or otherwise compromised newborns. Transfused blood should have a low titer of anti-A and anti-B antibodies.

(g) The risk of acid-base disorders, hyperkalemia, and hypernatremia can be minimized by using centrifuged packed red cells under 72 hours old resuspended in thawed fresh-frozen AB plasma just before exchange.

(h) Whole blood less than 4 hours old has deficient platelet function.

(3) **Technique of exchange transfusion.** Hypoxia, hypoglycemia, acidosis, and temperature problems should all be corrected before exchange transfusion is performed.

(a) A *radiant heater,* a cardiac monitor, and a reliable peripheral IV line should be in place.

(b) The *umbilical vein* should be used if possible. If the umbilical vein cannot be accessed despite soaking in saline for 30 to 60 minutes, the safest route is a *central venous line* (CVL). Alternatively, a peripheral intravenous line and peripheral arterial line can be used.

(c) In sick, hydropic infants, maximum safety of exchange transfusion may be achieved through use of umbilical arterial *and* venous catheters, so that blood can be removed and replaced simultaneously.

(d) In sick infants who are anemic (hematocrit < 35%), a partial exchange transfusion can be given with packed red blood cells (25–80 ml/kg) to raise the hematocrit to 40%. After stabilization, further exchange transfusions can be performed as needed to treat hyperbilirubinemia. Component transfusion therapy (PRBCs, FFP) should be utilized, with reconstituted whole blood used if necessary.

(e) Administration of albumin (salt-poor albumin, 1 g/kg 1–2 hr before exchange) increases the amount of bilirubin removed by the exchange. Albumin is **contraindicated** in CHF or severe anemia and is not usually used in early exchanges, in which the goal is to remove sensitized red cells rather than bilirubin.

(f) An infant's blood volume is approximately 80 ml/kg, and exchange transfusion should use twice the infant's blood volume (160 ml/kg), in aliquots of 5 to 20 ml, depending on the infant's tolerance for the procedure. (An aliquot should never exceed 10% of the infant's estimated blood volume.) A useful approach is to start with 10-ml aliquots, increasing to 20-ml aliquots in infants who weigh over 2 kg if the vital signs remain stable. **A two-volume exchange removes 87% of the infant's red blood cells.**

(g) Small aliquots and a slower rate reduce the stress on cardiovascular adaptation. The recommended time for an exchange in a full-term infant is 1 hour.

(h) Blood should be maintained at 37°C by using a temperature-controlled water bath with an alarm to signal overheating.

(i) Transfused blood should be mixed frequently since the RBCs will settle rapidly.

(j) If **heparinized blood** is used, a Dextrostix *blood sugar should be obtained from the blood and from the baby during the exchange*; 10 ml of 5% dextrose can be given as an umbilical venous push after each 100 ml blood if necessary. If the catheter tip rests above the liver, a more concentrated sugar solution can be used. When **citrated blood** is used, the infant's blood sugar should be checked for several hours after the exchange, and oral feedings or parenteral glucose should be given once the infant's condition is stable.

(k) When using **CPD blood**, most infants will not require additional calcium; following cessation of exchange transfusion, the Ca^{2+} level rapidly returns to normal. If needed, 0.5 to 2.0 ml of 10% calcium gluconate can be given following each 100 ml exchanged blood. However, this measure increases the ionized calcium fraction only temporarily. **Calcium should be administered slowly IV to avoid bradycardia.**

(l) When the transfusion is finished, a silk purse-string suture should be placed around the vein, leaving a "tail," so that it will be easy to find the vein for the next exchange.

(m) When the catheter is removed, the cord tie should be tightened for up to an hour. If it is not subsequently removed, skin necrosis can occur.

(n) Although their use is controversial, short-term ($\leq$ 48 hours) prophylactic antibiotics (penicillinase-resistant penicillin and an aminoglycoside) are recommended if a catheter was passed through an old, dirty cord; if there is great difficulty in passing the catheter; or if there are multiple exchanges.

(o) Subsequent exchange is indicated as for the initial transfusion.

(4) Complications of exchange transfusions

(a) Vascular. Embolization with air or clots.

(b) Cardiac. Arrhythmias, volume overload, and cardiac arrest.

(c) Electrolytes. Hyperkalemia, hypokalemia, hypernatremia, hypocalcemia, and acidosis.

(d) Coagulation. Thrombosis, thrombocytopenia.

(e) Infections. Bacteremia, viral hepatitis, cytomegalovirus, human immunodeficiency virus (HIV).

(f) Miscellaneous. Hypoglycemia, perforation of vessels, hypothermia, and, rarely, necrotizing enterocolitis.

e. Long-term treatment. Phenobarbital, 5 to 8 mg/kg/day, will increase bile flow and bilirubin excretion. Its therapeutic effect may not be seen for 3 to 7 days. It is most useful in cases of direct hyperbilirubinemia and Crigler-Najjar syndrome type II.

B. Anemia (see also Chap. 15)

1. The **causes** of anemia include extravascular blood loss, intravascular hemolysis, and decreased RBC production.

a. Blood loss

(1) Etiology

(a) Hemorrhage from the fetal to the maternal circulation.

(b) Twin-twin transfusion.

(c) Placenta previa, placental abruption.

(d) Umbilical cord rupture or hematoma.

(e) Incision of the placenta or cord.
(f) Traumatic amniocentesis.
(g) Rupture of anomalous placental vessels.
(h) Intracranial bleeding.
(i) Rupture of the liver or spleen.
(j) Gastrointestinal bleeding due to ulcer or enterocolitis.
(k) Iatrogenic anemia due to phlebotomy.

(2) **Evaluation**
(a) **Acute.** Manifestations are
  (i) Shock.
  (ii) Tachycardia.
  (iii) Tachypnea.
  (iv) Low venous pressure.
  (v) Weak pulses.
  (vi) Pallor.
  (vii) The hematocrit may initially be normal.
(b) **Chronic:** Manifestations are
  (i) Extreme pallor and a low hematocrit.
  (ii) Compensatory normovolemia and therefore minimal distress.
  (iii) CHF or hydrops at birth.

(3) **Laboratory evaluation**
(a) A Kleihauer-Betke smear of maternal blood to detect fetal red cells in the maternal circulation.
(b) The Apt test for fetal hemoglobin in gastric aspirate or stool.
(c) Intracranial and abdominal ultrasound if indicated.

b. **Hemolysis**
(1) **Etiology**
(a) Isoimmune anemias: Rh incompatibility, ABO incompatibility, minor blood group incompatibility (e.g., Kell, "e," "c," "E").
(b) Acquired hemolytic anemias: infection, DIC, vitamin E deficiency, drug reactions.
(c) Hereditary hemolytic anemias: red cell membrane defects (spherocytosis), enzyme defects (pyruvate kinase [PK] and G6PD deficiency).
(d) Hemoglobinopathies, for example, alpha and beta thalassemia syndromes.

(2) **Evaluation.** Manifestations include jaundice, hepatosplenomegaly, pallor, and hydrops.

(3) **Laboratory evaluation**
(a) Hematocrit, serum bilirubin, and reticulocyte count.
(b) Examination of a peripheral blood smear for red blood cell morphology.
(c) Direct Coombs test on an infant's red cells, with identification of the antibody if positive; antibody screen of maternal serum.
(d) Enzyme screen of infant's or parents' red cells (G6PD or PK deficiency).
(e) Screening for infection, with appropriate cultures.

c. **Decreased RBC production:** Blackfan-Diamond syndrome, Fanconi's anemia, hemoglobinopathies such as thalassemia, reactions to drugs, viral infections (e.g., parvovirus), and infiltrative diseases, such as leukemia, neuroblastoma, and storage diseases.

d. **Physiologic anemia of full-term and premature infants** reflects reduced erythropoiesis secondary to diminished erythropoietin production.

(1) **Physiologic nadir**
(a) *Full-term infants:* hemoglobin, 9.5 to 11.0 g/dl at 6 to 12 weeks.
(b) *Premature infants* (body weight 1,200–2,400 g): hemoglobin, 8 to 10 g/dl at 5 to 10 weeks.

(c) *Small premature infants* (body weight < 1,200 g): hemoglobin, 6.5 to 9.0 g/dl at 4 to 8 weeks.

(2) **Laboratory manifestations** of physiologic anemia include a decreased hematocrit and a low reticulocyte count. This transient state resolves when erythropoietin secretion, the reticulocyte count, and hemoglobin concentration all increase.

2. **Transfusion therapy**
   a. If an infant appears to have had **acute blood loss** at birth, immediate **vascular access** should be obtained. Blood should be drawn for laboratory evaluation including cross-matching.
      (1) If hypovolemic shock is present (decreased central venous pressure, pallor, tachycardia), 20 ml/kg of a **volume expander** should be given. Unmatched type O, Rh-negative blood should be kept available for this purpose. Albumin (5%), plasma, and normal saline are the secondary choices, in that order.
      (2) If blood loss was acute and limited, as in a fetal-maternal hemorrhage, volume expansion will provide immediate improvement. If there is continuing internal hemorrhage, the improvement will be less rapid and/or sustained. Infants in shock from asphyxia will have little response.
      (3) A repeat transfusion of 10 to 20 ml/kg can be given if signs of hypovolemic shock persist. If plasma or albumin was given initially, packed red cells are given in the second transfusion.
   b. **Chronic** fetal blood loss results in compensated anemia without evidence of hypovolemia. Packed red cells (10–15 ml/kg) should be given if the hematocrit is less than 30. If the hematocrit is less than 25 in a normovolemic or hypervolemic infant who may be in failure, a partial exchange transfusion with packed RBCs may be indicated.
   c. The condition of premature infants may be stable with a hemoglobin concentration of 6.5 to 8.0 g/dl. The level itself is **not** an indication for transfusion. However, if any other coexisting condition (e.g., sepsis, apnea, pneumonia, bronchopulmonary dysplasia) requires increased oxygen-carrying capacity, transfusion is indicated.
   d. Cumulative blood loss from phlebotomy must be carefully recorded. Blood replacement as packed red cells should be considered when 10% of the volume has been removed over a short time interval.
   e. **Transfusion volume** to replace red blood cells with packed RBCs (PRBCs) is calculated using the formula

$$\text{PRBC volume to be transfused} = \frac{\text{Hct desired} - \text{Hct observed}}{\text{Hct of PRBCs}}$$
$$\times \text{ weight (kg)} \times 80 \text{ ml/kg}$$

   (The average hematocrit [Hct] of packed red cells is 70.) In most circumstances, the volume to be transfused is about 10 ml/kg, usually administered intravenously over 1 to 3 hours. Infants should be monitored during transfusion.

3. **Prevention or amelioration of the anemia of prematurity**
   a. Premature infants should receive 25 IU water-soluble vitamin E daily as supplement or in premature formula until they are 2 to 3 months of age.
   b. Formulas similar to mother's milk, low in linoleic acid, should be used to maintain a low content of red blood cell polyunsaturated fatty acids.
   c. Iron supplements of elemental iron, 6 mg/kg/day, decrease the late anemia of prematurity. Iron therapy should be instituted when the infant is tolerating full-volume feedings.
   d. Conservative phlebotomy and transfusion practice are encouraged.

C. **Bleeding disorders**
   1. **Etiology, evaluation, and diagnosis** (see Chap. 15).
   2. **Treatment** (see also sec. **B** above)

    a. Treat underlying disease, such as shock, asphyxia, or infection.

    b. Place reliable IV line.

    c. After blood is drawn for studies, give 1.0 mg vitamin K_1 oxide (AquaME-PHYTON) IV over 2 to 3 minutes. The onset of action may be 2 to 3 hours. If liver disease is present, the onset of action may be longer.

    d. Fresh-frozen plasma, 10 ml/kg IV q8–12h, provides immediate replacement of clotting factors.

    e. If thrombocytopenia (platelet count < 20,000; < 50,000 if bleeding) is present, give 0.5 to 1.0 unit of irradiated platelets IV. **Platelets must not be given through an arterial line.** This should elevate the platelet count above 100,000/mm³ unless ongoing platelet destruction exists. In isoimmune thrombocytopenia, transfer compatible maternal or donor platelets if severe thrombocytopenia or bleeding develops.

    f. Packed red cells, plasma, and platelets are generally administered as component transfusion therapy. Occasionally, fresh whole blood will be used to replace platelets and clotting factors and to provide red blood cells.

    g. Clotting factor concentrates are used if a known factor deficiency is present.

    h. **Disseminated intravascular coagulation** should be treated by treating the underlying cause (sepsis, necrotizing enterocolitis) and giving fresh-frozen plasma and platelets to keep the platelet count above approximately 50,000. If bleeding continues, an exchange transfusion with fresh citrated blood may be helpful. If DIC is associated with gangrenous thrombosis of the large vessels, anticoagulation with heparin should be considered.

  3. Prevention

    a. Infants should be given vitamin K_1, 1 mg IM, at birth.

    b. Mothers who are taking phenytoin should be given 10 mg vitamin K_1 IM 24 hours before delivery. Their newborns should have prothrombin time (PT), partial thromboplastin time (PTT), and platelet counts monitored if any signs of bleeding occur. If these levels are prolonged, the infants should be given fresh-frozen plasma, 20 ml/kg. The usual 1-mg dose of vitamin K_1 (1 mg) should be given to the baby postpartum and repeated in 24 hours.

    c. Mothers should refrain from taking aspirin for 1 week before delivery.

D. Polycythemia

  1. Etiology

    a. Placental overtransfusion.

    b. Uteroplacental insufficiency.

    c. Other causes include maternal diabetes, congenital adrenal hyperplasia, Beckwith-Wiedemann syndrome, neonatal thyrotoxicosis, and congenital hypothyroidism.

  2. Evaluation and diagnosis

    a. Most infants with polycythemia are asymptomatic.

    b. Possible signs of polycythemia include cyanosis (due to increased unsaturated hemoglobin), jaundice, lethargy, jitteriness, hypotonia, seizures, and hypoglycemia priapism. Hyperviscosity syndromes can lead to CNS vascular thrombosis.

    c. **Central** hematocrits are the most reliable index of polycythemia and peak 2 to 3 hours after birth.

  3. Treatment

    a. Any central hematocrit above 60 warrants observation and possible treatment.

    b. Any symptomatic child should have a partial exchange transfusion if the central hematocrit exceeds 65.

    c. Asymptomatic infants with a central hematocrit of 60 to 70 can usually be managed by increasing fluid intake to reduce blood viscosity.

    d. **Exchange transfusion** is probably indicated with a central hematocrit of more than 70 in the absence of symptoms. Exchange is done with 5% albumin to bring hematocrit to 60 by the following calculation:

$$\text{Volume of exchange (ml)} = \frac{\text{Hct observed} - \text{Hct desired}}{\text{Hct observed}}$$
$$\times \text{ weight (kg)} \times 80 \text{ ml/kg}$$

VII. Metabolic problems (see also Chap. 12)

   A. Metabolic disorders. Genetic metabolic disorders are seen in 1 of every 200 infants.

   1. Etiology (see Chap. 12).

   2. Evaluation and diagnosis

   a. History. Suspect metabolic disease for

   (1) A positive family history of any such disorder.

   (2) A history of unexplained neonatal deaths in the family.

   b. Physical examination

   (1) Early neonatal symptoms and signs can include tachypnea, vomiting, diarrhea, temperature instability, hypotonia, lethargy, seizures, and coma. Later signs and symptoms include jaundice, unusual odor of urine or sweat, cataracts, coarse facial features, and developmental delay.

   (2) Progressive symptoms in an infant who was well at birth.

   (3) New symptoms after a change in diet.

   (4) Appearance of symptoms without evidence of asphyxia, infection, CNS hemorrhage, or other congenital defects.

   c. Laboratory signs of these disorders include hypoglycemia, elevated anion gap, metabolic acidosis, lactic acidosis, ketosis, hyperammonemia, hyperbilirubinemia, abnormal amino acid pattern in the blood, ketonuria, positive ferric chloride test of the urine, and presence of reducing substances in the urine.

   d. For purposes of **genetic counseling,** it is important to make an accurate diagnosis even if the affected infant dies. Infants who die with symptoms that may be caused by a metabolic disorder should receive a genetics consult, and special tissue samples should be archived.

   3. Treatment

   a. Transfer of the newborn to a unit with specialized metabolic laboratory capability should be considered because many of these disorders are rapidly fatal or cause permanent CNS damage unless they are properly treated.

   b. Exchange transfusion or peritoneal dialysis should be considered.

   c. An attempt must be made to prevent protein catabolism with possible accumulation of toxic by-products. The infant should be given oral or parenteral glucose. Specific dietary or vitamin therapy should be started after a diagnosis is achieved.

   4. Specific disorders with catastrophic presentations in the newborn period include

   a. Galactosemia

   (1) Signs and symptoms. Indirect (early) or direct (late) hyperbilirubinemia, hepatomegaly, lethargy, weight loss, gram-negative sepsis, cataracts, and hypoglycemia.

   (2) Diagnosis. Reducing substance in the urine (positive Clinitest) with negative urine for glucose (negative glucose oxidase dipstick test); assay of blood for galactose 1-phosphate uridyl transferase (Beutler test) on filter paper blood specimen; assay of urine for galactose; abnormal liver function tests (SGOT, SGPT, PT, PTT).

   (3) Treatment. Elimination of lactose from the diet.

   b. Organic acidemias. Methylmalonic acidemia, propionic acidemia, and isovaleric acidemia

   (1) Signs and symptoms. Poor feeding, vomiting, lethargy, tachypnea, coma, hypotonia, spasticity, and seizures.

   (2) Diagnosis. Metabolic acidosis, ketoacidosis, hyperammonemia, hypoglycemia, ammonia odor from sweat or urine, urine methylmalonic acid by paper chromatography, gas or thin-layer chromatography, plasma and urine amino acid analysis to detect increased glycine.

(3) Treatment. Reversal of metabolic acidosis, dietary therapy, and vitamin administration appropriate for the disorder.

c. **Hyperammonemia syndromes:** the organic acidemias (see above); urea cycle disorders: carbamyl phosphate synthetase deficiency, ornithine transcarbamylase deficiency, citrullinemia, argininosuccinic acidemia, argininemia, ornithine transaminase deficiency, orotic acidurias, hyperornithinemia, and hyperlysinemia.

(1) Symptoms and signs. Sluggish feeding, lethargy, irritability, hypertonicity, hypotonicity, tachypnea, coma, and convulsions.

(2) Diagnosis. Metabolic acidosis, hyperammonemia, gas or thin-layer chromatography, and high-voltage electrophoresis.

(3) Treatment. Production of ammonia can be reduced by restricting protein intake and providing sufficient calories to reduce catabolism. Excess ammonia can be removed by hemodialysis, peritoneal dialysis, or exchange transfusion. Alternate pathways for nitrogen excretion are provided by administering sodium benzoate, sodium phenylacetate, or arginine.

B. **Infants of diabetic mothers** (IDM) are at elevated risk for the following: perinatal asphyxia, birth trauma, congenital anomalies, hypoglycemia, hypocalcemia, hyperbilirubinemia, RDS, polycythemia, feeding problems, and renal vein thrombosis.

1. Etiology: maternal hyperglycemia and fetal hyperinsulinemia.

2. Evaluation

a. Physical examination. Special attention is directed toward the manifestations and complications of IDM, especially

(1) Macrosomia: asphyxia, birth trauma.

(2) Hypoglycemia: lethargy, jitteriness.

(3) Hypocalcemia: jitteriness, seizures.

(4) Polycythemia: ruddy skin, lethargy.

(5) Hyperbilirubinemia: jaundice.

3. Laboratory

a. Blood sugar.

b. Calcium if lethargic, jittery with normal blood sugar, or otherwise indicated.

c. Hematocrit if polycythemia suspected.

4. Diagnosis. None, some, or all of the above complications may be present in an IDM.

5. Therapy

a. Infants should receive 10% glucose and water or formula by mouth or gavage hourly starting at 1 hour of age until the blood glucose is stabilized. Breast feeding will not supply sufficient glucose. Parenteral glucose should be infused if hypoglycemia is refractory to feeding.

b. If the infant is hypoglycemic and there is difficulty in achieving vascular access, **glucagon** (300 µg/kg SQ, to a maximum dose of 1.0 mg) can be used to temporarily increase the blood sugar.

c. Rapid infusions of concentrated dextrose solutions may stimulate insulin release in hyperinsulinemic infants. This hyperinsulinemic state may provoke rebound hypoglycemia (see below).

C. **Hypoglycemia** in the neonate is defined as a blood sugar of less than 30 to 40 mg/dl. A blood glucose of less than 40 mg/dl should be evaluated, and a blood glucose under 30 mg/dl requires treatment.

1. Etiology (see Table 6-7).

2. Evaluation and diagnosis

a. Physical examination: lethargy, apathy, hypotonia, tremors, apnea, hypothermia, cyanosis, seizures, weak or high-pitched cry, and poor feeding.

b. Laboratory. In the newborn, utilize glucose oxidase methods that measure true glucose.

Table 6-7. Etiology of neonatal hypoglycemia

Decreased hepatic glucose stores, production, or release
  Prematurity
  Intrauterine growth retardation
  Hypoxia
  Asphyxia
  Hypothermia
  Sepsis
  Congenital heart disease
  Glucagon deficiency
  Glycogen storage disease (type I)
  Galactosemia
  Fructose intolerance
  Adrenal insufficiency
Increased utilization of glucose (hyperinsulinism)
  Infant of diabetic mother
  Erythroblastosis fetalis
  Exchange transfusions (intraexchange hypoglycemia if heparinized blood is used,
    postexchange hypoglycemia if citrated blood is used)
  Beckwith-Wiedemann syndrome
  Nesidioblastosis
  Islet cell adenoma
  Leucine sensitivity
  Maternal chlorpropamide therapy
  Maternal benzothiadizide therapy
Other causes
  Maternal therapy with beta-sympathomimetics
  Maternal or neonatal salicylate therapy

---

3. **Treatment.** To avoid hypoglycemic encephalopathy, maintain blood glucose level over 40 mg/dl.
   a. **Anticipation and prevention** are cornerstones to successful management.
   b. **Mild symptomatic hypoglycemia** (blood sugar 20–40 mg/dl) in infants over 2,000 g can often be successfully treated with oral glucose and water or formula.
      (1) Infants who cannot maintain normoglycemia for 2 hours should then be treated with **parenteral glucose.**
      (2) **Hydrocortisone,** 5 mg/kg/day IM, in two divided doses, can be used in cases that do not respond to glucose infusions. Glucocorticoid therapy is rarely instituted before 24 hours' postnatal age.
      (3) **Epinephrine, diazoxide, and growth hormone** are occasionally useful in special cases of chronic intractable hypoglycemia. *Endocrine consultation is required in these cases.*
D. **Hypocalcemia:** serum total calcium concentration less than 7.0 mg/dl or ionized calcium concentration below 4.0 mg/dl (1 mmole/liter).
   1. **Etiology.** Hypocalcemia results from decreased calcium intake and mobilization due to transient neonatal hypoparathyroidism.
      a. **Onset in first 3 days**
         (1) **Maternal factors.** Diabetes, toxemia, obstetric complications, severe dietary calcium deficiency, or maternal hyperparathyroidism.
         (2) **Intrapartum factors.** Asphyxia, prematurity, or maternal magnesium treatment.
         (3) **Postnatal factors.** Hypoxia, shock, asphyxia, poor intake, RDS, sepsis, respiratory or metabolic alkalosis, or exchange transfusion.

b. Onset after 3 days (see Chaps. 4 and 13). In addition to the above, a high-phosphate diet (milk, cereals), magnesium deficiency, intestinal malabsorption, renal disease, hypoparathyroidism, and vitamin D deficiency or a metabolic defect can result in hypocalcemia.

2. Evaluation and diagnosis

a. Physical examination. Findings may be nonspecific: irritability, jitteriness, hypertonia, a high-pitched cry, apnea, and seizures.

b. Laboratory

(1) Calcium should be measured regularly in infants with the preceding conditions and substantiated if necessary with ECG measurement of the QT (corrected QT interval) or Q-T interval.

(2) Evaluation of persistent hypocalcemia should include determination of ionized calcium, serum phosphorus, magnesium, BUN, creatinine, parathyroid hormone, and calcitonin.

3. Treatment (see also p. 400)

a. Preparations. It is preferable to use only one calcium salt (gluconate) for either IV or PO administration, for example, calcium gluconate 10% PO or IV (1 ml of 10% calcium gluconate = 100 mg calcium gluconate = 9 mg elemental calcium or 0.45 mEq/ml).

b. Dosage

(1) For asymptomatic hypocalcemia (Ca < 7 mg/dl without symptoms), when formula for premature infants is not available, give 5 to 10 ml/kg/day of 10% calcium gluconate PO or IV. This should provide maintenance calcium requirements (45–90 mg/kg/day elemental calcium). Start with a low dose and increase as needed. The oral dose is mixed in with the total day's feeding. The IV dose is given by slow continuous infusion over 24 hours. After hypocalcemia resolves, the dose can be gradually decreased over 48 hours.

(2) Acute symptomatic hypocalcemia with significant symptoms such as seizures or cardiac arrhythmias

(a) Give 1.0 to 1.5 ml/kg of 10% calcium gluconate IV immediately in a secure IV site.

(b) The dose should be given slowly IV (1 ml/min), with careful observation of the heart rate and the vein if a peripheral IV is being used, and repeated in 15 minutes.

c. Maintenance

(1) Following the acute dose, maintenance calcium, 45 to 90 mg/kg/day elemental calcium, should be given IV or PO.

(2) Treatment of hypocalcemia is rarely necessary for more than 4 to 5 days unless other complications are present.

d. Most hypocalcemia causes no symptoms and does not need rapid correction. **Aggressive, rapid therapy of asymptomatic hypocalcemia provokes excessive treatment risks.**

e. Persistent hypocalcemia. If the infant remains hypocalcemic despite adequate calcium supplementation and normal magnesium levels, a search for other causes of hypocalcemia must be initiated (see Chap. 13).

f. Associated hypomagnesemia

(1) Symptomatic hypocalcemia that is unresponsive to calcium therapy may be due to concomitant hypomagnesemia and will not respond unless the hypomagnesemia is treated.

(2) Treatment of symptomatic acute hypomagnesemia should include 0.1 to 0.2 ml/kg of 50% $MgSO_4$ IV (infuse slowly and monitor heart rate) or IM (can cause local tissue necrosis), repeated if necessary q6–12h. Maintenance magnesium therapy consists of oral administration of 50% $MgSO_4$, 100 mg or 0.2 mg/kg/day. If significant malabsorption is present, the dose can be increased two- to fivefold.

VIII. Infection. Infection accounts for 10 to 20% of neonatal deaths.

A. Congenital and prenatal infections

1. TORCH

  a. Etiology: classically includes toxoplasmosis, rubella, CMV, and herpes simplex virus (HSV). Syphilis, hepatitis B virus (HBV), and AIDS virus (see sec. **3** below) are also often included.

  b. Evaluation and diagnosis

    (1) Maternal history. Most prenatal maternal infections with these agents are asymptomatic.

      (a) Known history of congenital infection.

      (b) Habitual abortion.

      (c) Infertility.

      (d) Contact with cats or mice.

      (e) Ingestion of raw meat.

      (f) Immunosuppressive therapy.

      (g) Exanthem during pregnancy.

      (h) Unexplained adenopathy.

      (i) Unexplained illness during pregnancy.

      (j) Oral or genital lesions.

      (k) Occupational exposure to congenital infection (e.g., neonatal nurses, dialysis workers).

    (2) Maternal diagnosis. All mothers should be screened early in pregnancy for antibodies to syphilis, rubella, and hepatitis B surface antigen. Serologic testing is available for HSV, CMV, HBV, and HIV. Viral cultures are available for HSV, rubella, CMV, and enterovirus. Polymerase chain reaction (PCR)–based DNA testing for certain viruses is available in some centers. Maternal vaginal cultures are used to diagnose maternal gonorrhea and group B streptococcal colonization.

    (3) Neonatal manifestations include prematurity, intrauterine growth retardation, failure to thrive, and hepatomegaly with hepatitis and elevated direct bilirubin. **Disease-specific manifestations** include

      (a) Syphilis. Mucocutaneous lesions (snuffles), periostitis, osteochondritis, hepatomegaly, and rash.

      (b) Toxoplasmosis. Chorioretinitis, hydrocephalus, and intracranial calcifications.

      (c) Cytomegalovirus. Microcephaly with periventricular calcifications, thrombocytopenia, and hepatosplenomegaly.

      (d) Rubella. Retinopathy, cataracts, patent ductus arteriosus, pulmonary artery stenosis, deafness, and thrombocytopenia.

      (e) Herpes simplex virus. Skin vesicles, hepatitis, pneumonia, encephalitis, and DIC.

      (f) Hepatitis B virus. Hepatitis between 1 and 6 months of age.

      (g) Enterovirus. Encephalitis, sepsis-like syndrome, hepatitis, and DIC.

      (h) Parvovirus, anemia, hydrops fetalis.

      (i) HIV (see sec. **3** below for complete discussion).

    (4) Laboratory examination (see also Chap. 5)

      (a) Draw sera for a serology screen (5–10 ml blood; before **transfusions**) or use cord blood (serum). Samples should be paired with a maternal sample drawn at the same time. This should include an assessment of maternal immunoglobulin M (IgM)–specific antibodies. Convalescent serum from the mother and baby must be sent in 2 to 8 weeks.

      (b) Measure total cord blood IgM (normal < 20 mg/ml).

      (c) Send viral cultures (HSV, rubella, CMV, enterovirus).

      (d) Prepare Tzanck smear of vesicles from the infant or mother to assess for HSV, varicella.

      (e) Urine antigen and culture assay for CMV.

      (f) Send placenta for pathologic examination, including histology.

      (g) If appropriate, determine HBsAg, antibody to surface antigen (anti-HBs), hepatitis B core antigen (HB_cAg), and antibody to hepatitis B core antigen (anti-HB$_c$), as well as liver enzymes and bilirubin.

(h) Measure platelet count and PT, PTT.

c. Treatment (see also Chap. 5, p. 159)

(1) Treatment is available for toxoplasmosis (see Chap. 5).

(2) No specific treatment is available for rubella. Symptomatic therapy of congestive heart failure from PDA and surgical correction of cataracts may be indicated.

(3) Severe systemic CMV may require treatment with ganciclovir.

(4) Herpes simplex virus has been successfully treated with both vidarabine and acyclovir (see Chap. 5). Topical idoxuridine Ara-A ophthalmic eyedrops are recommended.

(5) If varicella develops in the mother less than 5 days before delivery or 2 days postpartum, there will be insufficient time for transfer of maternal antibody to the fetus. To ameliorate disease in the newborn, infants should receive 125 units varicella-zoster immune globulin (VZIG) IM. In both cases the infant should be isolated from the mother until she is no longer infectious. Other possible household contacts must be investigated.

d. Prevention

(1) Toxoplasmosis (see Chap. 5) incidence may be reduced by avoiding cats and the eating of raw meat during pregnancy, thus reducing incidence of primary maternal infection.

(2) Congenital **rubella** can be prevented by adequate immunization of childbearing women.

(3) Because the majority of neonatal **HSV** infections are acquired at the time of vaginal delivery, the infants of mothers with active genital herpes should be delivered by cesarean section. If the membranes are ruptured, the baby should be delivered by cesarean section as soon as possible. Postnatal infection can be acquired from mothers with active lesions. If the mother has a primary HSV infection or positive cultures at the time of delivery, or both, cultures should be obtained from the oropharynx/nasopharynx and conjunctivae at 24 hours of age. Infants with positive cultures or in whom symptoms of infection develop should have their culture repeated and antiviral treatment (acyclovir, 8–10 mg/kg IV q8h) initiated.

(4) Infants born to mothers in whom **hepatitis A** develops within 2 weeks of delivery should be given immune serum globulin (ISG), 0.15 ml/kg IM. Infants born to mothers who are HBsAg positive should receive both hepatitis B immune globulin (HBIG) and hepatitis B vaccine at birth. The hepatitis B vaccine is repeated at 1 and 6 months. Recommendations for routine immunization for HBV are covered in Chapter. 3.

2. Syphilis (see also Chap. 5, p. 125)

a. Etiology. Transplacental transmission of *Treponema pallidum.*

b. Evaluation

(1) Perinatal clinical signs include stillbirth, fetal hydrops, and prematurity.

(2) Postnatal manifestations include failure to thrive, persistent rhinitis, lymphadenopathy, exanthema, jaundice, anemia, hepatosplenomegaly, nephrosis, and meningoencephalitis.

c. Diagnosis

(1) Mother. Rapid plasma reagin with titers and fluorescent-treponemal antibody absorption test (FTA-ABS) with titers. Test at first antenatal visit and in third trimester.

(2) Infant

(a) Rapid plasma reagin with titer and FTA-ABS with titer.

(b) If available, IgM–FTA-ABS is most specific for fetal infection.

(c) X-rays of long bones may provide evidence of demineralization of periosteal new bone formation in the metaphyses.

    (d) Dark-field examination of any nasal discharge.

    (e) Cerebrospinal fluid (CSF) examination to evaluate for meningoencephalitis.

  d. Treatment (see also Chap. 5, p. 125)

    (1) If the infant's serologic test results are negative and he or she has no disease, *no* treatment is necessary.

    (2) If the serologic test results are positive, treat the **symptomatic** infant. Treat the **asymptomatic** infant for any of the following situations.

      (a) The titer is three to four times higher than the mother's.

      (b) The FTA is 3 to 4+.

      (c) The mother was inadequately treated or was untreated.

      (d) The mother is unreliable, and follow-up is doubtful.

      (e) The mother's infection was treated with a drug other than penicillin.

      (f) The mother had a recent sexual exposure to an infected person.

      (g) The mother was treated in the last month of pregnancy.

      (h) The mother has HIV and was treated for syphilis with less than neurosyphilis regimen.

    (3) If the baby has a positive RPR or FTA, or both, and the history and clinical findings (including x-ray) make infection unlikely, it is safe to await the IgM report and repeat RPR and FTA titers. Any significant rise in titer or any clinical signs require treatment. If the antibodies are transferred maternal antibodies, the baby should have a falling titer and be negative by 4 months. Treat if the serology is not negative by 6 months of age.

    (4) For infants with no evidence of CNS infection, give procaine penicillin G in aqueous suspension, 50,000 units/kg IM in one daily dose for 10 to 14 days, or aqueous crystalline penicillin G, 100,000 to 150,000 units/kg/day q8–12h IM or IV for 10 to 14 days (see Chap. 5, sec. **III.G.4.c**). Infants with CNS infection (CSF pleocytosis, elevated CSF protein, positive CSF serology) should be treated with aqueous procaine penicillin, 50,000 units/kg/day IM for 3 weeks, or aqueous crystalline penicillin, 150,000 units/kg/day q8–12h for 2 to 3 weeks. For infants at low risk for infection for whom follow-up is doubtful, treatment with benzathine penicillin G, 50,000 units/kg/day IM as a one-time dose, can be given.

3. Acquired immunodeficiency syndrome (see also Chap. 5, p. 151)

  a. Etiology. Maternal infection and transplacental passage of HIV.

  b. Evaluation. Consider the diagnosis in an infant when the mother or mother's partner is in a high-risk group.

    (1) Intravenous drug abuser.

    (2) Prostitute.

    (3) Sexual partner of HIV-positive man.

    (4) Sexual partner of hemophiliac.

    (5) Recipient of blood transfusion between 1979 and 1985.

  c. Diagnosis

    (1) Informed consent is required for testing of mother or baby.

    (2) Maternal HIV antibody status should be tested using an enzyme-linked immunosorbent assay (ELISA) with confirmation by Western blot analysis.

    (3) If the mother is positive, the **infant** may test positive for HIV antibody because of passive placental transfer of maternal antibody without transfer of HIV. Referral of such infants to a pediatric HIV program as soon as possible after birth is recommended. A combination of clinical, virologic, and serologic parameters can be used for early detection of HIV infection, including HIV culture and assay for p24 antigen. At 18 months of age, HIV antibody testing represents the child's own, rather than maternal, antibodies.

d. Treatment. Pre- and perinatal maternal treatment with zidovudine, combined with neonatal treatment, can reduce vertical perinatal transmission to less than 10%.

e. Breast feeding. Postnatal transmission of HIV from infected mothers to infants by means of breast milk is well documented. Although the risk for postnatal infection is small, HIV-positive mothers in developed countries should not breast feed.

f. Universal precautions

(1) Gloves, gowns, and eye protection should be worn in the delivery room.

(2) Never suction for meconium with direct endotracheal suction. DeLee suction trap or a special suction device should be used.

(3) Infants should be bathed carefully on admission.

(4) Linens and disposables should be placed in separate marked containers.

(5) Laboratory and phenylketonuria (PKU) tests should be specially labeled and enclosed.

4. Gonorrhea

a. Etiology. Intrapartum infection with Neisseria gonorrhoeae.

b. Evaluation

(1) Gonococcal ophthalmia usually presents within 3 days of birth. If the eyes are infected before birth in association with premature rupture of the membranes, symptoms may be present at birth. Usually, a watery, then mucopurulent, then bloody conjunctival discharge develops. Prominent edema of the conjunctiva and lids develops, followed by corneal edema and ulceration. Perforation of the globe with panophthalmitis may evolve.

(2) Other gonococcal infections include rhinitis, anorectal infection, arthritis, sepsis, and meningoencephalitis.

(3) Conjunctivitis from silver nitrate, HSV, staphylococci, pneumococci, *Escherichia coli*, and *Chlamydia* should be considered in the differential diagnosis.

c. Diagnosis

(1) A presumptive diagnosis is made by demonstration of gram-negative diplococci on Gram's stain of the exudate.

(2) Definitive diagnosis requires bacterial culture.

d. Treatment (see Chap. 5, p. 127)

(1) Asymptomatic infants. If a Gram's stain or culture from a maternal or neonatal source is positive for *N. gonorrhoeae*, the infant should be treated with one dose of aqueous crystalline penicillin G (50,000 units for term and 20,000 units for preterm infants) IM or IV, or ceftriaxone, 125 mg (50 mg/kg for preterm infants) IV or IM, in addition to ocular prophylaxis.

(2) Symptomatic infants (ophthalmia, arthritis, sepsis) should be treated with 100,000 units/kg/day q12h of aqueous crystalline penicillin G for 7 days.

(3) Frequent saline irrigations of conjunctivae will help remove inflammatory exudate.

(4) The possibility of penicillin-resistant gonococcus should be considered. Sensitivity testing should be done on all positive cultures. Cefotaxime, 100 mg/kg/day divided q8h (q12h for preterm infants) for 7 days, may be a more appropriate therapy until antibiotic sensitivities are obtained.

e. Prevention

(1) Pregnant women should have endocervical cultures for gonorrhea. Cultures should be repeated at delivery for high-risk women.

(2) Application of erythromycin 0.5% ophthalmic ointment, tetracycline 1% ophthalmic ointment, or 1% silver nitrate to the infant's eyes at the time of birth will usually prevent gonococcal ophthalmia.

Table 6-8. Bacterial and fungal organisms associated with newborn infection

Early infection
  Group B streptococci
  Escherichia coli
  Klebsiella-Aerobacter
  Enterococcus
  Listeria monocytogenes
  Streptococcus (Diplococcus) pneumoniae
  Group A streptococci
  Haemophilus influenzae
  Neisseria gonorrhoeae
  Anaerobes: *Clostridium, Bacteroides*
Late nursery infection (>5 d of age)*
  Staphylococcus aureus
  E. coli
  Klebsiella-Aerobacter
  Candida albicans
  Pseudomonas
  Serratia
  Staphylococcus epidermidis

*The causative organisms vary with the flora of the nursery and with its personnel.

B. Acquired bacterial infections (see also Chap. 5). The incidence of sepsis in the newborn is 2 in 1,000. A meningoencephalitis will also develop in approximately 25% of the cases of neonatal bacteremia and sepsis.
  1. Sepsis
    a. Etiology. Bacterial and fungal organisms associated with neonatal infections are listed in Table 6-8.
    b. Evaluation and diagnosis
      (1) Predisposing factors include
        (a) Premature onset of labor.
        (b) Prolonged rupture of membranes.
        (c) Maternal fever or other signs of chorioamnionitis.
        (d) Maternal colonization with group B streptococci.
        (e) Intravascular catheters in the neonate.
        (f) Tracheal intubation.
      (2) History. Sepsis may manifest as
        (a) Any sudden clinical deterioration.
        (b) Temperature instability or signs of metabolic acidosis.
        (c) Nonspecific signs, such as poor feeding, lethargy, vomiting, or diarrhea.
      (3) Physical examination
        (a) Cardiopulmonary findings include cyanosis, apnea, tachypnea, and respiratory distress.
        (b) Other findings include abdominal distention, ileus, pustules, petechiae, purpura, omphalitis, and seizures.
      (4) Laboratory and radiographic evaluation
        (a) Leukopenia below 5,000/mm^3, a total neutrophil count under 1,000/mm^3, and a ratio of immature (band) to total neutrophils of greater than 0.2 all correlate with an increased risk of bacterial infection.
        (b) Cultures. Blood cultures should be obtained from a peripheral site. Cerebrospinal fluid cultures should be obtained in infants who are believed to be at high risk for meningitis. Urine cultures are generally not helpful in the immediate perinatal period.

Table 6-9. Recommended antibiotic regimens for neonatal sepsis and meningitis

Organism	Site of infection	Antibiotic therapy[a]	Duration of therapy
GBS	Blood	Penicillin, 200,000 units/kg/d	10–14 d
	CNS	Penicillin, 400,000 units/kg/d	Complete 14–21 d
E. coli K1	Blood	Cefotaxime, 50–100 mg/kg/d or other third-generation drug	Complete 14 d
	CNS	Cefotaxime, 100 mg/kg/d (? gentamicin,[b] 5 mg/kg/d for 5–10 d for synergy)	Complete 21 d
Listeria	Blood	Ampicillin, 200–400 mg/kg/d (? gentamicin,[b] 5 mg/kg/d for up to 1 wk for synergy)	Complete 14 d
	CNS	Ampicillin, 400 mg/kg/d (? gentamicin,[b] 5 mg/kg/d for up to 1 wk for synergy)	Complete 14–21 d

[a]In all cases, therapy with ampicillin (300 mg/kg/d) and gentamicin (5 mg/kg/d) is initiated until an organism has been identified and antibiotic sensitivities are determined. Doses are divided q12h for term newborn infants and should be adjusted for increased renal clearance beyond the first week of life.
[b]Gentamicin is always 2.5 mg/kg/dose, with the interval adjusted based on gestational age and serum levels. In general, the intervals are q24h for infants <1,000 g, q18h for infants <35 wk gestation, and q12h for infants >35 wk.
Source: JP Cloherty, AR Stark (eds). *Manual of Neonatal Care* (3rd ed). Boston: Little, Brown, 1991.

    (c) Chest x-ray in infants with abnormal respiratory signs may reveal an infiltrate.

    (d) Antigen detection methods, for example, for group B streptococci, such as latex agglutination assays, may be helpful, especially in the setting of antenatal maternal antibiotic treatment or parenchymal lung disease with negative blood cultures. There is, however, a significant false-positive rate.

  c. Treatment of sepsis (see Chap. 7, p. 238; see also Table 5-2, p. 81).

    (1) When sepsis is suspected, initiate antibiotic treatment **before** culture results are available (Table 6-9).

    (2) Newborns at high risk for sepsis, or in whom the diagnosis of sepsis is suspected, should be treated for the pathogens of greatest concern— group B streptococcus (GBS), *E. coli* (*ECK1*), and *Listeria* (see Table 6-9). In this group, ampicillin and an aminoglycoside, such as gentamicin, are recommended for initial therapy. Ampicillin is used for initial therapy because of its effectiveness against streptococci, *Listeria monocytogenes*, enterococci, and some gram-negative bacteria. Third-generation cephalosporins may be useful in the treatment of gram-negative infections. However, they have limited activity against *Listeria* and may place neonates with significant hyperbilirubinemia at increased risk for kernicterus because they displace bilirubin from albumin-binding sites.

    (3) Although ampicillin and gentamicin provide excellent broad coverage for perinatal pathogens, this combination may not be preferred for neonates at risk for nosocomial infections (usually > 1 wk in the nursery or neonatal intensive care unit [NICU]). These pathogens include *E. coli, Klebsiella-Aerobacter, Pseudomonas, Serratia,* and *Staphylococcus epidermidis*. **The pattern of antibiotic susceptibility of the**

common pathogens causing nosocomial infections in the nursery is important. Given the predominance of coagulase-negative staphylococci as the principal cause of nosocomial sepsis, vancomycin has become a principal agent for presumptive nosocomial gram-positive bacterial coverage. Presumptive gram-negative coverage can continue to be provided with an aminoglycoside. Ampicillin and an aminoglycoside remain the antibiotics of choice when meningitis or a urinary tract infection is suspected.

    (4) Antibiotic therapy should be refined to accommodate the sensitivities of organism(s) recovered.

    (5) Drug levels (peak and trough) should be obtained around the third to fifth dose for aminoglycosides and vancomycin in order to ensure therapeutic levels and avoid toxicity.

2. Meningitis

  a. Etiology. Group B streptococci and *E. coli* account for 70% of all cases of neonatal meningitis in North America. *Listeria monocytogenes*, miscellaneous gram-positive and gram-negative organisms, *Haemophilus influenzae*, and anaerobes account for the remainder.

  b. Evaluation

    (1) Neonatal meningitis can be rapidly fatal, despite subtle initial clinical signs. Lethargy, irritability, seizures, or encephalopathy can develop.

    (2) A full fontanel is a late sign of meningitis.

    (3) Temperature instability or fever may be present.

    (4) Laboratory studies (see p. 208).

  c. Diagnosis

    (1) Any infant suspected of having sepsis should be considered for a lumbar puncture.

    (2) The diagnosis is suspected when more than 20 to 25 WBC/mm^3 are present in CSF and this is confirmed by a positive CSF culture.

  d. Treatment (see also Chap. 5, p. 137)

    (1) The initial empiric therapy for meningitis is ampicillin (300 mg/kg/day) and gentamicin (2.5 mg/kg/dose) (see Table 6-9).

    (2) The Gram's stain of CSF or recovery of specific bacterial antigens may guide initial therapy.

    (3) Isolation of an organism from cultures and antibiotic sensitivities guide subsequent therapy.

    (4) For meningitis in low-birth-weight infants who have been in the nursery for several weeks and in those infants with central intravascular catheters, a penicillinase-resistant penicillin or vancomycin should be added to the regimen or substituted for ampicillin because of the risk of *Staphylococcus aureus* or *epidermidis* infection.

    (5) The morbidity and mortality in gram-negative neonatal meningitis caused by penicillin-resistant organisms remain so high that early, aggressive therapy must be instituted. The poor penetration of systemically administered gentamicin into the cerebrospinal space can result in an inadequate bactericidal activity against gram-negative organisms.

    (6) To assess sterilization of the blood and CSF, repeat cultures should be performed.

    (7) Intravenous antibiotic therapy of meningitis should continue for 14 to 21 days. Gram-negative meningitis requires 21 days of treatment.

3. Group B streptococcal infection. Group B streptococcus (GBS) is the most common cause of sepsis in most nurseries in the United States.

  a. Etiology. Group B streptococci are recovered from the vaginal cultures of 25% of American mothers at the time of delivery. Of their infants, 25% have positive skin or nasopharyngeal cultures, or both. Yet, for every 100 colonized infants, only 1 will develop invasive disease.

  b. Evaluation

(1) Early-onset group B streptococcal sepsis can progress rapidly from mild respiratory distress, mimicking "transient tachypnea of the newborn," to shock and death. If the disease presents within a few hours of birth, the mortality is high, irrespective of therapy.

(2) Late infection presents as meningitis or sepsis, or both, at 2 to 4 weeks of age.

(3) **Laboratory evaluation** includes CBC, chest radiograph, blood culture, urinalysis and culture, lumbar puncture, and gastric aspirate.

c. Diagnosis

(1) **Diagnosis** is confirmed by positive blood, urine, or CSF cultures.

(2) The chest x-ray may show alveolar or interstitial infiltrates, or a pattern similar to that of HMD.

(3) Gram's stain of gastric aspirate may show chains of gram-positive bacteria and neutrophils.

(4) The latex agglutination test may be helpful in cases in which the mother was treated with antibiotics before delivery. Because of the high false-positive rate associated with urine latex agglutination tests, a positive result must be interpreted in the context of the clinical picture.

d. Treatment

(1) Infants with documented group B streptococcal pneumonia should be treated with aqueous penicillin, 200,000 units/kg/day divided into three to four doses for up to 14 days (see Table 6-9). One week of treatment with gentamicin often supplements penicillin therapy.

(2) In documented meningitis, treatment with penicillin G should be carried out for 14 to 21 days at 400,000 units/kg/day.

e. Prevention

(1) Polyvalent **group B streptococcus vaccine** is being evaluated for use in nonimmune pregnant women.

(2) Administration of **ampicillin** to colonized pregnant women with fever, a history of previously GBS-infected newborns, preterm labor, or prolonged rupture of membranes (>12 to 18 hr), at any gestational age, effectively reduces the incidence of neonatal group B streptococcal infection.

4. Pneumonia (see also Chap. 5, p. 102)

a. Etiology

(1) **Congenital pneumonia.** Transplacental agents include TORCH agents, enteroviruses, *T. pallidum, L. monocytogenes, Mycobacterium tuberculosis, Mycoplasma, Ureaplasma, and Candida albicans.*

(2) **Perinatally acquired pneumonia** is associated with inhalation of infected amniotic fluid (often caused by prolonged rupture of the membranes) or hematogenous miliary seeding of the lungs. These pneumonias are due to maternal vaginal flora, including group B streptococci, *E. coli,* other gram-negative enteric bacteria, staphylococci, pneumococci, anaerobic organisms, *Chlamydia, Mycoplasma, Ureaplasma,* and HSV.

(3) **Nosocomial pneumonia** acquired after birth can come from nursery personnel, other infants in the nursery, or nursery equipment. Staphylococci, gram-negative enteric bacteria, enteroviruses, respiratory syncytial virus, adenovirus, parainfluenza virus, *Chlamydia,* and HSV are common agents.

b. Evaluation

(1) **A history** of maternal fever, premature delivery, prolonged rupture of membranes, obstetric manipulation, or foul-smelling amniotic fluid should increase suspicion of neonatal bacteremia or pneumonia.

(2) **Physical examination.** Fever, lethargy, tachypnea, grunting, flaring of nasal alae, retractions, irregular breathing, rales, and cyanosis may be present.

    (3) Laboratory tests should include a CBC, and a chest x-ray for evidence of pulmonary infiltrate or pleural effusion. Cultures of the blood, urine, CSF, and tracheal aspirate (if intubated), should be obtained.

    (4) If large amounts of pleural fluid are present, thoracentesis should be performed. Direct lung aspiration or lung biopsy is indicated in cases that are unresponsive to standard therapy.

  c. Diagnosis. A chest radiograph shows a pulmonary infiltrate.

  d. Treatment

    (1) General supportive measures

    (2) Respiratory support

    (3) Antibiotic therapy should be instituted as detailed in the treatment of sepsis, above.

5. Omphalitis

  a. Etiology. Infection with streptococci and staphylococci is common. An ascending thrombophlebitis may indicate that the infection has spread to the liver, with resultant liver abscess or thrombosis of the hepatic vein.

  b. Evaluation and diagnosis

    (1) If true omphalitis is present, the infant should have a full evaluation for sepsis, including blood, urine, and CSF cultures.

    (2) Infection can cause peritonitis and septic emboli to the liver, lungs, pancreas, kidney, skin, and bone.

  c. Treatment

    (1) As for sepsis, IV antibiotics should be administered before culture results are available. Because *Staphylococcus* is a common agent, oxacillin and gentamicin should be continued for 7 to 10 days.

    (2) Any catheter in the umbilicus should be removed.

6. Tuberculosis in the newborn (see Chap. 5, p. 147).

7. Urinary tract infection is due to an ascending or hematogenous source. The diagnosis is made by examination and culture of urine obtained by a bladder tap or sterile catheterization. Initial systemic treatment with ampicillin and an aminoglycoside is indicated. Duration of parenteral treatment is 14 days. Ultrasound and contrast studies of the urinary tract are indicated after treatment in order to evaluate for anomalies and reflux. (see also Chap. 5, p. 121)

8. Skin pustules

  a. Etiology. Staphylococci and, less commonly, streptococci, are the most common causative organisms, followed by maternal group 6 streptococci, coliforms, and anaerobic organisms. Wounds from scalp monitors or abrasions related to delivery can cause both local and systemic infection.

  b. Evaluation and diagnosis. Gram's staining will show gram-positive cocci.

  c. Therapy

    (1) When only a few staphylococcae pustules are present, bathing with antibacterial soap and local application of bacitracin ointment may suffice.

    (2) If there are multiple pustules or the infant appears sick, a sepsis evaluation and systemic treatment with oxacillin are indicated. Systemic illness or local spread in spite of topical therapy requires the use of systemic parenteral antibiotics and occasionally incision and drainage.

9. Septic arthritis or osteomyelitis (see Chap. 5, pp. 134, 136).

  a. Etiology. Can result from bacteremia or local trauma (heel sticks).

  b. Evaluation and diagnosis require clinical examination, joint ultrasound and aspiration of fluid, and occasionally bone scan. Radiographic changes usually occur late in illness.

  c. Treatment is administration of systemic antibiotics for 3 to 4 weeks after local signs resolve (see Chap. 5). Open surgical drainage is recommended for diagnosis and relief of pressure in some joints (e.g., hip, shoulder), but needle aspiration may be sufficient for others (e.g., knee, wrist). Immobilization of joints is recommended until local signs have resolved and physical therapy can be initiated.

C. Isolation guidelines. Guidelines for obstetric-neonatal isolation procedures can be found in the American Academy of Pediatrics and the American College of Obstetricians and Gynecologists' *Guidelines for Perinatal Care*, 1994.

IX. Fluid and electrolyte management (see also Chap. 4)
  A. Electrolytes
    1. Sodium
      a. The usual maintenance requirement for sodium is 2 to 3 mEq/kg/day starting on the second or third day of life. Preterm infants may require 4 to 8 mEq/kg/day because of sodium wasting secondary to immature renal function. As the kidney matures over the first few weeks, this requirement will gradually decrease.
      b. Hyponatremia can result from sodium deficiency or free-water excess.
      c. Hypernatremia is caused by sodium overload, free-water loss secondary to diarrhea and vomiting, or failure to provide adequate free water in immature infants with increased insensible water loss.
      d. Treatment of hyponatremia and hypernatremia (see Chap. 4, p. 73).
    2. Potassium
      a. The usual maintenance requirement for potassium is 2 to 3 mEq/kg/day starting on the second or third day of life.
      b. Hyperkalemia in the newborn may be caused by excessive potassium administration, adrenal insufficiency, or exchange transfusion with old blood. The ECG may show peaked T waves.
      c. Hypokalemia in the newborn can be due to insufficient replacement of ongoing potassium losses, recurrent vomiting (e.g., pyloric stenosis), or diuretic use. The ECG may show depressed T waves.
      d. Treatment of hypokalemia and hyperkalemia (see Chap. 9, p. 310).
    3. Calcium requirements are 30 to 45 mg/kg/day. Since IV infiltrates with calcium containing intravenous fluids (IVF) can cause severe tissue damage, calcium should not be added to peripheral IVF unless necessary.
  B. Fluid and electrolyte monitoring. Fluid and electrolyte balance must be assessed frequently.
    1. History of intake and output.
    2. Physical examination and weight.
    3. Blood: serum electrolytes and osmolality.
    4. Urine: urinalysis and urine electrolytes.
  C. Fluid and electrolyte requirements
    1. Term infants
      a. Fluid requirement is approximately 60 to 80 ml/kg on the first day of life. Subsequently, add 20 ml/kg/day each day until total input peaks at about 150 ml/kg/day. Requirements are **decreased** in the setting of renal failure, cardiac failure, decreased insensible water loss (IWL), and increased antidiuretic hormone (ADH) states. Requirements are **increased** with excess IWL, low humidity, fever, activity, and increased renal loss.
    2. Premature infants
      a. Fluid requirements (ml/kg/day):

Body weight (g)	Days 1–2	Day 3	Days 15–20
>2,000	60–80	80–120	120–150
2,000–1,750	80	100	150
1,750–1,500	80	110	150
1,500–1,250	90	120	150
1,250–1,000	100	130	150
1,000–750	100–120	140	150

      b. Premature infants who weigh less than 1,000 g may require in excess of 200 ml/kg/day.
      c. Small premature infants who receive large volumes of IVF may require a glucose concentration of less than 10% D/W in order to avoid hyperglycemia and glucosuria.
      d. Electrolyte requirements

(1) Sodium. Premature infants require at least 2 to 3 mEq/kg/day starting on day 2 or 3. Many require up to 4 to 8 mEq/kg/day.

(2) Potassium intake should be initiated as 2 to 3 mEq/kg/day on day 2 or 3 if renal function is appropriate for gestational age.

X. Neurologic problems

A. Neonatal seizures (see also Chap. 20, p. 520)

1. **Etiology**
   a. **Asphyxia** (hypoxia, ischemia). The depressed newborn exhibits a **neonatal encephalopathy** that may be accompanied by seizures.
   b. **Intracranial hemorrhage.**
   c. **Infection.**
   d. **Metabolic or electrolyte disorders.**
   e. **Inborn errors of metabolism.**
   f. **Toxins.**
   g. **Cerebral dysgenesis.**
   h. **Benign familial seizures.**

2. **Evaluation**
   a. A full **perinatal history** and **neonatal examination** will help differentiate among the many causes of neonatal seizures.
   b. **Laboratory assessments** should include serum evaluation of blood sugar, sodium, calcium, magnesium, CBC and cultures, and a urine toxicology screen. A CSF examination, EEG with pyridoxine infusion, cranial ultrasound, and/or cranial CT scan can facilitate diagnosis, treatment, and determination of prognosis.

3. **Diagnosis.** Neonatal seizures can be divided into five categories: tonic, focal clonic, multifocal clonic, myoclonic, or, most commonly, subtle. Subtle seizures can include eye deviation, nystagmus, apnea, sucking movements, tongue thrusting, bicycling, and swimming movements.

4. **Therapy**
   a. **Treat neonatal seizures promptly.**
   b. Attention must first be directed to **vital signs**, with maintenance of airway, breathing, and circulation.
   c. Therapy should subsequently be directed at the treatable causes, such as hypoglycemia or pyridoxine deficiency (dose for pyridoxine administration is 50–100 mg IV).
   d. The cornerstone of antiepileptic therapy is **phenobarbital.**
      (1) The *loading dose* is 10 to 20 mg/kg administered over 5 to 10 minutes.
      (2) A dose of 10 mg/kg can be readministered one or two more times, if necessary, to control ongoing seizures.
      (3) The *maintenance dose* of phenobarbital is 4 to 5 mg/kg/day, administered qd or bid. Phenobarbital is well absorbed orally. The therapeutic range is 20 to 40 µg/ml. The half-life in newborns is 45 to 173 hours.
   e. **Phenytoin** is the usual second-line drug.
      (1) The *loading dose* is 20 mg/kg.
      (2) The *maintenance dose* for **IV phenytoin** is 5 to 8 mg/kg/day, usually divided bid. Doses of phenytoin that exceed 10 mg/kg/day are occasionally necessary to maintain therapeutic serum levels.
      (3) Phenytoin is very poorly absorbed orally and has an exceedingly short half-life in the first months of life. Long-term use should be avoided if possible.
   f. After administering phenobarbital and phenytoin, rectal **paraldehyde** is the usual next drug of choice. Rectal **valproate** is used on rare occasions.
   g. **Duration of therapy** is determined by the risk of recurrent seizures.
   h. Treatment with antiepileptic medications can sometimes suppress clinically evident seizures; in these cases, EEG monitoring will reveal persistent, clinically silent epileptic activity. It is controversial as to whether or not anticonvulsant levels should be increased to suppress these EEG findings.
   i. Long-term anticonvulsant therapy should be reassessed and modified if recurrent seizures develop or new side effects emerge.

B. Intraventricular hemorrhage (IVH)
1. **Etiology.** Multifactorial.
2. **Evaluation and diagnosis.** Presentation of IVH depends on the severity of hemorrhage.
   a. **Physical examination**
      (1) An infant with IVH may be asymptomatic or in extremis. In particular, though, premature infants with any abnormal neurologic signs have increased relative risk of IVH.
      (2) **Specific signs:** temperature instability, apnea, bradycardia, a full fontanel, shock, coma, tonic seizures, decerebrate posturing, quadriparesis, and dilated pupils (pupils may not constrict to light until 34 wk gestational age).
   b. **Laboratory**
      (1) **Real-time ultrasound** delineates the IVH.
      (2) Lumbar puncture often reveals xanthochromia, elevated protein, and late hypoglycorrhachia. Meningeal irritation from blood can cause a CSF pleocytosis.
      (3) A fall in hematocrit may be noted.
      (4) Metabolic acidosis can occur.
      (5) Most intracranial hemorrhages are clinically inapparent. Although 90% of IVHs occur in the first 3 days of life, hemorrhage can progress for several more days. All infants at risk for IVH (wt < 1,500 g, gestational age < 32 wk) should have a routine head ultrasound on day of life 1 to 3 and 7 to 10. Follow-up scans should be obtained as indicated.
3. **Classification.** It is most accurate to describe the anatomic distribution of an IVH.
4. **Prevention.** Prevention of preterm delivery is the most effective way to decrease the incidence of IVH.
5. **Therapy**
   a. General supportive care and measures should be instituted.
   b. Blood pressure should be maintained in a narrow, normal range.
   c. Excess cerebral perfusion may increase severity of cerebral hemorrhage and therefore should be avoided.
   d. Daily head circumference measurements and weekly ultrasound assessment of extent of hemorrhage and ventricular size should be obtained.
   e. Minor hemorrhages have a good prognosis and usually need only supportive care.
   f. If progressive ventriculomegaly develops with evidence of increased intracranial pressure, serial lumbar punctures can postpone definitive shunting. Furosemide (Lasix), 1 to 2 mg/kg/day, and acetazolamide (Diamox), 50 to 100 mg/kg/day, are used as ancillary treatments to reduce CSF production.
   g. In acute hydrocephalus that is unresponsive to serial lumbar punctures and diuretic therapy, a temporary ventriculostomy may be necessary.
   h. If progressive hydrocephalus recurs, the patient will require a ventriculoperitoneal (VP) shunt.
C. Periventricular leukomalacia (PVL). White matter injury can result in spastic diplegia, and other cognitive, motor, and sensory defects, including reduced visual fields.
XI. Necrotizing enterocolitis (NEC)
A. Etiology is multifactorial.
1. Impaired intestinal epithelial barrier function allows bacterial invasion of the bowel wall, with subsequent sepsis and perforation.
2. Factors that can exacerbate mucosal damage include ischemia, feeding of hypertonic formulas or medications, and local bacterial or viral infection.
B. Evaluation
1. **Physical examination.** Temperature instability, apnea, lethargy, shock, or nonspecific signs may be present. Signs of hypomotility (bilious gastric aspi-

rates), ischemia, and DIC (heme-positive stool, gastric aspirates) may also be present.

2. **Laboratory evaluation** should include ABGs; CBC (with WBC differential and platelet count); electrolytes; glucose; BUN; creatinine; PT and PTT; cultures of blood, stool, and CSF (if stable); kidneys, ureters, bladder (KUB), and crosstable lateral abdominal x-ray.

C. Diagnosis

1. The presence of pneumatosis intestinalis on abdominal x-ray confirms the diagnosis. Free peritoneal gas or gas in the portal venous system may be seen. Both are ominous signs.

2. **Laboratory abnormalities** include neutropenia, thrombocytopenia, acidosis, hyponatremia, hyperkalemia, hypoglycemia, and abnormal presence of reducing substances in stool.

D. Treatment

1. The infant should receive nothing by mouth.

2. A nasogastric tube should be placed to suction.

3. After appropriate cultures have been obtained, the infant should be started on broad-spectrum systemic antibiotics, including ampicillin, gentamicin, and clindamycin.

4. Treatment of shock, acidosis, hyponatremia, thrombocytopenia, or DIC should be instituted.

5. Frequent vital signs, examinations, serial abdominal x-rays, CBC with platelet count, electrolytes, and pH q6h determine the need for surgical intervention.

6. Early surgical consultation is recommended. Indications for surgery include perforation or persistent clinical deterioration.

7. Peripheral or central hyperalimentation should be instituted.

8. Bowel rest and antibiotics should be continued for 10 to 14 days.

9. Intestinal strictures or recrudescent NEC can complicate the convalescent phase of NEC.

XII. Drug withdrawal in the newborn

A. Etiology. Withdrawal symptoms may be seen in infants born to mothers who take narcotics, methadone, diazepam, phenobarbital, alcohol, ethchlorvynol, pentazocine, chlordiazepoxide, or other drugs of abuse.

B. Evaluation and diagnosis

1. **Maternal history**

2. The **infant's symptoms** include disturbed patterns of sleeping and waking rhythms, nasal congestion, sneezing, yawning, high-pitched cry, increased sucking, ravenous appetite, irritability, jitteriness, hypertonicity, hyperreflexia, clonus, sweating, tachypnea, vomiting, diarrhea, dehydration, fever, and seizures or tremors.

3. **Infants of methadone-treated mothers** may have severe, prolonged, or "late" withdrawal.

4. **Maternal cocaine addiction** has significant effects on the developing fetus and newborn, including intrauterine growth retardation, prenatal ischemic events in the CNS and GI tract, premature labor, and placental abruption following acute intoxication. Infants may be irritable and jittery for weeks after birth.

5. **Diagnosis** can be made from blood, urine, or stool.

C. Treatment. The goal of treatment is to minimize irritability, vomiting, and diarrhea, while promoting growth and sleep between feedings. Heavy sedation should be avoided.

1. Swaddling, holding, and rocking may comfort infants with mild symptoms.

2. **Drugs.** More severely affected infants will require medication.
    a. **Phenobarbital,** 5 to 8 mg/kg/day IM or PO in three divided doses, and tapered over 2 weeks, can ameliorate withdrawal.
    b. **Neonatal opiate solution** diluted to a concentration of 0.4 mg/ml morphine is given as 0.05 ml/kg dose q4–6h.
    c. Methadone should not be routinely used until more data on toxicity are available. **Methadone is excreted in breast milk.**

3. Proper disposition and follow-up of these infants should be arranged.

XIII. Surgical emergencies
  A. Tracheoesophageal fistula (TEF) with or without esophageal atresia (EA)
    1. Etiology. Esophageal anomalies in the newborn are classified based on anatomy.
    2. Evaluation. Symptoms may include excessive salivation, regurgitation of feedings, coughing from aspiration of feedings or gastric contents, abdominal distention, or a scaphoid, airless abdomen.
    3. Diagnosis
      a. Esophageal atresia is diagnosed by the inability to pass a catheter from the nose or mouth into the stomach. A plain chest radiograph may show a dilated upper esophageal pouch with a catheter coiled in the upper pouch.
      b. The absence of abdominal gas on radiograph suggests EA without a distal TEF.
      c. Tracheoesophageal fistula without EA may be suspected because of recurrent aspiration with feeding and excessive gas in the bowel.
    4. Treatment. The goal is to prevent aspiration and to provide nutrition and support before definitive surgical therapy.
      a. Sump catheter drainage of the upper pouch.
      b. Provision of a reliable IV line for nutrition and fluids.
      c. Thirty-degree head-up position.
      d. Close monitoring for signs of infection.
      e. Provision of adequate respiratory support.
      f. A **gastrostomy** is indicated to decompress the abdomen and prevent aspiration of gastric contents, particularly if mechanical ventilation becomes necessary. Definitive repair can be early, delayed, or staged.
  B. Omphalocele and gastroschisis
    1. Omphalocele
      a. Etiology. Omphalocele may be associated with other anomalies, including cardiac, genitourinary, anorectal, and limb anomalies, or may be part of a syndrome such as Beckwith-Wiedemann or trisomies 13, 18, and 21.
      b. Emergency medical treatment includes
        (1) Decompress the GI tract via nasogastric tube.
        (2) Protect an **intact** sac or intestines in a ruptured sac with saline-moistened Kling gauze and plastic wrap to support the intestinal viscera.
        (3) Provide IV fluids.
        (4) Initiate antibiotics (ampicillin and gentamicin).
        (5) Monitor temperature and blood pressure.
        (6) Provide immediate surgical treatment.
    2. Gastroschisis. Medical management of gastroschisis is similar to that of omphalocele. Infants with gastroschisis should be evaluated for malformation of the colon and intestinal atresia.
  C. Intestinal obstruction
    1. Etiology. The causes are listed in Table 6-10.
    2. Evaluation
      a. The **symptoms** of intestinal obstruction vary with the site of the lesion. Lesions distal to the pylorus present with bile-stained vomiting. Lesions high in the bowel such as malrotation with midgut volvulus will present with little abdominal distention, while lesions low in the bowel such as ileal atresia will cause distention. The patient may have a history of polyhydramnios.
      b. Laboratory evaluation may include hematocrit, CBC, electrolytes, ABGs and pH, a radiograph of the abdomen taken with the infant in the left lateral decubitus and flat positions, a barium swallow or enema, and a sweat test to assess cystic fibrosis in cases of meconium ileus.
    3. Diagnosis
      a. Pyloric stenosis.
      b. Duodenal atresia.
      c. Jejunoileal atresia.
      d. Volvulus with or without malrotation of the bowel is an emergency. It

Table 6-10. Etiology of intestinal obstruction in newborn

Mechanical obstruction (congenital)

Intrinsic
Pyloric stenosis
Duodenal atresia
Jejunoileal atresia or stenosis
Imperforate anus
Intraluminal cysts
Meconium ileus with or without
   cystic fibrosis

Extrinsic
Malrotation with or without midgut
   volvulus
Volvulus without malrotation
Peritoneal bands
Incarcerated hernia (premature infants)
Annular pancreas
Duplications
Aberrant vessels
Hydrometrocolpos

Acquired
Intussusception
Adhesions
Mesenteric artery thrombosis
Formation of intestinal concretions (lactobezoars)
Stenosis secondary to healed necrotizing enterocolitis

Functional obstruction

Prematurity

Defective innervation (Hirschsprung's
   disease)

Drugs
Hypermagnesemia
Heroin
Hexamethonium bromide

Sepsis

Enteritis
CNS disease

Necrotizing enterocolitis
Endocrine disorders such as hypothyroidism and adrenal insufficiency

---

may present as bile-stained vomiting without much abdominal distention in an infant who has previously been passing stools. Abdominal tenderness may be present. Radiographs may show duodenal obstruction with little air in the rest of the bowel. A barium enema may show the cecum in the upper right or central abdomen. Demonstration of absent or abnormal position of the ligament of Treitz confirms the diagnosis of malrotation.

    e. Meconium ileus.

    f. Functional obstruction due to conditions such as prematurity, meconium plug syndrome, hypermagnesemia, and Hirschsprung's disease.

  4. Treatment of intestinal obstruction includes

    a. Nasogastric suction.

    b. Fluid and electrolyte therapy; volume replacement (colloid) if indicated.

    c. Antibiotics if the integrity of the bowel is questionable or the infant appears sick.

    d. Surgical consultation.

D. Diaphragmatic hernia

  1. Evaluation. Mortality from this disease is high due to the associated hypoplastic lungs, abnormal pulmonary vasculature, and persistent pulmonary hypertension.

  2. Diagnosis. The diagnosis is confirmed by chest radiograph.

  3. Treatment. When a diaphragmatic hernia is suspected, the following measures should be employed.

    a. A large nasogastric tube should be inserted and put to suction.

    b. The infant should receive oxygen and respiratory support as needed. Any positive pressure should be administered through an endotracheal tube.

    c. An IV line should be placed.

    d. Hypoxia and acidosis should be treated.

    e. Prompt surgical correction should be carried out.

    f. Extracorporeal membrane oxygenation (ECMO) may be required.

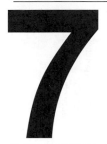

Emergency and Intensive Care

Anne Stack, Michael McManus, and Baruch Krauss

I. Cardiopulmonary resuscitation

  A. The **diagnosis** of cardiorespiratory arrest must be made rapidly (absent pulse and respirations). Prompt and orderly resuscitative efforts are essential, and **rapid assignment of responsibilities is mandatory.**

  1. The **first person** at a cardiorespiratory arrest must establish the diagnosis. **If the patient is unresponsive, call for help.** If the patient is not breathing, a patent **airway** is established via a chin lift or jaw thrust; two slow breaths are given, and then the **carotid** pulse is palpated. If there is no pulse, the first cycle of compressions and ventilations is begun (see below).

  2. **The resuscitation team** includes the following:

    a. The **leader** (the most experienced person) assigns others their roles, makes **all** therapeutic decisions, and **continually reassesses** the quality of the resuscitative efforts.

    b. **The airway is managed to ensure patency and adequacy of respirations.**

    c. **Cardiac compressions** are performed at an *age-appropriate* rate and depth.

    d. **Vascular access** should be accomplished by the next available person.

    e. Age- and weight-appropriate doses of **medications** are prepared.

    f. The **dose** and **time** of medication administration are recorded, as are **procedures** or **diagnostic tests**.

    g. The **float/circulator** monitors chest movement during ventilation and adequacy of cardiac compressions, places ECG leads, measures the blood pressure, and assists wherever help is needed.

    h. One person must obtain a **history** from the parents or caretakers and *keep them informed of events.*

  B. The following equipment and medications **must** be available.

  1. **Airway.** Oxygen, suction, and Yankauer suction catheters; adult and pediatric sized masks; oral and nasal airways; flow-dependent anesthesia or self-inflating bags; endotracheal tubes (ETT); laryngoscopes with pediatric and adult blades; McGill forceps; stylets; benzoin; and tape.

  2. **Drugs** (Table 7-1).

  3. **Vascular access.** Intravascular catheters, syringes, intraosseous needles, cutdown tray, tourniquet, and tape.

  4. **Other.** Blood pressure cuff, thermometer, glucose-specific coated strips (Dextrostix, Chemstrip), ECG machine and leads, defibrillator, chest tubes and Pleurivacs, Foley catheter, nasogastric tubes, and cardiac pacemaker.

  C. **The ABCs of resuscitation** (adapted from the American Heart Association recommendations)

  1. **Airway (A)**

    a. **Immobilize the cervical spine if spinal cord injury is a possibility.**

    b. Clear the oropharynx with a Yankauer suction or bulb suction. **Avoid blind finger sweeps.**

    c. The jaw-thrust or chin-lift maneuver removes obstruction caused by the tongue and soft tissues of the neck.

Table 7-1. Drugs used in a resuscitation*

Drug	Dose (adult dose)	Preparation	Route	Indication
Atropine	0.02 mg/kg (0.4 mg); 1.0 mg maximum	0.4 mg/ml	IV, IM, ETT	To treat bradycardia and to block vagally mediated bradycardia
Bicarbonate	1–2 mEq/kg (same)	1 mEq/ml; 0.5 mEq/ml available for infants	IV	Metabolic acidosis
Elemental calcium	10–20 mg/kg (300 mg)	CaCl = 27 mg/ml; calcium gluconate = 9 mg/ml	IV	Electromechanical dissociation: for positive inotropy and to increase vasomotor tone
Dextrose	0.5 g/kg (same)	25% D/W and 50% D/W	IV	Presumed hypoglycemia
Epinephrine	0.1 ml/kg (10 ml)	Epinephrine 1 : 10,000 (10 ml = 1 mg)	IV, ETT	Asystole, bradycardia, hypotension, to coarsen ventricular fibrillation before countershock
Lidocaine	1–2 mg/kg (50–100 mg)	100 mg/10 ml	IV, ETT	Ventricular ectopy
Naloxone hydrochloride (Narcan)	0.01 mg/kg (0.4 mg)	0.4 mg/ml	IV	Opiate intoxication

ETT = via endotracheal tube; D/W = dextrose in water.
*See sec. II for a discussion of cardiotonic infusions.

d. The head must be in the midline. Because the larynx in a child is more anterior and superior than that of an adult, the child can be put in the "sniffing" position to optimize patency; avoid hyperextension of the neck, as this can obstruct the airway.

e. Oral or nasopharyngeal airway placement may improve patency.

2. **Breathing (B).** Begin mouth-to-mouth or bag-to-mouth ventilation with 100% oxygen. **Assess the adequacy of the ventilation by observing chest wall excursion.** If chest wall excursion is insufficient despite airway patency, **prompt endotracheal tube placement** is indicated.

3. **Circulation (C)**

   a. The patient is placed on a hard, solid surface, and external cardiac compressions are started **immediately.**

   b. **Ventilation-compression.** The ventilation-compression ratio is 1 : 5 with a 1- to 1.5-second pause for ventilations to allow for adequate inspiratory time. The rate of compressions is at least 100 per minute for the infant and older child. The rate of compressions in the newborn is at least 120 per minute, with a 1 : 3 ventilation-compression ratio.

   c. **Technique.** Compressions for the **infant** are performed using one of two methods.

      (1) The **two-finger** technique utilizes two fingers of one hand for sternal compressions.

      (2) The preferred **hand-encircling** technique is performed using two hands; the infant is grasped with the fingers supporting the back and the thumbs over the middle third of the sternum.

      (3) Compressions in the **infant** are done *one* fingerbreadth below the nipple line. For the **toddler,** the heel of one hand is used and in the **older child,** two hands interlaced are used; in both cases, compressions are done *two* fingerbreadths above the xiphoid.

   d. The **adequacy** of cardiac compressions is assessed by palpating femoral or brachial pulses, or both. Counting aloud should be done by the rescuer who is doing chest compressions.

   e. An ECG **monitor** can be attached when help arrives. Temperature, blood glucose (e.g., Chemstrip, Dextrostix), and hematocrit are measured.

4. **Drugs (see Table 7-1)**

   a. **Route**

      (1) **Peripheral venous access** should be attempted percutaneously.

      (2) If peripheral access requires more than 1 to 2 minutes, proceed quickly to **intraosseous (IO) needle placement** at the proximal tibia or distal femur.

      (3) **Central access (femoral)** is best achieved using the Seldinger catheter-over-a-guidewire technique.

      (4) Several drugs can be delivered **via the endotracheal tube.** The dose should be doubled if using this route.

   b. **Specific problems and therapies**

      (1) **Asystole:** epinephrine and atropine.

      (2) **Bradycardia:** atropine or transcutaneous pacer.

      (3) **Hypoglycemia:** intravenous glucose.

      (4) **Hyperkalemia or acidemia:** sodium bicarbonate.

      (5) **Hypocalcemia:** intravenous calcium.

5. **Electrical energy**

   a. **Cardioversion and defibrillation**

      (1) **Supraventricular tachycardia (unstable)**

         (a) **Adenosine,** 0.1 to 0.2 mg/kg rapid IV push, can be attempted first (×2), followed by

         (b) **Synchronized cardioversion** at a dose of 0.25 to 0.50 joule/kg; double the dose if unsuccessful.

      (2) **Ventricular tachycardia (with a pulse)**

         (a) **Lidocaine,** 1 to 2 mg/kg IV 5–10min (maximum 3 mg/kg), followed by **procainamide,** 5 to 15 mg/kg slow IV (up to 30 mg/min to a total dose of 17 mg/kg), followed by **bretylium,** 5 to 10 mg/kg over 8 to 10 minutes (to a maximum of 30–35 mg/kg).

(b) If unsuccessful, **synchronized cardioversion;** dose, 1 joule/kg; double the dose if unsuccessful.

(3) **Ventricular fibrillation/pulseless ventricular tachycardia**

(a) **Nonsynchronized defibrillation,** 2 joules/kg. Repeat at twice the dose if unsuccessful two times.

(b) **Epinephrine,** 10 μg/kg IV, IO, or double the dose via endotracheal tube, and continue CPR.

(c) Precede subsequent defibrillation attempts with intravenous **lidocaine,** then **bretylium.** Maximum dose is 360 joules.

b. **Paddle placement**

(1) **Interface.** Electrode cream, electrode paste, and saline-soaked gauze can all be used; **do not use alcohol pads.**

(2) **Paddle placement:** one paddle at the right parasternum at the second intercostal space, one paddle in the left midaxillary line at the level of the xiphoid.

(3) **Safety. Announce "clear the table"** and be sure operator is clear before discharge.

(c) Resume cardiopulmonary resuscitation **immediately** until effective cardiac output is achieved.

D. **If pulseless electrical activity** is present, the patient should be evaluated and immediately treated for correctable mechanical or metabolic derangements. These include

1. Profound hypovolemia—the most common cause.
2. Hypoxia.
3. Cardiac tamponade.
4. Tension pneumothorax or hemothorax.
5. Hypothermia. (see p. 253).
6. Toxin ingestion (see Chap. 8).
7. Profound metabolic imbalance—hyperkalemia and acidosis (see Chap. 12).
8. Massive pulmonary embolus.

E. **Iatrogenic complications** include

1. Rib fracture.
2. Splenic or hepatic damage.
3. Pneumothorax from subclavian and internal jugular cannulation, positive pressure ventilation, or rib fracture.
4. Cardiac muscle damage or pericardial tamponade.

F. After successful resuscitation the patient must be closely monitored.

1. **Cardiovascular system**

a. Twelve-lead ECG and continuous ECG monitoring.

b. Blood pressure via indwelling arterial catheter.

c. Central venous pressure (CVP) to assess intravascular volume.

2. **Pulmonary system**

a. Arterial blood gas (ABG) to document the adequacy of ventilation and oxygenation.

b. Chest x-ray for ETT placement and evidence of aspiration, pneumothorax, or rib fracture.

3. **Central nervous system.** Observe for seizures, focal neurologic deficits, or signs of increased intracranial pressure.

4. **Renal system.** Electrolytes. The renal lesion most commonly seen is acute tubular necrosis (see Chap. 9).

5. **Gastrointestinal system.** Hypoperfusion injuries to the GI tract may be detected as abnormal liver function tests and blood in the stool.

6. **Other considerations**

a. Disseminated intravascular coagulation (see Chap. 15).

b. If trauma is suspected, evaluate with appropriate radiographs and serial hematocrits.

c. Sepsis or serious local infection may be a cause of the original arrest or a result of emergency procedures (see Chap. 5).

II. Shock is defined as failure of the cardiovascular system to provide oxygen and nutrients to the body's tissues. Shock in children may be subtle but early recognition and treatment are paramount. The diagnosis requires a careful history and physical examination for signs of compromised cardiac output. Compensatory mechanisms in the child are extraordinarily effective and *blood pressure is often maintained until very late.* **Consequently, normal blood pressure should not necessarily be reassuring.**

A. Etiology

1. **Hypovolemic shock** is due either to loss of intravascular volume or loss of vascular resistance.

   a. Hemorrhage.

   b. Severe gastroenteritis.

   c. Sepsis.

   d. Anaphylaxis.

   e. CNS injury.

   f. Burns.

2. **Hypervolemic or normovolemic shock** may be due to myocardial failure, outflow obstructive lesions, rhythm disturbances, or increased metabolic demands.

B. Evaluation

1. The **history** should include specific details of the acute illness, hydration status (fever, intake, and losses), past medical history, and medications taken.

2. **Physical examination.** An accurate weight and temperature must be obtained. Particular attention should be paid to the cardiopulmonary systems: respiratory rate and lung examination, pulse and cardiac exam, blood pressure with orthostatic changes, and peripheral perfusion. Neurologic status should be assessed, including level of consciousness and pupillary response. Serial observations are important to assess status and effectiveness of treatment.

3. **Laboratory studies** include

   a. Arterial blood gas.

   b. Complete blood count.

   c. Electrolytes, blood sugar, calcium, BUN, creatinine, cardiac enzymes, liver function tests, toxic screen, prothrombin time, partial thromboplastin time, and fibrin split products.

   d. A chest x-ray to evaluate cardiac size and pulmonary vasculature.

C. Diagnosis is confirmed by evidence of ineffective tachycardia, poor perfusion, and depressed mental status.

D. Treatment of shock

1. Establish and maintain an adequate **airway;** oxygen should be administered to every patient with signs of shock. Intubation and ventilatory support may be necessary.

2. **Volume resuscitation.** In shock without congestive heart failure, rapidly give a 20-ml/kg intravenous or intraosseous bolus of isotonic fluid (normal saline or lactated Ringer's solution). A second 20-ml/kg bolus is indicated if clinical improvement is not noted.

   a. If this volume replacement produces no clinical improvement, a CVP catheter can guide further therapy.

      (1) If the CVP is less than 5 mm Hg, further volume resuscitation is continued until the CVP is greater than 5 mm Hg.

      (2) If the CVP is greater than 5 mm Hg with no clinical improvement, the following should be considered.

         (a) Pharmacologic support (Table 7-2).

         (b) An ECG to evaluate the possibilities of myocarditis, pericardial tamponade, metabolic imbalance, or arrhythmias.

         (c) An echocardiogram to evaluate ventricular function or pericardial effusion.

         (d) A Swan-Ganz catheter.

Table 7-2. Drugs used in the treatment of shock

Drug	Dose	Maximum adult dose	Mechanisms of action	Indications	Limitations
Epinephrine	0.1–1.0 µg/kg/min	1–4 µg/min	α- and β-adrenergic, increases heart rate, increases systemic vascular resistance, positive inotropy	Anaphylaxis, hypotension, diminished cardiac contractility, bradycardia	Ventricular arrhythmias, decreases coronary blood flow, decreases renal blood flow
Norepinephrine	0.1–1.0 µg/kg/min	1–4 µg/min	α-adrenergic, increases heart rate, increases systemic vascular resistance	Hypotension without pre-existing vasoconstriction	Ventricular arrhythmias, decreases coronary blood flow, decreases renal blood flow
Isoproterenol	0.1–1.0 µg/kg/min	1–4 µg/min	β-adrenergic, increases heart rate, positive inotropy, decreases vasomotor tone	Bradycardia, diminished cardiac contractility	Ventricular arrhythmias, hypotension if the patient was hypovolemic
Dopamine	1–5 µg/kg/min	Same	Delta, increases renal, coronary, splanchnic flow	Poor tissue perfusion, to attempt to increase renal perfusion	Ventricular arrhythmias
	5–15 µg/kg/min	Same	β-adrenergic, increases heart rate, positive inotropy	Bradycardia, decreased myocardial contractility	Ventricular arrhythmias
	15–20 µg/kg/min	Same	α- and β-adrenergic, increases heart rate, increases systemic vascular resistance, positive inotropy	Hypotension, bradycardia, decreased myocardial contractility	Ventricular arrhythmias, decreases coronary blood flow, decreases renal blood flow
Dobutamine	1–20 µg/kg/min	Same	Similar to dopamine, but no delta effect; less alpha effect, possibly less chronotropic	Diminished myocardial contractility	Ventricular arrhythmias

3. Monitoring
   a. Vital signs. The following must be continuously monitored and recorded.
      (1) Temperature.
      (2) Respiratory rate.
      (3) Heart rate with cardiac monitoring.
      (4) Blood pressure. In infants and children, the best way to monitor
         blood pressure is by an indwelling arterial catheter. If this method is
         not possible, blood pressure can be monitored closely by frequent
         manual or other noninvasive measurements; a Doppler may be re-
         quired for auscultation.
      (5) Intake and output records. Intake, including crystalloid and colloid,
         and output, including urine via Foley catheter, nasogastric, wound,
         stool, and blood losses, should be recorded hourly.
III. Respiratory emergencies
   A. Upper airway obstruction
      1. Etiology
         a. Swelling of normal tissues (as in traumatic, infectious, and allergic
            processes).
         b. Aspiration of foreign objects.
         c. Anatomic abnormalities.
         d. Loss of **neurologic function** and soft tissue **tone.**
      2. Evaluation
         a. History
            (1) Onset. Acute or gradual.
            (2) The nature and course of **symptoms,** including fever, dyspnea, stri-
               dor, wheezing, dysphagia, dysphonia or aphonia, and cough.
            (3) Precipitating event or condition, including choking on a foreign body,
               trauma to the upper airway, and an acquired or congenital abnormality
               of the airway.
            (4) Current **medications.**
            (5) Allergies.
         b. The **physical examination** should quickly assess the adequacy of venti-
            lation and oxygenation and identify the cause and site of airway obstruc-
            tion.
            (1) General appearance, including alertness, distress, anxiety. Restless-
               ness, altered mental status, pallor, or cyanosis suggests **hypoxia.**
            (2) Vital signs.
            (3) Cardiorespiratory findings. The nature and adequacy of air move-
               ment and adventitious sounds, including stridor, dysphonia, and
               wheezing. *Tachycardia out of proportion to the level of anxiety* is of-
               ten present in the child with a compromised airway. **Bradycardia
               and hypotension occur in association with severe impairment of
               air movement.**
      3. Specific conditions
         a. Epiglottitis-supraglottitis is a rapidly progressive bacterial cellutitis of
            the supraglottic tissues that can result in total airway obstruction. **It is a
            true medical emergency.** Epiglottitis is most often seen in children 3 to 6
            years old; children under 2 years of age may occasionally become infected
            and the diagnosis confused with croup.
            (1) Etiology. *Haemophilus influenzae* type b (Hib) has traditionally been
               the cause of 95% of cases. The overall incidence has declined sharply
               with the advent of effective immunization against Hib. Group A strep-
               tococci, pneumococci, and, more rarely, *Corynebacterium diphthe-
               riae* or *Mycobacterium tuberculosis* are isolated as causal agents.
            (2) Evaluation
               **(a) To prevent death, the diagnosis must be made and defini-
                  tive airway maintenance established quickly.**
               (b) History usually reveals acute onset of respiratory difficulty with
                  rapid progression over several hours.

(c) **Physical examination** reveals drooling, dysphagia, fever, toxicity, inspiratory stridor, protruding jaw, and extended neck.

(d) Rarely, other hematogenous foci of infection may be present, including otitis, pneumonia, and meningitis. These must be ruled out.

(3) **Diagnosis**

(a) *Definitive diagnosis* is obtained via direct or fiberoptic visualization of the epiglottis conducted in the emergency room by experienced personnel. Under most conditions, however, **no attempt should be made to visualize the epiglottis or to carry out any other procedure until the airway has been secured.** Any manipulation, including aggressive physical examination or venipuncture, **can precipitate complete obstruction.**

(b) The *presumptive* diagnosis can be made on clinical grounds alone when needed, and if the child is in little distress, lateral neck x-rays may assist in the diagnosis. These should be done under controlled conditions, with the required staff and equipment for **immediate** intubation or tracheostomy in attendance. In younger children, special care must be taken that the film is truly lateral, as even slight rotation can produce "smudging" of the epiglottic shadow.

(4) **Therapy**

(a) Oxygen should be administered at the first sign of airway compromise. Care should be taken so as to not disturb the child. Slow, deep breaths improve laminar airflow and gas exchange.

(b) **Initial stabilization** requires placement of a secure artificial airway under controlled conditions (i.e., in the operating room after inhalation induction of general anesthesia). Intubation may be required for 1 to 3 days.

(c) **Nasotracheal intubation** is preferred over oral intubation as being more secure and comfortable for the patient. An oral endotracheal tube is initially placed and then changed if this can be done easily.

(d) *Very rarely,* when intubation cannot be carried out, **tracheostomy** is indicated.

(e) **After intubation,** the epiglottis can be examined and swabs for culture can be taken. At the same time, blood cultures can be drawn and IV fluids begun.

(f) **Antibiotic therapy** (see also Chap. 5). Ampicillin-sulbactam (Unasyn), 200 mg/kg/day, should be started immediately. Alternatively, ceftriaxone, 50 mg/kg/day, or cefotaxime, 150 to 200 mg/kg/day, can be used.

(g) Evaluation for other foci of infection should be continued and the patient maintained in respiratory isolation for 24 hours after initiation of antibiotic therapy.

b. **Croup,** or **viral laryngotracheobronchitis,** is marked by glottic and subglottic edema, resulting in loss of voice and airway narrowing. Inflammation and obstruction to airflow result in characteristic barking cough, and stridor.

(1) **Etiology.** Parainfluenza, influenza, respiratory syncytial virus, and, less commonly, adenovirus are typical causes. Bacterial infection has been increasingly recognized but remains unusual.

(2) **Evaluation and diagnosis**

(a) **History.** A coryzal prodrome is common, with increasing barking cough and hoarseness. Often, it is worse at night and usually occurs in children under 3 years of age.

(b) **Physical examination** is directed at assessing the extent of airway narrowing. **Inspiratory stridor, tachypnea, retractions, and diminished breath sounds indicate critical narrowing.**

Restlessness, tachycardia, altered mental status, or cyanosis suggests **hypoxia.**

(c) **Laboratory data.** A lateral neck x-ray will rule out epiglottitis. An anteroposterior neck film will show subglottal narrowing (the classic *steeple* sign). In serious cases, arterial oxygen saturation can be monitored continuously by pulse oximetry and adequacy of ventilation by ABG.

(3) **Therapy**

(a) **Home care.** Most cases of croup are mild and can be managed at home. Therapeutic measures include a cool-mist vaporizer, increased fluids, and careful observation. Parents should be instructed to call their physician if the child's respiratory distress worsens.

(b) **Hospital care.** Humidified oxygen should be administered in a quiet room where parents can stay with the child. Elimination of all but the most necessary procedures will help reduce the child's anxiety and associated increased respiratory work. If tachypnea is present, continuous pulse oximetry is desirable.

(c) Aerosolized **racemic epinephrine** is usually sufficient: 0.25 to 0.75 ml diluted with 2 ml normal saline (2.25%) and administered by standard passive aerosol equipment. However, rebound worsening may occur approximately 30 to 60 minutes after use. Therefore, its use **requires** observation for up to 4 hours.

(d) Steroid administration is now generally accepted as helpful in reducing the severity of croup and diminishing the need for intubation. Dexamethasone (0.5–0.6 mg/kg IM) can be used in moderate to severe cases.

(e) When respiratory compromise is severe and respiratory failure is present or imminent, **intubation** under controlled conditions is indicated. **The need for frequent administration of racemic epinephrine may indicate impending respiratory failure.**

(f) The decision to discharge is based on reduction in severity, the family's capacity for home care, and reduced need for observation.

c. **Foreign body aspiration** is the leading cause of accidental deaths in toddlers. The neurologic sequelae of aspiration depend on the relative compromise of air movement. The respiratory sequelae depend on the material aspirated and the extent and character of associated inflammation.

(1) **Etiology.** Poorly designed or age-inappropriate toys or food products, including peanuts, hard candy, and gum, are usually involved. **Balloons** are a particular hazard in younger children, who may bite the inflated toy and aspirate fragments as they startle at its rupture.

(2) **Evaluation and diagnosis** are directed at assessing the adequacy of air movement and locating the site of obstruction and type of offending material.

(a) The **history** should identify the acuteness of onset and the circumstances surrounding aspiration. Choking, gagging, high-pitched wheezing, dysphonia, or aphonia may be noted. A history of fever and the clinical course will help differentiate acute aspiration from an infectious obstructive process (epiglottitis, croup, bacterial tracheitis).

(b) The **physical examination** should first establish the adequacy of the airway and location of the obstruction.

(c) **Laboratory data.** Anteroposterior and lateral neck and chest roentgenograms will reveal radiopaque foreign bodies and occasionally provide clues as to the location of radiolucent objects. Obstruction of the upper airway from foreign bodies usually occurs at the laryngeal level. Inspiratory and expiratory films and fluoroscopy are sometimes very useful in patients with negative radiographic findings.

(3) Therapy depends on the acuteness and severity of the obstruction.

    (a) A conscious, actively choking, aphonic child with minimal air movement requires immediate noninvasive procedures.

    (b) If the child is in stable condition, pink, coughing, and vocalizing well, attempts to remove the foreign body (laryngoscopy or bronchoscopy) should await controlled conditions.

        (i) If the victim is an infant, (< 1 yr), **the Heimlich maneuver should be avoided because of potential intraabdominal injury.** In this age group, a combination of up to five back blows and five chest thrusts is recommended.

        (ii) If the victim is a child (> 1 yr), the **Heimlich maneuver** (4–6 subdiaphragmatic abdominal thrusts) is recommended.

        (iii) Blind finger sweeps are contraindicated in the infant and child because they can advance a foreign body further down the airway.

        (iv) An unconscious child with inadequate respirations should receive 100% oxygen by face mask. When staff members experienced in laryngoscopy are present, immediate direct **laryngoscopy** may allow visualization and removal of the foreign body. When this is not possible, or if laryngoscopy is difficult or prolonged, then **emergency cricothyrotomy** with a large-bore (e.g., 14-gauge) catheter (for insufflation of 100% oxygen), or tracheostomy, is indicated. Occasionally, **endotracheal intubation** will bypass a soft foreign body or move the object into a main-stem bronchus and permit ventilation of the contralateral lung.

  d. Bacterial tracheitis is an acute, infectious airway disease with clinical features common to both croup and epiglottitis.

    (1) Etiology. *Staphylococcus aureus* is the most common pathogen. Streptococcus and *H. influenzae* are other common pathogens.

    (2) Evaluation and diagnosis

      (a) History. Upper respiratory symptoms are usually present; then progress within hours or days to *severe* respiratory distress.

      (b) Physical examination reveals fever, barking cough, and inspiratory stridor.

      (c) Laboratory examination. A lateral neck **radiograph** obtained to rule out epiglottitis may show irregular tracheal margins with a blurring of the tracheal air column or a ribbon of mucosa lifting into the tracheal lumen. **Culture** of tracheal secretions should be positive. Blood cultures are usually negative.

    (3) Treatment

      (a) Humidified **oxygen** in a croup tent.

      (b) Antibiotics with adequate staphylococcal coverage (see Table 5-2).

      (c) Endotracheal intubation may be required for pulmonary toilet and relief of obstruction.

B. Lower airway disease may result in impaired gas exchange in the lung caused by viral and bacterial infections, foreign bodies, or intrinsic bronchospastic disease.

  1. Acute asthma (see also Chap. 16, p. 461) is a condition in which bronchospasm, mucosal edema, and mucous secretion and plugging contribute to significant narrowing of the large airways and subsequent impaired gas exchange.

    a. Evaluation and diagnosis

      (1) The **history** should include age, duration, and course of the present attack; course and severity of previous attacks; and a list of all medications (with doses) previously administered. Foreign body aspiration and anaphylaxis should be ruled out.

      (2) The **physical examination** should assess the adequacy of air exchange.

    (a) Altered mental status is a sign of marked impairment of gas exchange.

    (b) Vital signs should be measured often. Tachypnea and tachycardia are common. **An abrupt decline in respiratory rate may indicate impending respiratory failure.**

    (c) Measure and follow **peak expiratory flow rate (PEFR)**, if possible.

    (d) Assess the quality of breath sounds, prolongation of the expiratory phase, degree of dyspnea, and retractions. *Pallor* and *cyanosis* may be observed in severe cases. Paradoxically, as air exchange diminishes, audible wheezing may cease.

    (e) Assess hydration.

    (f) Palpate for subcutaneous emphysema in the neck and upper chest.

(3) Laboratory tests and ancillary studies should be done while starting therapy.

    (a) Measurement of **ABGs** is particularly helpful in evaluating response to therapy in patients with *severe symptoms*. **Pulse oximetry** confirms suspected desaturation.

    (b) Spirometry, particularly PEFR and 1-second forced expiratory volume (FEV_1), provides a good indication of the state of respiratory function in children.

    (c) Chest roentgenograms are useful **only** when the cause is in question (e.g., foreign body aspiration), when an associated pneumonia is considered likely, or when complications such as pneumothorax or pneumomediastinum are suspected.

    (d) Serum theophylline concentration in children taking theophylline should be assayed and followed.

b. Therapy

(1) Oxygen. Asthmatic patients are hypoxic. Give humidified oxygen by nasal cannula or face mask to deliver at least 30 to 40% oxygen, to maintain oxygen saturation greater than 94%.

(2) Inhalation therapy

    (a) Nebulized bronchodilators have surpassed subcutaneous agents as initial treatment of choice for reactive airway disease. Continuous or aggressive intermittent administration of beta-2 agonists often provides efficacy equal to or greater than parenteral therapy with fewer side effects.

    (b) Selective beta-2-specific bronchodilators such as **albuterol** and **terbutaline** are preferred over less selective agents such as **isoetharine,** yet individual patients may occasionally respond more favorably to the latter. **Isoproterenol,** though potent, has a narrow therapeutic index compared to more selective agents.

    (c) After initial assessment and administration of oxygen, begin **nebulized albuterol,** 0.1 to 0.25 mg/kg (up to 5 mg/dose) every 20 minutes three times or until measured peak flow normalizes or improves significantly.

    (d) Alternatively, nebulized terbutaline (IV preparation in nebulizer), 0.3 mg/kg up to 5 mg/dose, can be administered similarly.

    (e) Isoetharine and isoproterenol (1 : 200 preparation), 0.25 to 0.5 ml, can be diluted in 2 ml normal saline (NS) and delivered by an oxygen-driven nebulizer.

    (f) Albuterol (2 mg/5 ml) and terbutaline (1 mg/ml) can safely be given by *continuous nebulization* in a dosage of 0.3 mg/kg/hr to a maximum of 15 mg/hr.

    (g) Ipratropium bromide (Atrovent) is an anticholinergic bronchodilator with low absorption that lacks the systemic side effects of atropine. It is supplied as a metered-dose inhalation aerosol and can also be administered via an oxygen-driven nebulizer.

(3) Subcutaneous medication
   (a) Epinephrine is reserved for use in the *rare* patient who is unable to generate sufficient air movement to respond to nebulized bronchodilators. Give 0.01 ml/kg (1 : 1,000 dilution) SQ, with a maximum of 0.3 ml/dose. If a beneficial effect is obtained, the injection can be repeated twice at 20-minute intervals. **Excessive or inappropriate use of epinephrine can induce serious cardiac arrhythmias and cause increased restlessness and anxiety**, particularly in the presence of theophylline.
   (b) Terbutaline. When adverse effects of epinephrine are prohibitive for further use in older children, terbutaline, 0.01 ml/kg of 0.1% (1 mg/ml) solution SQ, with a maximum dose of 0.30 mg, can be used.

(4) Corticosteroids
   (a) Administration of steroids has become a first-line treatment for severe asthma and is indicated when there is no response to initial nebulized treatment or when response to repeated treatments is incomplete.
   (b) Oral or parenteral equivalents of methylprednisolone, 1 to 2 mg/kg/dose, are begun and repeated every 6 hours.
   (c) Inhaled corticosteroids are useful in maintenance therapy, but not appropriate as therapy for acute exacerbations.

(5) Hydration. The acutely ill asthmatic child has increased fluid requirements.
   (a) Oral fluids are usually adequate in mild attacks.
   (b) In severe attacks, oral fluid may precipitate vomiting, and a stable IV line should be placed. Generally, an infusion of 5% dextrose in ½ NS with 20 to 40 mEq/liter KCl at 1.5 times maintenance for the first 12 hours is adequate. Adjustments should be made depending on clinical status.

(6) Intravenous infusions of bronchodilators are indicated when the initial clinical presentation is one of severe distress, when oral medications are not tolerated, or when SQ or aerosol treatment has failed.
   (a) Aminophylline. Methylxanthines, once the mainstay of asthma treatment, have been largely replaced by inhalation therapies, steroids, and intravenous beta agonists. Drawbacks include low therapeutic index and side effects such as nausea, vomiting, and seizures. Theophylline preparations do not enhance the effects of continuous or frequently repeated beta-2 agonists, yet may sometimes produce additive bronchodilation.
      (i) Before starting aminophylline it is important to document any recent oral theophylline administration. A theophylline level may be useful.
      (ii) Intravenous aminophylline can be given as a **bolus** or a **constant infusion.** In **bolus** therapy, 5 to 8 mg/kg is infused over 20 minutes and is repeated every 6 hours. Further dosage can be adjusted after measuring postinfusion peak serum levels 30 to 60 minutes after the bolus. A **constant infusion** can be started following a routine loading dose. The usual dosage range for an infusion is 0.9 to 1.2 mg/kg/hr.
      (iii) Serum levels can be measured any time during an infusion. All aminophylline doses should be tailored to achieve a serum theophylline level of 10 to 20 µg/ml. Generally, 1 mg/kg IV bolus will raise serum concentration 2 µg/ml.
      (iv) Theophylline **toxicity** includes severe headache, tachycardia, tremors, gastritis with frequent vomiting, and seizures

(for management, see Chap. 8). **Note: Rapid IV infusion of aminophylline can lead to cardiac arrhythmias, hypotension, and death. When aminophylline is administered in combination with beta agonists, constant cardiac monitoring is essential.**

(b) In severe cases, **intravenous beta-2 agonists** are indicated. **Such therapy is conducted in an intensive care setting with continuous cardiorespiratory and hemodynamic monitoring via arterial line.**

    (i) Terbutaline is administered IV using the bolus-infusion technique: 10 µg/kg over 10 minutes followed by 0.4 µg/kg/min. *Titrate incrementally by 0.4 µg/kg/min to keep heart rate at less than 200 beats per minute (bpm).*

    (ii) Complications of terbutaline therapy include tremulousness, tachycardia, and hypokalemia.

2. Bronchiolitis is a syndrome of acute, small airway obstruction in young infants.

  a. Etiology. It is usually viral in origin (commonly respiratory syncytial virus [RSV]).

  b. Evaluation should include assessment of hydration and respiratory distress.

  c. The **diagnosis** is suggested by the onset of coryza, cough, dyspnea, and wheezing. Fever may not be present. Chest radiography reveals hyperinflation and shifting atelectasis. Collapse of the right upper lobe is common.

  d. Therapy

    (1) Humidified **oxygen** (40% or more). In severe cases, oxygenation should be followed with transcutaneous oxygen tension (PO_2) monitors, pulse oximeters, or ABGs.

    (2) Adequate **hydration** is important. Whether fluids are administered PO or IV depends on the severity of the respiratory distress. Infants in severe respiratory distress often cannot adequately and safely hydrate themselves orally.

    (3) In severe cases, assisted **ventilation** may be required.

    (4) Antibiotics are not routinely given, but are indicated if associated otitis media or pneumonia is present.

    (5) Bronchodilators given by inhalation are sometimes helpful.

    (6) Use of **ribavirin** is controversial with no consensus regarding which patients should be treated. Suggested indications include patients with RSV infection who require mechanical ventilation, have underlying cardiopulmonary disease including bronchopulmonary dysplasia (BPD), or are immunosuppressed.

3. Foreign body aspiration (see also p. 227) must always be considered in children who have an initial episode of wheezing or recurrent or unresponsive pneumonia. **Note:** A foreign body in the esophagus can cause significant respiratory symptoms.

  a. Evaluation and diagnosis.

    (1) History should investigate use of small objects on food such as raisins, peanuts, plastic toys, and so forth.

    (2) Physical examination may reveal asymmetric air exchange.

    (3) Roentgenographic studies will identify radiopaque foreign bodies or suggest bronchial foreign bodies by paradoxical movement of the diaphragms or ipsilateral obstructive emphysema with a mediastinal shift to the contralateral side.

  b. Therapy. Aspirated foreign bodies must be removed emergently when air exchange is significantly compromised, when the foreign body may imminently migrate into a more dangerous position, or when associated chemical irritants may complicate later removal (for example, peanuts). Emergent mechanical efforts to dislodge a foreign body (i.e., back blows) **can**

cause migration with complete obstruction and therefore should be attempted **only** when air exchange is inadequate to sustain life.

(1) **Bronchoscopy** is the definitive therapy.

(2) **Antibiotics** are useful when infection is present (see Chap. 5).

(3) Persistent atelectasis, pneumonitis, pneumonia, or emphysema should raise the question of a remaining fragment or second foreign body.

4. **Pneumonia** may present with significant respiratory distress secondary to impaired gas exchange (see also Chap. 5, p. 102).

   a. General supportive measures include 30 to 40% oxygen by face mask, and intubation if respirations are inadequate.

   b. Monitoring of ABGs and pulse oximetry is advised.

   c. For specific therapy, see Chap. 5.

5. **Pneumothorax**

   a. **Etiology.** Spontaneous pneumothorax may be an idiopathic occurrence in a previously healthy person, or it may be a complication of underlying pulmonary disease.

   b. **Evaluation**

      (1) **History.** The onset of severe respiratory distress is usually acute and sometimes painful.

      (2) **Physical examination.** Decreased fremitus, decreased breath sounds, and hyperresonance are present on the affected side. Asymmetric chest movement and displaced point of maximal impulse may be noted. Percussion over the clavicles on opposite sides reveals minor differences in percussion tones. In patients with very abnormal lung compliance, such as severe cystic fibrosis, the physical findings may be minimal.

      (3) **Laboratory.** A chest roentgenogram should be obtained.

   c. **Diagnosis** is confirmed by radiography.

      (1) **Minor to moderate:** less than 30% collapse.

      (2) **Major:** 30 to 70% collapse.

      (3) **If complete collapse** occurs, the possibility of tension pneumothorax should be suspected.

      (4) Under positive pressure ventilation, pneumothorax may be preceded or accompanied by **pneumomediastinum** or **pneumoperitoneum.**

   d. **Treatment** (for infants, see Chap. 6)

      (1) **If the clinical condition is critical, immediate lifesaving maneuvers become more important than diagnostic procedures.**

      (2) If the leak is in the **visceral** pleura, **positive pressure breathing can aggravate the situation.** If there is a leak in the **parietal** pleura (flail chest), on the other hand, positive pressure may be lifesaving.

      (3) **Simple observation** will suffice if the clinical condition is stable and the radiologic diagnosis is "minor."

      (4) **Cough suppression.** If necessary, dextromethorphan, codeine, or morphine should be used to suppress coughing. **The use of respiratory depressants is dangerous and necessitates frequent ABGs.**

      (5) **Thoracentesis.** Needle aspiration of air at the second anterior intercostal space is lifesaving whenever tension pneumothorax is present. Under positive pressure ventilation, a sealed system is unnecessary. A closed thoracostomy drainage system is connected after initial stabilization.

      (6) **Thoracostomy.** Tube thoracostomy is indicated when the pneumothorax is likely to reaccumulate. The term **closed thoracostomy** is used to designate a thoracostomy tube connected to a water-seal bottle. With a water seal (which can be improvised by placing the end of the tube under the surface of sterile NS contained in any container with an air vent), air (and also fluid) drains from the chest. Air cannot reenter the submerged tube tip **if the end of the tube and water seal are below the level of the patient's chest.** It is customary to place the "bottle" on the floor. If the system is functioning well, the fluid will be lifted a few centimeters as the patient breathes and produces

negative (subatmospheric) inspiratory pressure. Later, when the visceral and parietal pleura are adherent, this will not be seen.

IV. Cardiac failure (see also Chap. 10)

A. Congestive heart failure (see Chap. 10, p. 319).

B. Pericardial tamponade is an accumulation of fluid in the pericardial space, producing cardiac compression and inadequate diastolic filling, leading to a small, fixed stroke volume and low-output heart failure.

1. **Etiology**

   a. Primary pericardial disease, including viral, bacterial, and rheumatic pericarditis.

   b. Systemic disease that can cause secondary pericardial tamponade, including congestive heart failure (CHF), uremia, tumor, or collagen vascular disease.

2. **Evaluation**

   a. History. Symptoms may include fever, fatigability, shortness of breath, and signs of congestive failure.

   b. Physical examination

     (1) Evidence of low-output cardiac failure includes tachycardia, tachypnea, hypotension, thready pulses, cool extremities, mottled gray skin, and oliguria.

     (2) Cardiac examination reveals muffled heart sounds, pericardial friction rub, jugular venous distention, and passive hepatic congestion.

     (3) Laboratory evaluation includes ECG, chest x-ray (CXR), and echocardiogram.

3. **Diagnosis**

   a. The chest radiograph demonstrates a bulbous cardiac silhouette.

   b. The **ECG** shows S-T segment elevation, low voltage, and T-wave inversion.

   c. An **echocardiogram** confirms the effusion.

4. **Therapy. Emergent decompression by pericardiocentesis** or surgery (pericardial window or pericardial stripping), or both, is lifesaving. **Cardiovascular status is fragile, and sedation or positive pressure ventilation can precipitate collapse. Pericardiocentesis should be performed by the most experienced person available.**

   a. The patient's ECG should be continuously monitored.

   b. Equipment. A 10-ml syringe and a 1-in. 20-gauge needle are adequate for an infant or toddler, whereas a 30-ml syringe and 3-in. spinal needle (20 gauge) should be used in an adult.

   c. Prepare the subxiphoid area with a povidone-iodine (Betadine) and alcohol wash.

   d. Using sterile technique, insert the needle in the subxiphoid area at a 30-degree angle, aiming for the left-mid scapula. Slight negative pressure should be maintained on the syringe. When the pericardium is entered, fluid will appear in the hub of the syringe; this fluid can be *distinguished from intracardiac blood by its lower hematocrit and absent clotting.*

   e. ECG monitoring shows ST changes with myocardial injury.

   f. Complications include pneumothorax, arrhythmias, coronary laceration, and myocardial puncture.

C. Tetralogy of Fallot spells (see Chap. 10, p. 323).

V. Central nervous system emergencies (see also Chap. 20)

A. Seizures. Acute management of seizures requires attention to the "ABCs" of resuscitation primarily, and to the cessation of seizure activity secondarily.

1. **Etiology** (see Chap. 20, p. 513 *ff.*).

2. **Evaluation and diagnosis**

   a. The **history** should identify any underlying disease process. Careful attention should be paid to the details of the seizure itself, along with a comprehensive history of events surrounding the seizure.

   b. Physical examination should assess the **extent** of impairment of cardiorespiratory status and illuminate a direct cause for the seizure activity. Include the following:

(1) Vital signs.
(2) Head and scalp inspection for trauma.
(3) Pupils for size, shape, reactivity, and equality.
(4) Fundi for evidence of papilledema or hemorrhage.
(5) Tympanic membranes for infection or hemotympanum.
(6) Mouth for airway patency and tongue biting.
(7) Neck for meningismus.
(8) Chest for adequacy of respirations.
(9) Extremities for evidence of trauma.
(10) **Neurologic** examination.
   c. **Laboratory tests.** The laboratory evaluation should be selective, based on the history and physical examination.
   (1) Blood for immediate bedside capillary glucose determination (Dextrostix), CBC, electrolytes, BUN, glucose, calcium, magnesium, toxic screen (including lead), pH and pCO_2, anticonvulsant levels when appropriate, and ABGs when indicated.
   (2) Urine for urinalysis, toxic screen, and an immediate pregnancy test when appropriate.
   (3) Lumbar puncture for cerebrospinal fluid (CSF) examination when signs of CNS infection are present and increased intracranial pressure (ICP) and mass effect have been ruled out (see sec. B.2 p. 236; see also Chap. 20, p. 513).
   (4) A **CT scan** is indicated when head trauma, increased ICP, or a mass lesion is suspected.
3. **Therapy. The goals of therapy are to maintain the "ABCs" of resuscitation; to stop and prevent further seizures; to prevent or treat complications, or both; and to treat underlying etiologies of seizures when possible.**
   a. **Airway management**
   (1) Establish a patent airway via a chin lift or jaw thrust; protect the cervical spine (C-spine) if trauma is suspected or known.
   (2) Administer 100% oxygen.
   (3) Place an oral or nasopharyngeal airway if obstruction due to soft tissues is present.
   (4) Suction as necessary.
   (5) Ventilation by bag and mask with **100% oxygen** is indicated if spontaneous respirations are absent or suboptimal. Intubation may be required when bag-and-mask ventilation is insufficient or when long-term ventilation seems probable.
   b. **Intravenous access.** *Normal saline is the preferred fluid since it is compatible with all anticonvulsant medications.* If increased ICP is suspected, fluid administration should be minimized, assuming adequate blood pressure.
   c. **Anticonvulsant therapy. Note if the patient is already taking anticonvulsants since this can influence choice of further medication.**
   (1) **Benzodiazepines**
      (a) **Lorazepam (Ativan):** rapid acting
         (i) The initial dose is 0.05 to 0.10 mg/kg with a maximum dose of 4 mg; give over 1 to 4 minutes. A second dose of 0.10 mg/kg can be given if there is no response to the initial dose.
         (ii) Respiratory depression is a possible side effect of benzodiazepines and usually is due to rapid administration; airway equipment and skilled personnel should be present before administration.
      (b) **Diazepam (Valium):** rapid acting, short half-life
         (i) The initial dose is 0.1 to 0.2 mg/kg, with a maximum dose of 10 mg; given over 1 to 4 minutes. A second dose of 0.25 to

0.4 mg/kg with a maximum dose of 15 mg can be given if there is no response to the initial dose.

(2) Phenytoin has a relatively long duration of action that makes it a useful adjunct to the first-line benzodiazepines. The onset of action is 10 to 30 minutes.

(a) Phenytoin should be infused as soon as a benzodiazepine has been given. The dose is 15 to 20 mg/kg IV *in NS only* (since it precipitates in dextrose solutions) over 20 minutes (not faster than 1 mg/kg/min).

(b) Cardiac arrhythmias and hypotension are the most important adverse effects. Take care that infusion is not too rapid. Cardiac monitoring is essential.

(3) Paraldehyde can be used as an adjunct to diazepam and phenytoin if further therapy is required. Because paraldehyde is administered rectally, it can be used when an IV line cannot be started. The dosage is 0.3 to 0.4 ml/kg (maximum 8 ml) mixed in an equal volume of peanut or corn oil and administered PR via rectal tube.

(4) Phenobarbital

(a) The dose is 10 mg/kg IV given slowly over 10 to 15 minutes. If no effect is evident after 20 to 30 minutes, this dose can be repeated twice.

(b) The combined respiratory depressant effect of phenobarbital and a benzodiazepine is greater than either drug alone, and care must be taken when giving these medicines in conjunction with one another.

d. With prolonged or refractory seizures, precipitating conditions must be ruled out.

4. Specific disorders

a. Febrile seizures (see Chap. 20).

b. Hypoglycemia (see also Chap. 13). **Hypoglycemic seizures are a medical emergency.**

(1) Provide general supportive measures as outlined in sec. **3** above.

(2) Look for Medic-Alert bracelet or other evidence of insulin use.

(3) After withdrawing an aliquot of blood for glucose and other determinations, give intravenous dextrose, 0.25 to 0.50 g/kg as 25% dextrose in water.

(4) Consider an IV infusion of 4 to 6 mg/kg/min glucose.

(5) Investigate the cause of the hypoglycemia.

c. Hypertension

(1) Provide the general supportive measures outlined previously.

(2) Rapid therapy for hypertension is required (see Chap. 9).

(3) Ongoing seizures can be treated acutely as outlined in sec. **3** above for general seizure disorders. Investigate the cause of the hypertension.

d. Meningitis or encephalitis

(1) Provide the general supportive measures outlined previously.

(2) Anticonvulsant therapy is that outlined for a general seizure disorder (see sec. **3.c** above).

(3) Rapid institution of antibiotic therapy is critical.

B. Increased ICP (see also Chap. 20, pp. 511 *ff.*)

1. The **etiology** includes

a. Cerebral edema due to infection, hypoxia, and ischemia, Reye's syndrome, or toxins (e.g., lead).

b. Increased CSF volume due to hydrocephalus or an obstructed ventricular shunt.

c. Increased intracranial blood volume due to infection (meningitis and encephalitis), trauma (intraparenchymal bleeding, subdural hematoma), or arteriovenous malformations.

d. Space-occupying lesions due to tumor or abscess.

2. Evaluation

a. A complete **history** should include any evidence of infection, trauma, hypoxic events, previous seizures, CNS insults, and medications. Neurologic symptoms should be carefully documented, with detailed accounts of the duration and progression.

b. **Physical examination**

(1) **Vital signs** should be monitored closely. The Cushing reflex (bradycardia, hypertension, slow and irregular respirations) is a late finding and uncommon in children.

(2) The **physical examination** should be directed toward finding the causes of the increased ICP.

(3) **Neurologic examination.** See **Table 7-3 (Glasgow Coma Scale).** Complete and serial neurologic examinations are essential. Include pupillary and fundoscopic examinations. Look for focal neurologic deficits and listen for intracranial bruits. In the infant and toddler, measure the head circumference, feel for split sutures, and transilluminate the head.

c. **Laboratory studies include**

(1) **A CT scan,** once the patient's condition has stabilized.

(2) **Skull x-rays** are helpful for eliciting splitting of the sutures, calcification, or bone erosion secondary to prolonged increased pressure.

Table 7-3. Glasgow Coma Scale[a]

Response	Score
Eyes	
Open	
Spontaneously	4
To verbal command	3
To pain	2
No response	1
Best motor response	
To verbal command	
Obeys	6
To painful stimulus[b]	
Localizes pain	5
Flexion withdrawal	4
Flexion abnormal (decorticate rigidity)	3
Extension (decerebrate rigidity)	2
No response	1
Best verbal response[c]	
Oriented and converses	5
Disoriented and converses	4
Inappropriate words	3
Incomprehensible sounds	2
No response	1
Total	3–15

[a]The Glasgow Coma Scale, based on eye opening and verbal and motor responses, is a practical means of monitoring changes in the level of consciousness. If the response on the scale is given a number, the responsiveness of the patient can be expressed by summation of the figures. The **lowest** score is 3; the **highest** is 15.
[b]Apply knuckles to sternum; observe arms.
[c]Arouse patient with painful stimulus if necessary.

(3) A **lumbar puncture** is done **after** the CT scan (to rule out a mass lesion) for pressure measurement, and to aid in the diagnosis of infection or hemorrhage. **A lumbar puncture carries a risk of central herniation in the patient with increased ICP.** At times, however, examination of the CSF is essential, and the benefits outweigh the risks of the procedure.

3. Therapy. The goal of therapy is to decrease the ICP by decreasing one or more of the component volumes.

  a. All correctable lesions are treated.

  b. The initial therapy includes

    (1) Position. To avoid venous obstruction the patient's head should be kept midline, with the head of the bed elevated 30 degrees.

    (2) Oxygen and airway. The arterial oxygen tension (PaO_2) should be maintained above 100 mm Hg.

    (3) Hypocapnia. Endotracheal intubation and hyperventilation to maintain a $PaCO_2$ of 25 to 30 mm Hg will cause cerebral vasoconstriction and hence a decrease in the intracranial blood volume. Some patients will hyperventilate spontaneously and may not require mechanical ventilation.

    (4) Osmotherapy. Attempt to achieve an osmolarity of 300 to 320 mOsm/liter, as follows:

      (a) Calculate osmolarity if direct laboratory measurement is not available (mOsm = $[2 \times Na^+]$ + BUN/2.8 + blood glucose/18). The calculated value will be falsely low if other osmotic agents are present in the blood (i.e., mannitol, glycerol; see also Chap. 4).

      (b) Limit the amount of fluid intake (PO and IV).

      (c) Give **mannitol**, 0.25 to 0.50 g/kg, as a bolus q2–4h.

      (d) Give **furosemide** (Lasix), 1 mg/kg q6–8h.

      (e) During osmotherapy urine output should not fall below 0.25 to 0.5 ml/kg/hr.

    (5) Seizure control is important to avoid a sudden, massive increase in cerebral metabolism.

    (6) Normothermia must be maintained to avoid increased blood flow and volume.

    (7) Corticosteroids are effective in reducing the edema that surrounds brain tumors, but their benefit in intracranial hypertension from other causes has not been demonstrated. Dexamethasone (Decadron), 1 mg/kg/day in three divided doses, has been used. **Corticosteroids are contraindicated in the treatment of Reye's syndrome because of their catabolic effects.**

  c. Maximum increased therapy. If the preceding maneuvers fail to control the increased ICP, more invasive monitoring in the form of a CVP line and an ICP monitoring device is required. The following therapeutic maneuvers can then be tried.

    (1) Muscle relaxation. Muscle relaxants (pancuronium [Pavulon], 0.1 mg/kg q1–2h) will prevent intracranial hypertension associated with movement and muscle strain.

    (2) Sedation. Sedation is helpful in controlling ICP spikes due to agitation or noxious stimuli. Sedation can be achieved with narcotic and benzodiazepine combinations; tolerance can occur, especially with short-acting agents.

      (a) Short-acting agents: fentanyl (2–5 µg/kg/hr) infusion and midazolam (0.05–0.3 mg/kg/hr) infusion, or intermittent doses of these agents.

      (b) Longer-acting agents: morphine (0.1 mg/kg/hr) infusion with lorazepam (0.05–0.10 mg/kg q2–6h).

    (3) The duration of maximum increased ICP therapy can extend to weeks. The process of weaning the patient from therapy is started when the ICP is consistently in a normal range. The patient is first weaned from sedation and then from pancuronium and mechanical hyperventilation; osmotherapy is the last to be discontinued. The pace of weaning is dictated by the ICP response.

C. Traumatic spinal cord injuries. The patient usually presents with neurologic dysfunction below the level of the lesion.

1. **Etiology:** usually the result of hyperextension, hyperflexion, or axial loading injuries. The fractures or dislocations most commonly occur at the level of T12–L1, C5-C6, and C1-C2.

2. **Evaluation and diagnosis.** Patients may experience a *total loss* of function distal to the lesion (as in cord transections), or **temporary and completely reversible** loss (as seen in localized edema or **hemorrhage**).

   a. **History** should note the nature of the injury and details of the progression and degree of neurologic loss.

   b. The **physical examination** should include

      (1) The adequacy of ventilation and cardiovascular status.

      (2) Examination for associated injuries.

      (3) The **neurologic examination** will usually demonstrate

         (a) Loss of **motor and sensory function** below the level of the lesion.

         (b) **Areflexia** for 2 to 6 weeks, often with a return to some reflex activity at a later date.

         (c) Total **flaccidity** is initially present; **spasticity** follows weeks after the insult.

         (d) Urinary retention can also be a feature.

   c. **Laboratory studies** include

      (1) Radiographs of the spine.

      (2) Computed tomographic scan of the affected region.

      (3) A myelogram may be indicated.

3. **Treatment of spinal injury**

   a. Locate the lesion and attempt to minimize any further damage.

   b. The neck should be immobilized in a neutral position.

   c. **Respiratory function** must be supported as required. Patients with a lesion at C1–C2 will require mechanical assistance.

   d. The **cardiovascular system** must be supported as required; hypovolemia can result from associated autonomic dysfunction.

   e. A Foley catheter is placed to avoid bladder distintion.

   f. Traction or surgical decompression, or both, is usually attempted in an effort to minimize any further damage.

VI. Special problems in the emergency department

A. Evaluation of the febrile infant 0 to 90 days of life (see also Chap. 6, p. 208). Elevated temperature (> 38.0°C) in the infant most commonly indicates infection, whether viral or bacterial in origin. This may signify sepsis (nonlocalized, widespread infection) in a host with an immature immune system. Overwhelming viral infection can be as devastating as bacterial infection in this age group.

1. **Etiology.** Viral causes are present in up to 95% of cases. In the infant 0 to 28 days of life, group B streptococci, *Escherichia coli*, and *Listeria monocytogenes* are the primary bacterial pathogens responsible for infection. In infants 29 to 90 days, encapsulated bacterial organisms account for the majority of infections of bacterial origin, especially pneumococcus.

2. **Evaluation and diagnosis**

   a. The **history** should include a detailed account of general signs of infection: lethargy, irritability, and pallor as well as specific symptoms (i.e., rash, cough). Deviations in feeding and sleeping behaviors should also be investigated. Onset and height of fever should be documented.

   b. **Physical examination**

      (1) General appearance. Note evidence of irritability, lethargy, or decreased response to the environment.

      (2) Vital signs. Document *rectal* temperature. Tachycardia may be due to crying, fever, hypovolemia, or shock. Tachypnea may be caused by fever, pneumonia, or a compensation for acidemia. Blood pressure should be measured on all patients. Hypotension is a late sign of shock.

   c. Laboratory data

     (1) Culture specimens. Cultures are obtained from blood, urine by suprapubic aspiration or catheterization, and CSF by lumbar puncture.

     (2) Hematologic. Cerebrospinal fluid cell count may reveal pleocytosis. Complete blood count may or may not show leukocytosis, and may reveal potentially ominous neutropenia (absolute neutrophil count [ANC] < 500/mm^3). Urinalysis may reveal evidence of infection.

     (3) Chemistry. Cerebrospinal fluid protein and glucose and blood glucose should be measured..

     (4) Radiography. Chest x-ray if symptomatic.

     (5) Latex agglutination assays are available for bacterial detection in CSF, urine, and blood.

  3. Therapy (see also Chaps. 5 and 6)

   a. Any truly febrile infant aged 0 to 28 days must be hospitalized and treated with parenteral antibiotics, that is, ampicillin, 200 to 300 mg/kg/day, and gentamicin, 2.5 mg/kg/dose. From 29 to 90 days of age, any infant who is ill appearing should be hospitalized and treated with parenteral antibiotics, that is, cefotaxime, 50 mg/kg q8h IV.

   b. Well-appearing infants 29 to 90 days of age without an identified focus of infection on physical or laboratory examination can be treated as outpatients if good follow-up can be ensured. Ceftriaxone, 50 mg/kg IM, is given after evaluation and then again in 20 to 28 hours on reexamination.

B. Evaluation of the febrile child 3 to 36 months of age. Fever greater than 39.0°C without obvious source on physical examination indicates a 3% risk of bacteremia.

  1. Etiology. Viral causes of fever are present in 95 to 97% of cases. The encapsulated organisms, *Streptococcus pneumoniae, H. influenzae, Neisseria meningitidis,* and *Salmonella* species, are responsible for nearly all cases of bacteremia.

  2. Evaluation and diagnosis

   a. History: should include a review of systems including those susceptible to invasion by bloodborne bacteria as well as the presence of irritability or lethargy, or both.

   b. Physical examination

     (1) General appearance. Children with bacteremia may be well appearing and active. Fever may be the only sign. Note **unusual compliance with physical examination for age,** or diminished response to stimuli.

     (2) Vital signs (see sec. **A.2.b.(2)** above).

     (3) A careful examination should include the presence or absence of meningismus, cough, rales or wheezing, peripheral perfusion and hydration state, abdominal pain, and/or evidence of bone or joint infections. **Meningismus is not always present, especially in children less than 18 to 24 months of age.**

   c. Laboratory data

     (1) Culture specimens. Blood and urine cultures should be obtained. Lumbar puncture should be performed based on clinical impression.

     (2) Hematologic. Cerebrospinal fluid cell count, peripheral blood smear, and urinalysis may show evidence of infection.

     (3) Chemistry. Cerebrospinal fluid protein and CSF and **serum glucose** should be measured if lumbar puncture (LP) is performed.

     (4) Radiologic. Chest radiography should be performed **if the child has respiratory symptoms.**

  3. Therapy. Although presumptive antibiotic therapy has been shown to reduce the complications of bacteremia, it remains controversial as to whether the risks outweigh the benefits. Therefore, options exist as to therapy for the febrile child without an obvious source of infection. Empiric treatment can be amoxicillin, 25 to 40 mg/kg/day, or ceftriaxone, one dose, 50 mg/kg IM, pending culture results.

C. Sudden infant death syndrome (SIDS) is the leading cause of death in infants between 1 week and 1 year of age, with a peak incidence from 2 to 4 months. In the United States the incidence is decreasing, now at 139 per 100,000 live births.
  1. **Etiology**
     a. Mechanism is unknown.
     b. Incidence is slightly higher in siblings, but there is no predictable genetic pattern. Twins are more susceptible than nontwins (3.87/1,000 live births), and triplets are probably at greater risk (8.33/1,000).
  2. The emergency room **evaluation and treatment** of SIDS should include
     a. A detailed history and physical examination to rule out other causes of death.
     b. Support of the parents and surviving siblings. (see also Chap. 2, p. 13)
     c. Report of the death to the medical examiner.
D. Apparent life-threatening event (ALTE, previously termed "near-miss SIDS"). An ALTE refers to any unexplained, sudden near death of a young child.
  1. **Etiology** may include hypothermia, sepsis, overwhelming pneumonitis, airway obstruction, trauma or abuse, seizure, adrenal crisis, or toxic ingestion.
  2. **Evaluation and diagnosis**
     a. **History** should be directed toward finding an etiology, including description of the surrounding events and observed episode. Underlying illnesses and medications should be elicited.
     b. The **physical examination** should ensure that the infant is in no imminent danger and should pay careful attention to identifying underlying disorders. Measurement of vital signs and a respiratory and neurologic examination are mandatory.
     c. **Laboratory tests should be tailored to the historical and physical examination clues.** Complete blood count with differential, electrolytes, calcium, BUN, creatinine, blood glucose (and Dextrostix), and urinalysis should be considered, as should electroencephalogram, lumbar puncture, and radiologic studies to evaluate swallowing and gastroesophageal reflux (see Chap. 11, p. 356).
  3. **General management** includes a period of inhospital observation and monitoring. If sepsis is suspected, antibiotics should be started pending negative cultures (see Chap. 5). After initial management, further evaluation, including pneumography, parental education and support, and arrangements for home monitoring, when appropriate, should be coordinated with a medical center that has an active program for infants who have an ALTE.
E. Child abuse and neglect
  1. **Etiology** is multifaceted and may include
     a. Family stress factors.
     b. Parenting factors.
     c. Social factors.
     d. Parental problems (behavioral/psychiatric disorders, drug/alcohol abuse).
  2. **Evaluation**
     a. If a social worker is available, he or she is called promptly at the time of the family's visit. The physician should introduce the social worker as someone who is interested and able to help them through this difficult period. After the interview, the physician and social worker should confer.
     b. **Interviewing the parents**
        (1) In the initial interviews and in subsequent contacts, **no direct or indirect attempt to draw out a confession from the parent is made.** Denial is a prominent ego defense in virtually all abusive parents. Their often bizarre stories of how their child was injured should not be taken as intentional falsifications. These odd accounts frequently indicate parents' profound distress in acknowledging infliction of an injury or failure to protect a child. In the face of such a threatening reality, they repress it and may offer a blatant fabrication that must be accepted for the moment.

(2) A good interview technique allows parent and child to maintain the integrity of ego and family. It is appropriate to emphasize the child's need for hospital care and protection from harm. At this time the clinician should demonstrate concern and the ability to help the **parents'** distress as well.

c. In some frequent behavior patterns of abusive or negligent parents, they may

(1) Use severe punishments.

(2) Give a past history of abuse in their own upbringing.

(3) Display suspicion and antagonism toward others.

(4) Lead isolated lives.

(5) Make pleas for help in indirect ways, such as

    (a) Bringing the child to the clinician or emergency room for no specific reason or for repeated minor medical complaints.

    (b) Insisting that the child be admitted to the hospital for a minor illness and expressing anxiety if he or she is not.

(6) Lean on their children for support, comfort, and reassurance.

(7) Sample a variety of health care facilities without establishing a relationship with any one in particular.

(8) Display poor impulse control or an openly hostile attitude toward the child.

(9) Be unable to carry out consistent discipline, yet threaten or punish the child if he or she does not live up to an expectation or whim.

(10) Understand little about normal child development and seem unable to integrate such information.

d. The physical manifestations of child abuse may be present in any body system. A *thorough* and well-documented physical examination is imperative.

3. Diagnosis. Suspect child abuse or neglect whenever a child presents with any one or a combination of the following **clinical** findings.

  a. Fractures that a simple fall would be unlikely to produce

    (1) Different stages of healing in multiple fractures.

    (2) Metaphyseal fractures.

    (3) Epiphyseal separations.

    (4) Subperiosteal calcifications.

  b. Subdural hematomas.

  c. Multiple ecchymoses that may resemble purpura.

  d. Intestinal injuries, ruptured viscera.

  e. Burns of any kind, especially in infants.

  f. Poor hygiene.

  g. Inadequate gain in weight or height.

  h. Marked passivity and watchfulness; fearful expression.

  i. Bizarre accidents, multiple ingestions.

  j. Malnutrition.

  k. Developmental retardation.

4. Axioms of management

  a. Once child abuse or neglect is diagnosed, the **child is at great risk of reinjury or continued neglect.**

  b. **Protection** of the child must be a principal goal of initial intervention, but this protection must go hand in hand with a program to help the family through its crisis.

  c. Traditional social casework cannot in itself protect an abused or neglected child in a dangerous environment. Medical follow-up is also necessary, and day-to-day contact with a child care center may help significantly to encourage the child's healthy development.

  d. Public social service agencies in both urban and rural areas do not have sufficient well-trained personnel, and the quality of administration and supervision in these agencies often is not high. These factors militate against their operating effectively in isolation from other social agencies. Simply reporting a case to the public agency mandated to receive child abuse case reports may not be sufficient to protect an abused or neglected child or to help the family.

e. Early attempts by the hospital staff to identify the agent of an injury or to determine if neglect was "intentional" may be ill advised. There is **rarely** a need to establish **precisely** who it was who injured or neglected a child and why. Clinical experience has shown that it is more important to establish confidence and trust in the hospital personnel. This may be jeopardized by overly aggressive attempts to ferret out the specific circumstances of the injury. On the other hand, lack of evidence for parental "guilt" is not a criterion for discharge of the patient.

f. If there is evidence that the child is at major risk, **hospitalization** to allow time for assessment of the home setting is appropriate. Children under the age of 3 are frequent victims; infants under 1 year of age with severe malnutrition or failure to thrive, fractures, burns, or bruises of any kind are especially at risk of reinjury or neglect. **Prompt and effective intervention is vital to ensure their survival.**

F. **Rape and sexual abuse of children** are now recognized to be extremely common in the United States, with an estimated one of four adolescent girls victimized before reaching adulthood. Fewer than half of these incidents are reported to medical and legal personnel.

1. **Definitions**

a. **Rape** is a legal conclusion defined by state law. Most states distinguish between statutory rape and common law rape, the latter being penetration without consent. **Rape** as a term is used to refer to a violent act initiated by an assailant in which a victim is subjected to sexual act(s) performed by force or the threat of force without the victim's consent. **Statutory rape** is intercourse with a female below the age of consent (usually 16 yrs). **Sexual molestation** is noncoital sexual contact without consent.

b. **Sexual abuse** refers to sexual activity involving a child that is inappropriate because of the child's age, level of development, or role within the family. Authority and power allow the perpetrator to coerce the child into compliance. Sexual abuse is more chronic than rape and usually involves an acquaintance or a relative of the child.

2. **Evaluation and diagnosis**

a. The **history** should gather information necessary to assess the need for protective care and support services and the nature of medical therapy. A review of the abuse may be traumatic for the child and family, who should be interviewed together and then separately if possible. Great care and sensitivity must be demonstrated, as with other forms of child abuse (see sec. **E** above). The assistance of an experienced social worker, rape counselor, or psychiatrist is helpful. Include

   (1) The time of the abuse and the circumstances surrounding it.

   (2) Identification, when possible, of the perpetrator, to assess the risk involved should the child return home.

   (3) The nature of the sexual contact—oral, rectal, penile, or vaginal.

   (4) Vaginal discharge or perineal complaints.

   (5) Nonspecific complaints that may reflect chronic abuse: abdominal pain, enuresis, encopresis, recent school problems.

b. The **physical examination** is directed at careful observation and recording evidence of abuse, associated injuries, the presence of ongoing medical problems, and the emotional status of the child (Table 7-4). In most cases of sexual abuse (especially chronic intrafamily abuse), there are no positive physical findings. Consequently, the likelihood of sexual abuse is best assessed by examining data from the history and psychologicval data as well as the results of the physical examination. The examination should be done gently and only after careful explanation to the child and the family. Consent forms and standard evidence collection procedures should be explained and utilized in all suspected cases. Some of these cases may be

Table 7-4. Collection of evidence during the examination for sexual abuse or rape, or both

Study	Procedure	Comments
Clothing	If still wearing same clothing, collect in paper bag	Plastic bags may alter evidence
Wood's light examination	Shine Wood's light over scalp, skin, and perineum	Fluorescent areas may indicate semen
Pubic hair	Comb out pubic hairs and collect in envelope	Foreign hairs may be identified
Acid-phosphatase test	Wipe perineum or suspected area with moistened gauze and apply gauze to acid-phosphatase tape	If tape turns purple in <60 sec, examination is consistent with sperm being present
Gonococcal cultures of genital area, throat, rectum	Routine (using cotton swabs and Thayer-Martin media); prepubertal—vaginal, pubertal—cervical, males—urethral	
Chlamydia culture of genital area	Routine (using Dacron swab, culture media, and immuno-fluorescence kit if available)	Important even for youngest children
Fixed slides	Swab of posterior fornix onto dry slide	For examination of sperm, blood group, acid phosphatase
Urinalysis	Routine	May reveal urologic injuries, and inflammation, and may be useful in ruling out pregnancy at time of examination
Blood sample	Send for VDRL and, if necessary, blood typing and pregnancy test	CBC may also be useful if infection or blood loss is suspected

prosecuted. A full physical examination is required. In addition, special attention should be paid to

(1) The general emotional state of the child (e.g., anxious, apathetic).
(2) The presence of bruises, abrasions, lacerations, and other cutaneous lesions.
(3) The presence of significant trauma, including fractures and abdominal injuries.
(4) The external genitalia, which should be carefully examined for ecchymoses, edema, lacerations, and erythema. The genital examination can best be visualized by placing the prepubertal child in the frog-leg or knee-chest position. Specula are not needed in prepubertal girls.
(5) An internal vaginal examination must be performed whenever
   (a) A history of vaginal or rectal penetration by a penis, finger, or foreign object is elicited or suspected.
   (b) The history reveals symptoms relating to the vaginal or perineal area (e.g., discharge, dysuria).
   (c) Abnormalities (even minor) are observed on the external genital examination.
   (d) There are questions as to the veracity or completeness of the history regarding the nature and scope of abuse.

(e) Rape is a crime of violence. More than 80% of rape victims suffer from associated injuries. Great care must be taken to rule out vaginal and internal trauma.

c. Laboratory studies should include examination of vaginal secretions for fungi, *Trichomonas*, *Neisseria gonorrhoeae*, and *Chlamydia*. Rectal and pharyngeal cultures should also be obtained when appropriate. Completion of a standardized specimen kit should be performed in all cases of alleged sexual abuse, misuse, or rape. Urine should be obtained for pregnancy testing when age appropriate, as well as for serology for syphilis. Human immunodeficiency virus testing should be offered to the victim along with sensitive consultation at the time the results are available.

3. Therapy consists of management of acute medical conditions, venereal disease prophylaxis, pregnancy prophylaxis when appropriate, psychiatric support, social service management, and medical follow-up.

a. The therapy of acute medical conditions should be directed by the history and physical findings. Abdominal and vaginal trauma are common in violent assaults.

b. Venereal disease prophylaxis is recommended for all adolescents and young adults who have had contact with the assailant's genitals. In young children, presumptive treatment is not widely recommended because girls appear to be at lower risk for ascending infection than adolescent or adult women, and regular follow-up can usually be assured. (see Chap. 5, p. 103; Table 5-3)

(1) Oral prophylaxis. Amoxicillin, 50 mg/kg (maximum 3.0 g) is given in one dose with probenecid, 25 mg/kg (maximum 1.0 g), or cefixime, 400 mg PO in one dose, or ciprofloxacin, 500 mg PO in one dose. **Contraindications** to oral therapy are

(a) Rectal or oral penetration, because oral medication is ineffective with pharyngeal or rectal gonorrhea.

(b) Uncertainty of follow-up VDRL determinations, as oral therapy does not adequately treat incubating syphilis.

(2) Intramuscular prophylaxis. Give ceftriaxone, 125 mg IM once.

(3) Chlamydia prophylaxis. Give a single dose of azithromycin, 1 g PO. Alternatively, doxycycline, 100 mg PO bid for 7 days, can be used but requires compliance. In the younger child at risk for dental staining secondary to tetracyclines, it is often more judicious to wait for culture results before initiating an alternative therapy.

(4) Bacterial vaginosis. Metronidazole, 2 g PO in a single dose.

(5) Hepatitis B vaccine should also be considered.

c. Pregnancy prophylaxis (see also p. 429)

(1) Indications. Pregnancy prophylaxis should be considered when the following conditions are met.

(a) There is documentation or strong suspicion that intercourse has occurred.

(b) The patient has experienced menarche and is not presently menstruating.

(c) The time of unprotected intercourse is less than 72 hours before treatment.

(2) Prophylaxis consists of conjugated estrogens, for example, Ovral, two tablets immediately and two more 12 hours later. This regimen is almost universally associated with nausea and vomiting. Therefore, prochlorperazine, 5 to 10 mg PO, given 2 hours before estrogen, is usually helpful.

d. Psychiatric evaluation and support are essential, both for child and family. Victims of sexual abuse, even those who initially display seeming tranquillity or aloofness, may suffer from deep emotional disturbances. Rape counselors provide critical support.

e. Social service evaluation is helpful in assessing the circumstances surrounding the abuse and the relative safety of the child if he or she returns home. As in other forms of child abuse, when the safety of the home is uncertain, admission to the hospital or alternative placement is indicated. Sexual abuse is considered a form of child abuse, and state reporting laws will thus apply.

f. Medical follow-up. While the follow-up care is multidisciplinary, it is usually most helpful when one health provider is identified to the child and family, and has the responsibility of coordinating the various services and explaining the medical data to them. Medical follow-up should be carefully arranged to encompass the following:

(1) Follow-up examination and assessment of healing injuries.

(2) Check of cultures and other laboratory data, including human immunodeficiency virus (HIV) test results.

(3) Management of adverse effects of prophylactic therapy.

(4) Emotional and social service support.

G. Psychiatric emergencies (see also pp. 549 *ff.*)

1. Acute psychosis encompasses a group of conditions in which there is a gross impairment in reality testing such that an individual incorrectly evaluates thoughts or perceptions.

a. Etiology

(1) Nonorganic psychosis includes the schizophrenic, paranoid, and major affective disorders. Specific organic causes have not been identified.

(2) Organic psychosis includes metabolic, infectious, neoplastic, cardiovascular, and traumatic conditions, as well as drug ingestion (see Table 8-1).

b. Diagnosis

(1) An organic cause should be ruled out first. Clues to an organic cause include

(a) Altered level of consciousness.

(b) Visual hallucinations.

(c) An acute mental status change.

(2) A psychiatric evaluation is necessary to assess the nature and course of the disease.

(3) Direct evidence of nonorganic psychosis includes delusions or hallucinations, or behavior so grossly disorganized that disturbed reality testing can be implied. Among other concerns are suicidal or homicidal intentions, medications or hospitalization, and social support services.

c. Therapy

(1) Indications for hospitalization include

(a) Suicidal or homicidal ideation.

(b) Confusion severe enough to impair daily self-care or family attempts to provide care.

(c) When familial support or understanding of the patient's condition is judged inadequate.

(d) When the cause or nature of the psychosis remains unclear.

(2) Medication. Emergency medication (**Table 7-5**) is indicated when aggression or agitation is severe and unresponsive to supportive reassurance. Ingestion of an anticholinergic agent should be ruled out before antipsychotic medication is administered because it may mimic psychotic agitation.

2. Suicide. In the United States, suicide represents the third leading cause of death in adolescents. Girls attempt suicide more commonly than boys, but attempts by males are more often successful.

a. Etiology and precipitating factors. Suicide attempts are most commonly related to family problems, depression, school problems, relationship discord, and pregnancy.

b. Evaluation and diagnosis. All suicide attempts should be taken seri-

Table 7-5. Medications for the acutely agitated child

Drug	Dose*
Chlorpromazine	0.5 mg/kg IM
Thioridazine	0.5 mg/kg PO
Haloperidol	0.05–0.15 mg/kg/d PO q8–12h

*Medication can be repeated after 1 hr if no improvement is seen.

ously. Although varying in intent and severity, all suicide attempts imply a significant breakdown of social communication and relationships. The following are related to the assessment of suicide risk.

  (1) **Depression.** Severe guilt, hopelessness, and vegetative signs reflect a serious disturbance and an increased risk of subsequent suicidal behavior.

  (2) **Previous thoughts, attempts, and careful planning of attempts** usually imply an increased risk of subsequent attempts and a greater requisite intervention.

  (3) **Social and family dynamics** that precipitated the attempt and show little evidence of potential for rapid amelioration.

  (4) **Psychosis.** Suicidal attempts or ideation secondary to delusions or hallucinatinos are extremely serious and require hospitalization.

  c. **Management**

  (1) **Hospitalization** is indicated if the risk of suicide seems imminent, particularly if the conditions outlined in sec. **b.(1)–(4)** above are evident or suspected.

  (2) **Home management** should be undertaken only after careful psychiatric evaluation and when a sustained follow-up plan can be assured.

  (a) The crucial goal must be to modify the home environment sufficiently to make it tolerable for the child.

  (b) Access to immediate telephone or other personal support or counseling can be an important way to defuse a situation that is potentially intolerable for the patient.

3. The violent patient

  a. **Etiology.** Aggression is common in children and usually takes developmentally appropriate and controllable forms. However, occasionally the clinician is confronted by an acutely violent or threatening patient. To prevent harm to the patient and others, rapid and purposeful control of the patient is imperative. There are generally two types of situations that require intervention.

  b. **Management**

  (1) **Verbal intervention** may be useful in younger children in whom violent behavior is part of stereotyped tantrums or rage displays.

  (2) **Physical restraint** should be instituted as quickly and humanely as possible **if verbal intervention is unsuccessful for the protection of the patient and caretakers.**

  (3) **Medications** should be used judiciously. In the actively violent patient, they should be prepared before the patient is restrained.

  (a) **Antipsychotics** are useful to control agitation or combative behavior. They may enhance the effects of anticholinergic and narcotic agents and may produce hypotension, extrapyramidal reactions, tachycardia, and laryngospasm. **Haloperidol** (0.05–0.10 mg/kg IM) or **chlorpromazine** (0.25–0.5 mg/kg IM) can be used.

  (b) **Benzodiazepines** are most effective for patients who are severely anxious rather than actively violent. Respiratory depression can occur with large doses and enhancement of the depressant effects of alcohol, monoamine oxidase inhibitors, phenothiazines, tricyclic antidepressants, and barbiturates. Give **diazepam,** 0.1 mg/kg IV or PO (maximum 10 mg).

(4) Continuing care involves appropriate psychiatric placement, social service, and psychiatric evaluation (see Chap. 22).

(5) Ethical considerations. It is **imperative** that the use of restraints or medication meets the needs of patients and not the needs of the treating facility. In addition, it is often difficult to determine which patients are violent because of primary psychiatric conditions or which patients come to violence in response to what they perceive as oppressive social inequities. The potential for the "medicalization" of what are in fact social problems is significant. Strong efforts must be made to prevent the use of psychiatric or medical therapy to subvert the civil rights of patients or undermine the redress of social grievances. **Note:** State laws regarding the medicating of patients against their wishes vary. Clinicians should be acquainted with local provisions.

VII. Surgical acute care
A. Appendicitis
1. **Evaluation and diagnosis**
   a. **History.** Establish the time of onset. The appendix commonly perforates within 36 hours after pain begins. The *pain* is periumbilical and is almost always the first symptom. *Vomiting* is present and always follows the onset of pain. After several hours, pain usually shifts to the right lower quadrant. In the infant, decreased appetite, fever, and vomiting are generally present. Diarrhea may occur, especially with retrocecal appendicitis.
   b. **Physical examination,** when right lower quadrant pain is present, will usually reveal *tenderness, guarding,* and *rebound.* **Rectal examination** is imperative to elicit tenderness.
   c. **Laboratory data**
      (1) Urinalysis, urine culture, and Gram's stain.
      (2) The **WBC** usually is elevated, but rarely above 20,000 in a child with a nonperforated appendix.
      (3) Abdominal x-rays will show concave curvature of the spine to the right due to the spasm of right-sided abdominal musculature. An air-fluid level may be seen in the cecum. A fecalith may be seen and increases the likelihood of a perforation. With perforation, decreased bowel gas in the right lower quadrant and free peritoneal fluid may be seen, especially in children under 2 years of age. A chest radiograph may be helpful, since lower-lobe pneumonia occasionally mimics appendicitis.
2. **Therapy**
   a. **Appendectomy**
   b. When a perforated appendix is suspected, a triple antibiotic regimen (ampicillin, gentamicin, and clindamycin or cefoxitin) is usually administered (see Chap. 5).
B. Obstruction
1. **Intussusception** usually occurs in children from 1 month to 2 years of age and occurs when a segment of intestine telescopes into itself, causing obstruction, ischemia, and necrosis.
   a. **Etiology.** The majority of cases are idiopathic, but a lead point such as Meckel's diverticulum or adenopathy is not uncommon. Henoch-Schönlein purpura can be associated with intussusception.
   b. **Evaluation and diagnosis**
      (1) History
         (a) Intermittent abdominal pain, vomiting, and bloody ("currant-jelly") stools.
         (b) Violent episodes of colicky, severe abdominal pain, causing the child to cry out and draw the legs into flexed position are interspersed with relatively normal periods.
      (2) Physical examination

       (a) The child may be quiet, listless, irritable, or normal appearing between episodes of pain.

       (b) When the process presents later in the course, the child may show signs of prostration, pallor, and altered mental status. Careful vital sign measurement is essential in this setting.

       (c) A vague, sausage-shaped mass is palpable, either abdominally or rectally, in most.

       (d) Fever is common, particularly in infants.

    (3) Laboratory data

       (a) A characteristic filling defect extending from the cecum to distal parts of the colon is observed in the **barium enema.**

       (b) Hematocrit.

       (c) Stools should be tested for occult blood.

  c. Therapy

    (1) Intravenous fluids resuscitation is always necessary.

    (2) Barium or air enema. Most intussusceptions can be reduced by hydrostatic or pneumatic pressure during the diagnostic enema. When done in a controlled manner, with close collaboration between the surgeon and radiologist, this procedure is safe and may obviate the need for surgery.

    (3) When enema reduction is unsuccessful, **laparotomy and direct reduction** are required.

2. Malrotation and volvulus (see also Chap. 6, p. 217)

  a. Etiology. Congenitally abnormal position of the small bowel and associated abnormal posterior fixation of the mesentery. The most common age of presentation is under 1 month.

  b. Evaluation and diagnosis

    (1) The **history** almost always includes vomiting, usually bile stained. In older children, a past history of attacks termed *cyclic vomiting* may be elicited.

    (2) Physical examination may reveal abdominal distention, jaundice, blood-stained vomitus or stools, and shock.

    (3) Laboratory data

       (a) Abdominal films may reveal gas in the stomach with a paucity of air in the small intestine.

       (b) An **upper GI series and small bowel follow-through** will confirm the diagnosis, defining the positions of the ligament of Treitz and the cecum.

       (c) Stool testing positive for blood is a poor prognostic sign, indicating significant bowel ischemia.

  c. Therapy

    (1) Nasogastric tube.

    (2) Operative relief of the obstruction should be attempted as rapidly as possible.

    (3) Intravenous fluids (see Chap. 4).

3. Pyloric stenosis is a cause of obstruction in the first 8 weeks of life, with a peak in 2 to 4 weeks. Boys are affected 4 : 1 over girls, and it occurs more frequently in infants with a family history of the condition.

  a. Etiology: unknown. Mechanism is narrowing of the pyloric canal due to muscular hypertrophy.

  b. Evaluation and diagnosis

    (1) The **history** reveals the onset of nonbilious vomiting of feedings, sometimes, but not always, "projectile."

    (2) Physical examination. The findings will vary with the severity of the obstruction.

       (a) Dehydration and weight loss are common.

       (b) Palpation of an **olive-sized muscular tumor** following vomiting occurs in the majority of cases.

       (c) Visible gastric peristaltic waves are also common.

(3) Laboratory data

    (a) Ultrasonography reveals the hypertrophic pylorus.

    (b) If ultrasonography is not available, roentgenographic studies after a barium meal reveal stenosis ("railroad-track sign").

    (c) Electrolytes, BUN, glucose, pH, and serum bicarbonate should be followed, since significant abnormalities, usually metabolic alkalosis, may accompany the vomiting (see Chap. 4).

c. Therapy

    (1) Nasogastric tube.

    (2) Correction of the dehydration, alkalosis, and electrolyte abnormalities is a critical aspect of initial therapy (see Chap. 4).

    (3) Surgical correction should take place as soon as the metabolic abnormalities have been satisfactorily corrected.

C. Blunt trauma to the abdomen can be a serious injury, yet may present with subtle symptoms and signs that mimic other causes of abdominal pain. A child with significant internal abdominal injury might present many hours or even days after the traumatic event.

  1. Evaluation and diagnosis

    a. A **history** of trauma, from even seemingly minor events, should raise this possibility.

    b. Physical examination may reveal abdominal tenderness, bruises, or hematuria. Serial observation for deterioration of vital signs or increasing abdominal tenderness is warranted.

    c. Laboratory studies should include CBC, urinalysis, prothrombin time, partial thromboplastin time, platelet count, and clot for type and crossmatch in case blood loss is significant or surgical intervention is required. Computed tomography of the abdomen may reveal free fluid in the abdomen and delineate injuries of the liver, spleen, kidney, or pancreas.

  2. Therapy

    a. Surgical consultation.

    b. Initial management should be directed at maintaining adequate blood volume. **Two large-bore IV lines should be placed if abdominal hemorrhaging is suspected.**

    c. While splenic or hepatic injuries may generally be treated conservatively, massive or persistent bleeding mandates surgical intervention.

D. Ectopic pregnancy has become an important diagnostic consideration in evaluating the acute abdomen in adolescent girls (see also Chap. 14, p. 429).

  1. Etiology. Ninety-eight percent of ectopic pregnancies occur in the fallopian tube.

  2. Evaluation and diagnosis. Ectopic pregnancy in an adolescent may present as an abdominal catastrophe or, more subtly, with colicky pain and mild vaginal bleeding.

    a. A **catastrophic** presentation demands a rapid yet careful evaluation.

      (1) The patient usually is in shock, with signs of peritoneal irritation, including tenderness and rigidity but *rarely* fever.

      (2) *Intraperitoneal blood* can be palpated as a doughy mass in the cul-de-sac.

      (3) Although an ultrasound can often be diagnostic, **laparoscopy** is the definitive study.

      (4) Culdocentesis can be performed to confirm hemoperitoneum.

      (5) Laboratory tests should include preoperative studies and type and cross-matching for at least 4 units of blood.

    b. Nonacute presentation

      (1) The history includes vaginal bleeding after a missed period and lower abdominal pain.

      (2) The **physical examination** may reveal an adnexal mass by palpation. Extreme sensitivity to cervical motion is an important finding.

      (3) Laboratory tests include CBC and erythrocyte sedimentation rate (ESR) with serial hematocrits. Urinalysis should help rule out alternative diagnoses, including urinary tract infection (UTI) and renal calculi.

(4) A urine pregnancy test is positive in only half of ectopic pregnancies. Serum human chorionic gonadotropin determinations are more reliable indicators of pregnancy.

3. Therapy

   a. The *catastrophic presentation*, with the patient in shock, requires rapid stabilization and transfer to the operating room for definitive **surgery.**

   b. In a *nonacute presentation*, surgery is performed when there is a high index of suspicion of ectopic pregnancy based on procedures that may include culdocentesis, pelvic ultrasound, examination under anesthesia, and laparoscopy.

E. Pelvic inflammatory disease is an important cause of abdominal pain in female adolescents. Its clinical presentation may be similar to that of *appendicitis, ectopic pregnancy*, and *menstrual cramps*. For a discussion of evaluation and therapy, see Chap. 5.

VIII. Environmental emergencies

A. Near-drowning implies survival of at least 24 hours following a submersion episode. CNS injury remains the most difficult problem facing caretakers of near-drowning accidents.

   1. Etiology

   a. Cold-versus warm-water drowning. Hypothermia associated with cold-water drowning may provide protection against CNS hypoxic damage. There are no protective mechanisms in warm-water immersions.

   b. Freshwater versus saltwater drownings. Both freshwater and saltwater near-drownings damage alveoli, destroy surfactant, and result in pulmonary edema and hypoxia.

      (1) Freshwater. If a large amount of freshwater is aspirated, hypervolemia and water intoxication can also result.

      (2) Saltwater. If a large volume of saltwater is aspirated, *hypovolemia, hemoconcentration*, and *hypernatremia* can occur. The **resultant** *pulmonary edema* can be massive.

   2. Evaluation and diagnosis

   a. A **precise history** of the event should be obtained, including

      (1) The **type of water**—whether cold or warm, fresh or salt—and an estimate of contamination. If drowning is in another liquid, determine the chemical composition.

      (2) Associated injuries.

      (3) Estimation of the time submerged.

      (4) Clinical status when rescued. Note if any spontaneous respiration or heartbeat occurred.

      (5) Type of CPR required and when it was begun, **and duration.**

   b. Physical examination

      (1) Vital signs: blood pressure, pulse, respirations, temperature and **oxygen saturation.**

      (2) Careful cardiopulmonary and neurologic evaluations, including a Glasgow Coma Scale assignment (see Table 7-3).

      (3) Associated injuries, with particular attention to signs of neck and spinal cord injury.

   c. Laboratory investigation includes a general screen for hypoxic and hypotensive injury.

      (1) Blood studies: ABG, electrolytes, blood sugar, calcium, CBC, prothrombin time, partial thromboplastin time, liver function tests. A toxic screen may also be indicated.

      (2) Chest x-ray and other radiographs (i.e., cervical spine films) as required to rule out associated injury.

      (3) Electrocardiography.

      (4) Urinalysis, with a flow chart showing the hourly output.

   3. Treatment

    a. All patients who are victims of near-drowning should be admitted for observation. This includes patients who revive spontaneously at the site of the accident.

    b. Initial therapy

        (1) The ABCs of resuscitation are of paramount importance. Attention to a patent airway includes suctioning and clearing the airway of waterborne debris and vomitus.

        (2) Immobilizing the cervical spine is vitally important until injury is ruled out.

        (3) Pulmonary support. Atelectasis and hypoxia are major problems. Intubation and early positive end-expiratory pressure (PEEP) may be indicated.

        (4) Temperature resuscitation must begin immediately (see sec. **C** below). CPR will often be unsuccessful until the victim's temperature normalizes.

    c. Subsequent therapy

        (1) Cardiovascular support is given as required (see sec. **II**, p. 223).

        (2) Recognition and treatment of increased ICP if it occurs (see sec. **V.B**, p. 235).

        (3) Prophylactic antibiotics and the use of corticosteroids have not been shown to be efficacious.

        (4) All associated injuries must be treated.

        (5) Antibiotics are used for aspiration pneumonitis.

        (6) Early and intense **social service intervention** is necessary for the family of the victim.

B. Heat-related injury

    1. Burns

        a. Etiologies: heat or flame, chemical, electrical.

        b. Evaluation of the burn patient

            (1) The **history** must include

                (a) The **type of heat exposure** (e.g., an open flame, scald burn, electrical or **chemical** burn, explosion).

                (b) How or why the patient was exposed. **Try to assess for inadequate supervision or evidence of child abuse.**

                (c) Note if there is any evidence of **associated injuries.**

                (d) Assess for the possibility of an **inhalation burn.** The possibility of pulmonary burns **and carbon monoxide poisoning** is increased in explosion or closed space burn.

            (2) The **physical examination** must be complete.

                (a) Immediate attention is directed to the airway.

                (b) Vital signs and **initial weight to help guide fluid therapy.**

                (c) Indications of **inhalation injury** include **cyanosis,** carbonaceous sputum, carbon deposits in the oropharynx, stridor or hoarseness, facial burns, and singed nasal hairs. If any of these are present, **intubation** should be performed before further physical assessment is completed.

                (d) A search for evidence of **associated injuries follows, with attention to possible cervical spine injury**

                (e) The **surface burn is assessed last**.

                    (i) Surface area. Charts are available to help estimate the size of the involved area. In children over 12 years of age, the "rule of nines" can be used; in younger patients, surface area can be estimated based on the child's hand as 1% body surface area (BSA).

                    (ii) The **depth of the burn** or level of tissue injury must be evaluated. **Superficial** (first-degree) burns involve the epithelium only. There is vasodilation and little edema. Superficial and deep partial-thickness (second-degree) burns involve destruction of the epithelium and part of the corium, with sparing of the dermal appendages. Capillary damage presents with blister formation. **Full-thickness** (third-degree) burns cause destruction of the entire dermis with loss of sensation. Clinically, these burn areas appear white, with no blister formation, and are anesthetic.

    (iii) The presence of circumferential burns must be noted and distal blood flow assessed.

  (3) The **laboratory examination** includes

    (a) **Blood studies:** ABG, CBC, electrolytes, blood sugar, BUN, creatinine, calcium, prothrombin time, partial thromboplastin time, total protein, carboxyhemoglobin, and, if it is an electrical burn, creatine phosphokinase (CPK).

    (b) Chest x-ray.

    (c) Urinalysis.

    (d) Selected radiographs to rule out associated injuries.

c. Therapy. The general goals of therapy are to maintain adequate ventilation and oxygenation, to support the cardiovascular system in the face of massive volume loss, and to minimize tissue loss with local care and infection control.

  (1) If there is evidence of an **airway** or pulmonary burn, the patient should be **intubated.** Supplemental oxygen should be administered as indicated.

  (2) **Apply cold sterile saline soaks** to the burn to stop any remaining thermal damage.

  (3) **Establish IV access.** If the burn is extensive, a CVP line should be placed.

  (4) **Volume replacement** should be started if the patient has second- or third-degree burns involving more than 10% of the BSA. Volume replacement can be calculated as follows (see also Chap. 4): **volume replacement (ml) = %BSA burn × 4 ml/kg. (For infants, maintenance fluid requirements must be added.)** Normal saline or lactated Ringer's solution is used for initial fluid therapy. One half is administered over the first 8 hours and the remainder over the next 16 hours. The most useful index of adequate vascular volume is hourly urine output; therefore, calculations should serve as guidelines only. CVP monitoring may be useful.

  (5) A **Foley catheter** is placed to monitor urine output. **Nasogastric tube** is placed for decompression.

  (6) Analgesia **should be titrated to the patient's pain:** morphine, 0.1 mg/kg **q1–2h.**

  (7) **Tetanus toxoid** (0.5 ml IM) is given if tetanus prophylaxis status is uncertain or if more than 5 years have elapsed since the last booster.

  (8) The use of prophylactic antibiotics is controversial.

  (9) **Topical care.** Silver sulfadiazine (Silvadene) or mafenide (Sulfamylon) cream can be used twice a day for all burn areas, except the face, where bacitracin is recommended. Antibiotic-impregnated (Xeroform) gauze can be used as well. Sterile, bulky, dry dressings may then be applied.

  (10) **Early escharotomies or fasciotomies, or both, should be performed in all circumferential burns** if any distal circulatory impairment is present.

d. Electrical burns: evaluation and treatment

  (1) The patient should be **examined carefully for** an **entrance** as well as an **exit** wound and any **associated injuries.**

  (2) **Laboratory evaluation** includes CPK and urine for hemoglobin and myoglobin, and an ECG **for rhythm disturbances.**

  (3) A very common burn injury in pediatrics is an **electrical burn to the mouth.** These patients must not be debrided, and must be followed closely for a minimum of 3 weeks because of the potential for slough

of eschar and hemorrhage at the site of the lesion. Plastic surgical **intervention is recommended.**

2. **Heat stroke**
   a. **Etiology.** Heat stroke is a life-threatening syndrome characterized by impaired heat dissipation secondary to high ambient temperature.
   b. **Evaluation**
      (1) The **history** may reveal the following predisposing factors: alcohol abuse, obesity, heart disease, or fever. A careful history must include the duration of the temperature elevation, the therapeutic maneuvers attempted at home, and a history of oral intake and urine output.
      (2) The **physical examination** will reveal the findings enumerated in sec. **c** below.
      (3) **Laboratory evaluation**
         (a) Blood studies: ABG, electrolytes, blood sugar, serum osmolarity, BUN, creatinine, calcium, prothrombin time, partial thromboplastin time, CBC, and CPK.
         (b) Urinalysis, urine for myoglobin.
   c. **Diagnosis**
      (1) Characteristic triad in heat stroke:
         (a) Hyperpyrexia, or a rectal temperature greater than 41°C (105.8°F).
         (b) Hot, dry skin.
         (c) Severe CNS disturbances manifested by coma, seizures, headache, agitation, or confusion.
      (2) Other clinical symptoms and findings include
         (a) Tachycardia and hypotension with eventual circulatory collapse.
         (b) Oliguria or anuria with acute tubular necrosis.
         (c) Rhabdomyolysis, which can compound renal injury.
   d. **Therapy**
      (1) **Assess airway and ventilation;** give oxygen for cardiorespiratory or neurologic compromise.
      (2) **Rapid cooling**
         (a) Remove **all clothing.**
         (b) Place the patient in **an ice bath** or use ice bags at the neck, femoral, and axillary areas until the rectal temperature is less than 38.3°C (101°F).
         (c) Phenothiazines can be given to decrease shivering (which is a heat-producing process), but be aware that they can cause hypotension.
         (d) Keep skin moist; use fans to increase convection and evaporative heat loss.
      (3) **Volume replacement** is usually required and possibly CVP monitoring and inotropic support (see sec. **II,** p. 223).
      (4) The **renal status** is monitored and an hourly record of the intake and output kept.
      (5) If **seizures** are present, the patient should receive a loading dose of phenytoin, 10 mg/kg IV, or phenobarbital, 10 mg/kg IV (see p. 234).
3. **Heat "cramps"** are muscle cramps secondary to an acute loss of electrolytes after severe exertion. Treatment includes rest and fluid and electrolyte replacement.
4. **Heat exhaustion** or prostration is a *hypovolemic or salt depletion* state that presents with progressive lassitude, headache, nausea and vomiting, tachycardia, and hypotension. Treatment includes rehydration with close electrolyte monitoring and rest in a cool room.
C. **Cold-related injury**
   1. **Hypothermia** is a core temperature of less than **35.5°C.** Hypothermia causes marked depression of all organ systems. The heart is most significantly affected, including decreased cardiac output and the following rhythm disturbances: 30 to 35°C, atrial fibrillation and flutter; 26 to 30°C, ventricular ectopy and fibrillation; less than 26°C, asystole.

a. **Etiology:** results from any cold exposure.
b. **Evaluation and diagnosis. Patients should be managed carefully** to avoid precipitation of dysrhythmias in the irritable myocardium.

(1) **The history** should document the patient's symptoms, the duration and type of exposure, any medical therapy, and **past medical history.**

(2) On **physical examination,** the patient will be pale or cyanotic.

(a) **Vital signs.** Temperature **must** be obtained rectally or by esophageal catheter with a special low-recording thermometer.

(b) The **cardiopulmonary systems** should be assessed for breathing, perfusion, and evidence of dysrhythmias.

(c) **Neurologic examination**

(i) **Above 35°C:** alert, conscious, shivering.

(ii) **35 to 30°C:** clouded mentation, dilated pupils with lower temperatures, decreased shivering.

(iii) **Below 30°C:** unconscious, diminished deep tendon reflexes, diminished respirations.

(iv) **26°C and below:** The patient appears dead. Respiration is barely detectable.

(d) The patient should be examined closely for localized tissue damage (frostbite) (see sec. **2** below) and associated injuries **or ingestions**.

(3) **Laboratory studies.** The requirements for laboratory testing increase with the severity of the hypothermia.

(a) Arterial blood gas, electrolytes, BUN, creatinine, CBC, clotting variables, liver function tests, and a toxic screen as needed.

(b) A **chest x-ray** should be obtained to ascertain if there was any aspiration during the acute event or resuscitation.

c. **Treatment:** supportive measures and rewarming techniques

(1) **Rewarming should be started immediately.** The methods for rewarming are dependent on core temperature.

(a) **External rewarming.** This has the advantage of ease, but the disadvantages of inefficiency and of temperature afterdrop and rewarming shock.

(i) **Passive external rewarming.** Used only if the core temperature is greater than 35°C. Remove all clothing, and place the patient in a warm room under warmed blankets.

(ii) **Active external rewarming** is not to be used if the temperature is less than 32°C. Heat is applied to the body surfaces: warming blankets, water baths (temperature 37–40°C), and hot water bottles over the femoral and axillary areas. **Caution should be taken to avoid burn injury.**

(b) **Core rewarming.** More effective than external rewarming, core rewarming methods include

(i) Heating IV infusions in a blood warmer to 40 to 43°C.

(ii) Colonic and bladder lavage with saline at 40 to 44°C.

(iii) Nasogastric lavage is contraindicated because of the risk of inducing dysrhythmias.

(iv) Airway rewarming with inspired gases warmed to 42 to 46°C.

(v) **Peritoneal dialysis.** The dialysate should be warmed to 43°C. This may require bathing the dialysate bottles in a 54°C bath. Pleural lavage may be helpful.

(vi) Cardiac bypass when available.

(2) **Meticulous cardiopulmonary resuscitation must accompany rewarming.**

(a) **A patient cannot be pronounced dead until he or she remains asystolic after rewarming to a core temperature of**

30°C or the patient cannot be rewarmed to 30°C even with invasive measures.

(b) If the patient is asystolic or in ventricular fibrillation, continue CPR while rewarming.

    (i) Countershock for ventricular fibrillation may be ineffective at less than 30°C. Medications are usually ineffective below 30°C.

    (ii) Avoid excess $NaHCO_3$; alkalosis can precipitate ventricular fibrillation. Monitor ABGs.

2. Frostbite and other cold injuries

  a. Etiology. Tissue damage from cold exposure is caused by vascular injury. Cold exposures can cause

    (1) Freezing injuries (*frostbite*) result from exposure to freezing temperatures that cause crystallization of tissue water.

    (2) Nonfreezing injuries (*chilblain, immersion foot, trench foot*). These generally occur after long exposure to **cold** temperatures above freezing, usually with very high humidity.

  b. Evaluation and diagnosis require the following:

    (1) The **core temperature must be obtained,** and if hypothermia is present, rewarming should be started immediately (see sec. **1** above).

    (2) The **level of tissue damage** should be assessed by using the following classification system.

      (a) First-degree injury presents with hyperemia and edema and is quite painful.

      (b) Second-degree injury also presents with hyperemia and pain, but has clear vesicle formation.

      (c) In **third-degree injury,** necrosis of the cutaneous tissue with dark vesicle formation develops.

      (d) Fourth-degree injury has complete necrosis and loss of tissue extending into and below the subcutaneous level. This is a painless lesion.

  c. Therapy. The goals of therapy are to stop the cold injury and minimize further tissue damage and loss.

    (1) The skin should be **rewarmed.**

      (a) Remove from the cold.

      (b) Remove any restrictive clothing.

      (c) Topical ointments should be **avoided.**

      (d) The patient should not be allowed to smoke cigarettes or drink alcohol, in order to avoid vascular reactivity.

      (e) If the area is still frozen when the patient presents (i.e., no sensation; white, hard, brittle skin), the involved skin should be warmed in a water bath of 40°C. **Warm only until the area is unfrozen. The water bath temperature should not exceed 42°C.**

    (2) Local care should include only loose, dry dressings. Third- or fourth-degree injury blisters should not be broken. Second-degree blisters can be broken, followed by application of aloe vera cream to help prevent thrombosis.

    (3) Tetanus toxoid, 0.5 ml IM, is given unless the patient has received tetanus within 5 years.

    (4) Pain medication may be required: Morphine, 0.1 mg/kg q4–6h, is adequate.

    (5) Antibiotics should be given if there is any evidence of infection.

    (6) Physical therapy is required if there is any tissue damage over a joint.

    (7) Amputation, if needed, should be delayed until optimal healing has occurred.

IX. Acute care procedures

  A. Bag-and-mask ventilation

1. **Bag-and-mask ventilation is the first line of support in respiratory failure or apnea.** Good gas exchange may be maintained in the vast majority of patients while preparations are made for intubation.

   a. In infants, small oronasal passages and a relatively large tongue predispose to obstruction during mask ventilation. It is therefore critical that the airway be made patent: open the mouth and extend the jaw, pulling the tongue down and away from the palate and pharynx. Do not overextend the neck; keep the mouth partially open at all times using an oral airway if necessary.

   b. Care should be taken so as not to insufflate the stomach; this can be prevented by applying *gentle* cricoid pressure. If gastric distention becomes significant, an oro- or nasogastric tube should be briefly passed.

B. Intubation

1. **Indications for tracheal intubation** include

   a. Airway protection.

   b. Pulmonary toilet.

   c. Respiratory support.

2. **Preparation**

   a. **Equipment:** oxygen, suction with "tonsil tip" catheter, breathing system (self-inflating Ambu type or oxygen-inflated Mapleson type), laryngoscope handles (check batteries and bulbs), and age-appropriate blades; appropriate-sized masks, oral airways, endotracheal tubes, and stylets. **Endotracheal tube** (ETT) size can be estimated as follows: ETT size = (16 + age in years) divided by 4. For example: if a child is 4 years old: ETT size = (16 + 4)/4 = 20/4 = 5.

      For all equipment, always have one size larger and one size smaller immediately available.

   b. **Medications.** Atropine, methohexital (Brevital), propofol, etomidate, thiopental, or ketamine; succinylcholine, midazolam (Versed), morphine or fentanyl, cocaine, lidocaine (Xylocaine), Cetacaine

3. **Monitoring** will require ECG, pulse oximetry, blood pressure cuff, and stethoscope.

4. **General instructions for intubation**

   a. **Assemble** all the necessary equipment within easy reach.

   b. **Pretreat** the child with atropine, 0.02 mg/kg IV or IM, to avoid a vagally induced bradycardia.

   c. **Preoxygenate** the child with 100% oxygen by face mask. *This will delay arterial desaturation if intubation proves difficult and requires more time than anticipated.*

   d. **Positioning.** The child's head should be in the midline; this position should be maintained by an assistant. Because the child's larynx is more anterior and cephalad than the adult's, head positioning is slightly different. The child should be put in the "sniffing position," which in the infant is provided naturally by the prominent occiput and in older children can be obtained by placing a small blanket, diaper, or towel under the occiput. **Placing a roll under the shoulders may, in fact, obscure the airway.**

   e. **Laryngoscopy.** The laryngoscope is held in the left hand, while the mouth is opened with the right. The blade of the laryngoscope is placed in the right side of the mouth near the tonsillar pillar and swept to the midline, carrying the tongue to the left side of the mouth and out of the way. When a straight blade (Miller or Wis-Hipple) is used, the tip of the epiglottis is lifted to reveal the larynx. When a curved (Macintosh) blade is used, its tip is placed in the vallecula (above the epiglottis) and lifting exposes the vocal cords. In both cases the blade is moved by *lifting* the laryngoscope handle along its axis. **Tilting the handle does not improve visualization and leads to oral damage.** Frequently, further positioning of the head, or application of gentle cricoid pressure, will help bring the larynx into better view. Suctioning may be necessary.

f. Intubation. The endotracheal tube is brought in from the right side of the mouth and placed between the cords under direct visualization. **Passage of the tube directly down the laryngoscope blade obscures the view of the vocal cords.** With the start of ventilation, position of the tube is confirmed by

(1) Symmetric chest rise.

(2) Fogging of the endotracheal tube.

(3) Absence of sounds over the stomach.

(4) Clear breath sounds on both sides of the chest.

The tube is then secured into place and a confirmational x-ray is obtained. When proper position is confirmed, the tube is taped securely. For oral intubations, the insertion depth at the lips typically equals three times the internal diameter of the tube. For example, a 4.0 ETT is typically taped at 12 cm.

g. Postintubation sedation and restraints. The pediatric patient will often attempt to remove the tube; therefore, every precaution should be made to protect the airway. This may require sedation (chloral hydrate, 30–50 mg/kg q6h) or morphine (0.1 mg/kg q2–4h) and restraints that can be applied as arm/elbow splints. The feet should also be secured. The need for this should be explained gently to parents.

5. Sedation and relaxation techniques. Awake intubation provides the important advantage of maintaining spontaneous ventilation, yet is a stressful and often difficult technique. When possible in infancy, in debilitated patients, or in cooperative older children after topical anesthesia and light sedation, it is usually unsuitable for others. When heavy sedation is used, the risk of apnea is present and, when paralysis is employed, it is essential that the practitioner be skilled in management of the airway.

a. Anesthetics and muscle relaxants. The patient is given an induction of intravenous anesthetic, such as *thiopental* (4–6 mg/kg IV), *methohexital* (1.0–1.5 mg/kg IV), or *ketamine* (1.0–1.5 mg/kg IV). When the stomach is empty, adequacy of the airway is assessed with bag-and-mask ventilation. If the airway can be maintained easily, succinylcholine (1 mg/kg IV) is given for muscle relaxation. When the child is fully relaxed, the intubation is completed. The following *limitations of this technique* must be considered.

(1) A muscle relaxant should only be given by a person who is competent with intubations, usually an anesthesiologist.

(2) A child who has an airway obstruction or is known to be difficult to intubate is only managed in the operating room by an anesthesiologist and otolaryngologist. Children with obstructed airways can, as a rule, maintain their own airway better than the physician can with bag-and-mask ventilation.

(3) A child with hypotension, hypovolemia, or evidence of myocardial compromise should not receive a barbiturate because it can cause cardiovascular collapse. In such children, *ketamine* is a reasonable choice.

(4) Any child with progressive myopathy, evolving neuromuscular disease, acute major denervation, or burn injury should not receive succinylcholine. In these conditions, succinylcholine can cause profound *hyperkalemia*. **Children who have renal failure and difficulty with high serum potassium levels should not receive succinylcholine. In patients with muscular dystrophy, succinylcholine is associated with malignant hyperthermia.** Alternatives include *pancuronium* (Pavulon) or *vecuronium* (Norcuron), 0.1 mg/kg IV.

(5) Any child who has a full stomach should be intubated awake or in "rapid-sequence" fashion with cricoid pressure to prevent gastric aspiration. In *rapid-sequence technique*, cricoid pressure is applied during preoxygenation and maintained until the endotracheal tube is in place. Medications are given in rapid succession and the patient is not ventilated by mask. Success must be swift and immediate; the technique is contraindicated in patients in whom any potential difficulty with intubation is suspected.

b. **Benzodiazepines, narcotics, and topical anesthetics (Table 7-6)**
   (1) For awake intubations, children can be sedated with *midazolam* (Versed) given in 0.05 mg/kg IV increments and *morphine* (0.05–0.1 mg/kg IV increments), or *fentanyl*, 2 μg/kg IV increments. The oropharynx is sprayed with lidocaine or Cetacaine.
   (2) As a vasoconstrictor and anesthetic, cocaine is ideal for *nasal* topicalization. Alternatively, use a combination of phenylephrine and lidocaine.

c. **Blind nasotracheal intubations.** In young children, this technique is exceedingly difficult but in the older child and adolescent, it is acceptable. The naso-oral airway is topically anesthetized. Then, with the child in a sitting position with the head forward, the tube is slowly advanced with each inspiration. As the tube approaches the glottis, louder breaths are heard through it.

d. **Laryngeal mask airways** may provide a rapid means for temporarily delivering positive pressure ventilation. Risk of serious aspiration is reduced, but not eliminated.

C. **Ventilators**
   1. **Definition of terms used in mechanical ventilation**
      a. **Controlled ventilation** is complete mechanical ventilation in which the patient does no spontaneous breathing.
      b. In **assisted ventilation** the patient initiates a breath that the ventilator completes. This is usually combined with an occasional mandatory breath.
      c. In **intermittent mandatory ventilation (IMV),** the patient receives breaths at a preset rate, but can spontaneously generate his or her own respirations at any rate.
      d. In **continuous positive airway pressure (CPAP),** no preset breaths are given, and the patient breathes against a constant distending pressure.
      e. In **pressure support ventilation,** patient-initiated breaths are supplemented by a preset pressure supplied to the airway.
      f. In **pressure control ventilation,** a preset pressure is maintained throughout inspiration.
      g. In **high-frequency ventilation (HFV),** extremely small tidal volumes are moved rapidly (>100/min), leading to alveolar exchange through bulk flow. HFV permits maintenance of alveolar volume without the barotrauma that accompanies phasic pressure changes and may be particularly helpful in management of air leak states.
   2. The **types of ventilators** available are outlined below and compared in Table 7-7. Ventilators are classified by the event that terminates ventilation.
      a. **Time-cycled ventilator.** Inspiration continues for a preset time.
      b. **Volume-cycled ventilator.** Inspiration continues until the preset volume is delivered. In both time-cycled and volume-cycled ventilators, pressure limits can be set to avoid the problems of overdistention and barotrauma.
   3. **Indications for ventilation therapy.** Mechanical ventilation is used to treat or to prevent respiratory failure, indicated by hypoxia, hypercapnia, and respiratory acidosis. Specific clinical situations include
      a. **Apnea.**
      b. **Fatigue** from increased work of breathing caused by dynamic airway disease, parenchymal disease, or mechanical obstruction that inhibits diaphragmatic movement. In these cases it is important both to assist ventilation and to decrease or prevent atelectasis.
      c. **Neuromuscular disease.**
      d. **Skeletal problems** that produce restrictive lung disease or an unstable thorax.
   4. **How to use the ventilator:**

    a. Specific therapy must be tailored to accommodate each clinical situation.

        (1) CPAP prevents or reverses small airway closure and alveolar collapse, decreasing the work of breathing and possibly any intrapulmonary right-to-left shunt.

        (2) IMV, assisted, or controlled ventilation is used when the physician cannot generate an adequate minute ventilation.

    b. Sedation is usually required for the patient to tolerate the endotracheal tube and ventilatory support.

    c. Muscle relaxation may be required when high inflating pressures are used or when ventilation is difficult because the patient "fights" the ventilator.

  5. Assessment of mechanical ventilation

    a. The patient's **tidal volume** should be evaluated by visual inspection, auscultation, and measurement of expired volume at the airway. Chosen initial tidal volumes are typically 10 to 15 ml/kg. Cyanosis, nasal flaring, retractions, and patient discomfort indicate *inadequate* mechanical ventilation.

    b. When a patient is started on mechanical ventilation, it is imperative to evaluate adequacy of oxygenation and ventilation with ABGs.

    c. When a patient continues on mechanical ventilation, continual monitoring of gas exchange can be done with pulse oximetry, end-tidal carbon dioxide monitors, and arterial or capillary blood gases.

  6. Complications of positive pressure ventilation

    a. Barotrauma from high airway pressure can produce lung injury, pneumothoraces, pneumomediastinum, and pneumoperitoneum.

    b. If CPAP or PEEP is too high or air trapping occurs, there will be overdistention of the alveoli and carbon dioxide retention.

    c. Decreased systemic venous return producing a decrease in cardiac output can occur in a patient on positive pressure ventilation. This is exaggerated in the patient who is hypovolemic, has poor myocardial function, or has tamponade.

    d. Stacking of breaths may occur when expiratory time is insufficient and new positive pressure breaths are superimposed on previous inspired volumes. Peak inspiratory and end-expiratory pressures increase while tidal volumes decrease giving the illusion of worsening intrinsic lung disease. Increasing auto-PEEP as assessed during an expiratory pause identifies this condition.

    e. The most common complication is the selection of inappropriate ventilator settings with inadequate monitoring.

D. Central venous pressure (CVP) monitors

  1. Definition. CVP lines are intrathoracic catheters used for the assessment of intravascular volume status and secure administration of medications.

  2. Placement is indicated in

    a. Any situation in which a CVP measurement will help to guide therapy

        (1) Shock.

        (2) Anuria or oliguria.

        (3) During vasoactive drug therapy.

        (4) During therapeutic osmotherapy.

        (5) Congestive heart failure.

        (6) Situations in which massive fluid shifts are anticipated, that is, sepsis, burns, major trauma, surgery.

    b. Any situation in which secure vascular access is necessary or irritating medications must be given

        (1) During cardiac arrest.

        (2) During chemotherapy.

        (3) For infusion of vasoactive medications.

        (4) For hyperalimentation.

        (5) For rapid electrolyte repletion.

        (6) For repeated "mixed-venous" blood sampling.

  3. Required equipment includes

    a. Sterile preparations. Betadine, alcohol, gloves, masks, sterile drapes.

Table 7-6. Medications used for conscious sedation

Route	Indications	Drug	Dosing (mg/kg)
Sedative agents			
Topical	IV placement, LP Laceration repair	EMLA	2.5%/2.5% lidocaine/ prilocaine
		LET (viscous, lidocaine, epinephrine, tetracaine)	L: 4.0% E: 0.1% T: 0.5%
Local	Laceration repair	Lidocaine Bupivacaine	0.5, 1, 2% 0.25, 0.5%
PO	Anxiolysis Radiologic imaging	Midazolam Chloral hydrate Pentobarbital	0.5–0.75 50–100 (max 2 g) 2–6 (max 100 mg)
PR	Conscious sedation Radiologic imaging	Midazolam Pentobarbital	0.25–0.5 <4 yr: 3–6 (max 100 mg) >4 yr: 1.5–3 (max 100 mg)
Intranasal	Conscious sedation	Midazolam Sufentanil	0.2–0.5 (max 5 mg) 0.7–1 µg/kg
Intramuscular	Conscious sedation Dissociative anesthesia	Midazolam Ketamine	0.05–0.15 2–4
Intravenous	Conscious sedation Dissociative anesthesia Radiologic imaging	Midazolam Fentanyl Ketamine Pentobarbital	0.05–0.1 1–5 µg/kg 0.5–1 2–6 (max 100 mg)
Inhalation agents	Conscious sedation	Nitrous oxide	50% N_2O/50% O_2 mixture
Combination agents	Conscious sedation Dissociative anesthesia	DPT (IM) (Demerol, Phenergan, Thorazine)	D:1–2.5 (max 50 mg) P/T: 0.25–1 (max 25 mg) Ratio: 2 : 1 : 1–4 : 1 : 1 (as D:P:T)
		Midazolam/fentanyl (IV)	Begin at low range for both
		Midazolam/ketamine (IM/IV)	Mid: .025–0.05, ket: as above
		Midazolam/sufentanil (IN)	Mid: 0.2, suf: 0.7 µg/kg

Pharmacology			
Onset (min)	Duration	Comments	Contraindications
45–60	1–2 hr	Available as cream or patch	Age < 6 mo
			Broken skin (ineffective)
15–30	45–60 min	Available in liquid or viscous form and in varying strengths	Age < 6 mo
			Intact skin (ineffective)
			Application to mucous membranes, nostrils, earlobes, digits, or glans penis (TAC and local anesthetics with epi)
1–2	60–90 min	5–7 mg/kg (max dose)	
3–5	4–6 hr	1.5–3 mg/kg (max dose)	
10–30	60–90 min	No analgesia, variable	~
15–60	1–2 hr	absorption	Hepatic/renal disease
15–60	1–4 hr		
10–30	60–90 min	No analgesia, variable	
15–60	1–4 hr	absorption	
15–60	1–4 hr		
10–15	45–60 min	No analgesia	
10–15	1–2 hr		
10–20	1–2 hr	No analgesia	URI/asthma, age < 3 mo, hypertension/cardiovascular disease, increased ICP, psychosis
2–10	60–90 min	Local anesthesia usually not needed for laceration repair	
		Use with atropine, 0.02 mg/kg	
2–3	30–60 min	No analgesia	
2–3	45–60 min		
1	5–15 min		
1	15–20 min	No analgesia	
3–5	3–5 min	*Preset mixture (50% N_2O/ 50% O_2) delivered via inhalational demand-valve mask.	Impaired mental status, opioids within 4 hr, pregnancy, pneumothorax, or bowel obstruction
		*Washout with 100% O_2 for 5 min postprocedure.	Full stomach (meal within 1 hr) is a relative contraindication
		*Age < 5 yr may be unable to cooperate	
15–60	1–3 hr	Wide variability in onset and duration	Age < 6 mo, neurologic disease
		Oversedation common	
		Use with atropine (0.02 mg/kg—min 0.1 mg, max 0.5 mg)	

Table 7-6 (continued)

Route	Indications	Drug	Dosing (mg/kg)
IM	Hypoventilation	Naloxone	0.1 (max 2 mg)
	Fentanyl-induced chest wall rigidity	Flumazenil	0.02 (max 0.2 mg)
IV	Hypoventilation	Naloxone	0.1 (max 2 mg)
	Fentanyl-induced chest wall rigidity	Flumazenil	0.02 (max 0.2 mg)

PO = oral administration; PR = rectal administration; URI = upper respiratory infection; OD = overdose.

Table 7-7. Comparison of time-cycled and volume-cycled ventilators*

	Time-cycled	Volume cycled
Examples	Baby Bird, Healthdyne, Seachrist, Biomed, BP 200	MAI, MAII, Emerson, Bear II, V, Hamilton
Modes	CPAP, IMV, control, cannot assist	CPAP, IMV, assist, control
Physiology	Tidal volume will change with compliance and resistance changes	In patients weighing > 10 kg, tidal volume is relatively stable despite changes in airway resistance and compliance. In smaller children the compressible volume of the tubing is relatively large in comparison with the set tidal volume, so that with changes in airway resistance or compliance, delivered tidal volume cannot be accurately predicted
Patients	Best used in patients weighing < 10–15 kg; in larger patients it is difficult to maintain a high enough flow rate to deliver an adequate tidal volume	For the reasons enumerated above, best used in patients weighing > 10 kg
How to start	Child is ventilated by hand with a manometer in line to predict the pressures necessary for adequate chest movement	Tidal volume is estimated to be 15–20 ml/kg, and a rate is selected between 10–20 cycles/min

*Whenever a patient is started on mechanical ventilation, it is imperative to evaluate the adequacy of oxygenation and ventilation with ABGs.

		Pharmacology	
Onset (min)	Duration (min)	Comments	Contraindications
5–10	60–90 min		
5–10	60–90 min		Chronic benzodiazepine use, tricyclic OD
1–2	20–40 min		
1–2	30–60 min		Chronic benzodiazepine use, tricyclic OD

    b. Long angiocatheters or other catheter.
    c. Cutdown tray.
    d. Lidocaine 0.5%, without epinephrine.
    e. Heparinized saline (1 unit/ml).
  4. How to place the line
    a. Technical line placement is similar in the adult and pediatric patient, but the degree of difficulty is usually inversely related to the size of the patient.
    b. Access sites include the following:
      (1) The *internal jugular vein* is a preferred site, but access can be difficult in infants.
      (2) The *external jugular vein* is an excellent access site, but it can be difficult to thread the catheter into the chest.
      (3) The *subclavian vein* is easier to cannulate in the older child than in the infant but is easy to secure once placed.
      (4) The *brachial vein* is another preferred site. In an older child, percutaneous cannulation can be done, whereas a cutdown is often required in an infant. Long catheters can usually, but not always, be threaded centrally.
      (5) The *femoral vein* offers an easy site for fast cannulation, particularly when other procedures such as intubation or CPR are in progress. *When properly dressed*, infection rate is similar to that of other sites.
      (6) The *umbilical vein* offers an easy access route in infants, but it can be difficult to thread the catheter through the liver and into the chest.
    c. All lines should be placed with sterile procedure.
    d. Before beginning the cannulation, *estimate the length of catheter* that will be required to reach the right atrium.
    e. The Seldinger technique is typically employed with the vein initially entered using a hollow needle, a J-wire introduced through the needle, and the catheter advanced over the guidewire.
    f. Once the vein is entered, the catheter should be advanced until the tip is, ideally, just above (or, for femoral lines, below) the right atrium. The position can be evaluated during the procedure by the transducer wave forms. A chest x-ray should be obtained to ascertain the specific location of the catheter.
    g. Once the line is placed, CVP is most accurately measured with an electrical transducer. A water column can be used, but the normal tachycardia of younger children tends to produce a falsely high CVP reading. Transducers are zeroed at the level of the right atrium and measurements taken at the end of exhalation.
  5. Complications of CVP placement include
    a. Infection. The line should be handled with sterile procedure at all times.
    b. Air embolism can occur. The system should be closed to air at all times.

    c. Arrhythmias can occur if the catheter advances into the right ventricle. If a right ventricular tracing is present on the monitor, the line should be pulled back into the correct position.

    d. Pneumothorax or hemothorax can result from line placement. The postplacement chest x-ray can rule out this complication.

E. Arterial lines

  1. Definition. An arterial line is a direct cannulation of a peripheral artery for the purpose of continuous pressure monitoring, frequent arterial blood sampling, or both.

  2. Indications for placement

    a. Blood pressure monitoring for any clinical situation characterized by blood pressure lability.

    b. Frequent ABG monitoring (e.g., respiratory failure, therapeutic hyperventilation).

    c. Vascular access for frequent **blood sampling.**

  3. Equipment. The general equipment requirements are

    a. Sterile preparations: Betadine, alcohol, gloves.

    b. Tape, arm board, tincture of benzoin.

    c. Short Medicuts or angiocatheters (20, 22, or 24 gauge).

    d. A 10-ml syringe with a flush solution of heparinized saline (1 unit heparin/ml).

    e. Pressure monitoring equipment with high-pressure tubing.

  4. How to place the arterial line:

    a. Any of the peripheral arteries can be used, but preferred sites include

      (1) Radial artery. The Allen test should be performed to demonstrate adequate ulnar flow.

      (2) Posterior tibial or dorsalis pedis. Both of these arteries can be used. A modified Allen test can be performed to evaluate the adequacy of the artery not being used.

      (3) Axillary artery. Collateral circulation around the shoulder may be unpredictable, particularly in infants. The catheter should be removed if ischemia of the arm appears.

      (4) Femoral artery. The lower extremity should be observed closely for signs of embolism or vascular insufficiency..

      (5) Use of the temporal artery is discouraged because of the potential for backflow to the internal carotid artery during flushing and reports of associated cerebrovascular accidents.

    b. The extremity should be securely taped to an arm or foot board for support and stabilization. Be certain that the distal toes or fingers are visible, so that blood flow can be constantly evaluated.

    c. Cannulation should be performed using sterile technique.

    d. Percutaneous cannulation or cutdown procedures are acceptable. The overlying skin is *anesthetized* with a wheal of 1% lidocaine and the skin broken with a 20-gauge needle. The angiocath is advanced at a shallow angle toward the palpated pulse. Entry of the vessel produces immediate flashback, on which the needle is advanced very slightly and the catheter threaded into the vessel. Alternatively, the artery can be transfixed, the needle removed, and the vessel cannulated by slow withdrawal of the catheter until blood return is seen and it can be advanced directly or over a spring wire.

    e. After the line is placed, it should be secured with tape and tincture of benzoin. The patient should be under constant visual supervision while the line is in place.

    f. Normal saline with 1 unit of heparin/ml is infused at a rate of 1 to 2 ml/hr. **This line should be clearly labeled and is not a medication line.**

  5. Complications of arterial lines

    a. The main complication is **vascular compromise distal to the site of insertion,** either from spasm or from thromboembolism. If there is any evidence of vascular compromise, the line should be removed.

b. Massive blood loss can occur if the line becomes disconnected. To prevent this, all lines should be taped securely, the patient kept in a monitored setting, and the site accessible for continuous visual observation at all times.

c. Infection is uncommon.

F. Intraosseous fluid administration

   1. **Definition.** An intraosseous line is a direct cannulation of the bone marrow to achieve emergency access when vascular access cannot be obtained after 1 to 5 minutes of percutaneous attempts.

   2. **Indications.** Vascular access for volume and pharmacologic support of a critically ill child. All IV fluids and medications (including intravenous anesthetic agents) can be given via this route.

   3. **Equipment.** Number 18- to 20-gauge spinal needle, bone marrow needle, or commercial intraosseous line kit; sterile preparations.

   4. **Placement.** The most common site is one to two fingerwidths below the tibial tubercle on the anteromedial aspect of the tibia (the tibial plateau). **The needle is directed inferiorly to avoid growth plate injury.** Bone is penetrated with continuous pressure and a screwing motion; marrow entry is signified by loss of resistance and confirmed by aspiration. Saline injection is met with mild resistance, and gravity flow is less than that in the usual IV line.

   5. **Stabilization.** Stabilization of the intraosseus line may be difficult, particularly during transport. Spinal needles can be stabilized with a surgical needle holder clamped at skin level and taped in place.

   6. **Complications** include

      a. Growth plate injury (uncommon if placed correctly).

      b. Infection if this route of access is maintained for greater than 24 to 48 hours.

      c. Clysis secondary to improper placement or displacement into the soft tissues.

X. Analgesia and conscious sedation

   A. Analgesia

   1. **General principles**

      a. If pain is present in multiple sites, only the *single* most severe source will be recognized by the patient.

      b. There is no evidence that infants (including the neonate) and children feel pain less deeply than adults; hence, local anesthesia should be provided for diagnostic and therapeutic procedures (including circumcision) whenever feasible.

      c. Postoperative pain, although generally of shorter duration in children than in adults, may still be severe enough to require medication for several days.

      d. **Opioids depress respiratory drive and their use therefore necessitates close observation and monitoring of vital signs.**

   2. **Specific therapeutics** (see Table 7–6)

      a. **Topical and local anesthetics** are administered before painful procedures.

         (1) Safe limits of infiltration

            (a) Lidocaine without epinephrine, 4 to 5 mg/kg (newborns 3 mg/kg); with epinephrine, 7 mg/kg (newborns 4 mg/kg).

            (b) Bupivacaine without epinephrine, 2 mg/kg (newborns 1.5 mg/kg); with epinephrine, 2.5 mg/kg (newborns 2 mg/kg).

            (c) Administration of topical agents onto mucosal surfaces can cause excessive systemic absorption.

         (2) Vasoconstrictive agents (epinephrine, cocaine) should not be used as a component of local/topical anesthesia near end-arterial blood supply (fingers, toes, pinnae, penis, nose).

      b. **Non-narcotic analgesics**

         (1) **Acetaminophen** is the drug of choice for mild pain and antipyresis in children.

    (2) Nonsteroidal anti-inflammatory agents have analgesic properties equal to those of acetaminophen and aspirin, but may be of superior benefit when inflammation is present.

    (3) Acetylsalicylic acid (aspirin) has analgesic and antipyretic effects equal to those of acetaminophen. **Because of the risk of Reye's syndrome, the use of aspirin is contraindicated in the management of influenza-like illnesses or varicella.**

  c. Narcotic analgesics

    (1) Common actions: analgesia, sedation, **respiratory depression.**

    (2) Common adverse effects: pruritus, nausea, constipation, ileus, urinary retention, dysphoria.

    (3) Tolerance to opiates may occur with repeated administration, though this is highly variable. A patient who chronically receives opiates may experience symptoms of withdrawal (agitation, tachycardia, nasal stuffiness, diarrhea, goose flesh) if medications are stopped abruptly. This can be prevented by gradual tapering of opioid doses over a period of days.

    (4) In contrast to dependence, tolerance, and withdrawal, narcotic **addiction** should be regarded as a largely psychological process characterized by drug-seeking, compulsive behavior. Addiction is extremely rare in children or adults who are given opiates for acute or cancer pain. There is no basis for giving opioids infrequently or in inadequate doses for acute pain because of a fear of addiction.

B. Conscious sedation, as opposed to **deep sedation** or **general anesthesia,** is a state of mild to moderately depressed wakefulness in which the ability to follow commands and maintain protective airway reflexes remains intact.

  1. Indications for conscious sedation include

    a. Laceration repair.

    b. Fracture or dislocation reduction.

    c. Incision and drainage of abscess or hematoma.

    d. Lumbar puncture in an uncooperative patient.

    e. Radiologic imaging (e.g., CT, MRI, barium or air enema).

  2. Historical considerations regarding the appropriateness of conscious sedation include mechanism of injury, concurrent medical conditions (particularly airway or respiratory problems and cardiac problems), current medications, medication allergies, prior anesthetic/anesthesia reactions (including family history of malignant hyperthermia), last meal, and medications taken during the previous 4 hours.

  3. Preparation

    a. Anticipate and prepare for adverse drug reactions. Have reversal agents **(see Table 7-6),** if available, at the bedside.

    b. Have equipment for airway management available at the bedside.

    c. Have appropriate monitoring and personnel available. All patients who are sedated should have vital signs monitored, including pulse, respirations, blood pressure, and oxygen saturation.

    d. Obtain consent.

    e. Only patients with an American Society of Anesthesiologists (ASA) Physical Status Classification of I or II (*Anesthesiology* 1978; 49:233–236) should be sedated without consultation with an anesthesiologist.

  4. Medications used for conscious sedation (see Table 7–6).

  5. Discharge criteria

    a. Airway patency is satisfactory and protective reflexes are intact.

    b. The patient is easily arousable.

    c. Cardiorespiratory function is stable and satisfactory, including normal or baseline oxygen saturation.

    d. The patient can sit up (if age appropriate).

    e. The patient can talk (if age appropriate).

    f. For the very young or impaired child, a level of consciousness as close to usual as possible should be achieved.

    g. Document level of consciousness at the time of discharge, and provide instructions for postprocedure care of follow-up.

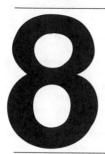

Poisoning

Carl Baum and Michael Shannon

Approximately 6,000,000 children ingest a potentially toxic substance annually. Children under 5 years of age account for 60 to 80% of recorded cases of poison ingestion; the majority of these poisonings result in low morbidity and mortality. Poisoning from plants, household products, cosmetics, and over-the-counter medications is most frequently encountered in children less than 5 years old. Although young children generally ingest single substances, adolescents and young adults frequently ingest multiple substances in a suicide gesture or an attempt to "get high."

I. Emergency management
A. Identification of the poison
1. Determine the product ingested, the amount taken, the time of ingestion, and the child's present condition. A regional poison center may be able to identify unknown pills.
2. In determining therapy, assume the **largest estimated amount** ingested.
3. **Physical examination** may reveal evidence for a particular ingestion. When the substance is unknown, consider common signs and symptoms (Table 8-1).
4. **Qualitative** analysis of blood or urine may confirm clinical suspicion. Gastric fluid analysis has no utility. **Quantitative** analysis of blood may be useful.

B. Supportive therapy.
While allowing normal renal and hepatic processes to detoxify the ingested toxin, observe general principles of supportive care.
1. **Respiratory support** (see also Chap. 7). Maintain a patent airway and provide oxygen, if necessary, to ensure adequate respiratory exchange. Endotracheal intubation may be required to prevent aspiration in patients with a depressed or absent gag reflex. Assisted ventilation is often necessary after exposure to CNS depressants.
2. **Cardiac support** (see also Chaps. 7 and 10). Provide intravenous crystalloid fluid to correct hypotension or shock. Vasopressors may be required with myocardial depressants (e.g., tricyclic antidepressants). Cardiac arrhythmias are managed according to advanced cardiac life support algorithms.
3. **Fluid homeostasis** (see Chap. 4). Replace previous and ongoing fluid losses while correcting electrolyte derangements.
4. **Hematologic** (see Chaps. 7 and 15). Correct hemolytic anemias with packed cell transfusions or exchange transfusions.
5. **Central nervous system** (see Chaps. 7 and 20). Toxicity may include CNS depression or seizures.
   a. An intravenous benzodiazepine (diazepam or lorazepam), phenytoin, and phenobarbital are the anticonvulsants of choice. Under select circumstances (e.g., isoniazid toxicity), a specific agent such as pyridoxine is indicated.
   b. **Provide** supportive measures for prolonged coma.
6. **Renal insufficiency** (see also Chap. 9) can result from use of ethylene glycol and nonsteroidal anti-inflammatory agents. Renal function should be monitored, with hemodialysis instituted as needed.

C. Gastrointestinal decontamination
1. **Gastric evacuation** is the first intervention to consider. However, efficacy falls dramatically when it is instituted more than 1 hour after ingestion. In such

Table 8-1. Common signs and symptoms of toxic exposures

System involved	Substances involved
Central nervous system	
Depression and coma	Sedative-hypnotics, narcotics, anticonvulsants, tranquilizers, tricyclic antidepressants, phenothiazines, hypoglycemic agents, alcohols, carbon monoxide, gases, solvents
Stimulation and/or convulsions	Amphetamines, sympathomimetic agents, cocaine, nicotine, salicylates, camphor, lead, strychnine, organophosphate, chlorinated insecticides, isoniazid methylxanthines
Hyperpyrexia	Salicylates, antihistamines, anticholinergics
Cardiovascular system	
Arrhythmias	Antihypertensives, digitalis, quinidine, antidepressants, cocaine
Tachycardia	Amphetamines and sympathomimetic agents, cocaine, tricyclic antidepressants, anticholinergics
Bradycardia	Beta blockers, cardiac glycosides, quinidine, calcium-channel blockers, clonidine
Hypotension	Narcotics, phenothiazines, antihypertensive agents, tricyclic antidepressants
Hypertension	Cocaine, sympathomimetics, anticholinergics
Gastrointestinal system	
Increased salivation	Organophosphate-carbonate insecticides, cholinomimetics
Decreased salivation	Antimuscarinic agents, antihistamines, organophosphates
Respiratory system	
Hypoventilation	CNS-depressant substances
Hyperventilation	Salicylates, cocaine, nicotine, methylxanthines
Abnormal odors on breath	
Alcohol	Alcohols, chloral hydrate
Acetone	Alcohol, acetone, lacquer
Wintergreen	Methyl salicylate
Garlic	Arsenic and organophosphate insecticides
Bitter almonds	Cyanide
Pears	Chloral hydrate
Ocular system	
Mydriasis	Antimuscarinic agents, sympathomimetric agents, psychotropic drugs, cocaine, amphetamines
Miosis	Narcotics, organophosphate insecticides, parasympathomimetic drugs, clonidine
Colored vision	Digitalis, quinine
Scotomas	Quinine, salicylates
Conjunctival injection	Marijuana, ethanol
Auditory system	
Tinnitus	Salicylates, streptomycin, ergot, quinines

Cutaneous system

Cyanosis	Nitrites, nitrobenzene, aniline dyes
Jaundice	Carbon tetrachloride, benzene, aniline dyes, chromates, phenothiazines, quinacrine
Discoloration of gums	Lead, bismuth, arsenic
Alopecia	Thallium, arsenic, colchicine, cobalt, radiation

cases, it should be deferred, especially if use will delay other decontamination measures.

  a. **Chemical methods**
    (1) **Ipecac syrup** is the method of choice for gastric emptying when ingestions are promptly recognized, because it induces emesis within 15 to 20 minutes in most patients after one dose. It removes approximately 30 to 40% of a substance when administered within 1 hour of ingestion. It is available without prescription and can be stored at home for emergency use. It is safe when taken in the recommended dosage.
      (a) For infants **9 to 12 months of age,** give 10 ml, then clear fluids.
      (b) For children **1 to 10 years of age,** give 15 ml (1 tbs), then clear fluids. Repeat once if vomiting does not occur within 20 minutes.
      (c) For children **10 years of age and older,** give 30 ml, then clear fluids. Repeat once if vomiting does not occur within 20 minutes.
    (2) Ipecac is **contraindicated** with caustics, hydrocarbons, or agents that cause rapid coma (relative contraindication) or in those who are comatose or having seizures.
  b. **Mechanical methods.** Orogastric lavage is as effective as ipecac and is the preferred means of gastric evacuation in children who arrive at the emergency department. It is faster and allows prompt administration of adsorbent and cathartic. **For the patient with depressed airway reflexes, intubation should be performed before passage of a lavage tube.**
    (1) **Equipment.** Number 18 to 40 French single-lumen lavage tube, 5-oz catheter-tip syringe.
    (2) For lavage, place the patient on the left side. A restraining papoose expedites the process.
    (3) Measure the distance to the stomach.
    (4) Use gel to facilitate insertion of tube; auscultate over the stomach for injected air to ensure proper placement.
    (5) Aspirate the gastric contents before lavage.
    (6) Lavage with normal saline, 10- to 20-ml/kg aliquots.
    (7) Perform saline lavage until the return is clear.
    (8) Leave activated charcoal or, if indicated, a specific antidote (e.g., *N*-acetylcysteine [Mucomyst]) in the stomach on completion.
    (9) Clamp the tube on removal to prevent aspiration.
2. **Adsorbents**
  a. **Activated charcoal,** an odorless, tasteless black powder, is the most effective means of gastrointestinal decontamination and can be administered without gastric evacuation.
    (1) **It should not be given before ipecac syrup. It is not effective against metals, alcohols, hydrocarbons, or caustics.**
    (2) The dose is 1 g/kg PO in 8 oz water or with cathartic (see sec. **3** below).
3. **Cathartics** hasten intestinal transit of gastrointestinal contents and theoretically decrease systemic absorption. Two common cathartics are sorbitol (2 ml/kg) and magnesium citrate (4–8 ml/kg, maximum 300 ml). Activated charcoal–cathartic mixtures provide a fixed dose of cathartic. **Sorbitol should be**

used with caution in children less than 2 years old since it can induce excessive fluid losses and dehydration. Whole bowel irrigation (WBI) employs 5 to 20 liters of an electrolyte-balanced solution (e.g., GoLYTELY) to clear the rectal effluent.

4. **Dilution** is a relatively ineffective method of gastrointestinal decontamination, but may ameliorate GI distress from gastric irritants.
5. **Neutralization** of ingested corrosives **is not advised. The resultant exothermic reaction can cause secondary tissue damage.**

D. **Elimination enhancement.** Use the following methods only in serious poisoning because they involve risk.

1. **Fluid diuresis** increases glomerular filtration and enhances elimination of drugs excreted primarily by the kidneys (e.g., lithium). Intravenous isotonic fluids at twice maintenance rate should sustain diuresis at two to three times normal.
2. **Ionized diuresis** maintains a drug in its ionized state. **Alkalinization** of the urine enhances excretion of acidic compounds, such as salicylates and phenobarbital. Alkalinize with 1 to 2 mg/kg sodium bicarbonate to attain a urine pH of greater than 7.
3. **Extracorporeal drug removal.** Exchange transfusions, peritoneal dialysis, hemodialysis, and hemoperfusion are reserved for the most severe cases.
   a. **Hemodialysis and hemoperfusion** are the most effective techniques of toxin removal. *Only substances with a small volume of distribution (<1 liter/kg), low protein binding, and a small molecular weight will benefit from hemodialysis; for hemoperfusion, protein binding and molecular weight are less important determinants of efficacy.* Hemodialysis permits correction of concomitant electrolyte or acid-base disturbances.
   b. **Peritoneal dialysis** is less effective and should be used only when hemodialysis or hemoperfusion cannot be performed (see Chap. 9, p. 313).
   c. **Exchange transfusion** is generally reserved for severe methemoglobinemia or hemolysis.

E. **Antidotes**

1. **N-Acetylcysteine,** for *acetaminophen intoxication:* 140 mg/kg PO as a loading dose and then 70 mg/kg q4h for 17 doses.
2. **Amyl and sodium nitrite followed by sodium thiosulfate,** for *cyanide:* sodium nitrite, 0.33 ml/kg of a 3% solution IV at 2.5 to 5.0 ml/min, followed in 15 minutes by sodium thiosulfate, 1.65 ml/kg of a 25% solution IV at 2.5 to 5.0 ml/min.
3. **Atropine sulfate** or **pralidoxime chloride** (Protopam), or both, for *organophosphate insecticides* (cholinesterase inhibitors)
   a. **Atropine:** 1 to 4 mg or 0.05 mg/kg IV, with repeat doses of 2 mg at intervals of 2 to 5 minutes to reverse muscarinic effects, and then as necessary to maintain atropinization.
   b. **Pralidoxime:** 20 to 50 mg/kg slowly IV, followed by continuous infusion of 10 to 20 mg/kg/hr to reactivate phosphorylated acetylcholinesterase.
4. **Deferoxamine,** for *iron:* 50 mg/kg IM (maximum 1 g) q4h, or 15 mg/kg/hr IV initially for severe intoxication. Do not exceed 6 g in 24 hours.
5. **Dimercaprol (British antilewisite [BAL]),** for *lead, arsenic, chromium, cobalt, and copper:* 2 to 4 mg/kg/dose IM at intervals of 4 to 8 hours for 5 days and then 3 mg/kg/dose q12h (see p. 284).
6. **Dimercaptosuccinic acid (DMSA;** Succimer) (see also p. 285) for *lead:* 30 mg/kg/day in three divided doses for 5 days followed immediately by 20 mg/kg/day in two divided doses for 14 days.
7. **Diphenhydramine (Benadryl),** for *dystonic reactions:* 1 to 2 mg/kg IV q6h for four doses (maximum single dose 50 mg IV).
8. **Ethanol,** for *methanol and ethylene glycol:* loading dose 600 mg/kg IV (10% solution) or PO (50% solution), then continuous infusion of 100 to 120 mg/kg/hr to maintain the blood ethanol level at 100 mg/dl. Higher doses are needed if the patient undergoes hemodialysis.
9. **Ethylenediaminetetraacetate (CaNa$_2$EDTA),** for *lead, mercury, copper,*

nickel, zinc, cobalt, beryllium, and manganese: 25 to 50 mg/kg/day IM in two to four divided doses or IV continuous infusion for 5 days. Add 0.5% procaine for IM use. **Only the calcium, disodium form, should be used to avoid severe hypocalcemia.**

10. **Flumazenil,** for *benzodiazepine* overdose: 0.02 mg/kg (maximum 0.2 mg) IV; repeat to 3 mg maximum. Flumazenil is **contraindicated in those who concomitantly ingest tricyclic antidepressants** or have received benzodiazepines for anticonvulsant therapy.

11. **Methylene blue,** for *methemoglobinemia:* 1 to 2 mg/kg IV as a 1% solution; repeat in 4 hours if needed. Infants should receive no more than 4 mg/kg/day.

12. **Naloxone hydrochloride (Narcan),** for *narcotics and propoxyphene:* 0.1 mg/kg/dose IV (2 mg in adolescents); 0.3 mg/kg IV if no response in 2 minutes. If there is a response, continue this therapy until a narcotic effect is no longer present.

13. **Oxygen,** for *carbon monoxide:* 100% O_2 for 30 minutes to 4 hours.

14. **Penicillamine,** for *lead, copper, arsenic, and mercury:* 15 to 30 mg/kg/day PO in divided doses. The maximum daily dose is 1 g (see sec. **III.D.1.c**).

15. **Vitamin K$_1$,** for *warfarin and bishydroxycoumarin:* 2 to 5 mg IM or IV. Its brief elimination half-life requires repeated administration.

F. Prevention. No course of therapy, no matter how trivial the ingestion, is complete without a discussion to ensure that the incident will not recur.

II. Specific ingestions. Table 8-2 lists certain common substances of low toxicity that require minimal intervention. The following are examples that require more complex management.

A. Acetaminophen. *Metabolites* of acetaminophen, rather than the parent compound, are hepatotoxic. In overdose, reactive intermediates bind to liver macromolecules, causing liver necrosis.

1. **Etiology.** Acetaminophen is frequently ingested by children and adolescents.

2. **Evaluation and diagnosis**

   a. **History. Timing** (when? acute or chronic?) is of critical importance. Initial nonspecific symptoms are not predictive of outcome. Although the history is often unreliable, a single ingested dose of approximately 150 mg/kg, **or** a dose greater than **7.5** g in an adolescent, may result in hepatic damage.

   b. **Physical examination.** Manifestations within the first 24 hours following acute ingestion include nausea, vomiting, and diaphoresis. Evidence of hepatotoxicity appears approximately 24 to 36 hours after ingestion.

   c. **Laboratory**

      (1) *A plasma acetaminophen level drawn 4 or more hours following ingestion is the best predictor of hepatotoxicity.* A plasma concentration greater than 150 μg/ml at 4 hours after ingestion is associated with possible **severe** hepatotoxicity (i.e., transaminases exceeding 1,000 IU/liter). Use the Rumack-Mathew nomogram (Fig. 8-1) to interpret other levels and times.

      (2) An increase in serum transaminases and prolongation of the prothrombin time may be seen after 24 hours, although these alterations can occur sooner. Serum transaminase activity peaks by 3 to 4 days after ingestion and returns to normal within a week in those who recover.

      (3) Hyperbilirubinemia and hyperammonemia can also result.

3. **Diagnosis.** Also consider Reye's syndrome, amino acid disorders, and alpha-1-antitrypsin deficiency in the child, and drug abuse (alcohol, heroin, volatile hydrocarbons) and Wilson's disease in the adolescent.

4. **Treatment**

   a. Remove the ingested dose with gastric lavage when the patient presents within 1 hour of ingestion.

   b. Activated charcoal should be administered if the patient presents within 4 hours after ingestion. After this interval, activated charcoal is warranted only if co-ingestants are suspected. Charcoal can be administered with *N*-acetylcysteine (Mucomyst) despite 10 to 39% adsorption of Mucomyst, be-

Table 8-2. Common ingestions of low toxicity

No treatment required	Removal necessary if large amounts ingested
Ballpoint inks	Aftershave lotion
Bar soap	Body conditioners
Bathtub floating toys	Colognes
Battery (dry cell)	Deodorants
Bubble bath soap	Fabric softeners
Candles	Hair dyes
Chalk	Hair sprays
Clay (modeling)	Hair tonic
Crayons with A.P., C.P., or C.S.	Indelible markers
130—46 designation	Matches (> 20 wooden matches or 2 books
Dehumidifying packets	of paper matches)
Detergents (anionic)	No Doz
Eye makeup	Oral contraceptives
Fishbowl additives	Perfumes
Golf balls	Suntan preparations
Hand lotion and cream	Toilet water
Ink (blue, black, red)	Toothpaste
Lipstick	
Newspaper	
Pencils (lead and coloring)	
Putty and Silly Putty	
Sachets	
Shampoo	
Shaving cream and shaving lotions	
Shoe polish (occasionally, aniline	
dyes are present)	
Striking surface materials of	
matchboxes	
Sweetening agents (saccharin,	
cyclamate)	
Teething rings	
Thermometers	

cause Mucomyst doses are far in excess of those needed for hepatoprotection.

   c. Avoid enzyme inducers such as phenobarbital.

   d. Avoid forcing fluids or ionized diuresis.

   e. Toxic metabolites of acetaminophen can deplete endogenous glutathione. *N*-Acetylcysteine provides a substitute for glutathione and is most effective when given within 8 to 10 hours. **It should not be withheld, however, even if the patient presents more than 24 hours following ingestion.** Once the need for *N*-acetylcysteine is determined, *all* doses must be given. *N*-Acetylcysteine should be diluted to a 5% solution before it is administered and repeated if vomiting occurs within 1 hour of administration. Placing the solution on ice with a lidded cup will inhibit the release of nauseating sulfurous fumes. An intravenous form is under investigation.

B. Alcohols. These CNS depressants also inhibit gluconeogenesis. Methanol and ethylene glycol are converted via alcohol dehydrogenase to toxic organic acid metabolites. Isopropyl alcohol is a gastrointestinal irritant; its metabolite, acetone, is not a toxic organic acid, and does not require the same aggressive management.

   1. Etiology. Most cases of acute intoxication are the result of ethanol ingestion.

   2. Evaluation and diagnosis

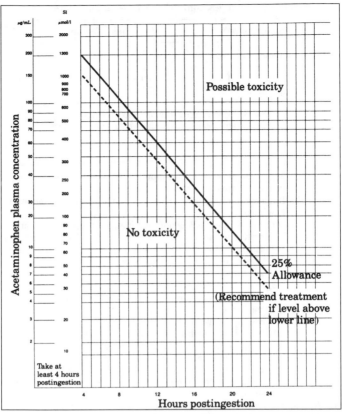

Fig. 8-1. Semilogarithmic plot of plasma acetaminophen concentration versus time based on data from adult patients. Patients with concentrations above the line at the corresponding times after ingestion may develop hepatotoxicity. Patients with concentrations below the line have a low probability of developing hepatotoxicity. (From BH Rumack, H Mathew. *Pediatrics* 55:871, 1975. Copyright © 1975 by the American Academy of Pediatrics.)

a. **History.** Consider other volatile alcohols (methanol, isopropyl alcohol) and glycols.

b. **Physical examination.** CNS depression is prominent, but, other CNS depressants may contribute to the clinical appearance (see p. 281). Isopropyl alcohol is a greater CNS depressant than ethanol.

c. **Laboratory**
   (1) Hypoglycemia can result from inhibition of gluconeogenesis. Younger children and infants are particularly susceptible.
   (2) Blood concentrations of specific alcohols or glycols may not be available rapidly. However, determination of the osmolal gap, the difference between measured and calculated osmolal concentration, allows an estimate of volatile concentration (see Table 8-3).
   (3) Confirm that the laboratory employs *freezing-point depression for the determination of osmolal concentration.* The boiling-point elevation technique vaporizes volatiles and leads to false-negative results.

Table 8-3. Volatiles: conversion of osmolal gap to level[a]

Alcohol or glycol	Conversion factor[b]
Methanol	2.8
Ethanol	4.3
Ethylene glycol	5.0
Isopropyl alcohol	5.9

[a]Level = conversion factor × osmolal gap (mOsm/L).
[b]Factors take into account molecular weight and specific gravity.

3. Treatment
 a. Management is generally supportive. Provide ventilatory support and intravenous dextrose as needed.
 b. If methanol or ethylene glycol is present, prevent metabolism to toxic metabolites.
  (1) Enzymatic block is possible if ethanol is present in sufficient concentration to saturate the enzyme alcohol dehydrogenase.
  (2) Ethanol block is recommended if the patient has a history of methanol or ethylene glycol ingestion *and* the osmolal gap technique (or a confirmatory level) suggests a concentration of greater than 20 mg/dl.
  (3) A bolus of 10% ethanol, followed by an appropriate infusion, should establish and maintain an ethanol concentration of 100 mg/dl (1,000 mg/liter), sufficient to saturate the enzyme (see p. 270).
 c. Consider hemodialysis for
  (1) Severe intoxication unresponsive to adequate supportive care or with serum ethanol or isopropyl alcohol concentrations above 500 mg/dl (5,000 mg/liter).
  (2) Suspected methanol or ethylene glycol ingestion, and the osmolal gap technique (or a confirmatory level) suggests a concentration of greater than 50 mg/dl.
C. Antidepressants exert their therapeutic effects via anticholinergic mechanisms, inhibition of neurotransmitter reuptake, or stabilization of membranes.
 1. Tricyclic antidepressants (TCA). The mechanisms listed above play a role in overdose. Additional mechanisms contribute to toxicity and complicate management. Inhibition of fast sodium channels causes membrane-depressant effects and cardiac toxicity.
  a. Etiology. TCAs are frequently implicated in serious overdoses.
  b. Evaluation and diagnosis
   (1) Physical examination. Decompensation may occur abruptly. Sedation, seizures, hypotension, tachycardia, and other dysrhythmias are common.
   (2) Laboratory
    (a) An ECG may reveal QRS prolongation greater than 0.1 seconds (100 msec), generally regarded as a predictor of toxicity, although other electrocardiographic abnormalities can occur.
    (b) Confirmatory levels of TCA parent compound and metabolites are not helpful in emergent situations.
  c. Treatment
   (1) Respiratory failure may occur, requiring airway protection and ventilatory support.
   (2) Do not administer ipecac. Rapid clinical progression may follow ingestion.
   (3) Despite the anticholinergic properties of TCAs, **physostigmine is not recommended.**
   (4) Lavage may be helpful in the first hour following ingestion. Its benefit

should be weighed against the possibility of decompensation and the associated risks of aspiration.

(5) Administer charcoal and cathartic.

(6) If QRS prolongation or refractory hypotension occurs, serum alkalinization (arterial pH from 7.45–7.55) should be maintained.

(7) Serum alkalinization, accomplished with boluses of sodium bicarbonate (1 to 2 mEq/kg IV), may increase extracellular Na concentrations, theoretically reversing membrane depression, while alkaline pH may directly stabilize cellular ion channels. Alkalinization through hyperventilation will not provide this theoretical dual mechanism.

(8) Excessive use of fluids can exacerbate respiratory complications such as acute respiratory distress syndrome (ARDS).

2. Lithium (Li). Although absorption following ingestion is complete by 6 to 8 hours, equilibration between blood and tissues is delayed. Toxicity tends to be more significant with chronic dosing.

   a. Etiology. Lithium is prescribed for bipolar disorders. Sustained-release formulations are available.

   b. Evaluation and diagnosis

   (1) Physical examination. Following acute ingestion, early signs may include nausea and emesis; as tissue levels rise, lethargy, tremor, and ataxia may appear.

   (2) Laboratory. Obtain Li levels, electrolytes, and renal function tests. Symptoms and signs lag behind peak Li blood levels. T-wave inversion may be seen on ECG.

   c. Treatment

   (1) Activated charcoal does not adsorb Li.

   (2) Lithium is excreted via the kidneys. Hydrate with isotonic fluid if clinically indicated. Hypotonic fluids should be instituted once the patient is euvolemic and has adequate urinary output to avoid hypernatremia.

   (3) Hemodialysis may be necessary. Indications include seizures and severe lethargy. Consultation with a toxicologist and nephrologist should be considered early if these symptoms occur, or if serial Li levels rise despite judicious hydration.

3. Monoamine oxidase inhibitors (MAOI). Irreversible inhibition of monoamine oxidase allows excess catecholamine release from neurons.

   a. Etiology. Significant interactions can occur with the selective serotonin reuptake inhibitors, meperidine (Demerol), and dextromethorphan, and with tryptophan-containing foods.

   b. Evaluation and diagnosis

   (1) History. The minimal toxic dose is 2 to 4 mg/kg. Symptoms may be delayed up to 24 hours (see p. 282).

   (2) Physical examination. Catecholamine release leads to sympathomimetic signs.

   (3) Laboratory. Levels are not available.

   c. Treatment

   (1) Emesis should not be induced, as it can worsen hypertension.

   (2) Hospitalization is required. Monitor and treat symptoms of sympathetic discharge. Alpha- and beta-blocking agents may be helpful.

D. Antipsychotics. Blockade of cholinergic, dopaminergic, and/or alpha-adrenergic receptors provides therapeutic effects, although side effects may be seen at therapeutic doses.

1. Etiology. Important classes of antipsychotics are

   a. Phenothiazine.

   b. Butyrophenone (haloperidol).

   c. Dibenzodiazepine (clozapine).

   d. Benzisoxazole (risperidone).

2. Evaluation and diagnosis

a. **Physical examination**

(1) Tachycardia and CNS depression result from anticholinergic effects, although other mechanisms may contribute to central sedation. Hypotension and miosis result from alpha-adrenergic blockade. Disturbances of temperature regulation may occur.

(2) Rigidity and hyperthermia characterize neuroleptic malignant syndrome (NMS), occasionally seen in patients maintained on antipsychotics.

(3) Extrapyramidal reactions may occur through blockade of dopaminergic receptors.

(4) Seizures may occur by unknown mechanisms.

b. **Laboratory**

(1) A CBC may reveal agranulocytosis associated with the dibenzodiazepine clozapine.

(2) Membrane-depressant effects may follow large overdoses, with prolongation of the QRS and especially the QT interval.

(3) Abdominal x-rays may reveal radiopaque tablets.

(4) Specific drug levels are not helpful in management of acute ingestions; butyrophenones (haloperidol) are not detected in routine toxicologic screens.

3. **Treatment**

a. Give charcoal and cathartic.

b. Treat membrane-depressant effects with sodium bicarbonate (1–2 mEq/kg IV).

c. Treat dystonic reactions with diphenhydramine (1 mg/kg).

d. Supportive management otherwise suffices.

E. **Cardiac drugs** (see Chap. 10, pp. 329 *ff.*). Table 8-4 summarizes toxicologic management of selected cardiac drugs.

F. **Caustics.** Severity of the caustic burn is related to pH, concentration, and duration of contact. A burn ensues during the first week, granulation tissue during the second week, and fibrosis during the third week.

1. **Etiology.** Typical **acids** ingested are toilet-bowl cleaners, metal-cleaning fluids, and industrial bleaching products. Typical **alkalis** ingested are powerful detergents, toilet-bowl cleaners, and dishwasher and laundry granules.

2. **Evaluation and diagnosis**

a. **History.** Pain in the mouth and retrosternal area may be experienced. Other symptoms include drooling, nausea, vomiting and abdominal pain.

b. **Physical examination.** Oropharyngeal burns may develop. **The absence of oral burns is not evidence against esophageal involvement.**

c. **Laboratory.** Esophagoscopy is best performed 12 to 24 hours after ingestion to determine the presence and extent of esophageal injury. Barium swallow may reveal esophageal mucosal injury.

d. **Diagnosis.** Esophageal perforation with mediastinitis and gastric perforation with peritonitis may occur. **Aspiration** can lead to pulmonary necrosis or glottic edema. Bacterial superinfection may occur during the first and second weeks, with esophageal stricture in later weeks.

3. **Treatment**

a. **Emesis and lavage are contraindicated.**

b. **Neutralization with acids or alkalis is contraindicated.**

c. Perforations, volume losses, and infection should be treated accordingly.

d. Prophylactic antibiotics are not indicated.

e. Steroids have a possible role in preventing stricture formation.

G. **Hydrocarbons. Aromatic** hydrocarbons affect mainly the CNS and pulmonary systems. The liver, kidney, myocardium, and bone marrow may also be involved. Organ toxicity results from *absorption.* **Aliphatic** hydrocarbons produce mainly pulmonary damage by *aspiration* (Table 8-5).

1. **Etiology**

a. **Aromatic** hydrocarbons include benzene, toluene, xylene, and styrene.

Table 8-4. Summary of cardiac drug toxicology

Drug or class	Mechanism	Signs of overdose	Treatment
Beta-adrenergic antagonists	Receptor blockade; membrane depression	Hypotension, bradycardia, conduction abnormalities, hypoglycemia, hyperkalemia	Charcoal, atropine, isoproterenol, glucagon, pacing; avoid vagal maneuvers
Calcium-channel antagonists	Receptor blockade; decreased vascular tone, cardiac conduction, excitation-contraction coupling	Hypotension, diminished contractility, bradycardia	Charcoal, ?calcium; glucagon can improve inotropy/chronotropy if hypotension persists; avoid vagal maneuvers
Clonidine	Alpha-2 adrenergic agonist; acts on central inhibitory receptors to decrease sympathetic outflow	Transient hypertension from initial stimulation of peripheral alpha receptors; later, hypotension, bradycardia, respiratory depression	Charcoal, supportive measures; ?naloxone; consider admission for 24 hr because of delayed symptoms
Cardiac glycosides (Digoxin)	Inhibition of ATP-ase-dependent Na-K pump	Tachyarrhythmias (usually ventricular); bradycardia, AV block, hyperkalemia	Treat hyperkalemia; charcoal; digoxin-specific antibodies for refractory hyperkalemia or life-threatening arrhythmias (digoxin levels following antibody administration cannot be reliably interpreted)

ATPase = adenosine triphosphatase; AV = atrioventricular.

   b. Aliphatic hydrocarbons include gasoline, naphtha, kerosene, and lighter fluid.
2. Evaluation and diagnosis
   a. History. Ingestion of hydrocarbons may induce **mucous membrane irritation,** nausea, vomiting, diarrhea, and perianal excoriation.
   b. Physical examination
      (1) Pulmonary involvement may be subclinical or evidenced by coughing, dyspnea, cyanosis, and rales. **Fever** and **leukocytosis** with or without pulmonary involvement are frequently present in the first 48 hours.
      (2) CNS manifestations include restlessness, confusion, drowsiness, and coma.
   c. Laboratory. Radiologic findings do not correlate with clinical status.

Table 8-5. Petroleum products: estimation of aspiration hazard versus systemic toxicity

Product	Source(s)	Systemic toxicity	Aspiration hazard*
Toluene, xylene, benzene, or ether	Industrial or rubber solvents	+++	+
Gasoline	Fuel	+	+++
Naphtha	Solvent, lighter fluid, dry cleaner, thinner	+	+++
Kerosene	Fuel, charcoal lighter fluid, thinner, pesticide solvent	+	+++
Mineral seal oil	Furniture polish	+	+++
Diesel oil	Fuel	+	++
Mineral oil		−	+
Lubricating oil	Motor oil, cutting oil, transmission fluid	−	−

+ = low risk; ++ = moderate risk; +++ = high risk; − = no risk.
*Formulations with increased viscosity have decreased aspiration hazard.

Pneumatocele, pneumothorax, pleural effusion, and pneumonia may complicate the pulmonary picture.

3. **Treatment**
   a. Removal of **aromatic** hydrocarbons is indicated if an amount greater than 1 ml/kg has been ingested.
   b. For **aliphatic** hydrocarbons, aspiration is more dangerous than GI absorption. Removal is indicated only if large amounts (>5 ml/kg) have been ingested, or if a more toxic substance is ingested along with the hydrocarbon (metals, pesticides).
   c. In the **alert** patient, lavage may be a safe method of removal. In the **obtunded** patient, protect the lungs with a cuffed endotracheal tube before lavage.
   d. Activated charcoal is not indicated.
   e. Oxygen, humidity, and bronchodilators may be necessary. Antibiotics should be reserved for superinfection.
   f. Present evidence does not support the use of corticosteroids.
   g. Infiltrates may require weeks to resolve.
   h. Management of CNS, liver, and renal involvement is supportive.
   i. Avoid **sympathomimetic drugs in light of myocardial irritability.**

H. **Iron**
   1. **Etiology.** Iron tablets and vitamins with iron are ubiquitous, and ingestion is common.
   2. **Evaluation and diagnosis**
      a. **History.** Symptoms generally occur 30 minutes to 2 hours after ingestion. Early symptoms include vomiting, bloody diarrhea, abdominal cramps, and drowsiness.
      b. **Physical examination.** After the initial phase (6–24 hr after ingestion), fever, metabolic acidosis, hepatic impairment, restlessness, convulsions, shock, and coma may appear.
      c. **Laboratory**
         (1) Initial studies should include a CBC, serum electrolytes, and a serum iron.
         (2) A radiograph of the GI tract may detect the presence of radiopaque iron tablets.
   3. **Treatment**
      a. Early **emesis** with ipecac syrup is indicated if 20 mg/kg or more of elemental iron has been taken.

(1) **Obtain** an abdominal radiograph to ensure removal of all iron tablets.

(2) Activated charcoal is not indicated.

(3) **Perform** whole-bowel irrigation if a radiograph reveals a significant number of iron tablets.

  b. **Use** IV fluids, sodium, bicarbonate, and volume expanders to correct acidosis and fluid loss.

  c. **Deferoxamine**

    (1) **Chelation ("challenge") test**

      (a) **Indications** include

        (i) History of a large amount ingested, with symptoms other than minimal vomiting and diarrhea, *or*

        (ii) Serum iron level exceeding the total iron-binding capacity (TIBC).

      (b) **Administration.** Deferoxamine, 50 mg/kg (maximum 1 g), is given IM. The urine will turn burgundy red (vin rose) when the serum iron level exceeds the TIBC or serum iron is greater than 500 mg/dl.

    (2) **Deferoxamine therapy**

      (a) **Indications** include

        (i) Coma or shock.

        (ii) Serum iron level exceeding the TIBC.

        (iii) Positive deferoxamine challenge test.

      (b) **Administration**

        (i) The parenteral route, whether IM or IV, will depend on the clinical state of the patient and the serum concentration. The IM dose is 50 mg/kg (maximum 1 g) q4h.

        (ii) In case of coma, hypotension, or acidosis, the IV route should be used. Give by infusion at a rate of 15 mg/kg/hr. Higher doses may be necessary.

        (iii) Cessation of therapy is dictated by improvement in the patient's clinical condition, a serum iron concentration within normal range, and the disappearance of the color in the urine.

    (3) **Dialysis.** Iron is not dialyzable except when bound to deferoxamine. Dialysis is indicated for oliguria or anuria.

I. **Salicylates and other nonsteroidal anti-inflammatory drugs (NSAIDs).** Salicylates are the most toxic of the NSAIDs.

  1. **Etiology.** NSAIDs are in widespread use. Toxicity can result from accidental ingestion of excess salicylate, chronic use at therapeutic doses, or ingestion of small amounts of oil of wintergreen (methyl salicylate). Victims of chronic poisoning are at higher risk for seizures and metabolic acidosis than those with acute single overdoses.

  2. **Evaluation and diagnosis**

    a. **History.** The first symptoms seen after salicylate ingestion are deep, rapid respiration; thirst; vomiting; and profuse sweating. Ingestion of greater than 150 mg/kg can produce symptoms. The toxicity of NSAIDs other than salicylates is low.

    b. **Physical examination.** In the salicylate-poisoned patient, hyperventilation, renal solute loss, an increased metabolic rate, and vomiting contribute to dehydration and worsening acidosis. In severe intoxication, confusion, delirium, coma, convulsions, circulatory collapse, and oliguria may ensue.

    c. **Laboratory**

      (1) Salicylates stimulate ventilation centrally and produce an initial respiratory alkalosis. A state of metabolic acidosis, especially in young children, is quickly superimposed.

      (2) Salicylates prolong prothrombin times, cause platelet dysfunction, and induce either hyperglycemia or hypoglycemia. Peak serum levels occur 2 to 6 hours after ingestion.

      (3) Initial laboratory studies include a CBC, electrolytes, blood gases, blood glucose, prothrombin time, and serum salicylate level.

(4) A salicylate level of 50 mg/dl causes mild symptoms, 50 to 80 mg/dl produces symptoms of moderate severity, and 80 to 100 mg/dl causes severe symptoms.

3. Treatment

a. Gastrointestinal decontamination is indicated when a toxic dose (>150 mg/kg) has been ingested.

b. **Provide** IV fluids to replace losses (see Chap. 4, pp. 70 ff.) and adequate glucose to correct hypoglycemia

c. Lower temperature elevation with tepid sponging.

d. Vitamin K can treat bleeding due to hypoprothrombinemia (although other factors are involved in coagulopathy).

e. Alkalinization of the urine and monitoring of the urinary pH (maintain above 7.5) will enhance excretion of salicylates, and shorten serum half-lives from 24 to 36 hours to 6 to 8 hours. Generous amounts of potassium (3–5 mEq/kg/day) are necessary to replace potassium loss and *alkalinize the urine*. Systemic pH should be monitored and maintained below 7.55.

f. Potentially fatal serum levels (100–150 mg/dl), oliguria or anuria, cardiac disease, coma, seizures, and a poor response to $NaHCO_3$ are all indications for hemodialysis.

g. Repeated doses of charcoal can enhance elimination via "gastrointestinal dialysis" and are recommended for serum levels greater than 50 mg/dl. A level of 50 mg/dl or any symptoms (except mild hyperventilation) generally indicate that hospitalization is necessary.

J. Theophylline

1. Etiology. Theophylline is a widely used xanthine bronchodilator.

2. Evaluation and diagnosis

a. **History.** Symptoms are widely disparate depending on whether the intoxication is the result of acute or chronic ingestion. In general, chronic ingestion is associated with a greater risk of seizures and arrhythmias. **Prolonged absorption** (as long as 17–36 hr) may occur, especially with slow-release preparations.

b. **Physical examination**

(1) Gastrointestinal signs are the most frequent and include vomiting and hematemesis.

(2) CNS toxicity includes agitation, restlessness, irritability, or mild obtundation. **Seizures** may occur in severe poisonings.

c. **Laboratory**

(1) Mild supraventricular tachycardia occurs often, but life-threatening arrhythmias are less frequent than in adults.

(2) Hypokalemia is common, particularly in acute overdoses.

(3) Therapeutic serum concentrations range between 10 and 20 μg/ml. Life-threatening arrhythmias and seizures usually occur with serum concentrations greater than 80 to 100 μg/ml after acute overdose.

3. Treatment

a. Administer activated charcoal, 1 g/kg, immediately.

b. Repeated doses of activated charcoal and ionic cathartics are indicated (see p. 267).

c. Vomiting should be treated aggressively in order to permit administration of activated charcoal. Effective antiemetics include metoclopramide, 0.5 to 1.0 mg/kg, or ondansetron, 0.15 to 0.3 mg/kg. The H_2 antagonist ranitidine can reduce gastric upset. Avoid phenothiazines.

d. Theophylline serum concentrations should be followed q4h to evaluate the effectiveness of treatment.

e. Do not induce fluid diuresis.

f. **Use** diazepam or phenobarbital, or both, to treat seizures (see Chap. 7, pp. 233 ff.). Avoid phenytoin.

g. Monitor for cardiac arrhythmias.

h. **Consider hemodialysis or hemoperfusion** in patients who are unresponsive to adequate supportive care or those who have serum concentrations above 80 to 100 μg/ml, or both groups.

K. Substances of abuse
1. CNS depressants
  a. Etiology. These include narcotics, hypnotic-sedative agents (barbiturates and nonbarbiturates), ethanol, and benzodiazepines (e.g., diazepam, clonazepam).
  b. Evaluation and diagnosis
    (1) History. All can produce physical and psychological dependence. Withdrawal symptoms can be expected with their abrupt cessation.
    (2) Physical examination
      (a) Following an acute overdose, all induce CNS (see Table 3) and cardiorespiratory depression.
      (b) Pupils are usually constricted.
      (c) Reflexes are diminished. Seizures are more frequent with propoxyphene, meperidine, and tramadol.
      (d) Seizures, delirium, cardiovascular collapse, and possibly death, are seen **only** in the case of alcohol and barbiturate withdrawal.
  c. Treatment
    (1) If the patient is comatose, administer naloxone, 0.1 mg/kg IV. If there is no response within 2 minutes, administer 0.3 mg/kg IV. If there is still no response, narcotic overdose is probably **ruled out.** If naloxone is successful in reducing coma, continue to administer it as needed. Flumazenil, 0.5 mg IV, can also be administered if the patient has no history of tricyclic antidepressant exposure.
    (2) Institute GI decontamination (see p. 267) and adequate supportive care.
2. CNS stimulants
  a. Etiology. These include amphetamines and amphetamine-like drugs, caffeine, and cocaine.
  b. Evaluation and diagnosis
    (1) History. These substances can induce psychological and physical dependence.
    (2) Physical examination
      (a) Increased CNS excitation may culminate in seizures.
      (b) Pulse rate and blood pressure are increased.
  c. Therapy
    (1) Following acute ingestion, institute GI decontamination measures (see p. 267).
    (2) Hypertension is usually of short duration and rarely necessitates treatment. If necessary, use phentolamine or nitroprusside.
    (3) Amphetamine psychotic reaction can be treated with chlorpromazine or haloperidol. Diazepam is the drug of choice for **hyperactivity** and **seizures.**
    (4) Acidification of the urine with ammonium chloride and ascorbic acid can enhance amphetamine elimination, but induces metabolic acidosis and is **not** recommended.
3. Substances that modify CNS perception
  a. Etiology. These include the hallucinogens phencyclidine (PCP), lysergic acid diethylamide (LSD), and mescaline; the cannabis group, including marijuana and hashish; and the volatile inhalants butyl nitrites and hydrocarbons (sniffing).
  b. Evaluation and diagnosis
    (1) History. Physical dependence does not develop. Psychological dependence is possible.
    (2) Physical examination
      (a) Hallucinogens induce euphoria, anxiety, or panic. The patient experiences time and visual distortion and visual hallucinations.

(b) Phencyclidine overdose produces extreme hyperactivity or cyclic coma, nystagmus, muscle rigidity, seizures, and hypertension. The pupils may be large or small. Flashbacks may occur.

(c) The cannabis group usually induces a state of euphoria and feeling of well-being. Hallucinations are rare. The pupils are unchanged but the conjunctivae are injected.

(d) Volatile inhalant users experience transient euphoria.

(3) Laboratory. Cardiac arrhythmias are the major acute complication of volatile inhalant users.

c. Therapy

(1) The patient with hallucinations or distorted perceptions needs a quiet and safe environment.

(2) Physical or chemical restraints should be avoided. If necessary, diazepam can be used (0.1 mg/kg PO or IV [maximum 10–20 mg]).

(3) Anticipate rhabdomyolysis in severely agitated patients.

L. Special cases

1. Lomotil

a. Etiology. This is an antidiarrheal agent that contains the anticholinergic agent atropine and the opioid diphenoxylate.

b. Evaluation and diagnosis

(1) History. Children are uniquely susceptible to the effects of Lomotil and may become symptomatic after ingestion of as little as one tablet; onset of toxicity may be delayed several hours.

(2) Physical examination. Central nervous system depression can recur after a period of apparent wellness.

c. Treatment. Young children who ingest Lomotil should be hospitalized for 24 hours of observation. Gastrointestinal decontamination should be performed. Ipecac should not be administered because of the risk of sudden central nervous system depression. Symptomatic CNS depression may respond to naloxone.

2. Oral hypoglycemic agents

a. Etiology. These agents stimulate insulin secretion.

b. Evaluation and diagnosis. Toxicity is exaggerated in young children, producing both late and recurrent hypoglycemia.

c. Treatment

(1) All children should be hospitalized for 24 hours of observation with frequent monitoring of blood sugar.

(2) Significant hypoglycemia should be treated with administration of 25% dextrose.

(3) Recalcitrant hypoglycemia is treated with intravenous glucagon, corticosteroids, and, if necessary, diazoxide.

III. Lead poisoning

A. Etiology. Lead poisoning in childhood results mainly from the ingestion of lead-based paint or dust. Infants are at risk when fed formula prepared with lead-contaminated water. The incidence is highest among the urban poor, but cases can be readily found among suburban, middle-class children, particularly when they reside in older homes (pre-1950) where renovation is occurring. Predisposing factors include iron, calcium, and zinc deficiency; older housing; low socioeconomic status; and pica. A number of lead-containing traditional cosmetics (kohl, surina) and folk remedies (greta, azarcon) are used in certain populations. Cookware may contain leaded glazes, and water may extract lead from solder in pipes or containers.

B. Evaluation and diagnosis

1. History

a. Emphasize the location, age, and condition of the home or other frequented areas.

b. Although common, the presence of **pica** is not a sine qua non in lead poisoning.

    c. Ask about the child's appetite, bowel habits, general behavior, and nutrition, as well as about signs of irritability and lethargy.

2. Physical examination. Include a thorough neurologic examination, a developmental assessment, and, if possible, a psychometric examination.

3. Laboratory

    a. Blood lead levels should be determined by **venous samples** whenever possible, to avoid the problem of skin contamination by lead-laden soil or dust. If a fingerstick sample is used, the finger should be carefully washed and rinsed. Elevated fingerstick lead levels should be confirmed promptly by follow-up venipuncture before intervention.

    b. Erythrocyte protoporphyrin (EP) is insensitive to Pb levels less than 20 μg/dl and is no longer recommended for screening. EP increasingly reflects lead toxicity when blood lead levels exceed 20 μg/dl, particularly when iron deficiency is present. Up to 35 μg EP/dl whole blood is considered acceptable in the absence of anemia. *Because 1 to 3 weeks of lead exposure is required to elevate protoporphyrin levels, it is possible for lead levels to be elevated acutely in the presence of normal EP.*

    c. Other blood tests. Blood tests in any child with elevated blood lead, EP, or both, should include a CBC, with attention to basophilic stippling of the erythrocyte; iron and iron-binding capacity; serum ferritin; BUN; and serum creatinine.

    d. X-ray films

        (1) Views of the **knees** are helpful in detecting widening and increased density of the zones of provisional calcification (chronic ingestion). Knee films in children 18 to 30 months of age should be interpreted by focusing on the proximal fibulae. In general, "lead lines" are associated with prolonged (i.e., >6 wk) Pb levels greater than 50 μg/dl.

        (2) Anteroposterior views of the **abdomen** should be obtained for radiopacities (acute ingestion).

    e. If encephalopathy is suspected, a CT scan of the brain should be obtained immediately to evaluate the possibility of cerebral edema.

    f. Lumbar puncture is contraindicated.

    g. Routine urinalysis may show pyuria, casts, glucosuria, or aminoaciduria, particularly when lead levels exceed 100 μg/dl.

C. Diagnosis (see Table 8-6).

D. Therapy. At all costs, the source of lead must be identified and removed.

    1. Commonly used **chelating agents** are EDTA, BAL (British antilewisite, dimercaprol), D-penicillamine, and DMSA.

    a. Ethylene diaminetetracetic acid (EDTA)

        (1) Mechanism of action. Urinary lead excretion is increased 20- to 50-fold. Bone pools of lead are reduced after multiple chelations with EDTA. EDTA crosses the blood-brain barrier poorly and enhances removal of other metals, notably zinc.

        (2) Route of administration. A continuous infusion gives the best results and is safest. EDTA can be given IM with procaine (0.5–2.0%). **Oral EDTA** can enhance GI absorption of lead and **is** contraindicated.

        (3) Dosage. A dosage of 50 mg/kg/day is administered for 3 to 5 days and then discontinued for at least 48 hours to permit clearance of the lead-EDTA complexes and reequilibration of lead stores. Further courses may be required. In severe lead poisoning (blood lead ≥70 μg/dl or symptoms present), EDTA should only be used in conjunction with BAL. In this case, the dose can be increased to 75 mg/kg/day, **although the risk of renal toxicity is increased.**

        (4) Toxicity. Renal toxicity can occur. Although hypocalcemia is avoided by the use of the calcium salt of EDTA, **hyper**calcemia can be seen with prolonged therapy. **Single doses of EDTA may actually increase brain lead, albeit transiently.** Other toxic effects include removal of zinc and other metals.

Table 8-6. Clinical and laboratory evidence of lead intoxication

Mild	Moderate	Severe
Clinical		
Lead exposure, usually to soil or dust	Probably paint exposure	Pica for paint
Asymptomatic	Predisposing iron deficiency	Secondary iron deficiency
May be predisposing iron deficiency	Positive family history	Abdominal pain, irritability, lethargy, fever, hepatosplenomegaly
Cognitive sequelae	Usually asymptomatic	Ataxia, seizures, coma, increased ICP, neurologic sequelae
	Loss of appetite and behavior changes	
	Behavioral and cognitive sequelae	
Laboratory		
Lead levels in whole blood 10–35 µg/dl	Lead levels 35–70 µg/dl	Lead levels > 70 µg/ml
EP in whole blood 35–125 µg/dl	EP in whole blood 125–250 µg/dl	EP levels > 250 µg/dl
KUB and knee x-rays usually negative	KUB x-rays negative	KUB x-rays positive
Serum iron/iron-binding capacity ≤ 16%	Knee x-rays positive	Knee films positive
Serum ferritin < 40 µg/ml	Serum iron/iron-binding capacity ≤ 16%	Serum iron/iron-binding capacity ≤ 16%
CBC normal	Ferritin < 20 µ/dl	Ferritin < 10 µg/dl
Lead mobilization test: ≤ or ≅ 1 µg Pb/mg EDTA/24 hr	CBC shows mild anemia	CBC shows basophilic stippling, anemia
	Lead mobilization test: ≅ 1 µg Pb/mg EDTA/24 hr	Decreased nerve conduction time
		CT scan shows increased ICP
		Aminoaciduria, glycosuria
		Lead mobilization test: > 1 µg Pb/mg EDTA/24 hr

ICP = intracranial pressure; KUB = kidneys, ureters, bladder.

    b. BAL

      (1) Mechanism of action. Two molecules of BAL combine with one of heavy metal to form a stable complex. Fecal as well as urinary excretion of lead is enhanced.

      (2) Route of administration. BAL in peanut oil is available only for IM administration.

      (3) Dosage. The usual dosage is **3 to 5** mg/kg/dose, three to six times a day. Since BAL is mainly used to lower the blood lead rapidly, it need not be given for a full 5 days with EDTA; 48 to 72 hours may suffice, **provided EDTA is continued.**

      (4) Toxicity. Toxic reactions may occur in as many as 50% of patients. A febrile reaction peculiar to children occurs in 30%, and a transient granulocytopenia may be present. **Discontinue iron** (the BAL-iron complex is toxic). BAL is **contraindicated in patients who are sensitive to peanuts.**

    c. d-Penicillamine, an oral chelating agent, is particularly useful in the treatment of low-level lead poisoning (i.e., blood Pb 20–35 µg/dl).

      (1) Mechanism of action. D-Penicillamine enhances the urinary excretion of lead.

      (2) Route of administration. It is currently available as both 125- and 250-mg capsules and scored 250-mg tablets. The capsules can be opened or the tablets crushed and suspended in liquid, if necessary. Strong fruit flavor masks the bitter taste. It should not be given with dairy products or iron.

      (3) The usual **oral dose** is 20 to 40 mg/kg/day in two to three divided doses. Side effects can be minimized by initiating therapy with small doses; for example, 25% of the expected dose, increasing after 1 week to 50%, and again after 1 week to the full dose, as well as by monitoring for toxicity.

(4) **Toxicity and side effects.** Mild toxicity usually resembles that of penicillin sensitivity, including rashes, transient leukopenia, and eosinophilia. Anorexia, nausea, and vomiting are infrequent. Isolated reports exist of nephrotoxicity, possibly from hypersensitivity reactions. Reversible hematuria, frequency, and enuresis occur in a few patients. **D-Penicillamine should not be administered to patients with known penicillin allergy.**

d. **Dimercaptosuccinic acid (DMSA; Succimer)** is an oral, water-soluble congener of BAL, indicated for treatment of children when lead levels exceed 45 µg/dl. It should not be used in symptomatic patients, or in those with ongoing exposure. DMSA is also effective in children with lead levels greater than 25 µg/dl.

(1) **Mechanisms of action.** DMSA dramatically lowers blood lead, but several courses of therapy may be required to adequately deplete the body burden of lead. It is specific for removing lead alone, in contrast to other chelators. Iron can be given concurrently.

(2) **Route of administration.** DMSA is presently available in 100-mg pelletized capsules that can be opened and sprinkled on food or in juice.

(3) The usual oral dosage is 30 mg/kg/day in three divided doses (q8h) for 5 days followed by 20 mg/kg/day in two divided doses (q12h) for 14 days. Although blood lead is initially lowered dramatically, "rebound" values 1 to 2 weeks after completion of a course of therapy reach 70 to 80% of the original value. Multiple courses may be needed.

(4) **Toxicity and side effects.** The principal toxicity is to the liver, producing mild, transient elevations of aspartate aminotransferase (AST) and alanine aminotransferase (ALT). Marked changes in alkaline phosphatase may occur. Cutaneous urticaria-like reactions have been reported.

2. **Monitoring chelation therapy.** Blood Pb should be followed closely during therapy (q48–72h for inpatients and q2–4 wk for outpatients).

a. During chelation therapy with EDTA, serum calcium, BUN, creatinine, and lead, as well as urinalyses, are monitored for evidence of hypocalcemia or renal toxicity. If such evidence is present, EDTA can be reduced or discontinued, and renal function usually returns to normal.

b. In encephalopathic patients, symptoms may worsen during therapy. Removal of lead with BAL should continue, with attention to CNS changes suggestive of cerebral edema (see p. 286). It may be wise to discontinue EDTA temporarily in such situations to reduce fluid requirements.

c. Patients who receive DMSA should have baseline liver function tests.

d. EDTA is administered for 3 to 5 days at a time. In general, urinary lead excretion tends to fall off after the fourth day regardless of the lead burden, while the risk of EDTA nephrotoxicity increases after the fifth day. For this reason, EDTA chelation is interrupted after 5 days. If the initial lead burden is very high, chelation is again begun after 48 to 72 hours. Therapy is then discontinued and long-term follow-up begun.

e. Because of the "rebound" phenomenon during reequilibration of body lead stores, blood lead and EP are best obtained 1 to 2 weeks after therapy.

f. The goal of therapy is to reduce body lead burden to safe levels (i.e., blood lead <15 µg/dl) and EP to normal (i.e., <35 µg/dl), although chelation therapy tends to be less efficient as the body burden is lowered. In general, the most complete therapy should be applied to children under 3 years of age.

E. **Management of plumbism.** Important management variables include age, duration of exposure, and risk factors such as iron deficiency, sickle cell disease, and developmental levels.

1. **Mild lead poisoning** (Pb <35 µg/dl)

    a. Identify and remove the **lead source.** Parents can help by wet-mopping the home to reduce lead dust.

    b. Administer **oral iron** (6 mg elemental iron/kg/24 hr) to correct iron deficiency and reduce further lead absorption. (see p. 433; Table 15-3)

    c. Repeat lead and EP determination monthly or more frequently. If values remain greater than 20 µg/dl longer than 2 months, consider D-penicillamine.

    d. D-Penicillamine (20–40 mg/kg/day PO) may be useful in reducing a low-level lead burden.

  2. Moderate lead poisoning (35–50 µg/dl)

    a. Identify and remove the **lead source.** If "deleading" is undertaken, remove the child **completely** from the home during the process and until a thorough cleanup is completed.

    b. Administer oral iron for 1 month or until EP stabilizes.

    c. After chelation therapy, restart iron therapy until both lead and EP values have returned to normal.

    d. It is likely that more than one course of chelation therapy will be needed.

    e. Mild, transient elevations of blood lead following chelation therapy are commonly due to "rebound" rather than reexposure, but significant increases in EP values usually accompany the latter.

    f. If the lead level is greater than 35 µg/dl *and* the lead source has been identified *and* the child is in safe housing, begin a course of DMSA as described in sec. **D.1.d** above.

    g. Iron therapy can be continued *during* therapy with DMSA.

    h. Monitor Pb, CBC, liver function tests (LFTs), BUN, and creatinine and urine sediment on days 14 and 21.

    i. Check for rebound at 14 and at 28 days' postchelation.

  3. Severe lead poisoning without encephalopathy

    a. Identify and remove the lead source.

    b. Hospitalize the child.

    c. Give 1.5 times the usual **maintenance fluids** (see Chap. 4).

    d. If the blood lead level exceeds 70 µg/dl, begin BAL IM in three divided doses of 5 mg/kg/24 hr for 48 to 72 hours.

    e. Administer EDTA IV if possible in continuous infusion or IM in three divided doses. If the IM route is chosen, the dose can be given bid or even in a single injection, *or*

    f. If the blood lead is less than 70 µg/dl, a course of DMSA can be begun, provided that the child is in the hospital. After 5 days of therapy, if *safe housing has been found*, the child can be discharged to receive the remaining 2 weeks of therapy on an ambulatory basis.

    g. Monitor BUN, creatinine, blood lead, LFTs (DMSA), and urinalyses.

    h. After chelation is completed, administer iron if it was not already given.

  4. Severe lead intoxication with encephalopathy

    a. This is a medical emergency. Treatment should be administered in an intensive care unit, if possible.

    b. Give maintenance fluids.

    c. Begin BAL IM, in six divided doses.

    d. Begin EDTA by continuous infusion.

    e. Treat cerebral edema with mannitol and dexamethasone (Decadron) (see Chap. 7).

    f. Continue chelation therapy at all costs, because cerebral edema will not respond to therapy until the lead burden is reduced.

    g. Treat seizures with anticonvulsants (see Table 20-2).

    h. After 5 days, discontinue therapy for 48 hours and restart.

    i. Monitor BUN, creatinine, calcium, electroencephalograms, urinalyses, and blood lead.

    j. Several courses of chelation will be needed.

  5. Sequelae. Both symptomatic **and** asymptomatic lead poisoning produce sequelae. All children with histories of significant lead poisoning should undergo thorough neuropsychological evaluation before entering school, ideally at ages 3 to 4.

F. Prevention. Lead poisoning is a preventable disease. Federal law prohibits the sale of leaded paint. Many states now have strong penalties for nonremoval of lead from houses in cases of plumbism. **Proper precautions are needed during deleading and renovation of old housing. Children should be removed completely from homes undergoing such work. Heating and sanding of lead paint are particularly dangerous** and should be avoided; scraping or chemical stripping are preferable. Intensive screening of children to identify those at risk, widespread inspection of housing, and stringent enforcement of sanitary and housing codes can reduce morbidity in this disease.

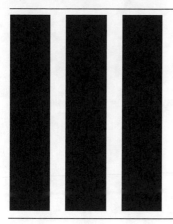

Disorders of Organ Systems

9

Renal Disorders

Kathy Jabs and Michelle Baum

I. Proteinuria

A. Etiology. Significant proteinuria can occur *with or without* intrinsic renal disease.

1. **Benign proteinuria** may be seen transiently with fever, dehydration, exercise, cold exposure, hypermetabolic states, seizures, heart failure, constrictive pericarditis, or urinary tract infection.

2. **Orthostatic (postural) proteinuria** is an exaggeration in the normal increase in protein excretion in the erect position compared to the recumbent position. It is not associated with serious renal disease or the risk of progressive decline in renal function.

3. **Glomerular diseases** are usually associated with proteinuria. In glomerulonephritis, proteinuria **and** hematuria are typically evident. The degree of proteinuria varies from the mild to the nephrotic range.

   a. Primary glomerular causes of proteinuria: minimal change disease, focal segmental glomerulosclerosis (FSGS), membranous glomerulopathy, and membranoproliferative glomerulonephritis (MPGN).

   b. Secondary causes

   (1) Infections: poststreptococcal glomerulonephritis, endocarditis, shunt (ventriculo-atrial) nephritis, hepatitis.

   (2) Autoimmune: systemic lupus erythematosus (SLE), Goodpasture's syndrome, Henoch-Schönlein purpura (HSP), polyarteritis nodosa.

   (3) Other: diabetes, Alport's syndrome, multiple myeloma, amyloidosis, renal vein thrombosis.

   (4) Tubulointerstitial processes such as tubulointerstitial nephritis or drug toxicity can cause mild to moderate proteinuria.

B. Evaluation and diagnosis. In children, protein excretion varies with age and body surface area. Significant proteinuria is defined as greater than 150 mg/day in adults, greater than 3 mg/hr/m^2 in children, or, if more than 10 years old, greater than 100 mg/day. Nephrotic range proteinuria is defined as greater than 50 mg/kg/day or 40 mg/m^2/hr or greater, and indicates significant glomerular disease. Alternatively, for patients with stable renal function, the **ratio** of protein to creatinine in a spot urine sample can be useful in identifying significant proteinuria. The normal urine protein-creatinine ratio is less than 0.2. Nephrotic range proteinuria is indicated by a ratio greater than 3. (Fig. 9-1).

1. Note how the sample was collected; look for fever, metabolic stress, and so forth, which might cause proteinuria. Check the urine on two or more occasions to confirm the presence of proteinuria.

2. Look for orthostatic (postural) proteinuria: Check a first AM and a PM urine with a dipstick; AM should be negative.

3. **Urinalysis** and **culture** are necessary. If proteinuria is detected in the context of a urinary tract infection, recheck the urine after completion of appropriate treatment.

4. Persistent, constant proteinuria may require referral to a nephrologist for further evaluation.

C. Treatment. No therapy is needed for orthostatic proteinuria. The treatment of proteinuria due to other causes depends on the diagnosis.

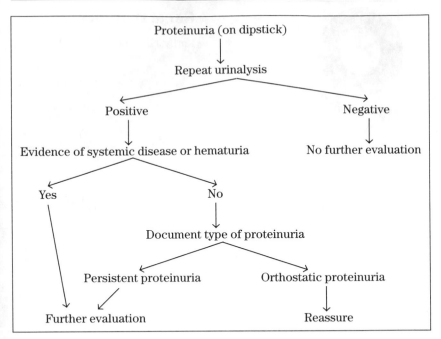

Fig. 9-1. Evaluation of proteinuria.

II. **Nephrotic syndrome.** The nephrotic syndrome is characterized by massive proteinuria, edema, hypoalbuminemia (albumin ≤2.5 mg/dl), and hyperlipidemia. The nephrotic syndrome occurs in 2 to 3 in 100,000 children less than 16 years of age per year. The peak incidence is between 2 and 4 years (75% of cases occur in children <5 yr of age). Boys are affected slightly more frequently than girls. Minimal change disease is the most common form of nephrotic syndrome. Of all patients with nephrotic syndrome, about 75% will have minimal change syndrome, 6 to 12% FSGS, 5 to 8% MPGN, and 8% other causes. The incidences of these diseases varies with the age at presentation.

A. **Etiology.** The nephrotic syndrome can occur as an isolated entity or as part of a progressive glomerulonephritis. The pathogenesis remains incompletely understood.

B. **Evaluation**

1. **History.** A history of antecedent infection is common.

2. **Physical examination.** A careful assessment should include weight, blood pressure, skin examination for rashes or other lesions, sites and extent of edema, and respiratory and cardiac status.

3. **Laboratory evaluation** includes a good urinalysis including microscopic evaluation, quantitative 24-hour urine protein excretion or spot protein to creatinine ratio, and selective protein index (urinary immunoglobulin G [IgG]/serum IgG divided by urinary transferrin/serum transferrin). Serum studies should include creatinine, electrolytes, cholesterol, C3, and albumin.

4. The presence of gross hematuria, elevated blood pressure, a low C3, nonselective proteinuria (selective protein index >0.2), age at presentation below 1 year or over 10 years, or failure to respond to corticosteroids suggests diagnoses other than minimal change nephrotic syndrome and a renal biopsy should be considered.

C. **Diagnosis.** A combination of the defined clinical features with nephrotic range proteinuria confirms the diagnosis. **However, all features need not be present,** especially early in relapse.

D. Treatment of minimal change nephrotic syndrome
1. **Immunomodulation**
   a. **Corticosteroids** are the treatment of choice, usually 2 mg/kg/day prednisone PO in divided doses (usual maximum dose 60 mg/day). This regimen is continued until the urine is protein free for 5 to 7 days. Following
   this, a further alternate-day regimen is generally given in a reduced dosage
   (1.0–1.5 mg/kg/day as one dose q48h) for a month; after that the steroids
   are tapered over 2 to 3 weeks and discontinued. Lack of response by 8
   weeks suggests corticosteroid resistance.
   b. **Cytotoxic therapy.** Cytotoxic therapy with agents such as cyclophosphamide has been shown to be effective in prolonging remission in patients
   who are "frequent relapsers" and require multiple or prolonged courses of
   prednisone; it appears less effective in those who show no response to corticosteroids. **Cytotoxic therapy should only be undertaken in consultation with a pediatric nephrologist.**
   c. **Cyclosporine** has been used recently in patients who are not responsive
   to steroids or who are frequent relapsers and have steroid side effects.
   Consultation with a pediatric nephrologist is recommended.
2. **Diuretics and albumin**
   a. **The use of a diuretic alone can be hazardous in the presence of a low
   serum albumin,** because this can aggravate existing contraction of the circulating blood volume and the risk of venous thrombosis.
   b. When accumulation of edema fluid is severe, as in marked ascites, pulmonary edema, inability to void due to penile or labial edema, scrotal edema,
   or skin breakdown due to marked peripheral edema, or when the nephrotic
   patient has a concomitant infection, diuresis can be prompted by administration of 25% albumin in a dosage of 0.5 to 1.0 g/kg IV slowly (over several
   hours) daily or q12h, followed by IV furosemide, 1 mg/kg. The patient's response should be reassessed after each dose. If the administration of albumin does not result in a diuresis, continued dosing can lead to volume
   overload and pulmonary edema. **Caution:** Too-rapid administration of albumin can cause pulmonary edema and congestive heart failure (CHF).
3. **General measures**
   a. **Diet.** A no-added-salt diet is advised for edematous patients. Strict fluid restriction should be prescribed in exact ounce amounts. For very edematous patients, fluid can be restricted to insensible losses plus urine output
   until remission is induced.
   b. **Activity.** No restriction of activity is required.
   c. **Instruction of family.** Parents and child should be well informed about
   nephrosis and should be taught to test urine for albumin with dipsticks. A
   written diary of urine protein, weight, and fluid input should be kept.
E. Complications
1. **Infection.** Early and vigorous treatment of **bacterial** infection is important. Infections with encapsulated bacterial organisms are more common. Patients
   with abdominal pain should be evaluated for spontaneous bacterial peritonitis,
   which is commonly caused by *Streptococcus pneumoniae.* Since **viral** infections can lead to relapse, the urine should be monitored closely during such infections. *Nonimmune patients who are exposed to varicella while receiving
   steroids should receive prompt administration of zoster immune globulin.*
   Patients in whom varicella develops should be hospitalized for administration
   of IV acyclovir and further monitoring for signs of systemic infection.
2. **Hypercoagulable state.** In patients with nephrotic syndrome, deep vein
   thrombosis (DVT), renal vein thrombosis, or even pulmonary embolus or
   thrombosis may develop. This is uncommon in the pediatric population.
3. **Complications of therapy.** Immunosuppression, gastritis, cushingoid habitus,
   hypertension, cataracts, and growth failure can occur secondary to steroid use.
F. Prognosis
1. In minimal change nephrotic syndrome, 80 to 90% of children show an initial response to corticosteroids. Of these, 80% will have further relapses.

2. The rate of relapse in a group of children tends to decrease after the first 10 years. A child who remains relapse free for up to 3 to 4 years has a 95% chance of remaining in remission thereafter. However, after one relapse, the subsequent course cannot be predicted, and the number of relapses per se does not affect the ultimate outcome.

3. Some children who are initially steroid responsive may subsequently become steroid nonresponsive. In addition, FSGS may develop in some children who initially have a clinical response and renal biopsy findings typical of minimal change nephrotic syndrome. In these children both a poor response to steroids and progressive renal insufficiency can develop.

III. **Hematuria.** Normal children excrete 200,000 to 500,000 red blood cells each day. Based on average urinary volumes, hematuria is defined as the presence of more than five red blood cells per high-power microscopic field on at least two properly performed urinalyses. While it is sensitive, the urine dipstick test has a high false-positive rate. Thus, red urine or a positive urine dipstick test, or both, mandate microscopic examination of the urine.

A. **Etiology**

1. **More than five red blood cells per high-power field** may be caused by any lesion from the renal artery to the tip of the urethra. In addition, high fever and vigorous exercise can cause a transient, benign increase in red cell excretion rate.

2. **Positive dipstick in the absence of red cells** on microscopic examination suggests cells that were lysed in transit to the laboratory, free hemoglobinuria, or myoglobinuria. Both pigments, hemoglobin and myoglobin, may be associated with nephrotoxicity, and full evaluation should proceed.

B. **Evaluation** should include a complete history, physical examination, and initial laboratory profile.

1. **History.** Any possible precipitating event is noted.

a. Particular attention is focused on possible antecedent streptococcal infection, symptoms of cystitis, or renal colic.

b. The **past medical history** focuses on hemoglobinopathies or any previous hemorrhagic tendencies and details of any drug or travel history.

c. Any **family history** of hematuria, renal disease, renal failure, collagen vascular diseases, nephrolithiasis, or deafness is delineated.

d. A **review of systems** includes recent rashes, arthralgias, arthritis, and abdominal pain, and notes fevers, malaise, anorexia, weight loss, exercise pattern, and trauma.

2. A thorough **physical examination** is required, with careful attention to height, weight, blood pressure, rashes, and edema. Anomalous features on abdominal or perineal examination are noted.

3. **Initial laboratory profile.** Basic laboratory tests include a urinalysis with complete microscopic examination and a urine culture. If hematuria is persistent, further evaluation should include CBC, erythrocyte sedimentation rate, platelet count, prothrombin time, partial thromboplastin time, creatinine, C3, and a spot urine calcium to creatinine ratio.

C. **Differential diagnosis.** The baseline investigations may provide the diagnosis **without further evaluation.** If not, the causes of hematuria can be separated into the following categories: **painless hematuria, painful hematuria, and gross hematuria.** For discussion of hematuria associated with primary glomerular diseases or with serious underlying systemic disease, see sec. IV.

1. **Etiology can be suggested by initial evaluation.**

a. An abdominal mass with hematuria requires exclusion of **Wilms' tumor, cystic kidney disease,** or **hydronephrosis.**

b. Perineal excoriation or meatal inflammation implicates **local factors.**

c. Hematuria occurs in association with **sickle cell disease or trait** and S-C **hemoglobin.**

d. A family history of asymptomatic hematuria suggests **benign familial hematuria or hypercalciuria,** whereas a family history of hematuria, deafness, and renal insufficiency suggests **Alport's hereditary nephritis.** Family history of stones or hypercalciuria should also be elicited.

   e. Hematuria with casts and proteinuria can occur in the critically ill child with **acute tubular necrosis (ATN), renal infarction, renal cortical necrosis, or renal vein thrombosis** (see p. 313).

   f. A **coagulopathy** is suggested by a history of bleeding.

2. **Painless hematuria**

   a. The most likely etiology is **benign hematuria** (familial or sporadic) or **hypercalciuria.** Family members should be screened with urinalyses to rule out **benign familial hematuria,** which is inherited as an autosomal dominant trait. **Hypercalciuria** may also be a familial condition and may be associated with a family history of nephrolithiasis. Hypercalciuria is defined as a spot calcium to creatinine ratio of greater than 0.2.

   b. **Glomerulonephritis** should be a consideration in asymptomatic hematuria, particularly when accompanied by proteinuria (see sec. **IV**).

   c. In **subacute bacterial endocarditis** and **neurologic ventriculo-atrial shunt infection,** hematuria is immunologically mediated and represents focal areas of glomerulonephritis.

   d. **Extraglomerular hematuria** may be asymptomatic; anatomic lesions can be detected by renal ultrasound or an intravenous pyelogram (IVP). An arteriovenous malformation can also cause hematuria.

   e. In a large number of patients, asymptomatic microscopic hematuria may persist without serologic or radiologic abnormalities. Follow-up of such children with **idiopathic hematuria** has shown no deterioration in renal function. Such patients should be followed regularly, with periodic examinations, urinalyses, serum creatinine (Cr), and blood pressures. During the follow-up period, the appearance of proteinuria, active urinary sediment with casts, deterioration in renal function, or development of hypertension suggests the need for further evaluation.

3. **Painful hematuria**

   a. A clinical picture of **cystitis** accompanied by hematuria, mild proteinuria (trace to 1+ unless hematuria is gross), and leukocyturia suggests bacterial, viral, or traumatic involvement of the bladder or lower urinary tract. A **Gram's stain** of the unspun urine and culture should be done. When bacterial infection is documented, **a voiding cystourethrogram** and a renal ultrasound should be performed in all children less than 3 years of age and in all boys after successful antimicrobial therapy. An ultrasound should be obtained in older girls.

   b. Culture-negative cystitis may be secondary to **viral infection.** Adenoviruses 11 and 21, influenza virus, and a papovavirus-like organism have been implicated. Viral cystitis with resolution of hematuria and normal findings on urinalysis at follow-up requires no further investigation.

   c. Culture-negative cystitis can also be caused by **tuberculosis** and **schistosomiasis,** and should be suspected in the appropriate clinical and endemic settings.

   d. In addition to **gonococcal** or **chlamydial urethritis,** vigorous masturbation and mechanical trauma to the urethra can also cause symptomatic hematuria with urethritis.

   e. In younger children with apparent cystitis, particularly girls aged 2 to 6, urethral or vaginal **foreign bodies** may be present.

   f. Hematuria accompanied by moderate to severe abdominal pain is characteristic of **nephrolithiasis.** True renal colic is rare in the pediatric age group.

   g. Microscopic hematuria following abdominal or flank **trauma** is common and often benign. However, if gross hematuria occurs or if microscopic hematuria is detected following seemingly minor trauma, an IVP or CT should be obtained to determine the extent of renal damage as well as to identify structural abnormalities that might predispose to bleeding with minor trauma.

4. **Gross hematuria**
   a. Both acute and recurrent **glomerulonephritis** can present with gross hematuria (e.g., IgA nephropathy).
   b. Evidence for **coagulopathy** should be sought.
   c. **Nonglomerular causes** of gross hematuria include **urinary tract infection, trauma, perineal irritation, nephrolithiasis, ureteropelvic junction (UPJ) obstruction, meatal stenosis, epididymitis, and tumor.**

IV. **Glomerulonephritis.** When asymptomatic hematuria occurs in the context of hypertension, active urinary sediment with casts, or proteinuria, glomerulonephritis should be suspected.

A. **Etiology.** Glomerulopathies can be divided into acute, rapidly progressive, and chronic processes (Table 9-1).

1. **Acute glomerulonephritis (AGN).** Usually, the patient has had an **antecedent streptococcal infection** manifest as pharyngitis, cellulitis, or impetigo. **Other infectious agents** include staphylococcus, pneumococcus, influenza A, Epstein-Barr virus, and Coxsackie virus. In addition, **chronic glomerulonephritides may present with a clinical picture suggesting AGN.** These entities include primary glomerular diseases such as MPGN and Immunoglobulin A (IgA) nephropathy, as well as secondary glomerular lesions associated with lupus nephritis, infective endocarditis, HSP, and hemolytic-uremic syndrome (HUS).

2. **Rapidly progressive glomerulonephritis (RPGN)** is typically associated with extensive glomerular crescent formation and thus is also referred to as **crescentic glomerulonephritis.**
   a. RPGN can occur as an idiopathic process associated with deposition of **anti–glomerular basement membrane** (anti-GBM) **antibodies** (Goodpasture's disease) or **immune complexes.** In RPGN with neither finding, circulating **antineutrophil cytoplasmic antibody (ANCA)** may be detectable (e.g., Wegener's granulomatosis).
   b. Diffuse crescent formation can be superimposed on other primary glomerular diseases such as MPGN and IgA nephropathy.
   c. RPGN can be associated with glomerular lesions that are secondary either to infectious processes (poststreptococcal glomerulonephritis, infective endocarditis, hepatitis) or to systemic processes, such as lupus, HSP, and vasculitis.

3. **Chronic glomerulonephritis** (e.g., MPGN and FSGS) should be considered in patients with persistent microscopic hematuria, particularly in the context of hypertension, active urinary sediment with casts, or proteinuria.

B. **Evaluation**
   1. A thorough **physical examination** is required, with careful attention to height,

Table 9-1. Diagnosis of Acute Glomerulonephritis

Low complement	Normal complement
Systemic disease	
Systemic lupus erythematosus	Polyarteritis nodosa
Infective endocarditis	Wegener's granulomatosis
Ventriculo-atrial shunt nephritis	Henoch-Schönlein purpura
Cryoglobulinemia	Goodpasture's disease
Isolated renal disease	
Postinfectious glomerulonephritis	IgA nephropathy
Membranoproliferative glomerulonephritis	Rapidly progressive glomerulonephritis
	Anti–glomerular basement membrane disease
	Immune complex disease

weight, blood pressure, rashes, joint involvement, and edema. The patient's respiratory and cardiac status should also be carefully assessed.

2. **Laboratory evaluation** should include creatinine, anti-streptolysin O (ASLO) titer, antideoxyribonuclease (DNAase) B titer or streptozyme profile, serum albumin, and complement levels (C3 and C4). An antinuclear antibody (ANA) test should be considered to aide in the diagnosis of lupus nephritis, particularly in the setting of depressed complement levels. **Renal biopsy** may be indicated to identify the histopathologic lesion and provide prognostic information.

C. **Diagnosis**
1. **Acute poststreptococcal (postinfectious) glomerulonephritis (APSGN)** is suggested by a history of antecedent infection, elevations in ASLO titer and anti-DNAase B titer, and depression of the C3 level for 4 to 8 weeks.
2. **Persistent hypocomplementemia** suggests MPGN, SLE nephritis, nephritis associated with infective endocarditis, or shunt infection.
3. **Henoch-Schönlein purpura** should be readily diagnosed by the typical rash of purpura on the buttocks and lower extremities, and by the other constellation of symptoms, including abdominal pain, bloody stools, joint involvement, and renal involvement. Renal biopsy is reserved for atypical or recurrent cases.
4. **Immunoglobulin nephropathy (Berger's disease)** is characterized by baseline microscopic hematuria punctuated by recurrent episodes of macroscopic hematuria that are typically precipitated by intercurrent respiratory illnesses.
5. **Focal and segmental glomerulosclerosis** is suggested by significant proteinuria often in the nephrotic range, microscopic hematuria, a nonselective protein index (>0.2), and failure to respond to corticosteroid treatment.

D. **Treatment**
1. For **APSGN**, the treatment is entirely symptomatic.
   a. Appropriate antibiotics are given to eradicate the streptococcal infection (see Chap. 5, Table 5-2, p. 81).
   b. Salt and fluid retention are common and can lead to edema. Frank nephrotic syndrome is uncommon. A no-added-salt diet is prescribed until the patient is asymptomatic. Then a normal diet is resumed. Fluid restriction is also helpful to decrease edema.
   c. **Hypertension** (see p. 298, Chap. 10, p. 321). Hypertension is often fluid and renin mediated. Mild hypertension often responds to salt and fluid restriction alone. When antihypertensive agents are indicated, the medication(s) chosen should have a rapid onset of action and be easily discontinued since they are usually necessary only for a short time.
2. Patients with **RPGN, chronic glomerulonephritis, or nephritis associated with a systemic disease** should be managed in consultation with a pediatric nephrologist.

E. **Prognosis**
1. In **APSGN**, the usual course ends in complete recovery. The urine sediment of patients with **APSGN** may remain abnormal for a prolonged period. Proteinuria often resolves before hematuria, which can persist for up to 2 to 3 years following the illness. The complement levels should return to normal in 8 to 12 weeks. In those children with persistently depressed complement levels, other glomerular processes such as membranoproliferative glomerulonephritis or lupus nephritis should be considered. Up to 5% of patients who appear clinically to have acute poststreptococcal glomerulonephritis have a continuously downhill course and progress to renal insufficiency. Renal biopsy in such patients usually reveals evidence of an underlying chronic glomerular disease.
2. **Membranoproliferative glomerulonephritis, focal and segmental glomerulosclerosis, and IgA nephropathy** are chronic renal diseases. They are characterized by occasional clinical remissions, but may progress to renal insufficiency. Poor prognostic signs include nephrotic syndrome and hypertension.

V. **Hemolytic-uremic syndrome.** The triad of acute nephropathy, hemolytic anemia with fragmented red cells, and thrombocytopenia constitutes one of the most common syndromes of acute renal failure seen in childhood. It is endemic in Argentina, California,

South Africa, and the Netherlands. It is often preceded by gastroenteritis or, much less commonly, an upper respiratory tract infection (URI).

A. Etiology. Most patients with diarrhea-associated (enteropathic) HUS have evidence of exposure to *Escherichia coli* 0157:H7. Shiga-like toxins are believed to cause the endothelial cell injury, which is central to the pathogenesis of HUS. Injury to endothelial cells in the renal microvasculature, for example, leads to a microangiopathic hemolytic anemia and subsequent glomerular and cellular injury.

B. Evaluation. Evaluate as for acute renal failure (see p. 307).
1. Do a CBC with a smear in any patient with acute renal failure.
2. Suspect HUS if a gastroenteritis precedes marked hematuria or renal failure, or both. Send stool culture for *E. coli* 0157:H7.
3. Assess renal function with a urinalysis, creatinine.
4. Complete neurologic examination.
5. Assess blood pressure.

C. Diagnosis
1. The patient usually has a history of a prodromal illness.
2. Microangiopathic hemolytic anemia is found, including low hematocrit, increased reticulocytes, burr cells and helmet cells on smear, and thrombocytopenia.
3. HUS may involve the GI tract (abdominal pain, vomiting, bloody diarrhea), renal (hematuria, oligoanuria, renal failure, hypertension), hematologic (anemia, thrombocytopenia), and neurologic (irritability, lethargy, seizures, stroke) systems.

D. Treatment is as for acute renal failure (see p. 307). At this time there is no definitive therapy for **HUS.** Treatment is solely supportive. In addition, note the following:
1. Fluid management is important. Once it is established that the child is euvolemic or volume expanded, fluid should be restricted to insensible losses and output (see p. 307).
2. Control hypertension (see sec. **VI**).
3. **Transfuse with only washed, white cell–poor blood, because these patients may be renal transplant candidates in the future.** Directed donation from family members who are potential kidney donors if the child develops end-stage renal disease should also be avoided.
4. Dialysis when indicated for fluid retention, uremia, hyperkalemia, acidosis.
5. Therapies utilized in some centers include plasma infusion and plasmapheresis, which are still controversial. There has been no benefit shown from the use of heparin, streptokinase, or antiplatelet agents.

E. Prognosis. Mildly affected patients tend to do well, with little or no long-term proteinuria, hypertension, or azotemia. Some patients with severe HUS will have long-term sequelae, such as hypertension, hematuria, proteinuria, and/or progressive renal insufficiency. Therefore, regular follow-up is recommended, which should include at least yearly blood pressure measurement, urinalysis, and serum creatinine.

VI. Hypertension. Hypertension is not a common pediatric problem. It is estimated to occur in 1 to 3% of children. Blood pressure should be measured annually in all children over 3 years of age, in children with symptoms consistent with hypertension, and in all hospitalized children. Most children who have mild elevations in their blood pressure have essential or primary hypertension. The younger the child and the more elevated the blood pressure, the more likely it is that there is a secondary cause of hypertension.

A. Etiology (Table 9-2)
1. **Transient hypertension** may be due to acute renal parenchymal disease, following surgery or trauma, excessive volume expansion, drug overdose (e.g., amphetamines), lead poisoning, and CNS disease.
2. **Essential or primary hypertension** can begin in childhood, generally in children greater than 10 years old. The pathogenesis is not firmly established; however, sodium and water retention, and increased vascular reactivity to circulat-

Table 9-2. Diagnosis of hypertension

Etiologic group	Examples
Cardiovascular	Coarctation
Renal disease	Glomerulonephritis, reflux nephropathy, pyelonephritis, polycystic kidney disease
Renovascular	Renal artery stenosis, ischemia secondary to embolus
Catecholamine excess	Pheochromocytoma, neuroblastoma
Endocrine	Corticosteroid excess, hyperthyroidism
CNS disease	Tumor, trauma
"Essential hypertension"	
Medication related	Oral contraceptives, decongestants, cocaine, amphetamines, phencyclidine (PCP), exogenous steroids
Other	Burns, traction, urologic surgery

ing vasoconstrictors, may contribute. Genetic and racial factors appear to play a role.
3. **Secondary hypertension** is associated with a variety of conditions. The most common cause for secondary hypertension is a renal abnormality (78%).
   a. **Newborn infants:** renal artery thrombosis (particularly following umbilical artery lines), renal artery stenosis, congenital renal malformations, coarctation of the aorta, Wilms' tumor.
   b. **Infancy to 6 years:** renal artery stenosis, renal parenchymal diseases, coarctation of the aorta.
   c. **Children 6 to 10 years:** renal artery stenosis, parenchymal diseases.
   d. **Adolescence:** renal parenchymal diseases, pheochromocytoma, birth control pills.
B. **Evaluation.** The goals of this evaluation are to determine the severity and the etiology of the hypertension and whether there are end-organ consequences (e.g., cardiac, retinal).
   1. **History.** Careful attention should be given to the neonatal history, especially of an umbilical artery catheter, and family history regarding hypertension, cardiac disease, pheochromocytoma, and renal disease. Information about constitutional symptoms, abdominal pain, voiding abnormalities, muscle or joint complaints, edema, and rashes, as well as drug use or any symptoms suggestive of a pheochromocytoma (pallor, flushing, palpitations, or sweating) should be elicited.
   2. **Physical examination.** Blood pressure should be measured multiple times in a quiet room to confirm the presence of hypertension. An appropriate-sized cuff that covers two thirds of the upper arm should be employed. The stethoscope bell should be used. The fourth Korotkov sound (K_4) is best to use in children, because K_5 often does not occur clearly. When possible, K_1 (onset), K_4 (muffling), and K_5 (disappearance) should be recorded. Norms for blood pressure use the K_4 for children less than 13 years old and K_5 for children 13 to 18. Height and weight should be plotted on appropriate growth charts. Coexisting features suggestive of renal disease, collagen vascular disease, endocrine disorders, genetic syndromes, or cardiac or vascular disease should be sought. In addition, careful neurologic evaluation should determine whether sequelae of chronic hypertension are present. A good fundoscopic eye examination should be performed. Palpation of femoral pulses is important. Abdomen should be examined for a mass or a bruit. Skin should be examined for café au lait spots (increased risk of renal artery stenosis and pheochromocytoma in neurofibromatosis.).

3. **Laboratory evaluation** should include urinalysis, serum electrolytes, and serum creatinine. If the child is obese or if the family history is suggestive, a serum lipid profile should be considered. Ambulatory 24-hour blood pressure monitoring is often helpful in determining if the blood pressure is persistently elevated and in eliminating the "white coat" hypertension.

4. An **echocardiogram** provides information about the chronicity and the severity of the hypertension and serves as a useful marker to follow treatment efficacy.

5. Radiologic studies in selected patients include a renal ultrasound to assess for renal anatomic abnormalities, a dimercaptosuccinic acid (DMSA)–radionuclide scan to evaluate perfusion, or an arteriogram to assess for renovascular abnormalities.

6. Hormonal evaluation in selected patients includes urinary catecholamines and metabolites, peripheral renin, and peripheral aldosterone.

C. **Diagnosis.** Hypertension is suggested by blood pressure values that are above the 95th percentile for age. The weight and height of the child should be kept in mind when interpreting the aged-based normals. Values for various age groups are depicted in Figs. 9-2 through 9-4.

D. **Treatment.** Any **diastolic blood pressure** above the 95th percentile requires treatment. Acute control is necessary if blood pressure elevation is associated with signs of hypertensive encephalopathy (blurred vision, severe headache, irritability, seizures) or cardiac symptoms (CHF).

1. **Hypertensive crisis.** In acute, severe hypertension, the immediate goal is blood pressure control. Subsequently, there should be a program of investigation and treatment aimed at long-term control. In order to rapidly decrease the blood pressure, parenteral or sublingual treatment is indicated. It should be kept in mind that, following normalization of blood pressure, symptoms such as headache, abdominal pain, and nausea may develop from rapid vasodilatation.

    a. **Nifedipine (Procardia)** is a calcium-channel blocker that can be given sublingually and has an onset of action within 15 to 30 minutes.
        (1) **Dosage.** Use 0.25 to 0.50 mg/kg sublingually.
        (2) **Advantage.** Nifedipine can be administered immediately in a hypertensive crisis before the placement of intravenous access. It has a rapid onset of action.
        (3) **Disadvantage.** Sublingual dose is difficult to administer precisely to small children.

    b. **Labetalol** (Normodyne, Trandate) is an adrenergic receptor blocking agent with selective alpha and nonselective beta effects.
        (1) **Dosage.** Initial dose is 0.25 mg/kg, with an additional 0.5 mg/kg at 15-minute intervals up to a total cumulative dose of 4.0 mg/kg. It can also be given as an IV infusion of 1 to 3 mg/kg/hr.
        (2) **Advantages.** One of the drugs of choice for hypertensive crisis. Not associated with reflex tachycardia as with other vasodilators. Labetalol has no significant effect on glucose metabolism, as do other beta-blocking agents. The onset of action is rapid and the effect is easily titrated.
        (3) **Disadvantages.** Rare cases of hepatocellular injury are seen with both acute and chronic labetalol therapy. Injury is usually reversible, but hepatic necrosis has been reported. **Liver function tests (LFTs) need to be followed and at the first sign of hepatic injury, labetalol should be discontinued.** Relatively contraindicated in asthmatics.

    c. **Sodium nitroprusside (Nipride)** *must be used as an IV drip with constant intensive care unit monitoring.* It is universally effective, because it causes immediate vasodilatation. The effects are rapidly titratable.
        (1) The dose is 0.5 to 8.0 µg/kg/min. **Note:** The prepared solution is inactivated by light. **Do not use with other drugs in the same IV line.**
        (2) *Blood levels of thiocyanate must be checked daily,* because nitroprusside is converted to thiocyanate by the hepatic enzyme, rhodanase. **Caution** is necessary in the presence of hepatic insufficiency.

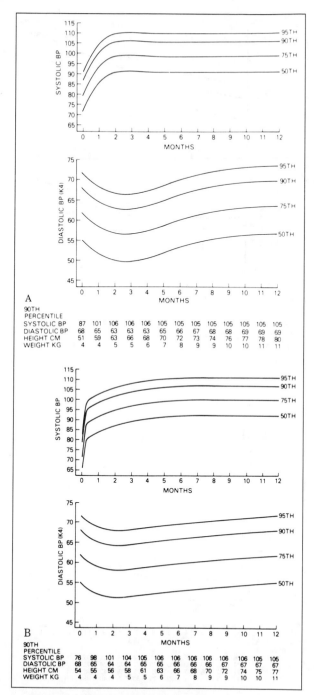

Fig. 9-2. Blood pressure in the first year of life in boys (A) and girls (B). (From Report of the Second Task Force on Blood Pressure Control in Children—1987. *Pediatrics* 79:1, 1987. Copyright 1987, American Academy of Pediatrics.)

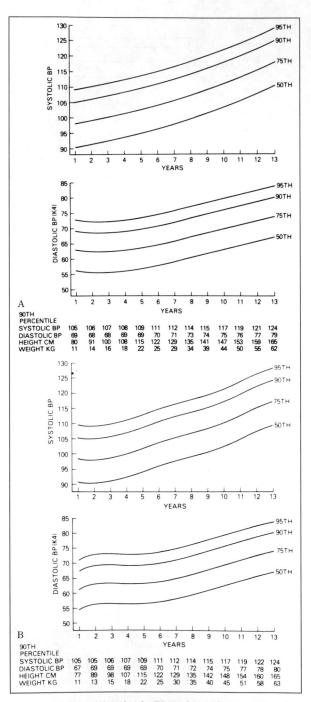

Fig. 9-3. Blood pressure in boys (A) and girls (B) aged 1 to 13 years. (From Report of the Second Task Force on Blood Pressure Control in Children—1987. *Pediatrics* 79:1, 1987. Copyright 1987, American Academy of Pediatrics.)

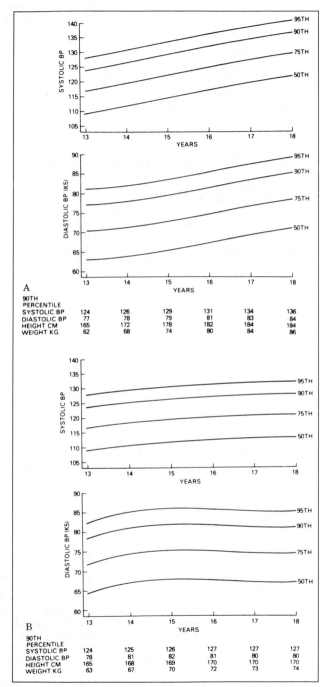

Fig. 9-4. Blood pressure in boys (A) and girls (B) aged 13 to 18 years. (From Report of the Second Task Force on Blood Pressure Control in Children—1987. *Pediatrics* 79:1, 1987. Copyright 1987, American Academy of Pediatrics.)

(3) Advantages. The onset of action is instantaneous and its effects are rapidly terminated on discontinuation. Nitroprusside is effective when all other drugs have failed. The rate of infusion can be titrated against desired blood pressure.

(4) Disadvantages. Nitroprusside requires constant supervision in the intensive care unit. Discontinuance of the IV drip means instantaneous loss of the pharmacologic effect.

d. Hydralazine (Apresoline) is a direct vasodilator. When it is given intramuscularly, the onset of action is within 15 to 30 minutes. Onset after IV administration is immediate.

(1) Dosage. Hydralazine is given parenterally at an initial dose of 0.1 to 0.2 mg/kg. This dose can be progressively increased q4h according to the response up to 10 times the initial dose.

(2) Advantages. Hydralazine does not reduce renal blood flow. It is effective fairly rapidly and has a short half-life. The dose is easily titrated and easily adjusted to patient size.

(3) Disadvantages. The most important side effects are tachycardia, nausea, vomiting, headache, diarrhea, and positive lupus erythematosus (LE) and rheumatoid factor reactions (very rare in children). The drug should be avoided in patients with arrhythmias and heart failure.

e. Diazoxide (Hyperstat) is a benzothiazide with no diuretic effect, which acts directly on the vascular smooth muscles. Diazoxide does not reduce renal blood flow. Its use has decreased with the advent of newer agents (e.g., labetalol, nifedipine).

(1) It is administered IV (1 mg/kg/dose) **as fast as possible** to achieve maximal action on the smooth muscle and minimal binding to serum protein. The effects last 3 to 15 hours. If the initial dose proves ineffective, further 1-mg/kg doses can be repeated at 10- to 15-minute intervals. The maximum dose is 5 mg/kg.

(2) Disadvantages. It produces hyperglycemia and can cause sodium and fluid retention. Transient tachycardia often follows administration.

f. Beta blockers. Esmolol (Brevibloc) is a selective beta-1 blocker with a very short duration of action (approximately 9 min). It is administered as a continuous infusion of 50 to 200 μg/kg/min, though experience in children is very limited. It is also rapidly titratable to desired effect. **Propranolol** is a nonselective beta blocker and is most safely given PO. The usual pediatric IV dose is 0.5 to 1.0 mg under careful monitoring conditions. Intravenous propranolol is reserved for life-threatening situations.

2. Mild or chronic hypertension, or both. It is important to identify children with essential hypertension, so as to optimize their diet and weight, control their hypertension, and educate them about the long-term implications of hypertension. For children with secondary causes of hypertension, it is important to identify the cause and to treat the hypertension. While epidemiologic data are inconclusive about the contribution of childhood hypertension to cardiovascular disease in adulthood, severe uncontrolled hypertension can cause significant end-organ damage in children. Several approaches to lowering blood pressure should be considered.

a. Nonpharmacologic therapy. Changes in diet, including sodium intake, and dynamic exercise and relaxation techniques, may be effective, especially in essential hypertension. Weight reduction may help lower blood pressure.

b. Diuretics can be used if mild hypertension fails to respond to diet (see p. 321).

c. Antihypertensive agents should be added if techniques in secs. **a** and **b** do not control blood pressure *or* if hypertension is moderately to severely elevated (see sec. **1** above). The general approach to pharmacologic therapy is to start with a single agent at a low dose; if no adverse effects occur, increase incrementally to the maximal dose; then add a second agent. In choosing a therapeutic regimen, the goals are to maximize compliance and to minimize adverse effects. The dosages of selected agents are shown in Table 9-3.

Table 9-3. Selected oral antihypertensive agents

Agent	Forms available	Initial daily dose	Dose interval	Comments
Vasodilators				
Hydralazine	10, 25, 50 mg	1 mg/kg	q6h	Diuretics frequently needed concomitantly
Minoxidil	2.5, 10 mg	0.1–0.2 mg/kg	qd or q12h	
Prazosin	1, 2, 5 mg	0.03 mg/kg	q8h	
Calcium-channel blockers				
Nifedipine	10, 20 mg	0.25–1 mg/kg	q6h or q8h	
Nifedipine XL	30, 60, 90 mg	30 mg	qd or q12h	The daily dose of the long-acting and regular forms are equivalent
Angiotensin-converting enzyme inhibitors				
Captopril	12.5, 25, 50, 100 mg	0.3–0.5 mg/kg	q8h	Risk of renal failure, hyperkalemia; contraindicated in pregnancy
Enalapril	2.5, 5, 10, 20 mg	0.15 mg/kg	qd or q12h	
Beta blockers				
Propranolol	10, 20, 40, 60, 80 mg	0.5–1.0 mg/kg	q6–q12h	Contraindicated in asthma, congestive heart failure, diabetes
Atenolol	25, 50, 100 mg	0.5–1.0 mg/kg	qd or q12h	Asthma not absolute contraindication

VII. Renal tubular acidosis (RTA). This syndrome is characterized by hyperchloremic metabolic acidosis secondary to defects in the renal tubular excretion of bicarbonate and acid. Generally, the glomerular filtration rate (GFR) is normal or mildly decreased.
  A. Proximal renal tubular acidosis (type II RTA)
    1. Etiology. Bicarbonate reabsorption in the proximal tubule is impaired, resulting in a lowered renal threshold for bicarbonate reabsorption.
    2. Evaluation and diagnosis
      a. Patients often present with failure to thrive, vomiting, and bone disease.
      b. Venous blood gases (VBG) and serum electrolytes reveal a hyperchloremic acidosis with low potassium.
      c. Urine pH varies with the degree of acidemia. Urine pH can be less than 5.5 with marked acidosis (serum $NaHCO_3 < 16–18$). Urine pH is inappropriately high in mild to moderate acidemia (serum $NaHCO_3 = 18–22$).
      d. Children with proximal RTA who also have phosphaturia, glycosuria, and aminoaciduria should be evaluated for Fanconi's syndrome.
    3. Treatment. Large doses of base (10–25 mEq/kg/day) are required to maintain the serum pH. Sodium bicarbonate tablets contain 4 to 8 mEq bicarbonate each. A bicarbonate solution can be made up, but has a short shelf life. Baking soda, which contains 44 mEq bicarbonate per teaspoon, can be added to food or formula, but is not very palatable. Citrate solutions are generally well tolerated and include Polycitra (1 mEq potassium citrate and 1 mEq sodium citrate per ml), Polycitra-K (2 mEq potassium citrate per ml), and Bicitra (1 mEq sodium citrate per ml). One mEq citrate is equivalent to 1 mEq bicarbonate. In primary proximal RTA, some patients may outgrow their bicarbonate requirement. This is often easiest to determine by allowing the child to outgrow his or her dose.
  B. Distal renal tubular acidosis (type I RTA)
    1. Etiology. A defect in the distal tubule results in an inability to excrete acid.
    2. Evaluation and diagnosis
      a. The presenting symptoms are usually growth failure, polyuria, and polydipsia.
      b. Venous blood gases and serum electrolytes reveal a hyperchloremic acidosis, with hypokalemia seen in a number of patients.
      c. The urine pH is rarely below 6.5, even in the face of severe acidemia.
      d. Urinary concentrating ability is frequently impaired.
      e. Nephrocalcinosis may be present due to increased urinary calcium excretion and decreased urinary citrate.
      f. Ammonium chloride loading test. To distinguish proximal from distal RTA, an ammonium chloride loading test can be done (Table 9-4). Ammonium chloride (75 mEq/m²) is administered PO followed by serial measurement of the urine pH, titratable acidity, and ammonium excretion. Concomitant blood pH and carbon dioxide should be checked hourly for 5 hours. The serum HCO_3 concentration should fall to 17 mEq/liter or less. If it does not, a larger dose of ammonium chloride (150 mEq/m²) should be given cautiously on a second test day. A **diagnosis** of distal RTA is confirmed by an inability to acidify the urine below 6.5, with depressed excretion rates of titratable acid and ammonium in the context of marked acidemia.

Table 9-4. Ammonium chloride loading test (normal values)

Age*	Urine pH	Titratable acid (μEq/min/1.73 m²)	Ammonium excretion (μEq/min/1.73 m²)
1–12 mo	5.0	62 (43–111)	56 (42–79)
4–15 yr	5.5	52 (33–71)	73 (46–100)

*Although current data are sparse, normal values for ages 1–4 years appear to approximate those of older children.
Source: Adapted from C Edelmann et al. *Pediatr Res* 1:452, 1967; *J Clin Invest* 46:1309, 1967.

3. Treatment

a. Bicarbonate or citrate in daily doses of 5 to 10 mEq/kg will correct the acidosis, minimize the risk of nephrocalcinosis, improve growth, and normalize the GFR.

b. There is no indication at present that children will recover spontaneously from distal tubular acidosis, and treatment must be continued for life.

c. The dosage of bicarbonate or citrate should be adjusted according to the blood pH. Daily urine calcium excretion should be kept below 2 mg/kg. Plasma potassium must be monitored. Some patients require all their bicarbonate as potassium bicarbonate.

C. Type IV RTA

1. Etiology. In this disorder, the aldosterone-mediated mechanisms for distal tubule acidification are defective. Thus, patients will have acidosis and hyperkalemia.

2. Evaluation and diagnosis

a. History includes significant urologic abnormalities or recurrent urinary tract infections.

b. Blood gases and serum electrolytes reveal a hyperchloremic acidosis, with **hyper**kalemia and hyponatremia.

c. The urine pH is usually less than 5.5 with severe acidemia.

d. In these patients, a careful urologic evaluation is indicated.

3. Treatment

a. Sodium chloride supplementation, potassium restriction, and/or furosemide (Lasix) treatment are frequently efficacious. Bicarbonate supplementation may be needed.

b. While surgery to correct urologic abnormalities and treatment of urinary infections should be pursued, the associated type IV RTA is usually not reversible.

VIII. Acute renal failure (ARF)

A. Prenal failure. All patients with apparent ARF must be assessed for a prerenal cause.

1. Etiology. Dehydration, hypovolemia, or hemodynamic factors can compromise renal perfusion and intrarenal blood flow.

2. Evaluation

a. Review the history and physical findings for evidence of volume depletion, episodes of hypotension or shock, decreased intravascular volume, and/or decreased cardiac output.

b. Measure the blood pressure and central venous pressure (CVP), if available.

3. The **diagnosis** of prerenal failure is suggested by

a. Urinary sodium less than 15 mEq/liter, fractional sodium excretion (FE_{Na}) less than 1.0 (FE_{Na} = urine/P_{Na} divided by U/P_{Cr} × 100).

b. Increased urine output in response to rehydration or increased intravascular volume, or both.

c. Improved renal function with improved cardiac function.

4. Treatment. Treatment is aimed at restoring renal blood flow and function.

a. Reestablish an effective circulating blood volume. In some patients, CVP monitoring is useful.

b. If, after restoration of extracellular fluid (ECF) volume, oliguria or anuria persists, fluid management should include insensible losses plus output replacement.

B. Intrinsic renal failure

1. Etiology. Renal parenchymal injury can result from a variety of causes. A history of severe and/or prolonged decreased renal perfusion suggests ARF due to ATN. Acute renal failure may be associated with acute glomerulonephritis, hemolytic-uremic syndrome, accelerated hypertension, uric acid nephropathy, exposure to nephrotoxic agents, or vasculitis.

2. Evaluation and diagnosis. First, assess the patient for prerenal or postrenal causes of ARF.

a. Stabilize the patient's condition **before** any invasive diagnostic procedures are performed.
b. Review history and laboratory evaluations for evidence of multisystem involvement (e.g., vasculitis, HUS).
c. Evaluate urinalysis for evidence of glomerular involvement (e.g., RBC casts).
d. Clarify nature of renal dysfunction.
   (1) Urinary sodium concentration less than 40, FE_{Na} greater than 2 if oligoanuria is present.
   (2) A radionuclide renal scan can be useful in assessing renal perfusion and function as well as in distinguishing intrinsic renal failure from cortical necrosis. Abdominal ultrasound is helpful in ruling out obstruction and shows characteristic patterns in chronic renal damage.
3. **Treatment**
   a. The use of an indwelling catheter **should be discontinued** as soon as possible in a severely oligoanuric patient in whom intrinsic renal failure is established.
   b. Weigh the patient bid (or use a metabolic bed with a scale).
   c. Measure intake and output.
   d. **Fluid management**
      (1) Fluid and electrolyte replacement should be calculated as insensible losses (400 ml/m^2/day) plus urine output and other losses.
      (2) Give as many calories as possible, orally if practical. A peripheral IV line can tolerate 10 to 15% glucose; a central line can tolerate up to 30% glucose.
      (3) When diuresis begins, increasing urine volume must be replaced with a solution containing approximately the same electrolytes as are being excreted. Therefore, it is helpful to follow urine sodium. If the patient has been hyperkalemic, **do not replace potassium until the serum potassium has returned to normal.**
   e. **Hyperkalemia**
      (1) If the serum potassium is 5.5 to 7.0 mEq/liter, sodium polystyrene sulfonate (Kayexalate) in sorbitol at a dose of 1 g/kg can be given PO or PR and repeated q4–6h until potassium is lowered. **Warning: 1 mEq sodium enters the body for each mEq potassium that is removed. Over time, hypernatremia can result.**
      (2) If the serum potassium is above 7 mEq/liter or if ECG changes are present (peaked T waves, widening of QRS complex, flattened P waves), or both, one or both of the following therapies are indicated immediately. Monitor the patient's ECG.
         (a) Give 10% calcium gluconate, 0.5 to 1.0 ml/kg IV over 5 to 10 minutes, with ECG monitoring. Calcium will decrease the cardiac sensitivity to the hyperkalemia.
         (b) Give sodium bicarbonate, 2 mEq/kg, as an IV push over 5 to 10 minutes. This will drive potassium into cells and decrease serum potassium without changing the total body load.
      (3) If hyperkalemia persists, administer insulin, 0.1 unit/kg IV with 25% glucose as 0.5 g/kg (2 ml/kg) over 30 minutes. This dosage can be repeated in 30 to 60 minutes if necessary. Monitor blood sugar. This approach will also drive potassium into cells and decrease serum potassium without changing the total body load. Prepare to dialyze the patient.
      (4) Acute dialysis is usually necessary if the potassium is above 7.5 mEq/liter, if the measures in **(2)** fail, or if **(3)** is needed.
   f. **Acidosis** can usually be alleviated by providing glucose for calories as well as 1 to 3 mEq/kg/day exogenous bicarbonate, citrate, or lactate. If the acidosis is severe and not adequately treated with base supplement or treatment is difficult due to fluid overload, dialysis is indicated.

g. Nutrition. The provision of optimal calories will help to decrease catabolism, lower BUN, and ameliorate the uremic state. With restricted fluids, limited calories can be given by a peripheral IV line.

(1) If the patient can take POs, optimize the calories of dietary solids and increase the caloric density of fluids with glucose polymers (Polycose). Many patients require more than the recommended daily allowance (RDA) for their height age to suppress catabolism. Appetite may be poor during an acute illness and often a combination of oral and IV nutrition is needed.

(2) If the patient will be NPO or cannot take enough calories orally, consider total parenteral nutrition.

h. Hypertension. If hypertension is acute and severe (greater than the 95th percentile for age), treat as outlined for hypertensive emergencies on p. 300. **Note:** In acute renal failure:

(1) Antihypertensive agents with rapid onset of action should be selected.

(2) Hemodialysis is indicated when hypertension is severe, related to fluid overload, and unresponsive to medical management.

i. Congestive heart failure

(1) Congestive heart failure can usually be prevented by proper **fluid restriction.**

(2) There is no place for diuretics in the anuric patient.

(3) Digitalis will not produce a dramatic effect. If CHF is severe, dialysis is indicated.

j. Drug therapy. Adjust the dosage or intervals of dosing of all drugs metabolized or excreted by the kidney.

k. Indications for dialysis

(1) Volume overload with severe hypertension or CHF.

(2) Hyperkalemia refractory to medical management.

(3) Severe acidosis refractory to medical management.

(4) Symptomatic uremia or rapidly rising BUN, Cr.

(5) Support for parenteral nutrition.

C. Postrenal failure

1. Etiology. Obstruction is usually due to congenital anomalies, urethral valves or stricture, hematuria with clots, tumor compression, or retroperitoneal fibrosis.

2. Evaluation and diagnosis. Obstruction is suggested by a history of genitourinary abnormalities, or lower abdominal trauma, or by the finding of flank masses or an enlarged bladder. Bilateral ureteral obstruction is suggested by absolute anuria. If a Foley catheter has been in place, obstruction of Foley can occur.

a. Check Foley catheter for patency and flush if obstructed.

b. Perform a renal ultrasound and a radionuclide scan.

c. Urologic consultation should be obtained.

3. Treatment consists of surgical correction or bypass, as required. Medical management as outlined in **B** above may also be needed.

IX. Uric acid nephropathy

A. Etiology. Uric acid nephropathy may be associated with the following:

1. Malignancies, especially leukemias and lymphomas **due to the large tumor burden and rapid cell turnover.** Uric acid nephropathy is a particular risk during induction chemotherapy.

2. Regional enteritis, due to increased intestinal absorption of uric acid.

B. Evaluation

1. Determine **uric acid levels** in all children with malignancies, especially before and during chemotherapy therapy. Measure uric acid levels in patients with regional enteritis.

2. Measure **renal function** in all at-risk patients. If acute renal failure is developing, evaluate as in sec. **VIII,** p. 307.

C. Treatment. The prevention of renal failure is the most important aspect of therapy.

1. Begin **allopurinol,** 10 mg/kg/day in three to four divided doses, in all children about to undergo massive cytoreductive therapy.
2. **Force fluids** to two to three times maintenance.
3. **Alkalinize the urine,** so that its pH is above 7.0, with IV sodium bicarbonate. Start with 1 to 2 mEq/kg/day and increase as needed. (Uric acid is more soluble in alkaline urine.)
4. If oliguria or anuria develops, **hemodialysis** is indicated.

X. Chronic renal failure (CRF) is an uncommon problem in childhood with an estimated incidence of 1 to 3 per million population less than 16 years of age.

A. Etiology
1. Approximately half have congenital lesions: obstructive uropathy, renal dysplasia, juvenile nephronophthisis, or polycystic kidney disease.
2. About a third of cases are due to glomerulopathy.
3. Chronic pyelonephritis leading to CRF occurs primarily in the presence of an obstructive congenital lesion or marked vesicoureteral reflux.
4. Other causes include hemolytic-uremic syndrome, malignant hypertension, interstitial nephritis, renal vein thrombosis, and nephrectomy for malignancy.

B. General therapeutic measures
1. **Water and salt balance** (see Chap. 4, pp. 70ff)
   a. **Fluid.** The aim is to replace insensible losses and urine output. For the patient with little or no urine output, a daily fluid restriction is necessary.
   b. **Sodium**
      (1) To avoid arterial hypertension, sodium intake should be limited except in patients with significant renal sodium wasting. A "no-added-salt" diet is usually sufficient, as it provides 40 to 90 mEq sodium per day (2 to 4 g sodium).
      (2) If salt wasting occurs, free salt intake may be necessary. Daily requirements are estimated by monitoring the patient's volume status (weight, blood pressure, and peripheral edema) and the urinary sodium excretion.
2. **Potassium** (see Chap. 4, p. 64)
   a. **Hyperkalemia.** Conditions that usually lead to hyperkalemia include
      (1) The onset of severe renal failure or sudden oliguria due to vomiting or diarrhea, or both, or to gastrointestinal bleeding.
      (2) The administration of aldosterone antagonists (spironolactone) or angiotensin-converting enzyme (ACE) inhibitors (captopril, enalapril) in selected patients.
      (3) **Massive hemolysis or tissue destruction.**
   b. **Treatment.** Serum potassium levels below 5.8 mEq/liter are usually well handled by further restrictions in potassium intake, using the following guidelines.
      (1) **Fruits high in potassium:** bananas, oranges (citrus), cantaloupe, apricots, raisins, prunes, and tomatoes.
      (2) **Vegetables high in potassium:** dark green leafy vegetables, potatoes, avocado, artichoke, lentils, beets, winter squash, and broccoli. Since cooking leaches out potassium, these vegetables should be cooked.
      (3) **Meats and fish.**
      (4) **Some breads and flours.**
      (5) **Miscellaneous foods high in potassium:** chocolate, cocoa, molasses, nuts, and dried beans. If serum levels are chronically above 5.8 mEq/liter, treatment with an exchange resin may be indicated to remove potassium from the body, and dialysis should be considered.
3. **Nutrition.** Growth failure can be marked with decreased GFR, but may be improved by appropriate dietary management.
   a. **Calories.** Chronic renal failure is complicated at some point by anorexia. This results in insufficient caloric intake and contributes to growth failure. A minimum caloric goal is 80% of the RDA. The RDA for height age is sufficient to determine the total calories and protein required. Sufficient non-

protein calories are needed to allow for protein sparing and to create an anabolic state. For infants, the appropriate caloric intake can be provided by supplementing proprietary formulas with carbohydrates and fats. Many infants will require nasogastric feedings to take in sufficient calories.

4. **Mineral metabolism in renal disease.** Secondary hyperparathyroidism and metabolic bone disease occur in renal insufficiency (GFR <25% of normal) unless vigorous measures are taken. The increase in the parathyroid hormone (PTH) is due to decreased renal phosphate excretion, decreased renal 1-alpha hydroxylation of 25-hydroxy vitamin D, and the resultant decrease in intestinal calcium absorption.

   a. **Hyperphosphatemia.** If the serum phosphate level is over 5 mEq/liter, or if alkaline phosphate is elevated, dietary phosphate must be restricted and oral phosphate binders administered. Once phosphate is normalized, vitamin D (as D_3 analogues or dihydrotachysterol) therapy should begin. Because of evidence that aluminum accumulation can cause osteomalacia and CNS problems in patients with CRF, aluminum-containing preparations are not recommended as oral phosphate binders. Similarly, because of the risk of hypermagnesemia, magnesium-containing preparations are not recommended. **Only calcium-containing preparations should be used as oral phosphate binders** (Table 9-5). Phosphate binders must be given with or just after all meals and snacks to bind the phosphate in the diet; otherwise, they are ineffective. Phosphate-containing enemas (Fleet) should be avoided.

   b. **Calcium balance.** In general, good control of serum phosphorus levels should precede the administration of supplemental calcium, but seizures or other complications make immediate treatment with calcium unavoidable (see also Chap. 4, p. 65).

      (1) **Hypocalcemia**
         (a) **Acute replacement** is needed only if the patient is symptomatic, that is, has hypocalcemic seizures, ECG changes, or tetany. Then 10 to 15 mg elemental calcium/kg is given IV q4h as 10% calcium gluconate. The correcting effects last only a few hours, and a new infusion or further PO administration is required.
         (b) **Oral preparations.** See Table 9-5 for the elemental calcium content of various oral calcium preparations. Therapy should be designed to provide the minimal allowance of 500 to 1,000 mg elemental calcium per day.

      (2) **Hypercalcemia.** Although hypercalcemia is not common in renal disease, it is a possible complication of the use of vitamin D, severe secondary hyperparathyroidism, prolonged immobilization, and supra-

Table 9-5. Phosphate binders

Trade name	Form	Elemental calcium	Active ingredients
Os-Cal*	500-mg tablet (chewable)	500 mg	Calcium carbonate
Phos-Ex	167-mg tablet	167 mg	Calcium acetate
	250-mg tablet	250 mg	
Phos-Lo	Tablet	169 mg	Calcium acetate
Titralac	Suspension	200 mg/5 ml	Calcium carbonate
Tums*	Regular tablet	200 mg	Calcium carbonate
	Extra strength	300 mg	
	Suspension	400 mg/5 ml	

*Nonprescription.
Source: Courtesy of Nancy Spinozzi, RD, Renal Nutritionist, The Children's Hospital, Boston, MA.

physiologic calcium concentration in dialysate. Clinical features of hypercalcemia include lethargy, confusion, headache, hyporeflexia, muscle weakness, ECG changes (decreased QTc interval), bradycardia, constipation, extraosseous calcifications, and nausea. If acute hypercalcemia occurs and immediate treatment is necessary, the following measures should be carried out.

(a) **Reduce calcium intake.** Discontinue the administration of vitamin D in any form (as in multivitamins). Review the patient's medications and diet.

(b) **Decrease the absorption of calcium.** Decrease gut absorption by administration of corticosteroids (prednisone, 1–2 mg/kg/day). This strategy requires days for optimal effect.

(c) **Hemodialysis** can be used to control severe hypercalcemia.

c. **Vitamin D.** The use of vitamin D preparations is recommended to improve intestinal calcium absorption and decrease PTH secretion, which will both decrease hyperparathyroid bone disease and the inappropriate hypertrophy of the parathyroid gland.

(1) 1,25-Dihydroxycholecalciferol (1,25-dihydroxy-vitamin D, calcitriol [Rocaltrol]) is recommended. The initial dosage is 0.15 μg/kg body weight per day; the exact dose required for metabolic control must be determined for each child. Follow-up should include following serum calcium and phosphate levels, alkaline phosphatase, and serum PTH. The advantage of calcitriol is its short half-life, with pharmacologic activity lasting 3 to 5 days per dose.

(2) Dihydrotachysterol. Initial dose should be conservative (0.10 mg/kg/day). The half-life is 2 to 3 weeks.

5. **Anemia in CRF.** In most children with CRF, anemia will develop by the time the GFR is reduced to 20% of normal. This is due to blood losses and the resultant iron deficiency and deficient erythropoietin synthesis by the kidney. **Recombinant human erythropoietin** is now widely administered to patients with CRF.

a. **Iron supplementation.** Iron stores should be regularly assessed by measurement of iron, total iron-binding capacity (TIBC), and ferritin. Iron supplementation with 2 to 6 mg/kg/day (elemental iron) should be initiated if the iron/TIBC is less than 20%.

b. **Recombinant human erythropoietin treatment** should be considered in children who require erythrocyte transfusions or are symptomatic with anemia. A typical starting dosage is 50 units/kg three times a week. The dose is administered subcutaneously to children who do not yet require dialysis or are receiving peritoneal dialysis and intravenously to children on hemodialysis. Erythropoietin must be used with care, in consultation with a physician experienced in its use.

6. **Growth retardation** is a significant problem for children with CRF.

a. **Nutrition and metabolic status.** Dietary intake must be optimized (see sec. **B.3,** p. 310 above). Metabolic abnormalities, including acidosis, hypocalcemia, and hyperphosphatemia must be adequately treated. Thyroid insufficiency should be ruled out (especially in cystinosis).

b. **Recombinant human growth hormone** treatment should be considered in children with adequate nutrition who are growing at a subnormal rate for age. The initial dose is 0.05 mg/kg administered subcutaneously each day. In addition to monitoring growth, careful attention should be paid to calcium and phosphate metabolism during treatment.

7. **Medications.** Water-soluble vitamins, most notably B vitamins and folate, are lost during dialysis and must be replaced. Daily administration of standard multivitamin tablets or equivalent liquid preparations with additional folate (1 mg/day) covers the basic requirements. Dosages of drugs excreted by kidneys must be adjusted.

8. **Hypertension** (see p. 298).

9. **Dialysis therapy.** There is no absolute level of urea nitrogen or creatinine at which renal replacement therapy, dialysis, or transplantation is indicated. Treatment should be initiated when subtle symptoms of uremia, such as weight loss, anorexia, or increasing fatigue, are present. In some cases dialysis is necessary to avoid overhydration and provide sufficient calories. Both hemodialysis and peritoneal dialysis are effective in children; however, the latter is technically easier in infants and small children. The choice of dialysis modality should be based on the preferences of the child and family, as there are lifestyle differences with the two types.

   a. **Peritoneal dialysis.** There are two types of peritoneal dialysis: continuous ambulatory peritoneal dialysis (CAPD) and continuous cycling peritoneal dialysis (CCPD). **CAPD,** the form of peritoneal dialysis in which the patient is dialyzed continually at a slow rate, offers the convenience of multiple exchanges throughout the day at home and at school. Episodes of peritonitis are a major complication. A variation of CAPD, **CCPD** is also available. In CCPD, overnight cycling of dialysis fluid is performed automatically by a machine and peritoneal infections tend to occur less frequently than in CAPD. CCPD requires hookup to the cycler for 12 hours at night. **Complications in peritoneal dialysis:**

   (1) **Infection** is usually due to **staphylococcus and gram-negative organisms.** Treatment should be initiated in a symptomatic patient even if culture results are not available. Intraperitoneal antibiotics are used. Systemic antimicrobial treatment and catheter removal are required for some infections, for example, fungal and *Pseudomonas.*

   (2) Skin breakdown can occur around the catheter exit or tunnel site. Umbilical, ventral, and inguinal hernias can develop.

   (3) **Hypoproteinemia** can occur as a result of protein losses in dialysis.

   b. **Hemodialysis** for childhood acute or chronic renal failure is practical. Even small infants and neonates can be dialyzed without difficulty by experienced personnel. It is more efficient than peritoneal dialysis, permitting control of both clearance and ultrafiltration within narrow limits. Vascular access is necessary. A catheter placed in the femoral or subclavian vein is sufficient for a temporary access in older children. Permanent access consists of a surgically created connection between an artery and vein (fistula). Children have been maintained on hemodialysis for years. Appropriate consultation and referral should be made.

10. **Transplantation** is preferable to chronic dialysis for most children with CRF. Any child with CRF should be considered a transplant candidate. Though transplantation cannot be regarded as curative, long-term survival is the rule and transplantation offers the optimal chance for rehabilitation from CRF. Referral should be made to a transplantation center.

XI. **Renal vein thrombosis (RVT).** Thrombosis within the intrarenal veins can occur in one or both kidneys as an acute, potentially life-threatening event. The process rarely begins in a main renal vein. Most patients are less than 1 year of age (90%), and 75% are under 1 month of age.

A. **Etiology.** The slow dual capillary circulation of the kidney is particularly vulnerable to thrombosis. The risk of RVT is heightened in the presence of hypoperfusion, hemoconcentration, hypercoagulability (e.g., in nephrotic syndrome with coagulation protein defects), or hyperosmolality. In the neonate, associated conditions include perinatal hypoxia, sepsis, prematurity, maternal diabetes mellitus, and maternal thiazide usage.

B. **Evaluation.** In any sick infant with compromised circulation, the clinician must be vigilant for RVT. Newborns often present with the classic constellation of hematuria (gross or microscopic), flank mass(es), anemia, and thrombocytopenia. A CBC and coagulation studies are indicated. Renal ultrasound and radionuclide studies can support the diagnosis of RVT without using contrast agents.

C. **Diagnosis** is suggested by positive findings during the above evaluation. The differential diagnosis includes that for flank masses (e.g., hydronephrosis, cystic kidneys, renal or adrenal tumors), vascular lesions (e.g., ATN, cortical or medullary necrosis, arterial thrombosis, HUS, adrenal hemorrhage), and infection.

D. Treatment

1. Treat supportively for intravascular coagulopathy; the utility of heparin or other anticoagulants is unproven. Thrombectomy even with bilateral RVT or caval thrombosis is controversial.
2. Treat acute renal failure if present.
3. Treat associated hypertension.

E. Prognosis. In several series, 30 to 40% survival is reported. Long-term sequelae can vary from clinical health with residual evidence of renal parenchymal loss to frank renal failure. Chronic hypertension may result.

XII. Congenital abnormalities of the kidney. Renal developmental abnormalities are diverse in their structural manifestations, physiologic consequences, and clinical findings. They may be characterized by renal maldevelopment, renal cyst formation, or both renal maldevelopment and cyst formation. Many patients present with abnormalities on renal ultrasound, such as cysts and abnormal echogenicity (Table 9-6).

A. Evaluation and diagnosis

1. Assess the patient for associated systemic abnormalities.
2. Assess renal function with BUN, creatinine.
3. Anatomic studies are indicated to define the abnormality and to determine if it is unilateral or bilateral.
   a. Ultrasound and radionuclide scan.

Table 9-6. Etiologic basis for renal ultrasound findings in the infant

Ultrasound finding	Renal abnormality	Additional abnormalities
Enlarged, echogenic kidneys	Cystic kidney disease (ARPKD, ADPKD, glomerulocystic disease) Multicystic kidneys Congenital nephrosis Obstruction Tumor Renal vein thrombosis Acute tubular necrosis, pyelonephritis Glycogen storage disease	ARPKD: occasional macrocysts, liver echogenic, intrahepatic biliary dilatation, may have hepatomegaly, splenomegaly
Renal parenchymal cysts	ARPKD ADPKD Glomerulocystic disease Hereditary syndromes, e.g., tuberous sclerosis Renal medullary cysts Simple renal cysts Cystic dysplasia	ADPKD: may have cysts in liver, pancreas, ovary, spleen; 4–5% of affected 30 yr old without renal cysts
Renal pelvic dilatation	Posterior urethral valves Ureteropelvic junction Obstruction Extrarenal pelvis Severe vesico-ureteral reflux Neurogenic bladder	

ADPKD = autosomal dominant polycystic kidney disease; ARPKD = autosomal recessive polycystic kidney disease.

b. Voiding cystourethrogram.

4. Consider early family counseling regarding genetics, end-stage renal disease (ESRD).

B. Treatment. For anomalies not associated with obstruction, factors known to hasten the decline in renal function (e.g., hypertension, urinary tract infection) should be minimized. With urinary tract obstructions, correction by a pediatric urologist or pediatric surgeon is critical. In general, conservative management of renal function or tubular impairment, or both, will permit the patient the best growth and development. Vigilance against urosepsis is important.

C. Prognosis: depends on the severity of the lesion, the prospect of surgical correction, and the reversibility of the associated renal damage.

10

Cardiac Disorders

Edward P. Walsh

I. Congenital heart disease

A. General principles

1. The major clinical signs/symptoms of congenital heart disease include cyanosis, cardiac murmur, and/or congestive heart failure (CHF). The specific lesions are extremely varied, and will often require consultation with a cardiologist for definitive diagnosis.
2. The most common congenital heart defects are listed in Table 10-1, arranged in order of prevalence.
3. Suspected congenital heart disease in the **neonate** requires prompt and aggressive evaluation. See Chapter 6 for detailed discussion.
4. Diagnostic evaluation for structural heart disease begins with history and physical examination, and includes chest x-ray, electrocardiogram, and measurement of transcutaneous oxygen saturation. Detailed testing includes echocardiogram and possible cardiac catheterization.
5. Definitive therapy for major cardiac malformations typically requires cardiac surgery. A growing number of lesions are now being corrected with interventional catheterization procedures, including patent ductus closure, atrioseptal defect closure, and relief of pulmonary-aortic-mitral stenosis.

II. Acquired heart disease

A. Myocarditis

1. **Etiology.** Infectious myocarditis is a potential cause of acute congestive cardiomyopathy and may be due to a variety of infectious agents with the exception of fungi. Myocardial damage is effected by either invasion of the myocardium (e.g., echoviruses or Coxsackie viruses), production of a myocardial toxin (e.g., diphtheria), or autoimmune mechanisms (e.g., rheumatic fever). In North America, the most common etiologic agents are viruses. Myocarditis can be either acute or chronic.
2. **Evaluation and diagnosis.** The clinical presentation ranges from asymptomatic to fulminant CHF, depending on severity.
   a. **Symptoms** include fatigue, dyspnea, palpitations, and chest pain (usually secondary to associated pericarditis). **Signs** include tachycardia, murmurs or gallops, and clinical evidence of CHF in severe cases.
   b. The **ECG** often shows S-T and T-wave changes, arrhythmias, conduction defects, and occasionally a pattern of reduced ventricular voltages.
   c. On **chest x-ray,** heart size ranges from normal to markedly enlarged.
   d. **Echocardiography** reveals dilated or hypocontractile ventricles, or both. Pericardial effusion may be present.
   e. **Infectious** etiology should be evaluated by appropriate cultures, including (for viruses) viral cultures of throat washings, blood, feces, and pericardial fluid, as well as by acute and convalescent sera.
   f. **Endomyocardial biopsy** and cardiac catheterization are performed in many cases to confirm diagnosis.
3. **Treatment**
   a. Treatment of infectious myocarditis begins with supportive measures, including treatment of CHF and maintenance of adequate oxygenation.

Table 10-1. Classic findings for the 10 most common congenital heart lesions

Lesion	Presentation	Physical examination	ECG	X-ray
Ventricular septal defect	Murmur, CHF	Pansystolic murmur	LVH, RVH	+CE, ↑PBF
Pulmonic stenosis	Murmur, ±cyanosis	Click, SEM	RVH	±CE, NL or ↓PBF
Tetralogy of Fallot	Murmur, cyanosis	SEM	RVH	±CE, ↓PBF
Aortic stenosis	Murmur, ±CHF	Click, SEM	LVH	±CE, NL PBF
Atrioseptal defect	Murmur	Fixed split S_2	Mild RVH	±CE, ↑PBF
Patent ductus	Murmur, ±CHF	Continuous murmur	LVH, ±RVH	±CE, ↑PBF
Coarctation of aorta	Hypertension	↓ Femoral pulses	LVH	±CE, NL PBF
Transposition	Cyanosis	Marked cyanosis	RVH	±CE, NL or ↑PBF
AV canal defect	Murmur, ±CHF	Pansystolic murmur	"Superior" axis	±CE, ↑PBF
Single ventricle	(Variable)	(Variable)	(Variable)	(Variable)

CE = cardiac enlargement; CHF = congestive heart failure; LVH = left ventricular hypertrophy; NL = normal; PBF = pulmonary blood flow; RVH = right ventricular hypertrophy; SEM = systolic ejection murmur; AV = atrioventricular.

    b. Monitoring and treatment, preferably in an intensive care unit, should be provided for arrhythmias, conduction abnormalities, and CHF.
    c. Since patients with myocarditis may be abnormally sensitive to digitalis glycosides, **digoxin should be administered cautiously.**
    d. Patients should remain at bed rest during the acute phase of their illness.
    e. **Corticosteroids are currently believed to be contraindicated in the acute phase of viral myocarditis.**
    f. Immunoglobulin G (IgG) therapy for viral myocarditis is now being used at some centers for acute treatment, on an investigational protocol.
B. Pericarditis (see also Chap. 5, p. 115)
    1. Etiology
        a. Bacterial. Bacterial pericarditis can occur by hematogenous or contiguous spread. The most common causative organisms are staphylococci, pneumococci, *Haemophilus influenzae*, meningococci, streptococci, and *Mycobacterium tuberculosis*.
        b. Viral. Viral pericarditis is often preceded by a history of upper respiratory tract infection and occurs as part of the spectrum of viral myopericarditis. The most common causative agents are Coxsackie virus, echovirus, adenovirus, influenza virus, mumps virus, varicella-zoster virus, vaccinia, or Epstein-Barr virus.
        c. Noninfectious causes include postoperative sterile inflammation after cardiac operations, collagen diseases, uremic fibrinous pericarditis, radiation-induced pericarditis, and malignant pericardial effusion.
    2. Evaluation and diagnosis
        a. Presenting clinical signs and symptoms depend on the etiology and presence or absence of tamponade. One sign of significant fluid collection is "pulsus paradoxus" of the systolic blood pressure. A "rub" may be present on auscultation.
        b. The **ECG** is characterized by diffuse S-T and T-wave abnormalities. The

QRS voltages may be decreased, and sometimes exhibit oscillation in amplitude (QRS "alternans"). *Echocardiography* establishes the presence of fluid in the pericardial space and is the most useful test to confirm the diagnosis and follow the response to therapy.

   c. The **chest x-ray** often shows an increase in the size of the cardiac silhouette with normal pulmonary vascular markings; associated infection of the lung or pleural space may be evident.

   d. **Pericardiocentesis** for culture and examination of pericardial fluid should be performed in all patients who appear toxic, or have evidence of tamponade.

   e. Additional studies should be done as appropriate to define the specific systemic cause.

3. **Treatment** (see also Chap. 7, p. 233)

   a. **General measures** include bed rest, analgesia, and observation for and treatment of tamponade with prompt pericardiocentesis.

   b. **Specific therapy** should be directed toward the etiology. In acute purulent pericarditis, antibiotic therapy appropriate to the sensitivities of the causative organism should be combined with effective pericardial drainage (see Chap. 5).

C. **Subacute bacterial endocarditis** (see Chap. 5, p. 113).

D. **Rheumatic fever** (see Chap. 5, p. 111).

E. **Kawasaki's disease** (see Chap. 18, p. 448).

III. **Recognition of the innocent murmur.** The innocent murmur is one that occurs in the absence of either anatomic or physiologic abnormalities of the heart and lacks association with future cardiovascular disease. Innocent murmurs are audible in 60% of school-aged children.

A. **Clinical characteristics of innocent murmurs**

1. **General**

   a. Systolic in time and of short duration.

   b. Loudest along the left sternal border; transmission is usually not widespread; loudness may change with position but not respiration and is usually grade III/VI or less and increases with exercise.

   c. Other heart sounds are normal (importantly, there is a *normal* split of the second sound).

   d. Thrills are absent.

   e. The ECG and chest x-ray are normal.

2. **Specific**

   a. **Still's murmur** is usually grade I–III. It is a vibratory, buzzing, or musical systolic ejection murmur, loudest in the second to fifth left intercostal spaces and maximal in the supine position. It may intensify with exercise, excitement, and fever.

   b. **Pulmonic systolic murmur.** A grade I–III, high-pitched, systolic ejection murmur, usually peaking in the first half of systole. It is maximal in the second left intercostal spaces, radiating upward and to the left. It is best heard in the supine position and more apt to be heard in persons with narrow anteroposterior chest diameter.

   c. **Cardiorespiratory murmurs** are of extracardiac origin; usually located at the heart-lung margin. They are not well transmitted. Their variable loudness and timing are associated with cardiac and respiratory cycles, and they often disappear in expiration. Their incidence is associated with thoracic cage deformities, and pleural or pericardial adhesions.

   d. **Cervical venous hum.** This is a grade I–VI continuous murmur with diastolic accentuation and is maximal in the supraclavicular fossa lateral to the sternocleidomastoid muscle. It may radiate below the clavicle, where it may be confused with the murmur of patent ductus arteriosus. It is elicited by turning the patient's head away from the side of the murmur and elevating the chin while he or she is in a sitting position. It is abolished by recumbency, turning the head to the ipsilateral side of the murmur, or digital compression of the ipsilateral internal jugular vein.

e. **Supraclavicular arterial bruit.** This is a crescendo-decrescendo early systolic ejection murmur. It is maximal over the supraclavicular fossa and prominent in the suprasternal notch. It can generate a carotid thrill. Radiation is better to the neck than to below the clavicles. The murmur is accentuated by exercise and abolished or diminished by hyperextension of the shoulders.

B. **Specific diagnosis.** The innocent murmur should be distinguished from the following lesions.

1. **Mitral valve prolapse**
   a. **Clinical evaluation.** Most commonly, mitral valve prolapse is characterized by an isolated variable mid- to late systolic click or a midsystolic click followed by a late systolic murmur at left lower sternal border. Since the click in mitral valve prolapse is not always evident, auscultation should be carried out in four positions: supine, left decubitus, sitting, and standing. The click and murmur occur earlier with maneuvers that decrease left ventricular volume or increase left ventricular contractility (e.g., inspiration, standing, a Valsalva maneuver, isoproterenol, amyl nitrate inhalation), or both. Opposite maneuvers (e.g., squatting, propranolol, phenylephrine) delay the onset of the click and murmur. **Regurgitant murmurs become louder with maneuvers that raise arterial pressure and diminish with those that decrease it.**
   b. **Laboratory data**
      (1) In approximately one third of patients with mitral valve prolapse seen by cardiologists, the **ECG** shows T-wave inversion with or without minimal S-T segment depression, characteristically noted in leads II, III, and aVf, with frequent additional involvement of the left precordial leads.
      (2) A **chest x-ray** reveals a normal heart size in the absence of mitral insufficiency.
      (3) The **echocardiogram** is abnormal in approximately 80% of cases.
   c. **Complications.** Although the prognosis in patients with mitral valve prolapse is generally excellent, rare complications include progression of mitral insufficiency, bacterial endocarditis, cardiac arrhythmias, cerebral ischemic events, and sudden death. Antibiotic prophylaxis against infective endocarditis should be used in patients with late or pansystolic murmurs (see Table 5-4).
   d. **Treatment.** Generally, no treatment is indicated unless mitral regurgitation advances or symptomatic arrhythmias are present. Beta blockers seem to be effective for the rare patient with chest pain or arrhythmias, or both, associated with mitral valve prolapse.

2. **Idiopathic hypertrophic subaortic stenosis (IHSS).** Auscultation is characterized by a harsh midsystolic ejection murmur that is maximal between the apex and left sternal border. Frequently, there is a separate pansystolic regurgitant murmur maximal at the apex, caused by mitral regurgitation. The systolic ejection murmur is augmented by maneuvers that increase contractility, decrease preload, or decrease afterload, that is, Valsalva maneuvers, standing, postextrasystole, or exercise. Conversely, the murmur diminishes with squatting or isometric hand grip. When IHSS is suspected, refer to a cardiologist because of the risk of sudden death.

IV. **Congestive heart failure.** Congestive heart failure (CHF) is a clinical syndrome in which the heart is unable to supply an output sufficient to meet the metabolic requirements of the tissues.

A. **Etiology** includes
1. **Congenital** diseases of the heart, usually with large left-to-right shunts or obstructive lesions of the left or right ventricle.
2. **Acquired** diseases of the heart (see p. 316).
3. **Arrhythmias,** including supraventricular tachycardia, or complete heart block.
4. **Iatrogenic** causes, including damage to the heart at surgery (ventriculotomy), fluid overload, or doxorubicin (Adriamycin) therapy.

5. **Noncardiac causes,** such as thyrotoxicosis, systemic arteriovenous fistula, acute or chronic lung disease, glycogen storage disease, or connective tissue or neuromuscular disorders.
B. **Clinical manifestations** fall into three categories.
   1. **Impaired myocardial performance.** These include growth failure, sweating, cardiac enlargement, gallop rhythm, and alterations in peripheral pulses, including pulsus paradoxus and pulsus alternans. Patients may complain of easy fatigue, dyspnea, and dizziness.
   2. **Pulmonary congestion** includes tachypnea, dyspnea with effort, cough, rales, wheezing, and cyanosis.
   3. **Systemic venous congestion** includes hepatomegaly, neck vein distention, and peripheral edema.
C. **Treatment.** Whenever possible, the precipitating causes (e.g., arrhythmia) and underlying causes (e.g., structural abnormalities) of CHF should be removed. Control of CHF can be achieved by (1) *increasing cardiac contractile performance*, (2) *reducing cardiac workload*, and (3) *reducing the volume overload* responsible for congestive symptoms.
   1. **Increasing cardiac contractile performance**
      a. **Digitalis** therapy increases cardiac output by directly enhancing the myocardial contractile state. Guidelines for digoxin use are detailed in sec. **VII.B.**
      b. **Other cardiotonic agents.** When CHF is associated with hypotension or is refractory to other modes of therapy, additional inotropic support can be achieved with the following:
         (1) **Dopamine.** The usual therapeutic dosage is 5 to 20 μg/kg/min by continuous IV infusion. Therapy is begun at a low dose (2 μg/kg/min) and gradually increased until the desired effect is achieved. At low doses (<5 μg/kg/min), dopamine causes renal vasodilation. At higher doses (>10 μg/kg/min), dopamine may have the undesirable effects of increasing total peripheral resistance and heart rate.
         (2) **Dobutamine.** The usual therapeutic dosage is 5 to 20 μg/kg/min, but should be titrated by the patient's response.
         (3) **Amrinone** improves cardiac performance by combined effects on contractility and afterload. The usual dosage is a 1 to 3 mg/kg load followed by an infusion of 5 to 20 μg/kg/min.
   2. **Reducing cardiac workload**
      a. **General measures**
         (1) **Restriction of physical activity** and periods of **bed rest** reduce metabolic requirements in older children and adolescents. Activity restriction is usually counterproductive in young children.
         (2) **Cool, humidified oxygen** by tent, mask, or nasal prongs may be useful in hypoxic patients.
      b. **Afterload reduction.** Vasodilator therapy decreases peripheral resistance and ventricular filling pressures. Agents that alter arteriolar resistance have the greatest effect on cardiac index, while agents that increase venous capacitance reduce congestive symptoms caused by elevated ventricular filling pressures.
         (1) **Acute therapy: Sodium nitroprusside** affects both arteriolar resistance and venous capacitance, thus treating both low output and congestive symptoms. Continuous IV infusion is usually begun at 0.5 μg/kg/min and increased until the desired effect is achieved or until arterial pressure falls by 10%. The average dose is 3 μg/kg/min. Sodium nitroprusside should be administered in an intensive care unit setting with monitoring by an arterial line. *Thiocyanate levels should be measured when the drug is used for an extended period.*
         (2) **Long-term maintenance: captopril and enalapril** are angiotensin converting enzyme inhibitors that block production of angiotensin II. They are "balanced" vasodilators with actions on both the arteriolar and venous beds. Dosages for captopril range from 0.5 to 3.0 mg/kg/day,

in three divided doses. Enalapril is generally used at a dosage of 2 to 10 mg bid.

3. Reducing volume overload

a. Sodium restriction. No-added-salt diets are used in children. Infants should receive a high-calorie, low-sodium formula.

b. Fluid restriction is necessary only when dilutional hyponatremia complicates far-advanced CHF. Formula intake should **not** be restricted in infants.

c. Diuretics. The effectiveness of a diuretic is dependent on renal perfusion, serum electrolytes, and acid-base balance. In the presence of shock or acute renal failure, diuretics will have little effect. Diuretic agents can cause profound changes in electrolyte composition, and therefore frequent electrolyte evaluations should be made. **Potassium depletion, especially in the digitalized patient, is dangerous and can be lethal.** The characteristics of commonly used diuretics are given in Table 10-2.

  (1) Thiazides are sulfonamide derivatives that share moderate potency and low toxicity. Those most commonly used in pediatrics are chlorothiazide (Diuril) and hydrochlorothiazide (HydroDIURIL).

    (a) Mechanism. The thiazide diuretics inhibit resorption of sodium and chloride at the cortical diluting site of the ascending loop of Henle and the early distal convoluted tubule.

    (b) Route of administration, absorption, and metabolism. The thiazides are rapidly absorbed from the GI tract and begin to have a diuretic effect within 1 hour. The duration of action of chlorothiazide is about 6 to 12 hours, while that of hydrochlorothiazide is 12 hours or more. Excretion is via the kidney, with some subsequent resorption.

    (c) Dosage. Give chlorothiazide, 20 to 30 mg/kg/day PO, in two divided doses, or give hydrochlorothiazide, 2 to 3 mg/kg/day PO, in two divided doses.

    (d) Toxicity

      (i) Potassium depletion can occur with long-term use. Alternate-day therapy, intake of foods high in potassium, administration of liquid potassium, or the addition of a potassium-sparing diuretic such as spironolactone can protect against potassium depletion. However, periodic measurements of serum potassium are necessary, especially early in therapy.

      (ii) Allergic reactions and side effects, such as thrombocytopenia, leukopenia, or vasculitis, are rarely seen. **Hyperglycemia** and **aggravation of preexisting diabetes or hyperuricemia** can occur.

  (2) Furosemide (Lasix). This loop diuretic should be used with careful observation of electrolytes, especially serum potassium.

    (a) Mechanism. Furosemide inhibits active chloride transport in the ascending limb of the loop of Henle, where 25% of sodium resorption occurs.

    (b) Route of administration, absorption, and metabolism

      (i) Lasix is well absorbed PO or can be given IV.

      (ii) When given PO, effects can be expected within 30 to 60 minutes. The onset of action after parenteral administration is within 5 minutes.

      (iii) The duration of action for the parenteral dose is 2 to 3 hours, and 6 to 8 hours for the PO dose.

      (iv) Both drugs are bound to plasma protein, with approximately two-thirds excreted by the kidney.

    (c) Dosage. Furosemide can be given as 1 mg/kg/dose over 1 to 2 minutes IV or 2 to 3 mg/kg/day PO.

Table 10-2. Dosages and characteristics of various diuretics

Drug	Dosage	Action				Adverse reactions	Mechanism of action
		Onset	Peak	Duration			
Furosemide	IV: 1.0 mg/kg/dose (over 1–2 min)	5 min	30 min	2 hr	Hypovolemia	Blocks resorption of Cl⁻ in ascending loop of Henle
(Lasix)	PO: 2–3 mg/kg/day	1 hr	1–2 hr	4–6 hr	Hypokalemia	
Chlorothiazide (Diuril)	PO: 20–30 mg/kg/day in 2 doses	2 hr	4 hr	6–12 hr	Hypokalemia	Blocks resorption of Na⁺ in ascending loop of Henle
Hydrochlorothiazide (HydroDIURIL)	PO: 2–3 mg/kg/day in 2 doses	2 hr	4 hr	6–12 hr	Hyperuricemia Hypersensitivity Dermatitis Photosensitivity	
Spironolactone (Aldactone)*	PO: 1–3 mg/kg/day in 2 doses	Several days			Headaches Gynecomastia Nausea and vomiting Rashes	Blocks aldosterone exchange of K⁺ for Na⁺

*Spironolactone is rarely given alone, but its potassium-sparing effect makes it useful in combination with other agents.

(d) **Toxicity.** Lasix is a potent medication, and clinical toxicity is usually manifested by **hypovolemia** or **hypokalemia.** It competitively inhibits urate secretion in the proximal tubule and can cause **hyperuricemia** and, in susceptible persons, gout. Transient or even permanent deafness has been reported. **Gastrointestinal disturbances, bone marrow suppression, skin rashes,** and **paresthesias** have been reported occasionally.

(3) **Spironolactone (Aldactone)** is a weak diuretic by itself but may be useful as an addition to diuretics previously discussed, both because of its different site of action and because of its potassium-sparing effects.

    (a) **Mechanism.** The diuretic properties of spironolactone result from its structural similarity to aldosterone. It is a competitive inhibitor of the mineralocorticoids that normally stimulate sodium resorption and potassium excretion in the distal tubules.

    (b) **Route of administration, absorption, and metabolism.** Spironolactone is absorbed orally. The diuretic effects may not be manifested for 2 to 3 days and its effects may persist for 2 to 3 days after cessation of therapy.

    (c) The **dosage** is 1 to 3 mg/kg/day PO.

    (d) **Toxicity.** The major complication is **hyperkalemia,** resulting from inhibition of potassium secretion with normal or increased potassium intake. Careful monitoring of serum potassium will avoid this problem. Gynecomastia may be seen in adolescents.

V. Hypoxic or cyanotic spells. Paroxysmal dyspnea with marked cyanosis often occurs in infants and young children with tetralogy of Fallot. Rarely, it occurs in other types of cyanotic congenital heart disease. It is characterized by increasing rate and depth of respirations with increased cyanosis, progressing to limpness, loss of consciousness, and, in the more severe cases, convulsions, cerebrovascular accidents, or even death.

A. Etiology

1. Cyanotic spells are due to an acute reduction of pulmonary blood flow, increased right-to-left shunting, and systemic hypoxemia.

2. "Spasm" of the infundibulum of the right ventricular outflow tract has been suggested. Other explanations include inadequate systemic venous return, decreased systemic vascular resistance, and a vicious cycle of arterial hypoxemia due to hyperpnea.

3. Anemia, either absolute or relative to the child's oxygen saturation, may predispose to cyanotic spells.

B. Diagnosis

1. **Signs and symptoms** include
    a. Reduction in intensity or disappearance of the pulmonary ejection murmur.
    b. Hyperpnea.
    c. Increased cyanosis.
    d. Irritability, often leading to unconsciousness and occasionally to convulsions due to cerebral anoxia.

2. **Laboratory findings** include
    a. Hypoxemia and acidosis.
    b. Diminished pulmonary blood flow on x-ray.
    c. Increased voltage of the P wave on the ECG.

C. Treatment

1. Place the child in a knee-chest position.
2. Give **oxygen** by hood or mask at 5 to 8 liters per minute.
3. Give **morphine sulfate,** 0.1 to 0.2 mg/kg IM or SQ.
4. If the spell is severe, give **sodium bicarbonate,** 1 mg/kg IV.
5. Volume expansion with crystalloid or blood should be given if cyanosis persists.
6. **Propranolol,** 0.1 mg/kg IV, may be effective in a protracted spell that does not respond to the preceding measures.
7. **Surgery** (corrective or palliative) may be necessary to increase pulmonary blood flow, or to prevent recurrence of spells.

VI. Arrhythmias
A. Etiology
1. **Arrhythmias** result from disorders of impulse formation, impulse conduction, or both.
   a. **Premature beats** and **tachyarrhythmias** are due to abnormal impulse formation caused either by enhanced automaticity, reentry, or triggered activity.
   b. **Bradyarrhythmias** are due to either depressed automaticity or block of an impulse.
2. Arrhythmias can be a manifestation of cardiac, metabolic, or acquired systemic disorder.
   a. Congenital heart disease (pre- and postrepair).
   b. Acquired heart disease.
   c. Electrolyte disturbances.
   d. Drug toxicity or poisoning.
   e. Disorders of endocrine, neurologic, or pulmonary systems.
   f. In association with inherited disorders of metabolism, collagen diseases, or infection.

B. Evaluation
1. Careful physical examination with attention to blood pressure, perfusion, and respiratory status.
2. Full **12-lead** ECG with long rhythm strip.
3. Additional information can be obtained by manipulating sympathetic tone during physical examination and during ECG.
   a. *Depress* tone with vagal maneuvers such as Valsalva or carotid massage, or use bag to face.
   b. *Enhance* tone with controlled exercise (treadmill testing).
4. Sporadic or infrequent arrhythmias can be studied with 24-hour ambulatory monitoring (Holter) or long-term event recorders.
5. If P waves are poorly seen on ECG, passage of an esophageal electrode can clarify atrial activity.
6. Complicated, drug-refractory, or potentially serious arrhythmias may require electrophysiology study (EPS) with intracardiac catheters, which record electrical activity directly from within the heart.

C. Diagnosis and treatment. Diagnosis is confirmed by demonstration of abnormal electrical activity as described above.
1. **Classification of arrhythmias**
   a. Premature beats.
   b. Tachycardias.
      (1) Narrow QRS complex (supraventricular tachycardia).
      (2) Wide QRS complex (ventricular or complex supraventricular tachycardia).
   c. Bradycardias
      (1) Depressed pacemaker activity.
      (2) Conduction block. Arrhythmias in an asymptomatic patient with a normal heart are generally benign. An arrhythmia should be diagnosed slowly and carefully, and should be judged to be an acute or potential danger to a patient before **any** therapy is undertaken. The toxicity of antiarrhythmic agents is generally high (see sec. **VII**).
2. **Premature beats**
   a. **Atrial premature beats (APBs)** may be an incidental finding in normal infants or children. If frequent, or if the patient is symptomatic, consider myopathy, hyperthyroidism, or the presence of an abnormal conduction pathway.
      (1) Diagnosis. Early beats with QRS similar to sinus beats, preceded by an abnormal P wave, followed by a noncompensatory pause.
      (2) Treatment. Not necessary in absence of underlying pathology.
   b. **Ventricular premature beats (VPBs)** are not uncommon in healthy normal patients, but could be a manifestation of serious cardiac pathology. Evaluation by a cardiologist is recommended for all children with VPBs.

(1) **Diagnosis.** Wide bizarre QRS without a preceding P wave, usually followed by full compensatory pause. Must be differentiated from APBs, which conduct to the ventricle with aberration.

(2) **Grading of VPBs.** Benign VPBs tend to be infrequent, of one morphology, and suppressed with exercise. If the VPBs are frequent, multiform, or occur as couplets or runs of ventricular tachycardia, serious pathology is more likely to be present.

(3) **Treatment.** The goal in treating VPBs is not to suppress every ectopic beat, but to prevent degeneration to sustained ventricular tachycardia or fibrillation.

(a) **Acute suppression.** Give IV lidocaine bolus (1.0 mg/kg); follow by infusion (10–50 µg/kg/min).

(b) **Chronic suppressive** therapy should be chosen after consultation with a cardiologist.

3. **Narrow complex tachycardia**

a. **General considerations**

(1) Narrow complex tachycardias have a QRS morphology similar or identical to that of normal sinus rhythm.

(2) Narrow complex tachycardias include most, but not all, supraventricular tachycardias (SVTs). (Some SVTs have a wide QRS complex.)

(3) Narrow complex tachycardias are relatively well tolerated (at least acutely).

b. **Sinus tachycardia (ST)** is a normal response to fever, stress, dehydration, and anemia, but can be exaggerated at times and confused with a primary arrhythmia.

(1) **Diagnosis.** Normal P wave preceding each QRS; some variability in rate.

(2) **Treatment.** Correct underlying cause.

c. **Automatic ectopic atrial tachycardia (EAT)** is an uncommon, but potentially serious, arrhythmia in children, caused by enhanced automaticity of a portion of atrial tissue. A cardiac consult is suggested to evaluate for myopathy and congestive failure.

(1) **Diagnosis.** Rapid atrial rate of 160 to 240/min, with unusual (ectopic) P wave; variable rate depending on activity; occasionally with blocked conduction of some beats to the ventricle.

(2) **Treatment**

(a) Often difficult! Cardioversion is **not effective.**

(b) Digoxin and beta blockers will slow the ventricular rate and occasionally stop the atrial tachycardia.

(c) Other drugs (e.g., amiodarone) can be tried if congestive failure is present.

(d) Eradication of the abnormal focus with radiofrequency catheter ablation **(RFCA)** is now being used successfully for this disorder.

d. **Atrial fibrillation** rarely occurs in a normal heart; if suspected, a cardiac consult is recommended.

(1) **Evaluation.** Consider myocarditis, valvular heart disease, hypertrophic myopathy, hyperthyroidism, and Wolff-Parkinson-White (WPW) syndrome.

(2) **Diagnosis.** The ECG shows irregular, rapid, low-amplitude atrial activity with a variable and irregular ventricular response. The QRS is normal, although occasional aberrant beats can occur (Ashman's phenomenon).

(3) **Treatment**

(a) If atrial fibrillation is present for more than a few days, anticoagulation is needed before converting the rhythm, to minimize the risk of embolization of atrial clots.

(b) Digoxin, beta blockers, or verapamil will increase atrioventricular (AV) block and slow the ventricular rate. Occasionally, these agents may convert fibrillation.

(c) Intravenous procainamide is often effective for acute conversion of atrial fibrillation. However, patients should be digitalized if possible before administration in an effort to offset the potential for enhanced rate of AV conduction due to procainamide.

(d) Synchronized cardioversion will convert most cases.

(e) Chronic therapy is needed to prevent recurrence.

e. Atrial flutter is uncommon in a normal heart, and pathology should be expected. A cardiologist should be consulted.

   (1) **Diagnosis.** Electrocardiography reveals regular atrial "sawtooth" waves at rates of 250 to 350/min, best seen in leads II, III, and avF. Conduction to the ventricle can vary (1 : 1, 2 : 1, etc.). The diagnosis is often hard during the 2 : 1 flutter, because every other flutter wave may be hidden in the QRS.

   (2) **Treatment**

   (a) Digoxin is effective in titrating the degree of AV block and in controlling the ventricular response rate. Rarely, digoxin will convert atrial flutter.

   (b) Quinidine and procainamide will frequently convert atrial flutter. If use of these drugs is contemplated, the patient should be **fully digitalized first,** because both drugs can acutely increase the ventricular response rate to flutter.

   (c) Synchronized cardioversion is almost always successful in converting atrial flutter.

   (d) Overdrive pacing with an esophageal or intracardiac pacing wire is frequently successful in terminating atrial flutter.

   (e) Maintenance therapy is necessary against recurrence.

   (f) Patients with refractory recurrent flutter can be considered for **RFCA** procedures.

f. AV node reentry is a common, narrow-complex SVT mechanism, accounting for about one-fourth of cases in children.

   (1) **Evaluation.** Atrioventricular node reentry usually occurs in patients with otherwise normal hearts. It is well tolerated acutely, although hypotension and congestive failure can occur if AV node reentry persists for many hours.

   (2) **Diagnosis.** The tachycardia rate is **strictly regular,** with normal QRS morphology. The P wave occurs quickly after the QRS (is sometimes buried in the QRS) and is inverted (retrograde P wave) in leads 2, 3 avF.

   (3) **Treatment.** The SVT due to AV node reentry is generally easy to convert. Enhancement of vagal tone will slow conduction within the AV node and frequently break the tachycardia. Carotid sinus massage, Valsalva maneuver, induced gag, or the application of ice to the face are all effective. **Ocular compression should be avoided because of reported retinal detachment.**

   (a) Intravenous **adenosine,** given by rapid push at a dose of 0.1 mg/kg, is highly effective if vagal maneuvers are not successful. The drug can be repeated at 0.2 mg/kg if the first dose fails.

   (b) **Alternate drug therapy** with digoxin (any age) or verapamil (>age 1 yr) can be used.

   (c) **Esophageal** or **intracardiac overdrive pacing** is very effective.

   (d) **Immediate synchronized cardioversion** is indicated in any patient with acute decompensation.

   (e) **Long-term treatment** can involve periodic vagal maneuvers, chronic medications (such as verapamil), or **RFCA** based on patient age and severity of symptoms.

g. Wolff-Parkinson-White syndrome (WPW) refers to the presence of an accessory AV conduction pathway outside the AV node. Congenital heart disease (particularly Epstein's disease) is fairly common.

   (1) **Evaluation.** Patients with WPW may be asymptomatic, but typically present with tachyarrhythmias. In very rare cases, patients with WPW

syndrome suffer cardiac arrest. Mechanisms of arrhythmia in WPW include narrow QRS complex reentry SVT ("orthodromic"), atrial flutter, atrial fibrillation, and wide QRS complex reentry SVT ("antidromic").

(2) Diagnosis. The sinus rhythm ECG of a patient with WPW reveals a short P-R interval and a slurred upstroke on the QRS (delta wave). Some patients with this disorder do not demonstrate a delta wave, in which case the pathway is said to be "concealed." The ECG in tachycardia is variable, depending on the SVT mechanism.

(3) Treatment of tachyarrhythmias in WPW depends on the SVT mechanism and **must be approached with some caution.** Cardiac consultation is recommended. If atrial flutter or fibrillation is present, digitalis and verapamil can produce serious ventricular tachycardia or arrhythmias, or both, and **should generally be avoided in WPW syndrome.**

(4) If the presenting arrhythmia is **narrow QRS** tachycardia ("orthodromic reentry"), intravenous **adenosine** is the preferred initial agent if vagal maneuvers fail.

(5) If the presenting arrhythmia has a **wide QRS** complex, one must be alert to the possibility that atrial flutter or fibrillation is present. In this setting, intravenous **procainamide** or electrical **cardioversion** is the preferred treatment.

(6) For chronic therapy in WPW syndrome, oral beta blockers, flecainide, and sotalol may be useful.

(7) If arrhythmia control is suboptimal in a patient with WPW, or if presenting symptoms are severe (e.g., syncope), intracardiac electrophysiologic studies are indicated. The accessory pathway can be localized, and **RFCA** can be carried out in the same setting. The success rates for RFCA in this disorder exceed 95%.

4. Wide complex tachycardia
  a. General considerations
    (1) Patients who present in wide QRS (>0.12 sec) tachycardia should be treated as an emergency.
    (2) In this arrhythmia, **the diagnosis is ventricular tachycardia (VT) until proved otherwise!**
  b. VT is generally associated with severe congenital or acquired heart disease.
    (1) Diagnosis. The ECG reveals rapid, wide, bizarre QRS complexes at regular rapid rates. Often the atrial rhythm is independent of the VT, and P waves can be seen to "march through" (AV dissociation).
    (2) Acute treatment. Any hypotensive or unresponsive patient should be treated immediately with synchronized electrical cardioversion. Thereafter, sinus rhythm can be maintained with IV lidocaine, procainamide, and/or bretylium.
    (3) Long-term management. Response to drugs can be evaluated with serial Holter monitoring or electrophysiologic studies with intracardiac catheters. Drugs commonly used for long-term therapy include procainamide, mexiletine, flecainide, beta blocker, sotalol, and amiodarone.
    (4) In high-risk patients, chronic protection from recurrent VT may require implantation of an internal automatic defibrillator device.

5. Bradycardia due to depressed pacemaker activity
  a. Sinus bradycardia is rarely a primary cardiac disorder and more often is associated with increased vagal tone, hypoxia, CNS disorder, hypothyroidism, hypothermia, anorexia nervosa, or drug intoxication. **It is a normal finding in healthy athletic teenagers.**
    (1) Diagnosis. The ECG reveals a normal P wave with normal AV conduction at rates less than 100 beats per minute in neonates or less than 60 beats per minute in older children. Escape rhythms of atrial or junctional origin may be seen.

(2) **Treatment.** No intervention is necessary if cardiac output is maintained. If needed, **atropine,** 0.01 mg/kg IV, will increase rate by reducing vagal tone.

b. **Sick sinus syndrome** refers to profound sinus node dysfunction, often with bursts of SVT (tachy-brady syndrome), seen most often several years after open heart surgery.

(1) **Diagnosis.** The ECG reveals slow atrial or junctional rhythm with frequent abrupt pauses. Episodic SVT (e.g., atrial fibrillation or flutter) can occur.

(2) **Treatment.** No acute treatment is required unless the patient is symptomatic. Bradycardia can be managed acutely with atropine or isoproterenol, but long-term management necessitates a pacemaker implant. If SVT episodes occur, a pacemaker is often necessary before beginning antiarrhythmic medications.

6. **Bradycardia due to conduction block**

a. **First-degree heart block** is associated with increased vagal tone, digitalis and beta blocker administration, inflammatory disease involving the conduction system, and congenital heart disease (especially atrioseptal defects, endocardial cushion defects, corrected transposition).

(1) **Diagnosis.** The ECG reveals a P-R interval prolonged for age: greater than 0.15 seconds in an infant, 0.18 seconds in a child, or 0.20 seconds in an adult.

(2) **Treatment.** None necessary.

b. **Second-degree heart block** refers to episodic interruption of AV conduction of one beat's duration.

(1) **Diagnosis**

(a) **Mobitz type 1 (Wenckebach) block** consists of a regular P wave with progressive prolongation of P-R interval and ultimately a dropped QRS. The R-R interval shortens progressively during a Wenckebach sequence, causing "grouped beating" of the QRS.

(b) **Mobitz type II block** has regular P waves, a typically normal or constant P-R interval, and an abrupt and unpredictable dropped QRS.

(2) **Treatment** for either form of second-degree heart block is generally unnecessary in absence of symptoms. Progression to third-degree heart block can occur, and close monitoring is needed in select patients.

c. **Third-degree (complete) heart block** can be congenital or acquired. The **congenital** form typically occurs in children born to mothers with connective tissue disease and results from the effects of maternal antibodies on the developing conduction system. **Acquired** AV block can be associated with inflammatory processes or structural heart disease. Acquired heart block can also result from direct trauma during cardiac catheterization or cardiac surgery.

(1) **Evaluation.** Complete heart block in a fetus or newborn suggests congenital heart disease or possible inflammation secondary to maternal connective tissue disease. All such infants should be evaluated with an echocardiogram, and maternal serum testing for antinuclear antibody (ANA) should be performed. Older children likewise should be screened for structural cardiac defects and inflammatory disease including endocarditis and vasculitis.

(2) **Diagnosis.** The ECG reveals a normal P-wave rate that is independent of the slower escape mechanism. The escape rhythm can be a narrow QRS complex junctional rhythm or a wide QRS complex ventricular rhythm.

(3) **Treatment** for complete heart block involves pacemaker implantation, depending on the cause of the conduction defect, the presence or absence of symptoms, and the rate and stability of the escape rhythm.

(a) Congenital complete heart block in the absence of structural heart disease is usually well tolerated in children. Pacing is indicated for symptomatic patients, those with slow escape rates, those with wide QRS complex escape rhythms, and patients with associated ventricular arrhythmias.

(b) Postoperative acquired complete heart block is generally an indication for pacing.

(c) Acquired heart block can be managed acutely with IV atropine, isoproterenol infusion, or temporary transvenous pacing.

(d) Permanent pacemakers are inserted transvenously in older children. Epicardial wires are placed via a thoracotomy in small infants or any patient with right-to-left intracardiac shunts.

(e) The ventricle alone may be paced (ventricular demand) or the pacemaker can be connected to both atrium and ventricle, thus allowing pacing and sensing in both chambers (AV sequential pacing).

VII. Antiarrhythmic therapy

A. Although the introduction of newer technologies has decreased reliance on **pharmacologic therapy** for cardiac arrhythmias, drug therapy still has a role in many patients, particularly very young children in whom invasive procedures may carry higher risk. Antiarrhythmic drugs are classified based on the mechanism of drug action at the cellular level. Only those agents in common use for the pediatric population are discussed here.

1. Class I agents are local anesthetics and act on the fast sodium current. They are subdivided as follows:

a. Class IA: quinidine, procainamide, disopyramide.

b. Class IB: lidocaine, mexiletine.

c. Class IC: flecainide.

2. Class II agents are beta-adrenergic blockers; propranolol is the prototype.

3. Class III agents are unique drugs that prolong action potential repolarization, and include amiodarone and sotalol.

4. Class IV agents are calcium-channel blockers. Verapamil is the prototype.

5. Digoxin and **adenosine** are classified separately.

B. Digoxin

1. General considerations

a. Although many digitalis glycosides are available, digoxin is the formulation of choice for infants and children.

b. Digoxin has a relatively narrow therapeutic index. **Care must be taken when digoxin dosage is ordered; avoidable disasters have occurred because of a misplaced decimal point!**

2. Indications

a. Control of ventricular rate in atrial fibrillation or atrial flutter.

b. Narrow QRS complex SVT (non-WPW).

c. Indirectly, for arrhythmias secondary to congestive heart failure.

3. Electrophysiology and ECG effects

a. Digoxin acts directly on cardiac cells and indirectly through the CNS.

b. Digoxin slows sinus node automaticity and prolongs the AV node refractory period.

c. Ventricular tissue refractory periods are decreased; the ECG may show a shortened Q-T interval and some abnormality of the S-T segment.

4. Digoxin pharmacology

a. Digoxin can be given PO, IM, or IV.

b. Orally, approximately 75% is absorbed, with onset of action within 15 to 30 minutes and peak effect at 1 to 5 hours.

c. "Total digitalizing doses" (TDD) are generally based on estimate of oral digoxin dosages. If digoxin is given IV (100% absorbed), the TDD should be reduced 25%.

d. Digoxin is excreted primarily by the kidney.

5. Digoxin dosage

    a. Before administration, a baseline ECG, serum electrolyte determination (particularly potassium), and some estimation of renal function are required.

    b. Digoxin is administered in two stages. Initial digitalization establishes the body stores, given over 24 hours in three divided doses: ½ TDD at time 0 hours, ¼ TDD at 12 hours, and ¼ TDD at 24 hours. Maintenance therapy is then administered, which is generally calculated as ⅛ TDD q12h (thus, ¼ TDD/day).

    c. Approximate total digitalizing doses (reduced 25% if IV)

      (1) Premature: 0.020 mg/kg PO.

      (2) Full-term newborn: 0.030 mg/kg PO.

      (3) Under 2 years: 0.040 mg/kg PO.

      (4) Over 2 years: 0.030 to 0.040 mg/kg PO.

      (5) Adult: maximum of 1.0 mg total PO.

    d. Digoxin is not removed with dialysis or cardiopulmonary bypass. Patients with renal failure must be monitored closely if digoxin is administered.

    e. Drug interaction occurs with quinidine, verapamil, and amiodarone, requiring a dosage reduction of approximately 50%.

6. Toxicity

    a. Digoxin elixir is a very **pleasant-tasting** preparation, quite appealing to toddlers, and families should be warned about the necessity for secure storage out of reach of children.

    b. Manifestations of digoxin toxicity

      (1) Arrhythmias. In children, sinus bradycardia and first- or second-degree AV block are the most common arrhythmias with mild to moderate intoxication. Severe acute overdose can precipitate SVT, complete heart block, and serious ventricular arrhythmias.

      (2) Gastrointestinal. Nausea and vomiting are common. Abdominal cramping and diarrhea can occur.

      (3) CNS. Hazy or blurred vision and perceptual color disturbances (yellow and green) may occur in patients with subacute or chronic intoxication. Lethargy and fatigue may be present.

    c. Treatment of intoxication

      (1) Stop the drug! Oral doses of digoxin, particularly the elixir, are rapidly absorbed. Cholestyramine resins can bind some digoxin in the GI tract and reduce absorption.

      (2) Check electrolytes and serum digoxin level. If serum potassium is significantly low, it should be replaced slowly and carefully because sensitivity to digoxin is much increased in hypokalemic states.

      (3) Lidocaine and phenytoin (Dilantin) are often effective in treating ventricular arrhythmias induced by digoxin toxicity.

      (4) Temporary transvenous pacing is indicated for a digoxin-induced, high-grade AV block.

      (5) Cardioversion is risky in digoxin-toxic patients; it can precipitate ventricular fibrillation, which may be impossible to correct. It should be reserved as a last resort.

      (6) A rapid and effective treatment for serious digoxin-induced rhythm disorders is digoxin-specific "Fab" antibody fragments (Digibind). Intravenous infusion generally corrects life-threatening arrhythmias within 30 minutes.

C. Quinidine (class IA)

  1. General considerations

    a. Quinidine is a potent but potentially dangerous agent. It should be used only with careful monitoring.

  2. Indications

    a. In conjunction with digoxin for atrial fibrillation or flutter.

    b. SVT in some patients with WPW syndrome.

    c. High-grade ventricular ectopy or VT in selected patients.

  3. Electrophysiology and ECG effects

a. Increases effective refractory period of atrial and ventricular tissue.
b. Vagolytic effects may enhance AV conduction.
c. In normal doses, the major ECG change is a moderate increase in Q-T interval. In sensitive or toxic patients, the QRS duration may increase, and the Q-T interval can be markedly increased (>30% from baseline).

4. Pharmacology
  a. Quinidine is available as the sulfate (half-life 6 hr) or gluconate (half-life 8 hr).
  b. Administer by oral route only. **The IV formulation can cause profound hypotension and is contraindicated.**
  c. Metabolism and excretion are via liver and kidney.

5. Dosage
  a. An initial test dose should be given with careful ECG monitoring. **If idiopathic QRS widening or profound Q-T prolongation occurs, the drug should be withheld.**
  b. Dosage for children: 15 to 60 mg/kg/day, divided q6h for sulfate, or q8h for gluconate.

6. Precautions and side effects
  a. Gastrointestinal symptoms of nausea and diarrhea are common and may necessitate discontinuation.
  b. A small percentage of patients experience a worsening of ventricular arrhythmias (including a specific form of polymorphic VT known as **torsade de pointes**), even at therapeutic serum levels.
  c. Hemolytic anemia and thrombocytopenia have been reported.

7. Drug interactions
  a. Reduces renal digoxin excretion by half.
  b. Reduces warfarin (Coumadin) requirements.
  c. Can shorten Dilantin half-life.

D. Procainamide (class IA)
  1. General considerations
    a. Procainamide is a synthetic local anesthetic.
    b. It has a potentially high number of side effects. Close monitoring is required.
    c. Procainamide, unlike quinidine, can be administered IV, although some hypotension can still occur (usually reversed easily with volume expansion).
  2. Indications
    a. Used in conjunction with digoxin for atrial flutter or fibrillation.
    b. Acute management of SVT, including WPW patients.
    c. High-grade ventricular ectopy and VT.
  3. Electrophysiology and ECG effects are similar to those of quinidine.
  4. Pharmacology
    a. Excretion and metabolism are both hepatic and renal.
    b. Procainamide has a short half-life (3–5 hr) and requires frequent dosing. A slow-release form is available for q6h dosing.
    c. Infants may need very large oral doses to obtain therapeutic serum levels, probably because of poor absorption.
  5. Dosage
    a. Intravenous dosage
      (1) Infants: 7 mg/kg over 1 hour.
      (2) Children: 7 to 15 mg/kg over 1 hour.
    b. Oral dosage: 15 to 50 mg/kg/day, divided q4–6h.
    c. Serum levels can be followed.
  6. Precautions and side effects
    a. Procainamide can be "proarrhythmic" and worsen ventricular arrhythmia or cause torsade de pointes.
    b. Drug-induced lupus syndrome is a well-recognized complication, particularly in adults, but may not require discontinuation of the drug.

E. Disopyramide (class IA)
  1. General considerations
    a. Disopyramide, as an IA agent, is similar to quinidine and procainamide.

With the exception perhaps of treatment of arrhythmias in hypertrophic myopathy, it has little advantage over these other IA drugs, but it is a useful substitute if patients develop intolerable side effects to them.

    b. Depression of myocardial contractility may be slightly greater with disopyramide than with other IA agents; it should be used with caution if at all in patients with poor ventricular function or renal failure, or both.

2. Indications

    a. Similar to those of quinidine and procainamide.

    b. Arrhythmias in patients with hypertrophic myopathy.

3. Electrophysiology and ECG effects are similar to those of quinidine and procainamide.

4. Pharmacology and dosage

    a. For oral use only.

    b. Infants: 10 to 20 mg/kg/day, divided q6h.

    c. Children: 5 to 15 mg/kg/day, divided q6h.

5. Precautions and side effects

    a. Not for use in patients with depressed ventricular function.

    b. Disopyramide may be "proarrhythmic," and careful monitoring is indicated.

    c. Anticholinergic side effects, such as dry mouth, blurred vision, and urinary retention, can occur.

F. Lidocaine (class IB)

1. General considerations

    a. An effective IV agent, quite well tolerated even in the face of myocardial dysfunction, with few side effects at standard doses.

    b. Local anesthetic.

2. Indications

    a. Acute suppression of ventricular arrhythmias.

    b. Before cardioversion as prophylaxis against ventricular arrhythmias for patients receiving digoxin.

    c. Possible predictor of response to oral IB agents.

3. Electrophysiology and ECG effects

    a. Lidocaine has its major effect on abnormal Purkinje and ventricular cells, where spontaneous automaticity is suppressed.

    b. Electrocardiography is unaffected.

4. Pharmacology

    a. Lidocaine is metabolized quickly on its first pass through the liver. An IV bolus will produce an acute effect within 5 minutes, but peak levels decay after only 30 minutes. Additional boluses or constant infusion are necessary to maintain levels.

    b. Patients with hepatic dysfunction may require lower infusion rates.

5. Dosage

    a. Intravenous bolus, 1.0 mg/kg, can be repeated q10 min for three doses.

    b. Constant infusion, 10 to 50 μg/kg/min.

    c. Monitor serum levels if prolonged infusion is required.

6. Precautions and side effects

    a. In patients with marked sick sinus syndrome or complete heart block, in which a ventricular rhythm serves as the "escape" rhythm, lidocaine is **not** indicated!

    b. At therapeutic serums levels, side effects (except mild nausea) are virtually nonexistent.

    c. Toxic levels can produce GI distress with nausea and vomiting, and CNS difficulties such as ataxia and seizures. Hypotension may occur at very elevated serum levels.

    d. Treatment for toxicity is to withhold the drug. Elimination is generally rapid.

G. Flecainide (class IC). This agent is a potent blocker at all levels of the conductive system, but its use in children is limited, and it should only be considered after consultation with a cardiologist.

H. Beta blockers (class II). Several beta blocker formulations are now available for routine use.

1. **General considerations**
   a. **Propranolol** is still the most widely used agent, but must be taken q6–8h. Longer-acting agents (**atenolol** and **nadolol**) are useful in older children, with doses given once or twice a day. Short-acting agents (**esmolol**) can be used for acute arrhythmia management.
   b. Noncardiac beta blockade side effects, such as aggravation of bronchospasm in asthmatic patients, may be reduced somewhat with "cardioselective" beta blockers. However, the "selectivity" is never absolute with any preparation.
   c. Occasional CNS side effects of fatigue and depression can be reduced somewhat by beta blockers with low CNS penetration.
   d. For the evaluation of drug efficacy in arrhythmia management, it is advisable to begin with a trial of **propranolol.** In older children, one can later switch to a once-a-day agent to simplify dosage and, on occasion, to reduce potential side effects.

2. **Indications**
   a. Effective for SVT (including WPW); acts by blocking reentry circuits involving AV node, and also by reducing spontaneous premature beats.
   b. Useful in acute and chronic treatment of ventricular arrhythmias, including arrhythmias associated with a long Q-T interval.

3. **Electrophysiology and ECG effects**
   a. At normal levels, beta blockers do not directly change cellular electrical activity. Their major action appears to be secondary to beta blockade.
   b. On the ECG, the slowing of sinus rate and a slight increase in P-R interval are noted.
   c. The heart rate response to exercise is blunted in patients receiving long-term beta blockade.

4. **Pharmacology and dosage**
   a. Intravenous **esmolol** dosage: 0.5 mg/kg rapid push.
   b. **Oral propranolol** dosage: 1 to 3 mg/kg/day, divided q6h.
   c. **Intravenous propranolol** dosage (for emergency use only): 0.025 mg/kg q15 min to maximum of four doses.
   d. Oral **atenolol** dosage: 1.0 mg/kg once a day.

5. **Precautions and side effects**
   a. **Intravenous administration can cause hypotension and bradycardia.** Whenever possible, oral administration is preferred.
   b. **Beta blockers are generally contraindicated in patients with asthma.**
   c. **Severe hypoglycemia** at times of stress can be caused by long-term beta blocker therapy.
   d. Beta blockers in combination with **verapamil** (IV *or* oral) are **contraindicated** because of profound additive myocardial suppression.
   e. Fatigue, depression, and decreased exercise tolerance can occur.

I. Amiodarone (class III)

1. **General considerations**
   a. Amiodarone is a potent antiarrhythmic agent that has proved quite useful in difficult arrhythmias when all conventional medications have been unsuccessful. The potential side effects are quite serious, and the drug should be reserved for refractory, life-threatening rhythm disturbances after consultation with a cardiologist.
   b. The pharmacology of amiodarone is not completely understood. The half-life is exceedingly long (several weeks). Giving oral loading doses for 10 days, followed by a once-a-day maintenance dose, is the usual method of administration. In the hospital, monitoring during the loading period is generally required.
   c. The ECG effects of amiodarone reflect its diffuse suppression of all elements of the conduction system. Sinus slowing, increased P-R interval, increased QRS duration, and prolongation of Q-T are all observed.

  d. Potential side effects include interstitial pneumonitis, hyperthyroidism or hypothyroidism, photosensitive skin rash, peripheral neuropathy, corneal microdeposits, hepatitis, and blue skin coloration. It enhances the effect of warfarin, and raises the concentration of digoxin, Dilantin, and several antiarrhythmic agents.

J. Sotalol (class III)

 1. General considerations

  a. Sotalol is among the newer antiarrhythmic agents to be introduced for pediatric use. It combines properties of class II and III agents.

  b. Sotalol is effective for both supraventricular and ventricular arrhythmias. Because of its beta blockade properties, use is not recommended in patients with depressed ventricular function unless no other effective therapy is found.

  c. Side effects in young patients include bradycardia, hypotension, headaches, and abdominal pain. It may be "proarrhythmic."

  d. Sotalol should be used only in consultation with a cardiologist.

K. Verapamil (class IV)

 1. General considerations

  a. Calcium-channel blocking agents act primarily on the cells of the sinoatrial (SA) and AV nodes. Verapamil is effective in interrupting and preventing SVT that involves the AV node in its circuit.

  b. Verapamil can speed up conduction over accessory pathways in patients with WPW syndrome and should be used with caution.

  c. Verapamil is contraindicated in children less than age 1 year. **Profound hypotension and circulatory collapse have been observed following its administration in infants.**

  d. Verapamil should not be administered to patients who are receiving quinidine or beta blockers because of the additive myocardial suppression of the drugs.

 2. Indications

  a. SVT, particularly AV node reentry.

  b. To slow ventricular response acutely to atrial fibrillation or flutter.

  c. Ventricular arrhythmias that may be due to automaticity.

 3. Electrophysiology and ECG effects

  a. Decreases automaticity of sinus node and slows conduction over AV node.

  b. Electrocardiography reveals sinus slowing and increased P-R interval.

 4. Pharmacology and dosage

  a. Metabolized by the liver.

  b. Intravenous administration of verapamil is usually effective within seconds for interrupting usual AV node reentry SVT. The dose is 0.05 to 0.10 mg/kg (maximum 5.0 mg) IV push. This dose can be repeated q15 min three times.

  c. Oral dosage is 4 to 15 mg/kg/day, divided q8h.

 5. Precautions and side effects (see also sec. **1.b** and **c** above).

  a. Intravenous verapamil can cause significant hypotension, bradycardia, and AV block even in older children with good myocardial function. This problem can often be corrected acutely with the administration of IV calcium, or isoproterenol, or both.

  b. Oral verapamil can worsen CHF in patients with poor ventricular function.

  c. Generally well tolerated; nausea is a rare side effect.

L. Adenosine has largely replaced verapamil, digoxin, and beta blockers in the acute management of supraventricular tachycardia.

 1. General considerations

  a. Adenosine is an endogenous nucleoside that can produce profound but transient block of the sinus and AV nodes when administered as a large rapid bolus.

  b. Because of rapid metabolism (<10 sec) this drug must be given as close to the central circulation as possible (e.g., antecubital vein

rather than a hand vein), and pushed quite rapidly followed by a saline flush.
2. **Indications**
   a. Reentry SVT involving the AV node as part of the circuit.
   b. As a diagnostic tool (e.g., to uncover atrial flutter waves by transiently slowing AV conduction).
3. **Dosage** is 0.1 mg/kg by rapid IV push. The dose can be doubled and repeated as a second IV push after 5 minutes. Maximum dose is 12 mg.
4. **Side effects** are few.
   a. Transient sinus bradycardia and AV block are seen, but last less than 15 seconds.
   b. Patients may complain of short-lived chest pain, facial flushing, shortness of breath, and dizziness.
M. **Cardioversion** is the use of a **synchronized,** direct-current shock applied to the heart to convert certain arrhythmias to normal sinus rhythm. Except under emergency conditions, it should be used only by a cardiologist.
   1. **Indications**
      a. **Atrial fibrillation.** Immediate cardioversion is indicated if atrial fibrillation is of short duration, if a rapid ventricular rate cannot be controlled, or if hemodynamic compromise exists. When cardioversion is elective, patients should receive anticoagulant therapy with a Coumadin derivative before cardioversion. Cardioversion may be unsuccessful in restoring normal sinus rhythm in occasional patients with a very enlarged left atrium (e.g., mitral stenosis).
      b. **Atrial flutter** converts often at low energy levels (0.5 W-sec/kg). For this condition, cardioversion should be performed as an emergency procedure only in hemodynamically compromised patients; otherwise, cardioversion can be performed electively.
      c. **SVT.** Vagotonic maneuvers and medical therapy should be used initially unless hypotension or CHF is present. Energy settings of 0.25 to 0.5 W-sec/kg should be sufficient.
      d. **VT.** Cardioversion is the treatment of choice for sustained VT. During preparation for cardioversion, a bolus of IV lidocaine (1–2 mg/kg) can be given. Cardioversion is usually accomplished with 1 to 2 W-sec/kg.
      e. **Ventricular fibrillation.** Immediate cardioversion with an **unsynchronized** discharge at an energy level of 2 to 6 W-sec/kg is required for ventricular fibrillation in children (see Chap. 7, pp. 221ff).
   2. **Contraindications** include sinus tachycardia, digitalis-induced arrhythmias, multifocal or automatic atrial tachycardia, and the supraventricular arrhythmias associated with hyperthyroidism. For patients with sick sinus syndrome, delayed recovery of sinus node function must be anticipated, with equipment on hand to provide temporary pacing if needed.
   3. **Techniques. One must be prepared for complications, and the procedure should only be done in a carefully monitored environment.** Cardioversion should be performed at the lowest possible energy level to minimize complications.
      a. Electrical cardioversion, even with low energies, is painful. Unless the patient already has altered consciousness from the arrhythmia, analgesia should be provided with IV administration of a short-acting barbiturate or benzodiazepine. These drugs for elective cardioversion should only be used in a carefully monitored environment by an individual experienced with respiratory support. The child should be preoxygenated before the procedure is performed. When the patient's lid reflex is lost, cardioversion can be attempted.
      b. The device should be synchronized on the R wave to avoid the ventricular vulnerable period. **For treating ventricular fibrillation, the synchronizing switch must be turned off.**
      c. The electrode paddles should be liberally covered with conductive paste

and placed in the second right intercostal space and the fifth left interspace in the anterior axillary line in older children and adults, or in the third space in the parasternal area or below the left scapula in younger children.

   d. Postconversion arrhythmias are not uncommon and include APBs, VPBs, and delayed recovery of the SA node, manifested by slow junctional rhythm or sinus bradycardia. Occasionally, these must be treated. Lidocaine (IV), atropine (IV), and isoproterenol (IV) should be drawn up in advance, accessible for rapid delivery if necessary.

N. Radiofrequency Catheter Ablation (RFCA) has become an increasingly common therapy for tachycardias in children since 1990. Transvenous electrode catheters are used to map local electrical activity to pinpoint the abnormal focus or pathway that is causing the rhythm disorder. Once located, high-frequency electrical current is passed through the tip of mapping catheter and creates a small burn on the endocardial surface (3–5 mm in diameter). If the catheter was correctly positioned, this will permanently eliminate the cause of tachycardia.

   1. Suitable "targets" for RFCA include

   a. Accessory pathways (WPW and "concealed").

   b. Selective modification of the AV node for AV nodal reentry.

   c. Ectopic atrial tachycardia.

   d. Atrial flutter.

   e. Some forms of ventricular tachycardia.

   2. Success rates for RFCA in children exceed 90%, but this must be balanced against risks of an invasive catheterization. The risk of potential complications may be higher during the first year of life.

   3. Indications for RFCA in the pediatric age group are still evolving. Generally accepted indications now include

   a. Any tachycardia that produces life-threatening symptoms, even if episodes are infrequent.

   b. Patients with ventricular dysfunction induced by chronic or incessant tachycardias.

   c. Patients with congenital heart disease who are scheduled for hemodynamic surgery, where the tachycardia could complicate intraoperative or postoperative management, or both.

   d. Older children with symptomatic (but not life threatening) tachycardia in whom conservative management has failed.

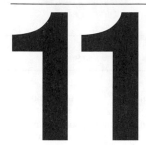

Gastroenterologic Disorders

Athos Bousvaros

I. General principles
A. Nutrition
1. **Evaluation** (see also sec. **II.R.**, p. 371)
   a. **Growth parameters** (specifically the following indices)
      (1) Weight/age.
      (2) Height/age.
      (3) Weight/height (see Chap. 3).
      (4) Head circumference.
   b. **Anthropometrics**
      (1) Triceps skin fold.
      (2) Arm circumference.
   c. **Blood tests**
      (1) Complete blood count with lymphocyte count.
      (2) Purified protein derivative (PPD) and *Candida* (skin tests).
      (3) Total protein, albumin, transferrin, and globulins.
      (4) Liver function tests and alkaline phosphatase.
      (5) Iron and total iron-binding capacity.
      (6) Calcium, phosphorus, magnesium, and zinc.
   d. **Urine tests**
      (1) Creatinine and creatinine-height index (*Pediatrics* 46:696, 1970).
      (2) Nitrogen balance study.
      (3) Calcium, phosphorus excretion.
2. **Diets** prescribed for the management of a specific nutritional deficiency can be obtained by writing to the Nutrition Department at the Children's Hospital Medical Center, Boston, MA 02115. For patients in whom the oral route is not appropriate, nasogastric (NG) or nasojejunal feedings are indicated, utilizing elemental formulas (Table 11-1). Indications for the selection of enteral formulas are found in Table 11-2.
3. **Therapy**
   a. **General approach.** Enteral nutrition is preferred if gastrointestinal function is intact or mildly impaired. Patience is an important principle in the management of malnourished patients. Remember that the severely malnourished patient is in a tenuous homeostatic state. Too rapid a disruption of this homeostasis can cause severe problems (e.g., cardiac arrhythmias, pulmonary edema). The following measures are suggested.
      (1) **Correct fluid and electrolyte disorders** (hyponatremia, hyposmolality, acidosis, hypomagnesemia, hypokalemia, hypophosphatemia). Watch for the development of hypophosphatemia with refeeding. Monitor cardiac rhythm and obtain daily electrolytes during initial refeeding.
      (2) Treat for infections.
      (3) **Protein load.** Start with 1 g/kg/day and increase as tolerated.
      (4) **Caloric load**
         (a) For **severely malnourished children,** start with 50 kcal/kg/day, and increase by 25 kcal/kg/day every 2 to 3 days as tolerated.

Table 11-1. Enteral hyperalimentation chart

Formula name	Instant Breakfast and milk	Ensure	Sustacal
Calories/ml	0.93	1.06	1.00
Carbohydrate source	Maltodextrin, sucrose, lactose	Corn syrup, sucrose	Corn syrup, sucrose
Protein source	Intact milk protein	Sodium and calcium caseinates, soy protein isolate	Sodium and calcium caseinates, soy protein isolate
Fat source	Butterfat from milk	Corn oil	Partially hydrogenated soy oil
Protein (g/liter)	48.00	37.00	61.00
Fat (g/liter)	20.00	37.00	23.00
Carbohydrate (g/liter)	160.00	145.00	140.00
MOsm/kg	600.00	470.00	625.00
Na/K (mEq/liter)	42/61	37/40	41/53
Dietary fiber (g/liter)	Minimal	Minimal	Minimal
Cost ($/8 oz)	0.60	1.44	1.73
Form	Powder	Liquid	Liquid
Similar products	Sustacal powder, Fortashake	Nutren 1.0, Isosource	Promote, Replete
Uses/features	Good-tasting supplement if patient tolerates lactose	Lactose-free caloric supplement	High-protein, polymeric, no MCT in Sustacal

*Formulas specifically designed for pediatric ages 1–10 yr.

    (b) For **mild to moderate malnutrition,** start with 80 to 100 calories/kg/day.
  (5) Formulas without lactose or sucrose to prevent diarrhea secondary to disaccharidase insufficiency are recommended in the moderate to severely malnourished child. **Polymeric formulas** contain intact milk or soy protein, and are usually adequate as a caloric supplement (for oral and tube feedings). In contrast, **elemental formulas** offer lower fat content and hydrolyzed protein and may be useful in patients with gut allergy or injury. The higher osmolarity of most elemental formulas will often cause loose stools. **Semi-elemental formulas** offer easier absorption than polymeric formulas, and lower osmolality than elemental formulas, but should not be used in patients who have a history of anaphylaxis to milk or soy. **Sucrose-containing formulas** (e.g., Pediasure) or flavored elemental formulas (e.g., Neocate) are generally more palatable for oral consumption by children.
  (6) If the infant is anorectic, initial **nasogastric feeding** should be considered. In children with chronic swallowing dysfunction, **gastrostomy** may allow supplemental feeding without affecting development of oral motor skills.

Osmolite	Ultracal	Nutren 1.5	Pediasure*
1.06	1.06	1.50	1.00
Corn syrup, sucrose	Maltodextrin	Maltodextrin	Hydrolyzed cornstarch, sucrose
Sodium and calcium caseinates, soy protein isolate	Sodium and calcium caseinates	Casein	Sodium caseinate, whey protein
Medium chain triglyceride (MCT), corn oil, soy oil	Soy oil, MCT	MCT, canola oil, corn oil, lecithin	Partially hydrogenated soybean oil
37.00	42.00	40.00	30.00
44.00	43.00	45.00	49.00
145.00	116.00	113.00	110.00
300.00	310.00	500.00	325.00
24/26	38/39	22/32	16/33
Minimal	13.6	Minimal	Minimal
1.69	2.07	1.45	1.79
Liquid	Liquid	Liquid	Liquid
Isocal, Isosource, Attain	Jevity, Nutren 1.0 with fiber, Fibersource	Ensure Plus, Resource Plus	Kindercal*
Low osmolality/ sodium	Supplemental soy fiber	High caloric density for fluid-restricted patients	Lactose-/gluten-free caloric supplement

    (7) Vitamin and mineral supplementation should aim to correct both general nutritional depletion and specific micronutrient deficiencies (e.g., rickets, folate, vitamin B_{12}, zinc, and selenium deficiencies).

  b. Total parenteral nutrition (TPN). Intravenous alimentation is delivery of a mixture of hypertonic dextrose and crystalline amino acid solutions utilizing a central high-flow vein. This method should be used if the enteral route is not possible. Intravenous alimentation should be used in all patients who will be nil per os (NPO) for 2 weeks or more. Periods of poor intake from 2 to 3 days to 2 weeks should be managed with peripheral IV alimentation.

    (1) Nitrogen sources are generally provided as pure crystalline amino acids. The usual daily requirement of each is 2 to 4 g/kg in infants and children. The bulk of the caloric content of hyperalimentation fluid is derived from glucose. The amount required in most infants is 25 to 30 g/kg/day. The rest of the metabolic needs (i.e., water, electrolytes, minerals, and vitamins) are provided in the customary amounts.

    (2) Intralipid (soybean oil), a fat emulsion that provides 1.1 calories/ml (10% solution) or 2.0 calories/ml (20% solution) is necessary to prevent essential fatty acid deficiency and should be given as at least 5 to 10% of the total calories. The following are the recommended rates.

Table 11-1 (continued)

Formula name	Next Step Soy*	Vital HN	Peptamen
Calories/ml	0.66	1.00	1.00
Carbohydrate source	Corn syrup solids, sucrose	Maltodextrin, tapioca, starch	Maltodextrin, starch
Protein source	Soy protein	Wheat, soy, meat protein hydrolysate, free amino acid	Enzymatically hydrolyzed whey
Fat source	Palm olein, soy, coconut, sunflower oil	MCT, sunflower oil	MCT, sunflower oil, lechithin
Protein (g/liter)	21.90	42.00	40.00
Fat (g/liter)	29.10	11.00	39.00
Carbohydrate (g/liter)	79.10	185.00	127.00
MOsm/kg	260.00	460.00	270.00
Na/K (mEq/liter)	13/26	20/34	22/32
Dietary fiber (g/liter)	Minimal	Minimal	Minimal
Cost ($/8 oz)	0.66	7.89	6.01
Form	Powder	Powder	Liquid
Similar products		Critacare HN (liquid)	Reabilan
Uses/features	For milk-protein–allergic toddlers, may be concentrated	Semielemental low fat	Semielemental, low osmolality

    (a) 5 to 10 ml/kg for the first 10 kg.
    (b) 2.5 to 5.0 ml/kg for the second 10 kg.
    (c) 1.25 to 2.5 ml/kg for all weights above 20 kg. The maximum infusion is 4 g/kg/day. We usually begin 0.5 g/kg (5 ml/kg) of 10% Intralipid the day of or the day after PN is started.
  (3) Caloric densities utilized
    (a) Amino acids, 4 calories/g.
    (b) 10% dextrose, 0.34 calories/ml.
    (c) 20% dextrose, 0.68 calories/ml.
    (d) 30% dextrose, 1.02 calories/ml.
  (4) **Peripheral venous hyperalimentation** is usually administered as a 10% glucose solution with 2% amino acids that contains water, electrolytes, minerals, and vitamins. If given at a rate of 150 ml/kg/day, 50 calories/kg/day are supplied, which is sufficient to prevent a negative nitrogen balance.
  (5) **Indications for TPN.** Any patient who is unable to maintain adequate nutrition via the enteral route is a candidate for TPN. Some specific disease states in which TPN is employed include chronic diarrheal states, inflammatory bowel disease with growth failure or fistulae, postoperative status, chronic pancreatitis and pseudocyst, short-bowel syndrome, and esophageal injury.

Peptamen Junior*	Tolerex	Vivonex Pediatric	Neocate One*
1.00	1.00	0.80	1.00
Maltodextrin, starch	Glucose, oligosaccharides	Maltodextrin, modified starch	Maltodextrin, sucrose
Enzymatically hydrolyzed whey	Free amino acids	Free amino acids	Free amino acids
MCT, canola oil, lechithin	Safflower oil	MCT, soybean oil	Coconut, canola, sunflower oil
30.00	21.00	24.00	30.00
39.00	1.50	24.00	35.00
137.00	230.00	130.00	146.00
260.00	550.00	360.00	835.00
20/33	20/31	17/31	9/24
Minimal	Minimal	Minimal	Minimal
5.94	5.26	4.50	2.75
Liquid	Powder	Powder	Liquid
	Vivonex TEN (higher protein)	Neocate One+*	Vivonex Pediatric*
Semielemental, low osmolality	Elemental—for gut allergy/ inflammation— monitor for fatty acid deficiency	Elemental—tube or oral feedings in gut allergy/inflammation	Elemental, palatable for oral feedings

(6) Management of hyperalimentation program

    (a) A central venous catheter is placed and its position checked radiographically.

    (b) A 10% glucose solution is given IV as maintenance fluid (see Chap. 4). Adequate electrolytes should be provided. Continue the infusion for 12 to 24 hours.

    (c) A 20% glucose–amino acid solution is then given as maintenance fluid for 12 hours.

    (d) The infusion rate is increased approximately 10% q12h until fluid intake is 135 ml/kg/day, irrespective of age. An infusate with 20% glucose and 3 g/day protein provides the equivalent of 110 calories/kg/day. Generally, no more than 200 ml/kg/day is used in infants. It may be necessary to decrease the protein content of the infusate at such rates. Higher dextrose concentrations can be utilized if the patient is fluid restricted.

    (e) Lipid infusion. Lipid is commonly administered by use of connector tubing (Y) proximal to the millipore filter so that lipid will join to the glucose–amino acid–electrolyte solution just before the infusion site.

    (f) Multiple-lumen catheters are used to safely permit administration of parenteral nutrition *and* IV medication.

Table 11-2. Indications for selecting enteral formulas

Conditions	Formula description	Suggested formulas Infants	Older children
Supplemental caloric needs (normal functioning intestine)	Nutritionally complete		Carnation Instant Breakfast
Lactose intolerance	Lactose free	Isomil Nursoy Prosobee	Pediasure Kindercal Nutren I-S Enrich Ensure Plus Isocal Osmolite
Abnormal nutrient digestion and absorption with starch, lactose, or sucrose malabsorption	Hydrolized protein, MCT oil, and glucose	Pregestimil	Vivonex Neocare One+ Peptamen Junior
Severe steatorrhea (e.g., bile acid deficiency)	Contains MCT oil	Alimentum Portagen Pregestimil	Osmolite Peptamin Reabilan HN Vital HN Vivonex Pediatric
Increased protein needs	High-protein formulation		Sustacal
Complete formula with fiber			Enrich Jevity
Caloric additives		Corn oil (fat) MCT oil (fat) Polycose (glucose)	Same as for infants

    (g) For patients on long-term support, the administration of parenteral nutrition is cycled to permit infusion at night, with capping of the central venous line during the day to permit freedom of movement.

(7) Monitoring the patient receiving TPN

    (a) Daily weights should be measured.

    (b) Intake and output, and qualitative sugar and acetone, are measured on all urine specimens.

    (c) Sodium, potassium, chloride, BUN, and glucose are determined daily while increasing fluid and then weekly when fluid requirements have been reached.

    (d) Complete blood count, magnesium, calcium, phosphorus, triglyceride levels, total protein, aspartate aminotransferase (AST; SGOT), alanine aminotransferase (ALT; SGPT), lactic dehydrogenase (LDH), alkaline phosphatase, bilirubin, and creatinine are measured initially and then weekly.

    (e) Copper, zinc, and iron levels are measured at the beginning of therapy and then monthly.

    (f) 24-hour urine for creatinine, Ca^{2+}, PO_4^{2+}, and Mg^{2+} is obtained every 2 weeks.

(8) Complications of TPN

(a) Infection is the most serious complication of TPN. Fungi (usually *Candida albicans*) and bacteria are the infecting agents.

    (i) Care of the central venous line must be scrupulous.

    (ii) Unexplained glycosuria may be the first clue. Blood cultures should be obtained from the patient and from the line.

    (iii) *When sepsis is documented, the central venous line should be removed if possible.*

(b) Hepatic complications

    (i) Abnormalities in liver function test results are common during the course of TPN. Hepatomegaly with elevations of serum transferases (often to high levels), with prolongation of prothrombin time (PT) and partial thromboplastin time (PTT), may be seen, and liver biopsy reveals a fatty liver.

    (ii) Cholestatic liver disease frequently develops in premature infants.

(c) Metabolic complications

    (i) Hyperglycemia is common in septic patients, premature infants, and patients with renal disease.

    (ii) Hypoglycemia is a common and severe complication **if TPN is stopped abruptly.** It is recommended that cycled PN patients have their infusion gradually reduced over 1 hour before the PN is stopped.

    (iii) Acidosis occurs in patients with renal compromise or prematurity when large (4 g/kg/day) protein loads are administered.

    (iv) Hypomagnesemia can occur in patients with low endogenous magnesium stores (e.g., those with chronic diarrhea).

    (v) Hyperlipidemia can occur with excess lipid administration or sepsis.

    (vi) Hyperammonemia. (see also Chap. 12, p. 280)

    (vii) Hypocalcemia.

    (viii) Carnitine and selenium deficiencies have been described.

(d) Trace metal deficiency

    (i) Copper deficiency is not uncommon and is manifested by anemia, neutropenia, and rash.

    (ii) Zinc deficiency is common and is manifested by an erythematous, maculopapular rash (acrodermatitis enteropathica) involving the face, trunk, metacarpophalangeal joints, and perineum. *Low* serum alkaline phosphatase is common.

(e) Mechanical complications

    (i) Arrhythmias can occur with an improperly placed catheter.

    (ii) Venous thrombosis is rare.

    (iii) Air embolus occurs only after accidental coupling of the IV line.

    (iv) Skin sloughs can occur from infiltration of peripheral venous infusions.

(f) Complications of Intralipid administration

    (i) Bilirubin. Lipid can displace bilirubin from albumin and may need to be held or infused at lower rates in jaundiced infants.

    (ii) Eosinophilia can occur.

(g) Contraindications to the use of Intralipid include sustained triglyceride levels above 400 and hyperlipidemic states.

B. Evaluation of gastrointestinal disease

  1. Examination of the stool

    a. Examine the stool for consistency, odor, blood, and mucus. The presence of gross blood and mucus indicates colitis. Use saline and Lugol's solution to look for parasites.

    b. Clinitest to detect the presence of reducing substances

(1) Mix one part **fresh** stool in two parts water. (To detect sucrose intolerance, hydrolyze with 1 N HCl, boiling for 30 sec.)

(2) Centrifuge and add 15 drops of supernatant to one Clinitest tablet.

(3) The test is positive if 0.5% or more of reducing substance is present. The presence of reducing substance is always abnormal and indicates sucrose or disaccharide intolerance, or both.

c. pH

(1) Normal stool pH is 7 to 8.

(2) A decreased pH suggests the presence of organic acids, as seen in disaccharide intolerance.

(3) An increased pH suggests secretory diarrhea.

d. Hemoccult or guaiac test for blood.

e. Sudan stain for fat. Place a representative sample on two slides. On the first slide, put two drops of 95% ethyl alcohol and several drops of Sudan black III. Place a cover slip and examine for neutral fats. On the second slide, put two to four drops of 35% acetic acid and several drops of Sudan black III. Place a cover slip, heat the slide to boil, and examine for split fats (*N Engl J Med* 264:85–87, 1961). The presence of fat (red) globules in the slide indicates a positive test. The amount of fat globules correlates with the 72-hour fecal fat assay.

f. Fecal leukocytes

(1) Stain with Loeffler's methylene blue, or Wright's or Gram's stains.

(2) Infections or inflammatory processes with leukocytes include *Campylobacter, Salmonella, Shigella,* typhoid fever, invasive *Escherichia coli, Clostridium difficile,* ulcerative colitis, and Crohn's disease. A predominance of band forms suggests shigellosis.

g. Cultures for ova and parasites. Commercially available preservative kits increase the rate of identification of parasites.

h. *Giardia* antigen enzyme-linked immunosorbent assay (ELISA). This assay offers increased sensitivity for detection of *Giardia* in the stool, but will not detect other parasites (e.g., *Blastocystis hominis*).

2. Fecal fat excretion. Although often distasteful to patient and clinician, this is the best method for detecting steatorrhea.

a. All stools are collected for 72 hours.

b. The patient must keep a diary of food intake during this period, so that the amount of fat in the diet can be estimated. *The diet should contain at least 35% fat.*

c. Coefficient of absorption (CA) = (dietary fat − fecal fat)/dietary fat × 100). **Normal values:** Values for breast-fed infants are lower but are not precisely known.

(1) Prematures: 60 to 75%.

(2) Newborns: 80 to 85%.

(3) 10 months to 3 years: 85 to 95%.

(4) Older than 3 years: 95%.

3. D-Xylose excretion. This test reflects enteric mucosal absorption. Its reliability for detecting mucosal disease is controversial, but it remains a useful screening test.

a. Give 14.5 g/m^2 after an overnight fast.

b. Measure serum xylose at 1 hour; above 25 mg/dl is normal.

c. Delayed gastric emptying can cause falsely low levels.

4. The **breath hydrogen test** is useful for detection of lactose and sucrose malabsorption.

a. After an overnight fast, the patient is given a loading dose of the disaccharide to be studied.

b. A breathing mask is placed over the nose and mouth, and 3 to 5 ml expired air is collected in a syringe at 30-minute intervals for 3 hours.

c. Hydrogen excreted is measured; excretion of more than 11 ppm H$_2$ indicates disaccharide malabsorption.

d. False positives and false negatives may be seen as a result of natural or antibiotic-induced changes in bacterial flora. *No antibiotics should be administered within 1 week before the test.*

5. The **Schilling test** measures the ability to absorb ingested vitamin B_{12}. It is used to evaluate patients with pernicious anemia, ileal dysfunction syndromes, malabsorption, pancreatic insufficiency, bacterial overgrowth, and Crohn's disease.

6. **Overnight pH monitoring** will evaluate for excessive gastroesophageal reflux. In patients with paroxysmal events suspected to be due to reflux (e.g., apnea or choking), the time of the acute event should correlate with a period of reflux to establish an association.

7. **Esophageal manometry** is designed to evaluate the motility characteristics of the esophagus and the upper and lower esophageal sphincter pressures. It provides information in diseases such as scleroderma, achalasia, diffuse esophageal spasm, and gastroesophageal reflux.

8. **Rectal manometry** is designed to evaluate the relaxation and pressure of the rectal sphincters. It is useful in the diagnosis of Hirschsprung's disease.

9. **Radiologic evaluation**
   a. Plain radiographs
      (1) Flat plate.
      (2) Upright—for air-fluid levels, pneumoperitoneum.
      (3) Decubitus—for pneumoperitoneum.
   b. An **upper GI series** and small bowel follow-through.
   c. **Barium enema.**
   d. **Oral cholecystogram.**
   e. Percutaneous transhepatic cholangiogram.
   f. Computed tomography and magnetic resonance imaging.

10. **Nuclear medicine and ultrasound**
   a. **Abdominal ultrasound** to evaluate liver parenchyma, biliary tree, and pancreas.
   b. **Technetium-99 scans** for evaluation of pathologic gastroesophageal reflux, aspiration pneumonia, or gastric emptying.
   c. **Hepatobiliary iminodiacetic acid (HIDA) scan** (or other iminodiacetic acid derivatives) for evaluation of bilirubin excretion.
   d. **A liver and spleen scan** to evaluate the liver and spleen size as well as filling defects.

11. **Endoscopy (plus biopsy)**
   a. Esophagogastroduodenoscopy.
   b. Proctosigmoidoscopy.
   c. Colonoscopy.
   d. Endoscopic retrograde cholangiopancreatography.

C. **Preparation for bowel procedures.** The following are standard bowel preparations utilized at our hospital. The duration of NPO varies with the age of the patient; the primary goal of NPO is to prevent vomiting or aspiration during a radiographic or endoscopic procedure. Proper bowel preparation is essential for colonoscopy, where mucosal defects or polyps may be obscured by fecal material.

1. **Upper gastrointestinal radiographic series with small bowel study:** NPO for 4 hours for infants under 1 year, NPO for 6 hours for patients over 1 year.

2. **Upper gastrointestinal endoscopy;** NPO for 6 to 8 hours.

3. **Percutaneous endoscopic gastrostomy:** as for upper endoscopy, with antibiotic prophylaxis (e.g., cefazolin, 30 mg/kg given on call to the procedure, with 2 more doses to follow).

4. **Flexible sigmoidoscopy**
   a. Bisacodyl, 5 mg PO the night before the procedure.
   b. 250 to 750 ml saline enema the night before and morning of the procedure.
   c. NPO past midnight.

5. **Colonoscopy:** preparation 1 (for infants, toddlers and uncooperative children)
   a. Clear liquids for 48 hours before the procedure.
   b. Bisacodyl, 5 mg the morning and night before the procedure.
   c. Saline enema, 250 to 750 ml the night before and morning of the procedure.
   d. NPO past midnight.

6. **Colonoscopy:** preparation 2 (for cooperative older children and teenagers)
   a. Regular diet until 5 PM the evening of the procedure.
   b. Beginning at 5 PM, 250 ml (1 cup) balanced electrolyte lavage solution (BEL; e.g., GoLYTELY, Colyte) q15 min for a minimum of 4 liters, until pure liquid is being passed from the rectum. Some older adolescents may require up to 6 liters of BEL. Note: As BEL can cause nausea, it is recommended that the physician premedicate the patient with 0.1 mg/kg metoclopramide (usual range 5–10 mg) 15 minutes before the first cup of BEL.
   c. NPO past midnight. If the patient is unable to take BEL by mouth, it can be administered through a nasogastric tube.
   d. NPO past midnight.
7. **Barium enema**. If searching for a mucosal defect or polyp, use colonoscopy preparation 1 or 2. However, no bowel preparation should be utilized in the patient with Hirschsprung's disease, as bowel preps can obscure the transition zone.
8. **24-hour esophageal pH monitoring**
   a. NPO for 4 to 6 hours.
   b. Discontinue all antireflux medications (including prokinetic agents, acid secretion inhibitors, and antacids) for at least 1 day before the test.
   c. If the patient is being fed by continuous gastric feedings, these should be changed to bolus feedings for the duration of the study. In addition, nasogastric tubes should not be left in for the duration of the study.

II. **Specific entities**
  A. **Malabsorption.** Because fat absorption depends on all the phases of digestion, the presence of *steatorrhea* (fat malabsorption) is the best indicator of a malabsorptive defect. Further tests will permit the localization of specific sites of abnormality (see sec. **I.B.**, p. 343)
  B. **Diarrheal disease.** Diarrhea is among the most common symptoms in pediatrics, and in underdeveloped countries it is the most common cause of morbidity and mortality in childhood. Evaluation of chronic diarrhea includes a history, with particular attention to blood or mucus in the stools, weight loss, failure to thrive, associated symptoms (fever, recurrent infection), drugs taken (particularly antibiotics), GI surgical procedures, family history, travel, age, and race. A physical examination should attend to nutritional status, hydration, edema, protuberant abdomen, abdominal masses, muscular habitus, rectal prolapse, and affect, particularly irritability. The hemodynamic and neurologic status should be carefully evaluated. Laboratory studies include a CBC, erythrocyte sedimentation rate (ESR), urinalysis, serum protein analysis (SPA), stool examination, and sweat test.
   1. **Acute gastroenteritis** (See also Chap. 3, p. 52)
      a. **Etiology.** This common condition has many causes. These are listed in Table 11-3.
      b. **Evaluation.** This condition is often manifested by a sudden onset of vomiting, followed by diarrhea. It is most often self-limited. Fever may or may

Table 11-3. Common causes of acute diarrhea in childhood

Viral enteritis (e.g., rotavirus in children <2 yr)
Bacterial enteritis
   Enterotoxin associated (*Escherichia coli, cholera, Clostridium perfringens, Staphylococcus*)
   Nonenterotoxin associated* (*Salmonella, Shigella, E. coli, Yersinia*)
Parasitic enteritis (amebiasis,* giardiasis, cryptosporidiosis)
Extraintestinal infection (e.g., otitis media, urinary tract infection, sepsis)
Antibiotic induced* (*Clostridium difficile*)
Hemolytic-uremic syndrome*
Inflammatory bowel disease* (ulcerative colitis, Crohn's disease)

*May be associated with blood in the stool.

not be present, but with a reduction of fluid intake and abnormal losses, dehydration can occur, especially in children under 3 years of age.

(1) History. Record the following: weight loss, duration, presence of blood or mucus, type and frequency of stools, type and amount of feedings, frequency of urination, presence or absence of tears, associated symptoms (e.g., fever, rash, vomiting, localized abdominal pain) and current family illnesses, source of water supply, attendance at a day care center, contact with animals, and travel history.

(2) Physical examination should include measurement of vital signs and weight, assessment of postural changes, and description of the skin turgor, mucous membranes, fontanels, eyes (presence or absence of tears), activity state, irritability, and associated rashes.

(3) Laboratory tests can be minimized in the milder clinical states, but a stool Wright's stain for neutrophils may be helpful, and urinary specific gravity can detect early dehydration. The yield from stool cultures is much higher when the Wright's stain is positive.

c. Therapy

(1) Children with acute diarrheal disease and minimal to moderate dehydration are treated most effectively with **oral rehydration therapy** (ORT; Table 11-4). In the initial vomiting stage, small volumes (5–15 ml) of ORT should be given frequently; large-volume feedings should be avoided.

(2) Boiled skim milk has a very high osmolar load and can cause hypernatremia. High osmolar fluids (e.g., cola, ginger ale, apple juice, chicken broth) should also be avoided.

(3) Once rehydration is accomplished (usually in 8–12 hr), easily absorbed foods from the regular diet should be started, for example, rice, rice cereal, bananas, dry cereal, crackers, and toast. Lactose- and sucrose-containing fluids can be diluted 1 : 1 with water if secondary disaccharidase deficiency is present.

(4) The value of drugs such as kaolin and belladonna-containing compounds remains unproved, and their use should be discouraged. An antispasmodic, such as diphenoxylate (Lomotil), camphorated opium tincture, or loperamide (Imodium), is not recommended for use in children (*MMWR* 41:1, 1992). Even when spasm is reduced, **fluid losses continue to occur into the lumen of the gut, but are not measurable and give a false sense of security.** In toxogenic diarrhea the elimination of the toxin is also delayed by these agents.

(5) Antiemetics such as promethazine (Phenergan) or dimenhydrinate (Dramamine) are not recommended for vomiting associated with acute diarrhea for use in children (*MMWR* 41:1, 1992). The side effects of these drugs preclude their long-term use. If vomiting persists, more vigorous evaluation and management are indicated.

(6) Close follow-up, including daily weights, is imperative, particularly in smaller infants, who can rapidly become dehydrated.

Table 11-4. Approximate electrolyte content for oral rehydration solution

Solution	Composition of oral rehydration fluids (mmole/liter)				
	Glucose	Na	K	Citrate	Osmolality
Pedialyte (Ross)	140	45	20	10	270
Ricelyte (Mead Johnson)	70	50	25	10	200
Rehydralyte (Ross)	140	75	20	10	305
WHO solution (ORS)	111	90	20	10	310

(7) Specific therapy for acute diarrhea
  (a) Enterotoxigenic *E. coli.* Bismuth subsalicylate (Pepto-Bismol).
  (b) *Shigella* species. Trimethoprim-sulfamethoxazole (Bactrim, Septra).
  (c) *Campylobacter jejuni.* Erythromycin, clarithromycin.
  (d) *Clostridium difficile.* Vancomycin, cholestyramine.
  (e) *Giardia.* Quinacrine, metronidazole (Flagyl), bacitracin.
  (f) *Entamoeba histolytica.* Metronidazole (Flagyl).
2. Chronic gastroenteritis. Diarrheal symptoms that last more than 2 weeks are chronic. The causes of chronic diarrhea are listed in Table 11-5.
  a. Nonspecific diarrhea is the most common cause of chronic diarrhea in childhood.
    (1) The **etiology** is unknown. Psychosocial and family stress are often implicated.
    (2) Evaluation and diagnosis. The classic history is of watery diarrhea with multiple formula and dietary changes in the age group 1 to 5 years. The physical findings and growth are normal. The findings of routine urinalysis and stool cultures are negative. The diagnosis is based on exclusion of other causes of diarrhea.
    (3) Therapy. The goal of therapy is to stop diarrhea (and to ensure that normal growth continues).
      (a) The family should be reassured that the illness is not too serious.
      (b) Often, past dietary manipulations may have contributed to the production of symptoms, and correction of the diet may result in relief of the diarrhea. A decrease in the intake of fructose and sucrose-containing drinks, or changing the diet, may function as a placebo.
      (c) Should reassurance and dietary adjustment fail, hospitalization may be necessary. The disappearance of diarrhea during hospitalization may help convince the family of the absence of significant disease and permit the examination of psychosocial factors.
      (d) Antidiarrheal medication is not indicated.
      (e) X-ray contrast studies should be done when it is necessary to rule out anatomic abnormalities.

Table 11-5. Causes of chronic diarrhea

Chronic nonspecific diarrhea (irritable bowel syndrome)
Chronic infections: *Yersinia, Escherichia coli, Giardia, Clostridium difficile, Cryptosporidium,* small bowel overgrowth
Cystic fibrosis
Gluten-sensitive enteropathy (celiac disease)
Disaccharide deficiency (particularly lactose intolerance)
Food allergy
Inflammatory bowel disease
Immunodeficiency states (including transient hypogammaglobulinemia)
Anatomic causes
  Short-bowel syndrome
  Malrotation
  Hirschsprung's disease
Endocrine
  Hyperthyroidism
  Addison's disease
  Congenital adrenal hyperplasia
Others
  Urinary tract infections
  Acrodermatitis enteropathica
  Neuroblastoma and ganglioneuroma

C. Constipation (See also Chap. 3, p. 53)
1. **Definition**—no clear criteria in children. In adults, the passage of three or fewer hard bowel movements a week or the inability to expel formed hard stool defines constipation. However, some infants may have one to two normal bowel movements a week.
2. **Encopresis**, or fecal incontinence, in the older child is almost always associated with constipation, loss of internal sphincter tone, and fecal overflow.
3. **Etiologies.** Though a wide variety of disorders can cause constipation (Table 11-6), 99% of constipation seen in a pediatrician's office is functional, and can be managed medically with the regimen below. In the neonate or infant, Hirschsprung's disease, neurogenic constipation (i.e., caused by myelomeningocele or tethered cord), hypothyroidism, and an anteriorly placed anus need to be considered; these entities become rarer in later childhood.
4. **Evaluation.** A careful history and physical examination are usually the only evaluation necessary in the toddler or older child.
   a. **History** should include time of passage of first meconium (passage in first 24 hr makes Hirschsprung's disease less likely), age of onset of problem, frequency of stools, size of bowel movements, presence of pain with defecation, presence of blood in stool, presence of rectal prolapse, time of toilet training, and presence of encopresis or enuresis. Usually, children with functional constipation have large, "softball-sized" bowel movements every 2 to 7 days.
   b. **Physical examination** should include careful abdominal examination (for stool or other abdominal masses), inspection of the anus (for its placement and for the presence of hemorrhoids or fissures), rectal examination, back inspection (for any sacral sinuses or hair tufts), and neurologic examination (including lower extremity reflexes).
   c. **Abdominal plain film** can help assess the quantity of stool in the colon and identify spina bifida occulta.
   d. **Rectal manometry** demonstrates relaxation of the internal anal sphincter, which is absent in Hirschsprung's disease. It can also be used for biofeedback in children with refractory constipation.
   e. **Barium enema** should be performed on an unprepped colon in constipated children. It is principally utilized to identify a transition zone in patients with suspected Hirschsprung's disease. Absence of a radiographic transition zone in the neonate or young infant does not exclude Hirschsprung's disease.
   f. **Rectal biopsy** demonstrates an absence of ganglion cells in Hirschsprung's disease. The absence of ganglion cells on a rectal suction biopsy should be confirmed by a surgical full-thickness biopsy.
   g. **Ultrasound or computed tomography** can identify abdominal masses causing obstruction.
   h. **Magnetic resonance imaging** should be performed in patients with suspected spinal cord lesions.
5. **Treatment of functional constipation**
   a. Infants under 6 months old often respond to increased fluid intake plus the addition of 15 ml of prune juice or 10 ml of Karo Syrup to 4 oz formula. In more severely constipated infants in whom Hirschsprung's disease is not suspected, lactulose (1ml/kg/day in the formula) can help. A glycerin suppository is usually adequate to help an acutely constipated infant.
   b. For older children
      (1) Cleanout stage—utilized in children older than 18 months with severe constipation and hard stool in the rectal vault. Either of the following:
         (a) **Bisacodyl** (Dulcolax)—5 mg for children 18 months to 10 yrs, 10 mg for children 10 to 18 years, PO given qAM for 3 consecutive days.
         (b) **Enemas**—10 ml/kg normal saline given daily for 3 consecutive days. Alternatively, one pediatric Fleet Enema qd for 3 days can be used in children over 5, or one adult Fleet Enema qd for 3 days

Table 11-6. Etiologies of pediatric constipation

Functional-predisposing factors
Developmental
    Cognitive handicaps
    Attention deficit
Situational
    Excessive parental interventions
    Coercive toilet training
    Toilet phobia
    School bathroom avoidance
Psychogenic
    Depression
    Anorexia nervosa
Constitutional
    Genetic predisposition
    Colonic inertia
Reduced volume and drying
    Low-fiber diet
    Dehydration
    Malnutrition, underfeeding
    Faulty diet—excessive milk

Altered anatomy and physiology
Structural
    Anal stenosis
    Imperforate anus
    Anterior displaced anus
Acquired inflammatory stricture
    Necrotizing enterocolitis
    Inflammatory bowel disease
Malrotation, congenital intestinal bands
Abdominal pelvic masses
    Anterior sacral meningomyelocele
    Sacral teratoma
Aganglionosis and abnormal myenteric plexus
    Hirschsprung's disease, congenital
    Chagas' disease, acquired
    Intestinal pseudo-obstruction
Abnormal abdominal musculature
    Prune belly
    Gastroschisis
Abnormal innervation
    Meningomyelocele
    Spinal cord tumor
Hypotonia
    Cerebral palsy
    Amyotonia congenita
    Familial visceral myopathy
Connective tissue disorder
    Scleroderma
    Amyloidosis
    Mixed connective tissue disease
    Lupus erythematosus

Table 11-6. (continued)

Metabolic or endocrine dysfunction
Hypothyroidism
Hypercalcemia
Lead ingestion
Diabetes mellitus
Panhypopituitarism

Drugs
Antacids, bismuth, anticholinergics, antihistamines, and opiates

Source: Adapted from AJ Rosenberg. Constipation and Encopresis. In R Wyllie, JS Hyams (eds). *Pediatric Gastrointestinal Disease*. Philadelphia: Saunders, 1993. P 199.

in children over 12. Disadvantages of enemas include difficulty of administration and risk of water intoxication (with tap water enemas) or phosphate overload (with Fleet Enemas).

(2) **Maintenance.** The maintenance phase usually needs to be continued for several months. Behavioral/lifestyle changes include sitting on the toilet twice a day after meals, and eating a diet high in fiber. The dose of medication should be adjusted to result in at least one soft bowel movement every other day. Use either

    (a) **Mineral oil (MO)**—1 to 2 ml/kg/dose (maximum 60 ml/dose) bid. Contraindicated in infants under 18 months of age, neurologically handicapped patients, or patients with swallowing dysfunction due to the concern of aspiration. A supplemental multivitamin is recommended in patients receiving chronic MO therapy due to the theoretical potential of MO to interfere with fat-soluble vitamin absorption.

    (b) **Lactulose**—1 ml/kg/dose qd or bid (maximum 60 ml bid). Lactulose is often more palatable to young children. Side effects include abdominal cramping.

D. **Hirschsprung's disease** (congenital, aganglionic megacolon). Congenital absence of the intrinsic ganglionic plexus of Auerbach and Meissner, which involves varying lengths of the rectum and colon. The incidence is estimated at 1 in 5,000. A family incidence exists in 10% of cases.

  1. **Etiology.** The cause is unknown.

  2. **Evaluation**

    a. The **neonatal history** includes failure to pass meconium in the first 24 hours of life or bile-stained vomiting in the first week of life. In late infancy and childhood, the history reports increasing constipation.

    b. **Rectal examination** classically reveals a tight anal sphincter and an empty rectum followed by an explosive gush of stool and gas. In the *neonatal period* abdominal distention is a prominent feature, whereas in the older child, fecal masses are palpable.

  3. **Diagnosis**

    a. **X-rays** of the abdomen reveal dilated loops of bowel on an anteroposterior film. Rectal air is absent.

    b. The **barium enema** may reveal a narrow aganglionic segment with a dilated colon above. (In the immediate neonatal period, this typical pattern may be absent.) An important clue will be a 24-hour film showing that the barium is still present. In young infants or "short segment" Hirschsprung's disease, the barium enema findings may be normal or nondiagnostic. The patient should not receive a preparatory enema.

    c. **Rectal manometry** may reveal absence of the normal relaxation reflex of the internal sphincter.

   d. Rectal biopsy is definitive. If a suction biopsy does not reveal ganglion cells, a full-thickness surgical biopsy is necessary. The biopsy may need to be repeated if symptoms persist when laboratory findings are normal.
4. **Treatment**
   a. The neonate with Hirschsprung's enterocolitis is often extremely ill, with shock and sepsis.
      (1) A nasogastric tube is passed for decompression.
      (2) Urgent intravenous rehydration is begun.
      (3) Antibiotics (e.g., ampicillin + gentamicin + clindamycin) are given.
      (4) An emergency colostomy is performed in an area of the colon where ganglion cells are seen.
      (5) Resection of the aganglionic segment is delayed for 6 months to 2 years.
   b. Surgical management. Three types of operations have been utilized.
      (1) Swenson. The aganglionic colon is resected, and the ganglion-containing bowel is anastomosed to the rectal stump.
      (2) Duhamel. A longer piece of rectum, usually 5 to 7 cm, is left and closed proximally. Ganglionic bowel is pulled down retrorectally to 1 cm from the mucocutaneous junction, leaving part of the internal sphincter intact. Colorectal anastomosis is achieved by clamping the posterior wall of the rectum to the anterior wall of the colon.
      (3) Soave. This operation leaves 10 to 20 cm of rectal stump. The mucosa is stripped and the ganglionic bowel pulled through.
   c. Surgical complications
      (1) Following colostomy
         (a) Circulatory collapse resulting in severe enterocolitis can occur after colostomy for decompression. Treatment is supportive, that is, fluid and electrolyte replacement and antibiotics.
         (b) Persistent diarrhea, which is often due to disaccharide deficiency, can occur. A Clinitest is positive. A change in the type of sugar in the formula will alleviate symptoms.
      (2) After definitive surgery. Segmental obstruction with overflow incontinence is often a problem, especially in the first few months after surgery.
E. Gastrointestinal hemorrhage
1. **Etiology.** The causes of upper and lower gastrointestinal hemorrhage are highly age dependent (Table 11-7).
2. **Evaluation** and **therapy** involves answering four questions. (Questions a–c can usually be answered in the clinic or emergency setting, while question d frequently requires further radiographic or endoscopic evaluation.)
   a. Is the patient hemodynamically stable?
   b. Is it really blood?
   c. Is the blood from the upper or lower intestinal tract?
   d. What is the site of bleeding?
3. **Diagnosis and management**
   a. Upper GI bleeding most commonly presents as melena (tarry stool) or hematemesis (vomiting of blood). A large-volume upper GI bleed can present with hematochezia (bright-red blood per rectum). Lower GI bleeding presents with maroon or bright-red bloody stool.
   b. The **history** should include any prior peptic ulcer disease, gastroesophageal reflux disease, liver disease, infection, vomiting of long duration, or nonsteroidal anti-inflammatory drug use. The patient/parent should describe the color of any vomitus, number of bowel movements, and amount of blood in the stool. Any change in skin color (pallor) or sensation of light-headedness (presyncope) suggests significant blood loss.
   c. Physical examination
      (1) Orthostatic vital signs—pulse, blood pressure. (If the patient is in shock, proceed directly to part e.)
      (2) Nasopharyngeal examination.

Table 11-7. Etiologies of gastrointestinal bleeding

Age group	Common	Less Common
Upper gastrointestinal bleeding		
Neonates (0–30 d)	Swallowed maternal blood Gastritis Duodenitis	Coagulopathy Vascular malformations Gastric-esophageal duplication Leiomyoma
Infants (30 d–1 yr)	Gastritis and gastric ulcer Esophagitis Duodenitis	Esophageal varices Foreign body Aortoesophageal fistula
Children (1–12 yr)	Esophagitis Esophageal varices Gastritis and gastric ulcer Duodenal ulcer Mallory-Weiss tear Nasopharyngeal bleeding	Leiomyoma Salicylates Vascular malformation Hematobilia
Adolescents (12 yr–adult)	Duodenal ulcer Esophagitis Esophageal varices Gastritis Mallory-Weiss tear	Thrombocytopenia Dieulafoy's ulcer Hematobilia
Lower gastrointestinal bleeding		
Neonates (0–30 d)	Anorectal lesions Swallowed maternal blood Milk allergy Necrotizing enterocolitis Midgut volvulus	Vascular malformations Hirschsprung's enterocolitis Intestinal duplication Coagulopathy
Infants (30 d–1 yr)	Anorectal lesions Midgut volvulus Intussusception (<3 yr) Meckel's diverticulum Infectious diarrhea Milk allergy (<4 yr)	Vascular malformations Intestinal duplication Acquired thrombocytopenia
Children (1–12 yr)	Juvenile polyps Meckel's diverticulum Intussusception (<3 yr) Infectious diarrhea Anal fissure Nodular lymphoid hyperplasia	Henoch-Schönlein purpura Hemolytic-uremic syndrome Vasculitis (SLE) Inflammatory bowel disease
Adolescents (12 yr–adult)	Inflammatory bowel disease Polyps Hemorrhoids Anal fissure Infectious diarrhea	Arteriovascular malformation Adenocarcinomas Henoch-Schönlein purpura Pseudomembranous colitis

SLE = systemic lupus erythematosus.
Source: AD Olson, CH Hillemeir. Gastrointestinal Hemorrhage. In R Wyllie, JS Hyams (eds). *Pediatric Gastrointestinal Disease*. Philadelphia: Saunders, 1993. P 259.

    (3) Skin examination (for hemangiomas, telangiectasias, caput medusa).
    (4) Abdominal examination
        (a) Epigastric tenderness suggests peptic ulcer disease.
        (b) Splenomegaly suggests portal hypertension.
    (5) Rectal examination and stool guaiac are mandatory in all cases of GI bleeding.

d. Nasogastric tube placement. This should be a tube sufficiently large to allow suction and lavage of gastric contents. Lavage should be performed until gastric contents are clear. Iced saline is no longer recommended as it will lower core temperature. The presence of esophageal varices does not contraindicate NG tube placement.

e. Hemodynamic stabilization
    (1) One or two large-bore intravenous lines.
    (2) In hemodynamically unstable patient, immediate infusion of 10 to 20 ml/kg isotonic crystalloid (normal saline, lactated Ringer's, or 5% albumin in NS or LR).
    (3) The best volume replacement when shock is due to hemorrhage is blood. In a patient in unstable condition, O-negative blood can be given while waiting for cross-matched blood. The hematocrit does not acutely reflect the patient's degree of hemorrhage.
    (4) Patients with massive GI bleeds will also need clotting factors (fresh-frozen plasma) and platelets.

f. Localization of the site of bleeding
    (1) Fiberoptic endoscopy is the procedure of choice to localize upper GI bleeding, and may also allow simultaneous therapeutic intervention (see part h). All patients with melena or vigorous hematochezia should undergo fiberoptic endoscopy, as 3 to 5% of duodenal ulcers will have a blood-free nasogastric lavage.
    (2) Lower GI bleeding is more difficult to localize, and techniques utilized include radiographic studies (radiolabeled red cell scan, Meckel's diverticulum scan, and arteriography), upper endoscopy, colonoscopy, and, in severe cases, laparotomy.

g. Pharmacotherapy
    (1) Vasopressin is used to treat variceal hemorrhage in children. A bolus dose of 20 units of vasopressin per 1.73 m^2 body surface area diluted in 10 ml/kg of 5% dextrose in water (D5W) is given over 15 minutes, followed by a continuous infusion of 0.2 units/1.73 m^2/min. The dose can be increased to a maximum of 0.8 units/m^2/min. Fluid overload, vasoconstriction, and hyponatremia are reported side effects.
    (2) Octreotide (a long-acting analogue of somatostatin) has also been utilized to treat variceal and gastric hemorrhage in adults, though limited experience with this drug exists in children, and a pediatric dose has not been established. A suggested starting dosage for adults is 50 to 100 µg q8h SC or IV; a suggested starting dosage for children is 2 µg/kg q8h SC or IV.
    (3) Intravenous **H$_2$ receptor antagonists** (cimetidine, 10 mg/kg/dose q6h) or ranitidine (1 mg/kg/dose q6h), with or without **antacids** (Maalox, Mylanta, Amphogel), 1 ml/kg/dose q2–4h, will treat gastritis, esophagitis, and ulcers.

h. Other therapeutic interventions depend on the etiology of the bleed.
    (1) Bleeding esophageal varices can be treated by the therapeutic endoscopist (sclerotherapy, rubber band ligation), interventional radiologist (transjugular intrahepatic portosystemic shunt), or pediatric surgeon (Sengstaken-Blakemore tube placement, emergency portosystemic shunt).
    (2) Bleeding gastric or duodenal ulcers not responsive to pharmacologic therapy can be treated via electrocautery, injection of epinephrine, embolization of blood vessels, or surgery.

(3) Some bleeding lesions require resection (e.g., colonic polyps, Meckel's diverticula).

F. Peptic ulcer disease and **gastritis** are being increasingly diagnosed in infants and children.

1. **Evaluation.** Vomiting is frequently seen, especially in small children, and the pain is often atypical when compared to peptic disease in adults.

   a. **History** should focus on vomiting, abdominal distention, hematemesis, melena, poor eating, abdominal pain (usually related to meals), medications, associated underlying illness, and family history.

   b. **Physical examination** may demonstrate epigastric tenderness and occult blood in the stool.

   c. **Laboratory studies** include a CBC, reticulocyte count, and stool guaiac. Fasting and 60-minute postprandial gastrin levels should be obtained if the Zollinger-Ellison syndrome is being considered.

   d. **Diagnostic procedures**
      (1) Upper GI series (50–60% sensitivity for ulcers).
      (2) Fiberoptic endoscopy (>95% sensitivity). The presence of **Helicobacter pylori** should be evaluated for in every patient undergoing endoscopy for gastritis or peptic ulcer disease. Pathologic examination of the hematoxylin and eosin stain is usually sufficient to identify *H. pylori*, but in some cases silver stain or *H. pylori* culture is helpful.

2. **Treatment**
   a. **Antacids.** The recommended dosage is 0.5 to 1.0 ml/kg 1 and 3 hours after each meal and at bedtime for 4 to 6 weeks. Alternating aluminum- and magnesium-containing antacids can reduce the incidence of diarrhea and constipation.

   b. **H$_2$ blockers include cimetidine, ranitidine, famotidine, and nizatidine.** Cimetidine is given in a dosage of 5 to 10 mg/kg/dose PO four times a day with meals and at bedtime for 6 weeks. Ranitidine is given in a dosage of 2 mg/kg/dose PO bid. Children with symptoms that persist longer than 6 weeks can be given a single dose of an H$_2$ blocker at bedtime for 3 to 12 months.

   c. **Sucralfate** is a nonabsorbed sulfated disaccharide, that acts locally to form a barrier for irritated mucosa. The recommended dose is 1 g/1.73 m^2, given ½ hour before meals and at bedtime for 4 to 6 weeks.

   d. **Proton pump antagonist. Omeprazole** inhibits hydrogen ion production by the parietal cell, and is the most potent blocker of gastric acid secretion. The recommended dosage is 20 mg/1.73 m^2 once a day. Use of this agent for more than 3 consecutive months is not recommended, and patients for whom long-term therapy is utilized should have their serum gastrin monitored.

   e. **Diet.** No form of diet (including bland) has been shown to be helpful in healing ulcers or in preventing their recurrence.

   f. **Misoprostol** is a synthetic prostaglandin analogue that may be useful for patients with gastritis or ulcers secondary to prolonged nonsteroidal use.

   g. **Antibiotics** are recommended for all cases of gastritis or peptic ulcers where *H. pylori* has been identified. Several antibiotic regimens exist for *H. pylori* eradication (*Am J Gastroenterol* 87:1716–1727, 1992), including the following combination regimens:
      (1) Children under 16 years: amoxicillin, 40 mg/kg/day divided tid (maximum 750 mg tid) for 14 days + metronidazole, 20 to 30 mg/kg/day divided tid (maximum 500 mg tid) for 14 days + Pepto-Bismol, 1 to 2 tablespoons PO tid for 6 weeks.
      (2) Children 16 years and older: tetracycline, 500 mg PO qid for 14 days + metronidazole, 20 to 30 mg/kg/day divided tid (maximum 500 mg tid) for 14 days + Pepto-Bismol, 2 tablespoons PO tid for 6 weeks.
      (3) Side effects of the above regimens are usually due to the metronidazole, and include nausea, vomiting, and a disulfiram reaction if a pa-

tient receiving metronidazole ingests alcohol. The success rate of the above regimens in clearing *H. pylori* is 80 to 90%, and can be increased by the addition of an H_2 blocker (e.g., ranitidine, 150 mg PO bid for adults) or omeprazole (20 mg PO bid for adults). Recurrence of *H. pylori* is common; endoscopy is still the gold standard for detecting recurrence, though serologies and radiolabeled breath tests are becoming increasingly available.

G. **Pathologic gastroesophageal reflux** is defined as the abnormal clearance of acid from the distal esophagus. It differs from functional gastroesophageal reflux of infancy, which is defined as the regurgitation of gastric contents into the esophagus *without* pathologic complications. Gastroesophageal reflux is never normal after 1 year of age.

1. **Etiology.** The causes include anatomic abnormalities (e.g., hiatus hernia, lower esophageal sphincter [LES] pressure, transient LES relaxation, and esophageal dysmotility).

2. **Clinical manifestations** include (see also *Gastroenterology* 81:376, 1981)
   a. Recurrent emesis.
   b. Recurrent pneumonia.
   c. Asthma.
   d. Choking or apnea.
   e. Failure to thrive.
   f. Sandifer syndrome (neck hyperextension).
   g. Heartburn (pyrosis).
   h. Dysphagia.
   i. Nocturnal cough and wheeze.
   j. Hematemesis.
   k. Rumination.
   l. Iron-deficiency anemia.

3. **Evaluation and diagnosis**
   a. **Upper GI series** to assess anatomy, the presence of strictures, and the gastric outlet.
   b. The **continuous intraesophageal pH probe** study is the best test to evaluate acid clearance. It should be obtained over an 18- to 24-hour period. Normal values for the normal amount of acid in the esophagus vary with age.
   c. A **technetium-99m (⁹⁹ᵐTc) scan** (milk scan) to assess regurgitation of gastric contents into the lungs, and gastric emptying.
   d. **Endoscopy** and **biopsy** to evaluate the presence of esophagitis (basal zone hyperplasia, infiltration of neutrophils, and the presence of intraepithelial eosinophils).
   e. **Esophageal manometry** to assess esophageal motility and lower esophageal sphincter pressure.

4. **Therapy**
   a. **Treatment for infants under 1 year of age with functional gastroesophageal reflux.** Children are fed small, thickened feedings and are placed prone with the head of the bed elevated after meals.
   b. For children with **abnormal acid clearance, heartburn, or esophagitis,** the following therapies are suggested.
      (1) **Antacid therapy** (alternating ALternaGEL and Mylanta). The dosage is 0.5 to 1.0 ml/kg 1 and 3 hours after meals and at bedtime.
      (2) **Therapy to block acid secretion.** Cimetidine, 5 to 10 mg/kg/dose q6h, ranitidine, 2 mg/kg/dose bid; or, in severe cases, omeprazole (20 mg/1.73m²/day qAM).
      (3) **Prokinetic agents.** Cisapride (Propulsid), 0.2 to 0.3 mg/kg/dose (maximum dose 20 mg) tid before meals; metoclopramide (Reglan), 0.1 to 0.2 mg/kg/dose qid before meals; or bethanechol chloride (Urecholine), 2.9 mg/m²/dose PO q8h. The maximum single dose is 50 mg.
      (4) If intensive medical therapy fails, **surgical intervention** (e.g., Nissen fundoplication) is indicated.

H. Chronic recurrent abdominal pain (RAP; (functional abdominal pain) is the most common cause of chronic abdominal pain in children. (See also Chap. 3, p. 57)

1. Apley's definition—at least one episode of abdominal pain per month for 3 consecutive months, severe enough to interfere with routine functioning.
2. Exists in up to 10% of school-aged children.
3. **History.** Paroxysmal episodes of crampy pain in the periumbilical or suprapubic area, usually lasting 5 to 30 minutes, with periods of wellness in between. Pallor during episodes is commonly reported.
4. **Physical examination** and growth curve are usually normal.
5. The presence of any of the following makes functional abdominal pain unlikely.
   a. Changes in frequency of bowel movements (constipation, incontinence).
   b. Direct relationship of pain to eating.
   c. Pain awakening child at night.
   d. Dysuria.
   e. Rectal bleeding or occult blood in the stool.
   f. Systemic symptoms (fever, weight loss, arthralgia).
   g. Focal pain or tenderness away from umbilicus.
   h. Vomiting.
   i. Physical findings of malnutrition or inflammatory bowel disease.
6. Functional abdominal pain should be differentiated from **psychogenic abdominal pain**, which is caused by stress or psychiatric disturbance, and is characterized by constant severe pain or pain behavior, inability to function, and extensive school absence. There may be psychological overlay to both organic and functional pain.
7. **Laboratory** evaluation should include CBC, differential, erythrocyte sedimentation rate, urinalysis, urine culture, and stool for occult blood. If indicated, stool for ova and parasites, lactose breath test, plain abdominal film, upper GI series, amylase, lipase, liver function test, and albumin should be obtained.
8. **Therapy**
   a. Description of the entity of functional abdominal pain, with emphasis on the differences between RAP, organic pain, and psychogenic pain. Reassurance that problem is benign.
   b. Identification of stress and anxiety.
   c. High-fiber diet.
   d. If lactose intolerance by history, trial of lactose-free diet.
   e. Regular follow-up.

I. Inflammatory bowel disease
1. **Ulcerative colitis**
   a. **Etiology.** Ulcerative colitis is a chronic, inflammatory mucosal disease of unknown origin. Genetic, environmental, psychological, infectious, and immunologic mechanisms have been implicated.
   b. **Evaluation**
      (1) The **history** usually includes bloody diarrhea and recurrent abdominal pain.
      (2) Systemic manifestations, including arthritis, erythema nodosum, uveitis, episcleritis, and liver disease, may precede or accompany the GI symptoms.
      (3) **Physical examination** of the abdomen is usually benign, unless local complications of toxic megacolon or perforation have occurred. Growth failure is present in fewer than 10% of patients.
      (4) **Laboratory** evaluation includes CBC, stool examination, sedimentation rate, albumin and total protein, cultures (for *Salmonella, Shigella, Yersinia, Campylobacter, E. coli* 0157:H7, *Aeromonas*, and *Plesiomonas*), *C. difficile* toxin, ova and parasites analysis, sigmoidoscopy, rectal biopsy, barium enema, and upper GI series with small bowel follow-through.
   c. **Diagnosis**
      (1) Stool examination reveals blood and fecal leukocytes.
      (2) Sigmoidoscopy or colonoscopy reveals biopsy-confirmed colitis.

(3) Stool cultures are negative, *C. difficile* toxin is absent, and ova and parasites are not present.

(4) The CBC may reveal anemia, leukocytosis with left shift, thrombocytosis, and elevated ESR.

(5) Serum albumin levels may be low or normal.

(6) A barium enema may reveal colitis, but is usually superfluous if colonoscopy is performed. Upper GI series is normal.

(7) A tuberculin skin test is negative.

d. Treatment depends on the severity of the symptoms and signs.

(1) Nonsteroidal anti-inflammatory agents. Sulfasalazine (Azulfidine) is usually the drug of choice in mild to moderate cases. Therapy is begun at 500 mg/day (10–15 mg/kg/day) and increased over 4 to 5 days to 2 to 3 g/day (40–50 mg/kg/day) in two divided doses. Side effects include leukopenia, agranulocytosis, hemolytic anemia, arthralgia, headache, rash, and, rarely, lower GI bleeding. Other 5-aminosalicylate derivatives are now available for patients who are allergic or intolerant of sulfasalazine, including olsalazine (Dipentum) and mesalazine (Pentasa, Asacol). In addition, 5-aminosalicylate enemas (Rowasa) are available for patients with ulcerative proctitis or left-sided ulcerative colitis.

(2) Corticosteroids are the mainstay of therapy in moderate to severe ulcerative colitis. In the moderate case in which sulfasalazine alone is inadequate, prednisone, 1 to 2 mg/kg/day in a daily dose, is given. In patients who require IV therapy, methylprednisolone sodium succinate (Solu-Medrol), 1 to 2 mg/kg/day in two to four divided doses, is indicated. In limited rectal disease, methylprednisolone (Medrol) enemas are preferred over systemic therapy.

(3) Immunosuppressive agents, including azathioprine and 6-mercaptopurine (1.5 mg/kg/day), are sometimes tried in patients who respond poorly to or cannot be weaned from corticosteroids. Side effects include immunosuppression, leukopenia, and a possible increased risk of malignancy. Cyclosporine (3–4 mg/kg/24 hr given as a continuous infusion) is effective in controlling severe colitis that is unresponsive to intravenous corticosteroid therapy.

(4) Parenteral alimentation should be used in all patients who require prolonged IV therapy.

(5) Enteral alimentation. Elemental diets, which usually must be administered by NG tube, can be an effective treatment for Crohn's disease.

(6) Psychiatric consultation may be required to assist the patient or the parents, or both, to cope with chronic ulcers.

(7) Surgery. Colectomy is curative. The indications are

(a) Perforation.

(b) Toxic megacolon.

(c) Massive bleeding.

(d) Severe corticosteroid side effects that preclude further use.

(e) Poor growth.

(f) Chronically disabling disease.

(g) Malignancy. Patients with long-standing ulcerative colitis have a definite risk of developing colon cancer. Appropriate screening, such as colonoscopy and rectal biopsy, should be performed annually on patients who have had the disease for more than 10 years. Any sign of dysplasia on biopsy is an absolute indication for colectomy.

2. Crohn's disease. This is a chronic transmural and predominantly submucosal inflammatory disease that can affect any part of the GI tract from mouth to anus; it most often affects the distal ileum and colon while sparing the rectum.

a. Etiology. The cause is unknown.

b. Evaluation

(1) The history commonly includes growth failure (which occurs in 50% of patients), recurrent fever, and abdominal pain. Diarrhea is less common than in ulcerative colitis. Systemic symptoms include arthritis, erythema nodosum, uveitis, oral aphthous ulcers, and perianal disease. Tuberculosis and parasitic disease (amebiasis, *Strongyloides*) should be considered if a travel history is present.

(2) Physical examination may reveal evidence of malnutrition, localized abdominal signs or perianal disease on rectal examination, and blood and mucus. The clinician should also consider Behçet's disease if genital ulceration occurs, and malacoplakia if extensive fistulizing disease is present.

(3) Laboratory tests include a CBC, ESR, SPA, electrolytes, iron, iron-binding capacity, folate, sigmoidoscopy or colonoscopy, barium enema, and upper GI series.

c. Diagnosis

(1) Stools. Cultures are negative for bacteria, ova, parasites, and *C. difficile*. The stool guaiac test may be positive.

(2) A CBC reveals anemia, leukocytosis with left shift, and thrombocytosis. The ESR is often elevated, but can be normal in up to one third of cases.

(3) A tuberculin skin test is negative.

(4) Serum iron and folate levels may be low, and iron-binding capacity is increased.

(5) SPA reveals a serum albumin level that may be low.

(6) Sigmoidoscopy may show colitis (if the colon is involved).

(7) An upper GI series with small bowel follow-through may show small bowel involvement, most commonly in the ileocecal area.

(8) Growth failure. Severe growth failure can occur even though fewer than 5% of patients have malabsorption. The causes of growth failure are believed to be lack of caloric intake and disease activity.

(9) Periodic flare-ups are common.

(10) An abnormal Schilling test suggests B_{12} malabsorption secondary to terminal ileal involvement.

d. Treatment

(1) Colonic Crohn's disease. Sulfasalazine (Azulfidine) and corticosteroids are given as in ulcerative colitis. Other 5-aminosalicylate preparations can be utilized for Crohn's colitis in the sulfasalazine-intolerant patient.

(2) Ileal Crohn's disease. Corticosteroids are the drug of choice. Sulfasalazine is not useful for this specific disease. Azathioprine (Imuran, 1.5–2 mg/kg/day) and 6-mercaptopurine (1.5 mg/kg/day) will bring about a remission in 60 to 70% of patients with steroid-refractory Crohn's disease, but take up to 3 months to work .

(3) Perianal disease. Metronidazole (Flagyl), 250 mg PO tid, has been used with benefit.

(4) Antispasmodics have no place in the management of acute disease. However, in chronic disease, with diarrhea and tenesmus, they may be useful. Loperamide hydrochloride (Imodium), 2 mg PO tid prn, is commonly utilized.

(5) The use of elemental formula supplementation has proved to be beneficial for patients with Crohn's disease and growth failure, and may induce a temporary disease remission.

(6) TPN also promotes growth and initiates puberty in those who fail to respond to corticosteroids, but it is rarely used because of the increased risk and lack of superiority over elemental formulas.

(7) Psychiatric consultation is useful for the patients and their families in managing this chronic, often debilitating, disease.

(8) The indications for surgery are less clear-cut than for ulcerative colitis because of the chronic nature of this disease. They include

      (a) Perforation.

      (b) Obstruction.

      (c) Extensive perianal or rectal disease unresponsive to other therapeutic modalities.

      (d) Severe growth failure, in which a localized segment can be removed.

J. Irritable bowel syndrome is the most common illness to prompt gastroenterology referral in adults. It is also seen in older school-aged children and teenagers, and may overlap with functional abdominal pain. The primary challenge in establishing the diagnosis is ruling out other illnesses.

  1. History includes crampy abdominal pain with intermittent wellness, relief of pain with defecation, frequent bowel movements, loose stool with or without mucus, and abdominal bloating. Eating can worsen the cramping. Dyspepsia may be present. There should be no weight loss or fever.

  2. The **physical examination** is normal. Stool guaiac is negative for occult blood.

  3. Screening **laboratory results** (including CBC, ESR, liver function tests, amylase, and urinalysis) are normal. Pathogenic bacteria and parasites are absent in the stool. Lactose breath hydrogen testing should be considered.

  4. Sigmoidoscopy to exclude colitis should be considered.

  5. Therapy involves

    a. Explanation of the diagnosis and reassurance that a life-threatening illness does not exist.

    b. Increasing fiber in the diet, or beginning a fiber supplement (Metamucil or Citrucel, 1 tablespoon PO bid).

    c. In patients with diarrhea, the addition of loperamide, 2 to 4 mg PO tid, or cholestyramine, 4 g bid, can help to alleviate symptoms.

    d. Patients whose lifestyle is affected by the symptoms (e.g., school or work absenteeism) can benefit from counseling, relaxation techniques, or biofeedback.

K. Gluten-sensitive enteropathy (GSE; celiac disease) is manifested clinically by malabsorption and morphologically by a flat intestinal mucosa. Both improve on a gluten-free diet and are exacerbated by the reintroduction of gluten into the diet. It is a lifelong disease that presents most frequently between 9 and 18 months of age (earlier in formula-fed infants), but can be seen at any age. The development of antibody screening for celiac disease in the past 5 years has improved the identification and monitoring of these patients.

  1. Etiology. The mechanism of gluten sensitivity is unknown. Genetic factors play an important role. It is more common in Ireland (1 : 200) than in the rest of the world (United States estimate is 1 : 3,000). Theories as to its cause include immune mediation of gluten toxicity and an enzymatic defect.

  2. Evaluation

    a. The **history** may include a family history of GSE, failure to thrive, irritability, anorexia, and chronic diarrhea.

    b. The **physical examination** classically reveals an irritable, malnourished child with a potbelly and proximal muscle wasting, characteristically including the buttocks. However, some patients present atypically with features only of a selective malabsorption, that is, only growth failure, anemia, and rickets.

    c. Laboratory investigations should include a blood count, serum albumin, immunoglobulin (Ig), folate, iron, iron-binding capacity, stool examination, and sweat test. Antigliadin and antiendomysial antibodies are now standard for screening and monitoring of celiac disease. The antiendomysial IgA antibody is the most useful screening test, with a sensitivity of greater than 90% and specificity of greater than 98%. The antigliadin IgG antibody has a higher sensitivity, but a much higher number of false-positive tests. As both antigliadin and antiendomysial antibodies have false-positive and false-negative tests, intestinal mucosal biopsy is mandatory for the diagnosis of GSE.

  3. Diagnosis

    a. The findings of stool examination, including cultures for ova and parasites, are negative. Clinitest findings are variable. Sudan stain and a 72-hour stool-fat test usually reveal steatorrhea.

b. The results of a D-xylose absorption test and lactose hydrogen breath tests may be abnormal.

c. A series of three jejunal biopsies associated with gluten elimination and reintroduction were recommended by the European Society for Pediatric Gastroenterology and Nutrition to establish the diagnosis.

(1) The *initial* biopsy reveals a flat, villous lesion; this is not a pathognomonic finding.

(2) Clinical improvement, including a return to normal growth, is demonstrated on a gluten-free diet for 6 months. A *second* jejunal biopsy demonstrates a return to normal morphology.

(3) A *gluten challenge* is done for up to 6 weeks. Gluten powder, where available, is sprinkled into food in a dosage of 10 g/day. In the absence of gluten powder, gluten-rich flour can be substituted. Gluten-containing foods can be reintroduced, but children who taste previously restricted foods may resist a return to gluten restriction. A positive gluten challenge is the only available confirmatory test for GSE.

(4) After 6 weeks of gluten challenge (or earlier if symptoms recur), a *third* jejunal biopsy is done. It is unusual for overt diarrheal symptoms to occur during the challenge period. Biopsy evidence of active enteritis confirms the diagnosis. A normal biopsy essentially rules out celiac disease, but a subsequent biopsy may be needed after 1 year on the normal diet if symptoms recur.

d. More recently, it has been demonstrated that antiendomysial antibody titers may fall to normal levels with a gluten-free diet, and rise when the patient is rechallenged. Therefore, it is controversial as to whether all patients with celiac disease still require three small bowel biopsies.

4. Treatment

a. A gluten-free diet is begun immediately. Rye, oats, and barley should also be excluded.

b. Lactose should be omitted for the first 6 weeks to ameliorate the secondary disaccharide intolerance that is usually associated with GSE. A soy-based or other lactose-free formula will accomplish this purpose in infants.

c. Irritability is the first symptom to respond to therapy; diarrheal symptoms may linger for up to 6 weeks. If diarrhea persists, it may be necessary to alter the sugar base of the formula prescribed.

d. Vitamins and minerals should be replaced according to specific losses. A multivitamin preparation and iron are usually administered for 2 to 3 months, after which resolution of malabsorption permits normal dietary replacement. Common specific deficiencies are vitamin D, folic acid, vitamin K, and iron.

e. A gluten-free diet is maintained for life. For this reason, confirmation of the diagnosis must be as clear as possible.

5. Prognosis

a. On adequate gluten restriction, patients achieve normal life expectancy and fertility.

b. Spontaneous remission does not occur.

c. Recent reports indicate that patients with GSE may have an increased incidence in the subsequent development of gastrointestinal lymphomas, and that compliance with a gluten-free diet helps reduce the risk.

L. Disaccharidase deficiency may be primary (genetic) or secondary to intestinal mucosal damage. The most commonly seen disaccharidase deficiency is primary acquired lactase deficiency (lactose intolerance). Congenital disaccharidase deficiencies (including congenital sucrase-isomaltase deficiency and lactase deficiency) are rare, and are characterized by chronic diarrhea and reducing sugars in the stool when the offending disaccharide is ingested. Primary lactase deficiency is extremely common in older children.

1. **Etiology.** The condition is hereditary; up to 20% of white adults, 80% of black adults, and 90% of Asians will have varying degrees of lactose intolerance.
2. **Evaluation**
   a. Lactase deficiency usually presents in children over 3 years of age. Detection of lactose intolerance *before* three years suggests a secondary lactose intolerance, except for the very rare congenital lactase deficiency.
   b. The history includes recurrent abdominal pain and flatulence or diarrhea, or both. Family history is usually positive.
   c. The physical examination is usually normal.
   d. Laboratory tests include a stool examination, including pH, reducing substances, and lactose breath hydrogen test.
3. **Diagnosis**
   a. The stool may be positive for reducing substances.
   b. The results of the lactose breath hydrogen test are almost always positive.
   c. Small bowel biopsy is usually not necessary. If performed, mucosal disaccharide levels are normal except for lactase.
   d. There is usually a dramatic response to milk withdrawal in both primary and secondary lactase deficiency. It does not distinguish one from the other.
4. **Therapy**
   a. A lactose-free diet is begun immediately.
   b. A calcium supplement may be needed for long-term therapy (see Food and Drug Administration requirements). This can be supplied in patients over 5 to 6 years of age by commercially available calcium-containing antacid tablets (e.g., Tums, Rolaids).
   c. Primary lactase deficiency persists for life. However, patients can reintroduce lactose in small amounts until symptoms supervene. LactAid, a commercially available lactase, appears to be of value in some patients who wish to ingest a limited amount of lactose. Lactose-free milk and foods are now widely available in many areas.
M. **Food sensitivity.** The most common food sensitivities associated with GI disease are cow's milk and soy protein. Except for double-blind placebo-controlled food challenge, there is no reliable diagnostic testing for gastrointestinal manifestations of food allergy. Diagnosis and therapy often involve withdrawal of the offending food antigen, with rechallenge at a future time.
1. **Cow's milk protein sensitivity.** The incidence of cow's milk protein sensitivity is estimated at 0.5 to 1.0% of infants under 6 months of age. Gastrointestinal involvement is usually limited to the upper GI tract or to the colon, with allergic colitis being the most common presentation.
   a. **Etiology.** Systemic sensitivity (e.g., anaphylaxis, wheezing) to cow's milk appears to be mediated by immediate (type I) hypersensitivity, whereas GI disease can be mediated by other immune mechanisms.
   b. **Evaluation.** Sensitivity to cow's milk usually presents in infants.
      (1) The **history** may include pallor, edema, irritability, vomiting, diarrhea, colic, failure to thrive, and hematochezia.
      (2) The **physical examination** may reveal a pale, edematous child. Some infants present with a colitis-like picture with profuse, bloody diarrhea.
      (3) **Laboratory tests** include a CBC, serum albumin and immunoglobulins, serum iron, iron-binding capacity, IgE, radioallergosorbent test (RAST) to milk sensitivity, gastric and intestinal biopsy, sigmoidoscopy, rectal biopsy (if the patient has grossly bloody diarrhea), and stool guaiac.
   c. **Diagnosis**
      (1) The CBC may show iron deficiency anemia and eosinophilia.
      (2) SPA may reveal low serum albumin and immunoglobulins.
      (3) Immunoglobulin E levels are usually normal and the RAST is negative in GI disease alone, but generally not in systemic allergic disease.
      (4) Gastric biopsy may reveal a gastritis with eosinophilic infiltration.

(5) Biopsy of the small intestine reveals a patchy, flat, villous lesion.

(6) In patients with allergic colitis, sigmoidoscopy reveals an eosinophilic infiltrate in the mucosa.

(7) Occult blood is present in the stool.

(8) Withdrawal of milk protein (not lactose) produces a dramatic clinical and morphologic response. Reintroduction of milk protein after remission exacerbates clinical and morphologic abnormalities. Unlike GSE, this disease is transient, and milk protein can be tolerated after the age of 1 to 2 years. A milk challenge should not be attempted in patients with a history of milk anaphylaxis. In other patients, the milk challenge should be performed in the presence of medical staff with resuscitation equipment available.

d. Therapy

(1) A milk-free diet is instituted immediately. Breast-feeding mothers whose infants develop allergic colitis may respond if mother restricts all milk products from her diet.

(2) In view of associated secondary disaccharidase deficiency, a disaccharide-free formula or diet is introduced.

(3) Since 30% of infants with documented milk allergy may also react to soy, we generally place such infants on a casein hydrolysate (Nutramigen, Alimentum, or Pregestemil)

(4) An iron supplement should be provided.

2. Soy protein sensitivity. The incidence of isolated soy sensitivity is unknown. It is estimated that 20 to 30% of patients with milk sensitivity have associated soy sensitivity.

a. Etiology. The cause is unknown.

b. Evaluation. The history, physical examination, and laboratory investigations are similar to those carried out in patients with cow's milk sensitivity. The syndrome is usually seen in infants for whom soy formulas have been prescribed.

c. Diagnosis

(1) The CBC may show iron-deficiency anemia and eosinophilia.

(2) The SPA may reveal low levels of serum albumin and immunoglobulins.

(3) Immunoglobulin E levels are generally normal. The RAST reaction is generally negative in GI disease alone, but positive in systemic allergic disease.

(4) Gastric biopsy may reveal a gastritis with eosinophilic infiltration.

(5) Biopsy of the small intestine reveals a patchy, flat, villous lesion.

(6) Sigmoidoscopy reveals colitis.

(7) Withdrawal of soy protein produces a dramatic clinical response.

(8) Rechallenge after remission will reproduce abnormalities in a manner similar to that occurring with milk challenge.

d. Therapy

(1) A soy protein–free diet is instituted.

(2) An iron supplement is indicated.

(3) Whether this lesion is transient or permanent is unknown.

3. Eosinophilic gastroenteritis

a. Etiology. The cause is unknown.

b. Evaluation

(1) The **history** often reveals the onset of systemic allergy (usually asthma) and abdominal pain.

(2) Growth failure is a prominent part of the syndrome. The physical findings may also include pallor and edema.

(3) **Laboratory** investigations include a stool guaiac test, CBC, SPA, IgE, serum iron, and skin and RAST test reactions to various foods (see Chap. 16).

c. Diagnosis

(1) The CBC may reveal peripheral eosinophilia and iron-deficiency anemia.

(2) The SPA may reveal hypoalbuminemia and hypogammaglobulinemia.
(3) Serum IgE may be elevated.
(4) RAST and skin test reactions to many foods are often positive.
(5) Gastric antral biopsy reveals gastritis with eosinophilic infiltration.
(6) Jejunal biopsy reveals an abnormal antrum and abnormal gastric mucosa.

d. Treatment
(1) Dietary manipulations can alleviate acute symptoms (anaphylaxis) but may not affect the long-term course of disease.
(2) Prednisone in a dosage of 1 to 2 mg/kg/day can be used if dietary management fails. Then, alternate-day corticosteroids can be used.
(3) Cromolyn sodium (Gastrocrom) has been used, though efficacy has not been proven. The suggested dosage is 20 mg/kg/day divided q6h.
(4) Vitamins and iron supplements are indicated.
(5) Unlike cow's milk sensitivity, eosinophilic gastritis (like GSE) can be a lifelong condition in some patients.

N. Pancreatitis
1. Etiologies (Table 11-8).
2. History includes abdominal pain, anorexia, nausea/vomiting, fever, and respiratory distress. The clinician should inquire about predisposing factors, including trauma, drug exposure, hyperlipidemia, cystic fibrosis, gallstone disease (including sickle cell anemia), and family history of pancreatitis.
3. Physical examination shows abdominal tenderness, rigidity, guarding, and diminished bowel sounds/ileus. In more severe cases, the following signs develop.
  a. Dehydration, hypotension, and intravascular volume depletion secondary to intraabdominal third spacing.
  b. Skin bruising including Cullen's sign (ecchymosis around navel) or Grey Turner's sign (ecchymosis of flanks).
  c. Pulmonary abnormalities—tachypnea, dyspnea, pleural effusions.
  d. Mild jaundice can occur in idiopathic pancreatitis, but moderate or severe jaundice suggests gallstone pancreatitis.
  e. Ascites—either secondary to liver disease or a ruptured pancreatic duct.
4. Laboratory tests—useful in diagnosis and in predicting severity.
  a. Serum amylase —elevated amylase (usually >160 IU/dl) has a sensitivity of 75 to 95% for acute pancreatitis. An amylase level greater than 500 has a specificity approaching 100%. Amylase may be elevated in other conditions, including salivary gland inflammation or duct trauma, ovarian cysts, ruptured ectopic pregnancy, diabetic ketoacidosis, cholecystitis, perforated ulcer, renal failure, and macroamylasemia. A normal amylase does not exclude pancreatitis.
  b. Lipase. Elevated lipase has a sensitivity and specificity greater than 90% for pancreatic inflammation, since the pancreas constitutes the primary source of serum lipase.
  c. Other laboratory tests to be obtained include hemogram with differential, coagulation studies, electrolytes, calcium, BUN, glucose, liver function, and urinalysis. Severe pancreatitis is characterized by anemia, thrombocytopenia, hypoalbuminemia, hypocalcemia, and decreased urine output. Tachypnea or respiratory distress should be assessed by blood gas.
5. Radiography
  a. Plain abdominal films—to look for obstruction or ileus.
  b. Ultrasound—to evaluate the biliary tree and gallbladder and to rule out any pancreatic pseudocysts.
  c. Chest radiograph.
  d. Computed tomography will identify necrotic regions of pancreas and pseudocysts.
  e. Endoscopic retrograde cholangiopancreatography (ERCP) is useful in imaging the biliary and pancreatic ducts in an acute severe pancreatitis, particularly when gallstones or pancreatic transection are suspected.

Table 11-8. Etiologies of pancreatitis

Trauma
  Accident
  Abuse
  Gallstones/choledocholithiasis
  Anatomic obstruction
    Ductal stenosis
    Choledochal cyst/choledochocele
    Pancreas divisum
    Gastrointestinal duplications
Infections
  Mumps
  Coxsackie B
  Herpes simplex
  Epstein-Barr virus
  Mycoplasma
  Escherichia coli 0157:H7 (hemolytic-uremic syndrome)
  Parasitic infections (including *Ascaris* and *Clonorchis*)
Drugs
  Thiazides
  Furosemide
  Sulfonamides
  L-Asparaginase
  Valproate
  Procainamide
  Estrogens
  Tetracycline
  Azathioprine
  6-Mercaptopurine
  5-Aminosalicylates
  Dideoxyinosine
  Steroids are a possible cause
Toxins
  Alcohol
  Organophosphates
  Carbamates
  Scorpion venom
  Acetaminophen overdose
Metabolic disease
  Cystic fibrosis
  Hypertriglyceridemia
  Hyperlipidemias types I, IV, V
  Hyperparathyroidism/hypercalcemia
  Renal disease
Vasculitis
  Kawasaki's disease
  Henoch-Schönlein purpura
  Polyarteritis nodosa
  Systemic lupus erythematosus
Iatrogenic
  Postoperative
  Post–endoscopic retrograde cholangiopancreatography
Nutritional/tropical and refeeding pancreatitis
Ischemia/shock
Hereditary
Idiopathic

6. Therapy

  a. General principles—fasting, bowel decompression, vigorous fluid and colloid replacement, respiratory support, early computed tomography in severe cases, surgical intervention if necessary.

  b. NPO. Nasogastric tube required if ileus or vomiting present.

  c. Pain control—meperidine, 1 to 2 mg/kg q4–6 h. Avoid morphine because of concerns of precipitating sphincter of Oddi spasm.

  d. Monitoring recommendations—in moderate to severe cases

   (1) Strict input and output—urine specific gravity q6h. Foley catheter if necessary. Aim to keep urine output greater than 1 ml/kg/hr.

   (2) Pulse oximetry if tachypnea present.

   (3) In severe cases intensive care is required.

  e. Laboratory studies (including serum calcium) every 12 hours in patients with fluid/electrolyte imbalance.

  f. Medical and fluid management

   (1) Anticipate third spacing/colloid sequestration into pancreas and retroperitoneal tissues.

   (2) Intravenous crystalloid fluid

    (a) Maintenance—D5 ¼ or D5 ½ NS + 20 mEq KCl/liter.

    (b) Nasogastric replacement ml/ml—D5 ½ NS + 20 mEq KCl/liter.

    (c) Third-space fluid (lactated Ringer's or NS with 5% albumin) should also be given if there is clinical evidence of hypovolemia or sequestration of fluid into the abdomen. This rarely occurs in mild pancreatitis.

  d. Hyperalimentation—may be useful in cases in which a prolonged course is predicted, or to treat hypocalcemia or hypomagnesemia. Use Intralipid solution with caution to avoid hypertriglyceridemia.

  e. Antibiotics are generally not needed unless sepsis or pancreatic abscess (necrotizing pancreatitis) is suspected.

  f. Respiratory. Supplemental oxygen is often helpful if there is evidence of hypoxemia or desaturation. Assisted ventilation may be necessary in severe cases.

  g. Consider H_2 antagonist (e.g., cimetidine, 10 mg/kg/dose q6h) or antacids (Mylanta, 1 ml/kg/dose q4h) as gastrointestinal bleeding prophylaxis.

  h. Endoscopic or surgical intervention may be needed in a minority of cases (e.g., with a common bile duct stone or with severe necrotizing pancreatitis).

O. Pancreatic insufficiency

 1. Etiology. Pancreatic insufficiency (PI) is rare in children. The most common cause is cystic fibrosis (CF). Less common causes include Schwachman-Diamond syndrome (PI and neutropenia); chronic mucocutaneous candidiasis with polyglandular endocrinopathy; isolated deficiencies of lipase, colipase, or enterokinase; Johanson-Blizzard syndrome (PI, developmental delay, facial dysmorphism); and Pearson's syndrome (PI and sideroblastic anemia).

 2. Diagnosis

  a. Spot stool fat.

  b. 72-hour fecal fat.

  c. D-Xylose and small bowel biopsy will be normal in most cases of PI, as they detect intestinal mucosal damage.

  d. Complete blood count.

  e. Sweat test.

  f. Genotyping for CF (if indicated).

  g. Bentiromide test (*Gastroenterology* 101:207–213, 1991).

  h. Pancreatic stimulation.

 3. Cystic fibrosis. Gastrointestinal complications include

  a. Pancreatic insufficiency, which occurs in 85% of patients with CF. These individuals usually have a history of chronic diarrhea, with foul-smelling stools and failure to thrive.

b. Meconium ileus presents with intestinal obstruction, often associated with ileal atresia, in the immediate neonatal period in 15% of patients.

c. Rectal prolapse is a common presenting feature.

d. Meconium ileus equivalent, distal intestinal obstruction in the older child or adult, presents with abdominal pain and may be associated with intussusception.

e. Growth failure is quite common despite current therapy.

f. Cirrhosis of the liver develops in 15 to 20% of patients. An elevated alkaline phosphatase is often the first sign of liver involvement. Subsequent development of portal hypertension is common.

g. Diabetes mellitus. Overt diabetes occurs in 1% of patients. Abnormal results on glucose tolerance tests are routinely found. Ketoacidosis is rare.

h. Gastroesophageal reflux. The incidence is increased in patients with CF.

i. Pancreatitis. Recurrent acute pancreatitis may develop in patients with residual pancreatic function.

j. Gallstones occur in nearly one third of all patients with CF, although acute cholecystitis develops in only a few.

4. Therapy

  a. Treatment of pancreatic insufficiency

  (1) Pancreatic enzyme preparations. All patients with cystic fibrosis who have steatorrhea (85%) require supplemental pancreatic enzymes. Although fat absorption improves with these agents, it does not return to normal. Various pancreatic preparations are available. Dose is titrated on stool frequency, degree of steatorrhea, and growth. Excessive dosage can result in the "meconium ileus equivalent," that is, recurrent abdominal pain, palpable fecal masses, and obstruction. High-dose pancreatic enzyme supplementation (>5,000 units lipase/kg/meal) has also been associated with the development of colonic strictures. The dosage of pancreatic enzymes is largely empiric. Lipase, 500 units/kg per meal, is a recommended starting dose, and the dosage is titrated to result in one to three formed or semi-formed stools per day, up to a maximum recommended dose of 1,500 units of lipase per kg/meal. Spot or 72-hour fecal fat is useful in assessing residual steatorrhea.

  (2) Diet should contain 130 to 150% of normal calorie needs based on weight, age, and activity level. Fat content should not be restricted and should approximate 30% of total calories. If weight gain and growth are inadequate, or if significant weight is lost due to exacerbation of disease, supplemental feeding should be considered via nasogastric or gastric tube as nighttime feedings. If GI involvement is significant in infants, a semi-elemental formula such as Pregestimil should be used.

  (3) Vitamins are indicated for patients with PI and fat malabsorption. A new multivitamin (ADEK) provides recommended amounts of vitamins A, D, E, and K for patients with CF. Alternatively, one can provide vitamins individually.

    (a) Vitamin A: 5,000 to 10,000 IU/day.

    (b) Vitamin E: 200 to 400 IU/day.

    (c) Vitamin K: 2.5 mg biweekly until age 1 year, then supplement only if liver disease is present or when PT is prolonged.

    (d) Vitamin D: 800 IU/day if serum levels of 25-hydroxy vitamin D are inadequate.

  (4) Calcium. Dietary or supplemental consumption should be 1,000 to 1,500 mg/day elemental calcium.

P. Hepatic failure

  1. Etiology. Acute hepatic failure is a clinical syndrome that results from severe hepatic dysfunction or massive hepatic necrosis and leads to derangement of all hepatic functions, including synthetic, excretory, and detoxifying functions.

    a. Infection: acute viral hepatitis, especially hepatitis B.

 b. Hepatotoxins: acetaminophen, ethanol, valproate, isoniazid, halothane, and mushrooms (*Amanita phalloides*).
 c. Hepatic ischemia: cardiopulmonary failure, Budd-Chiari syndrome, and hepatic artery ligation.
 d. Metabolic abnormalities: Reye's syndrome, Wilson's disease, and galactosemia.
2. **Evaluation**
 a. The **history** may reveal evidence of a previous viral infection; exposure to blood products, drugs, or chemicals; circulatory collapse; preexisting liver disease; or a family history of liver disease.
 b. The **physical examination** reveals progressive jaundice (except in Reye's syndrome), asterixis ("liver flap"), fetor hepaticus, mental confusion, or coma.
 c. Laboratory investigations
  (1) Initial evaluation should include urinalysis; CBC; platelet count; PT; PTT; BUN; electrolytes; glucose; creatinine; ammonia, AST (SGOT), ALT (SGPT), alkaline phosphatase; bilirubin; blood gases; serum albumin; serologic serologies for hepatitis A, B, C, D, and E, Epstein-Barr virus, herpes virus, and others; slit lamp examination for Kayser-Fleischer rings; serum copper; ceruloplasmin; 24-hour urine copper; alpha-1-antitrypsin level; antinuclear antibody; anti–smooth muscle antibody; anti–liver-kidney microsomal antibody; urine for organic and amino acids; and toxic screen.
  (2) Complete blood count, electrolytes, calcium, phosphorus, BUN and creatinine glucose, and clotting studies need to be performed daily in the critically ill patient.
3. **Diagnosis**
 a. The blood count may reveal leukocytosis or hemolytic anemia, or both. (Always rule out Wilson's disease when liver disease and hemolytic anemia occur.)
 b. Prothrombin time and PTT are prolonged. Serum albumin may be low.
 c. SGOT and SGPT are increased.
 d. Alkaline phosphatase may be normal or increased.
 e. Except in Reye's syndrome serum bilirubin is usually increased, both in direct and indirect fractions.
 f. Blood glucose may be low.
 g. Blood urea nitrogen and electrolytes may reflect hypokalemia and hyponatremia.
 h. Blood gases may reveal a metabolic alkalosis or, less commonly, acidosis.
 i. Serologic tests for hepatitis A, B, C, D, or E may be positive.
 j. If serum copper and ceruloplasmin are low, and 24-hour urinary copper excretion is increased, further diagnostic tests for Wilson's disease are needed (see sec. **Q.2.a**, p. 369).
 k. The findings of a toxic screen may be positive if ingestion has occurred.
 l. The occurrence of oliguria may be due to prerenal azotemia, hepatorenal syndrome, or acute tubular necrosis. The first two are characterized by low (<10) urinary sodium and fractional excretion of sodium, while the latter has a high urine sodium and sometimes casts in the urinalysis.
4. **Treatment.** The purpose of therapy is to alleviate the systemic effects of liver failure and promote liver cell regeneration. Supportive therapy is provided until liver function is recovered, or until liver damage is deemed irreversible, at which time transplantation should be considered.
 a. Prepare a flowsheet to record laboratory data and daily intake and output.
 b. Fluid and electrolyte disturbances
  (1) Monitor serum and urinary electrolytes at least daily (up to q6h in unstable patients).
  (2) Hypoglycemia is treated with a 10 to 15% glucose solution IV at a rate dependent on renal function.
  (3) Hypophosphatemia and hypokalemia should be treated.

(4) Hypoalbuminemia with intravascular hypovolemia is treated with 25% albumin, 1 g/kg.

(5) A central venous pressure line is needed to monitor volume status in patients with low urine output.

c. **Coagulopathy** is treated with

(1) Vitamin K, 5 to 10 mg/day (or 1 mg/year of age) IV, for 3 days or while PT remains prolonged. If therapy is needed for more than 3 days, reduce this vitamin K dosage to 1 to 2 mg/day.

(2) Fresh-frozen plasma (FFP) is given if active bleeding or severe coagulopathy exists. Indiscriminate use can result in fluid overload, and FFP provides only short-term correction of coagulopathy.

(3) Plasmapheresis may be required to control bleeding.

d. **Encephalopathy** and hyperammonemia are treated with

(1) Protein restriction to 10 g (or 1 g/kg) protein per day.

(2) Give lactulose, 1 ml/kg (maximum 30 ml) q6h, or neomycin, 50 mg/kg/day q6h, or both, to reduce the activity of endogenous flora.

(3) Avoidance of sedatives, especially benzodiazepines.

(4) Raised intracranial pressure and cerebral edema may occur. Diagnosis is established by CT scan, and managed by elevation of the head of the bed, fluid restriction, mannitol (0.25–0.5 g/kg/dose), and, in rare cases, hyperventilation and intracranial pressure monitoring.

e. **Infection** with bacteria and opportunistic organisms is common secondary to reticuloendothelial system dysfunction. Always culture urine, blood, and ascitic fluid.

f. **Gastrointestinal bleeding** is usually due to varices or gastritis (see p. 352). We recommend ranitidine (1.0–1.5 mg IV q8h) prophylactically.

g. If the liver failure is deemed irreversible, consider **transplantation.**

Q. **Chronic hepatitis**

1. **Definition**—persistence of elevated transaminases for greater than 6 months, with or without other signs of liver dysfunction.

2. **Differential diagnosis** of chronic hepatitis is given in Table 11-9. The emphasis should be on identification of *treatable causes* of chronic hepatitis, which include autoimmune chronic active hepatitis, Wilson's disease, hemochromatosis, drug-induced liver disease, and hepatitis B and C.

a. **Wilson's disease** is an autosomal recessive metabolic disorder, associated with consanguinity, and characterized by cirrhosis of the liver, bilateral softening of the basal ganglia of the brain, and greenish-brown

Table 11-9. Causes of chronic active hepatitis

Autoimmune—types I and II	Drug-Related
Virus associated	Alcoholic liver disease
Hepatitis B	Alpha-methyldopa
Hepatitis C	Isoniazid
Delta hepatitis	Phenothiazines
HIV	Oxyphenacetin
Metabolic	Nitrofurantoin
Hemochromatosis	Halothane
Wilson's disease	Sulfonamides
Alpha-1-antitrypsin deficiency	Propylthiouracil
Primary hepatobiliary disorders	Nonalcoholic steatohepatitis
Primary biliary cirrhosis	
Sclerosing cholangitis	

Source: From A Bousvaros, WA Walker. Gastrointestinal and Liver Disorders. In ER Stiehm (ed). *Immunologic disorders of infants and children.* Philadelphia: Saunders, 1995; 697–741.

pigmented rings in the periphery of the cornea (Kayser-Fleischer rings). Clinical manifestations include the following:

(1) Age of onset is usually between 6 and 20 years of age.

(2) Modes of presentation include acute hepatitis, fulminant hepatic failure, chronic active hepatitis, hemolytic anemia, renal tubular dysfunction, cholelithiasis, or neurologic disease. Acute and chronic hepatitis are common in children, while neurologic symptoms (tremor, dysarthria, or psychiatric disturbance) are unusual presenting features in childhood.

(3) Evaluation and diagnosis

(a) Clinical and family **history**, especially regarding psychiatric or neurologic disease and childhood deaths.

(b) Neurologic and general **physical examination**.

(c) Slit lamp examination for Kayser-Fleischer rings. Gross inspection is inadequate.

(d) Laboratory studies

(i) Complete blood count with differential, reticulocyte, and smear (for hemolysis).

(ii) Liver function tests.

(iii) 24-hour urinary copper.

(iv) Serum copper and ceruloplasmin.

(e) Diagnosis is established by performing a liver biopsy for histology and quantitative liver copper.

(4) Treatment

(a) Penicillamine (beta-1 beta-dimethylcysteine; see also Chap. 8 sec. **III, D.C.**, pp. 284–285) is the treatment of choice. The dosage is 250 mg D-penicillamine hydrochloride PO qid before meals. If no improvement is seen, the dosage can be increased to 2 g/day. The side effects of penicillamine include skin rashes, leukopenia, nephrotic syndrome, a lupus-like syndrome, and hemolytic anemia.

(b) Diet should limit copper intake to 1 mg/day by avoiding foods that are high in copper such as organ meats and chocolate. Measure tap water for copper.

b. Autoimmune chronic active hepatitis

(1) Definition. Autoimmune chronic active hepatitis is an idiopathic severe hepatitis that is now classified into two types.

(a) Type I typically presents in adolescent and young adult women, and is characterized by the presence of antinuclear and anti–smooth muscle antibodies.

(b) Type II frequently presents in young children, and is characterized by the presence of anti–liver-kidney microsomal antibodies.

(2) Clinical features. The patient is usually ill, with a greater than 2-week history of fatigue, malaise, jaundice, and anorexia. Fulminant liver failure may be the initial presentation. Transaminases are usually between 100 and 1,000 IU/ml, and serum bilirubin is elevated. Hypergammaglobulinemia is frequently present.

(3) Diagnosis is established by characteristic features on liver biopsy, and by positive antibodies.

(4) Therapy

(a) Prednisone, 2 mg/kg/day (maximum 60 mg) is given for one month, then gradually tapered to an alternate-day regimen.

(b) In patients who do not respond to prednisone, or who relapse, Imuran (1.5–2 mg/kg/day) is used.

(c) Therapy may be lifelong, as the relapse rate off medication is high.

c. Hemochromatosis. Idiopathic genetic hemochromatosis is rare in children, but is the most common genetic cause of liver disease in adults. Secondary hemochromatosis is seen in children receiving chronic transfusions (renal disease, thalassemia, sickle cell disease, etc.)

(1) Clinical features of advanced disease include hepatomegaly, elevated transaminases, cirrhosis, diabetes, cardiomyopathy, hypopituitarism, arthritis, and bronze skin complexion. Milder cases may simply have elevated transaminases and laboratory evidence of iron overload.

(2) Laboratory diagnosis involves demonstrating high serum iron (>180 µg/dl), high transferrin saturation (Fe/total iron-binding capacity [TIBC] ratio > 0.8), iron densities on MRI scan, and elevated liver iron levels on biopsy.

(3) Therapy for genetic hemochromatosis is weekly phlebotomies until laboratory studies normalize. Secondary hemochromatosis is treated with iron chelation (desferoxamine).

d. Chronic hepatitis B and C is defined as a condition with serologic evidence of hepatitis B or C accompanied by elevated transaminases for greater than 6 months. In 10% of patients with chronic hepatitis B and 50% of patients with chronic hepatitis C cirrhosis will develop if they are untreated.

(1) Diagnosis is established by documentation of elevated transaminases, serology, and liver biopsy. The typical chronic hepatitis B carrier will have a positive $HepB_sAg$, negative $HepB_s$ antibody, and sometimes a positive $HepB_eAg$. A patient with chronic hepatitis C will have a positive hepatitis C virus (HCV) antibody.

(2) Therapy with alpha interferon will result in clinical improvement in 30% of patients with chronic hepatitis B, and 50% of those with chronic hepatitis C. The improvement with hepatitis B patients is usually sustained, while 50% of those with hepatitis C will worsen when treatment is stopped. Side effects include flu-like symptoms, malaise, myelosuppression, and worsening of autoimmune disease. The drug is still investigational in children.

R. Protein-energy malnutrition. Sustained deficits in the daily intake of protein or energy in relationship to specific requirements for nitrogen–amino acids and calories will result in the clinical syndrome of protein-energy malnutrition. This broad spectrum of protein-energy deficiency is conditioned by several factors: the severity of the defieiency, the duration, the age of the host, the cause of the deficiency, and the relative severity of protein versus energy deficiency (*Am J Clin Nutr* 23:67, 1970). Adequate nutrition is the most important aspect of therapy in acute and chronic illness.

1. Classification

  a. A child with **marasmus** has a caloric deficiency and an expected weight for age of less than 60% of normal. The clinical characteristics include the following:

  (1) The age of maximal incidence is 6 to 18 months.

  (2) No clinical evidence of edema with normal serum albumin ("skin and bones").

  (3) Poor nitrogen retention.

  (4) No fatty infiltration of the liver.

  (5) A slow response to dietary therapy during the first 4 weeks.

  b. Kwashiorkor is predominantly a protein deficiency; usually, the child has a minimum weight not less than 60% of expected weight for age.

  (1) The age of maximal incidence is 12 to 48 months.

  (2) Clinical evidence of edema with low albumin.

  (3) Fatty infiltration of the liver.

  (4) Initial weight loss with delivery of edema.

  c. Intermediate protein-energy malnutrition occurs in children who weigh less than 60% of the expected weight, but without the salient features of either marasmus or kwashiorkor (see *Br Med J* 3:566, 1972).

2. Diagnosis. See sec. I.A.1, p. 337 for assessment of malnutrition.

3. Therapy. See sec. I.A.3.a, p. 337.

12 Metabolic Disorders

Mark Korson

I. **General features.** Metabolic diseases are generally inherited inborn errors of metabolism that can present in infancy, childhood, adolescence, or adulthood. Each is due to the absent or deficient activity of a specific enzyme necessary for the metabolism of an amino acid, carbohydrate, fatty acid, or more complex intermediate compound. The clinical presentation is the consequence of toxic metabolite accumulations, diminished production of necessary intermediary products, or both. Many patients can be effectively managed using dietary modification, vitamin or cofactor supplementation, and often specific innovative therapies. With *early* diagnosis and *rapid* implementation of effective therapy, the outcome for many metabolic disorders is favorable.

II. **Clinical presentations.** The **acute presentation** of a metabolic disease either in the newborn period or thereafter constitutes a **true medical emergency.** Clinical suspicion must be high, and intensive treatment must begin **without delay** to prevent potential mortality and reduce the chance of debilitating, long-term morbidity. A careful **family history** is essential, with particular attention toward fetal loss, previous neonatal or infant deaths or sudden infant death syndrome (SIDS), Reye's syndrome–like illnesses, unexplained neurologic symptoms or mental retardation in the patient or other family members, and parental consanguinity.

The possibility of a metabolic disease should be considered in an individual who has any of the following symptom complexes, with suspicion rising when a combination of these symptoms occurs.

A. **Neonatal catastrophe.** Presentation in the newborn period is often severe, usually after feeding has begun.
   1. **Signs and symptoms** may include the following: **tachypnea, seizures, lethargy and coma, altered muscle tone, and hepatomegaly and jaundice,** often associated with **poor feeding and vomiting.**
   2. **Acute biochemical disturbances** include metabolic acidosis, hypoglycemia, and/or hyperammonemia.

B. **Biochemical disturbances.** These include metabolic acidosis, hyperammonemia, and hypoglycemia.
   1. Patients who are *chronically* acidotic are tachypneic, feed poorly, and fail to thrive.
   2. Disorders associated with recurrent *acute* metabolic decompensation are often associated with a high anion gap acidosis (frequently with marked ketosis), hypoglycemia, and/or hyperammonemia. At these times, patients may demonstrate an unusual odor in the urine, sweat, earwax, and so forth.

C. **Liver disease**
   1. Metabolic liver disease may be associated with hepatomegaly and jaundice. The hyperbilirubinemia can be conjugated or unconjugated, or both, in nature.
   2. Hepatic dysfunction commonly occurs and often includes a coagulopathy, particularly when metabolic disease presents in the neonate and young infant (e.g., galactosemia and tyrosinemia).
   3. Hypoglycemia and hyperammonemia may reflect defective hepatic regulation by a damaged liver.

D. **Neurologic disease** (see also Chap. 20)

1. Because metabolic disorders tend to affect the central nervous system in a *diffuse* manner, neurologic symptoms are generally nonlateralizing and global, and include altered states of consciousness, altered muscle tone and reflexes, movement disorder, ataxia, and developmental delay.
2. When they occur, **seizures** are frequently multifocal in origin.
3. A genetic metabolic etiology should be considered in any child with unexplained neurologic symptoms.

E. **Myopathy or cardiomyopathy, or both.** Metabolic disease that affects muscle can be slow and subtle in onset, or can occur suddenly during a period of acute decompensation.
   1. **Symptoms** can include muscle weakness, exercise intolerance with easy fatigability, or muscle pain. Myoglobinuria may follow an infectious illness or period of intensive exercise.
   2. **Cardiomyopathy** presents with symptoms of heart failure, arrhythmia, or sudden death. With few exceptions, the type of cardiomyopathy (i.e., dilated or hypertrophic) is not helpful in discerning the specific metabolic etiology.

F. **Storage disease**
   1. Metabolic storage disorders are characterized **in early childhood** by the progressive development of coarsened facies, hepatosplenomegaly, kyphoscoliosis with joint contractures, cloudy corneaes or retinal "cherry-red spot" or both, and hearing loss (conductive or sensorineural). General development plateaus, and patients follow a **neurodegenerative clinical course.**
   2. Less severe **juvenile and older-onset** forms of these disorders do not present with the classic infantile phenotype but may present with a learning disorder, loss of cognitive skills, or frank dementia; muscle weakness, cramping, or difficulty in walking; ataxia; seizures; or a behavioral or psychiatric disorder.

III. **Evaluation of acute metabolic disease by clinical/biochemical presentation** (Tables 12-1 and 12-2).

IV. **Diagnostic laboratory evaluation** (Table 12-2)
A. **Newborn blood screening**
   1. Screening of newborn blood collected on a filter paper in the first few days of life ("PKU test") is routinely done in all states in the United States and Canada, and in most developed countries. Several metabolic diseases can be identified in this manner, including **congenital hypothyroidism, phenylketonuria (PKU), galactosemia, galactokinase deficiency, maple syrup urine disease (MSUD), homocystinuria, and biotinidase deficiency.** Although all states screen for PKU and congenital hypothyroidism, screening for the other disorders varies from state to state.
   2. **Newborn screening** allows early institution of **therapy** for a metabolic disease to occur before the onset of clinical symptoms or irreversible neurologic damage.
   3. Children with **positive newborn blood tests should be referred as soon as possible to a metabolic center** for diagnostic confirmation and institution of therapy. The degree of sensitivity and specificity for newborn screening tests is generally high. Those newborn screens obtained before 24 hours of age probably test positive in affected cases. However, as a precaution, **any child whose sample is obtained during the first 24 hours of life should have another screen repeated** within the first 7 to 10 days.
   4. **Any neonate who is transferred from one nursery to another should have a screen test performed at both the referring and receiving hospitals** to avoid mishaps when no specimen is obtained.
   5. Although a negative newborn screening result strongly suggests that a child does not have the disease in question, repeat definitive testing is indicated when a patient's clinical presentation supports the diagnosis.

B. **Urine "spot" tests.** The following are simple tests that can provide quick diagnostic information.
   1. **Urine ketones** (Acetest, Ketostix) test for acetoacetate and are positive in acute organic acid disorders, MSUD, and congenital lactic acidemias. An

Table 12-1. Common clinicobiochemical characteristics of some acutely presenting metabolic diseases

Disorders	Acid-base abnormalities		Hypogly-cemia	Hyperam-monemia	Liver dys-function	Ketonuria		Myoglo-binuria
	Primary metabolic acidosis	Primary respiratory alkalosis				Increased	Absent/decreased	
Amino acid disorders								
Urea cycle disorders	O			+	O			
Tyrosinemia type I		+	+	O	+			
Organic acid disorders								
Maple syrup urine disease	+		+	+		+		
Propionic acidemia	+		O	+		+		
Methylmalonic acidemia	+		O	+		+		
Multiple carboxylase deficiency (and biotinidase deficiency)	+		O	O		+		
Glutaric acidemia type I	+		O	O		+		
β-Ketothiolase deficiency	+		O	O		+		
Congenital lactic acidemias/mitochondrial disorders								
Pyruvate dehydrogenase deficiency	+					O		
Pyruvate carboxylase deficiency	+		O	O		+		
Respiratory chain defects	O		O	O	O	O		
Defects of carnitine metabolism and fatty acid β-oxidation			O	O	O			
Multiple acyl CoA dehydrogenase deficiency (glutaric acidemia type II)	O		O	O	O		+	

Long/medium/short (hydroxy-) acyl CoA dehydrogenase deficiency	O						
Primary carnitine deficiency	O	O	O	O			
Carnitine palmitoyl transferase deficiency	O	O	O	O			
Carbohydrate disorders							O
Glycogen storage disease type I	+	+		+			
Galactosemia	O	O		+			
Hereditary fructose intolerance	+	+		+			
Disorders of gluconeogenesis	+	+		O	O		
Peroxisomal disorders							
Zellweger disease				+		+	
Neonatal adrenoleukodystrophy				+		+	
Infantile Refsum disease				+	+		
Disorders of bile acid metabolism	O	O		O		+	
Disorders of metal metabolism							
Wilson disease	O		O				

+ = feature present in most cases; O = feature present occasionally.

Table 12-2. Initial laboratory evaluation of acutely presenting metabolic disease

	Blood test	Urine test	Other
All patients	Blood gas Bicarbonate Electrolytes BUN Glucose Calcium phosphate Ammonia AST/ALT Lactate Amino acids CBC	Urinalysis Ketones Reducing substances Amino acids Organic acids	

When considering more specific groups of metabolic disease, the following studies may need to be added:

	Blood test	Urine test	Other
Amino acid disorders	PT, PTT	Orotic acid	CSF amino acids
Organic acid disorders	Carnitine Biotinidase		
Congenital lactic acidemias/mito-chondrial disease	Lactate and pyruvate CK		CSF lactate and pyruvate CSF protein
Fatty acid oxidation defects	Uric acid CK Carnitine Acylcarnitines	Acylglycines	
Carbohydrate disorders	PT, PTT Triglycerides, cholesterol Uric acid		
Peroxisomal disorders	Very long-chain fatty acids Phytanic acid Pipecolic acid Red blood cell plasmalogens	Bile acids	
Disorders of bile acid metabolism	PT, PTT	Bile acids	

AST/ALT = aspartate aminotransferase (AST)/alanine aminotransferase (ALT); PT = prothrombin time; PTT = partial thromboplastin time; CK = creatine kinase; CBC = complete blood count with differential and platelets; BUN = blood urea nitrogen.

absent or hypoketotic response to documented hypoglycemia suggests a disorder of fatty acid beta-oxidation or glycogen storage disease type I.

2. **Reducing substances** (Clinitest) is positive in galactosemia, hereditary fructose intolerance (HFI), and any disorder with a renal Fanconi syndrome. Since glucose is a reducing substance, untreated galactosemia or HFI is characterized by a positive Clinitest response in the face of a negative dipstick for glucose.

C. **Blood tests**

1. **Amino acid quantitation** of blood (serum or plasma) should accompany urine testing for the diagnosis of amino acid, organic acid, and urea cycle disorders, as well as the congenital lactic acidemias and mitochondrial disorders.

2. **Serum carnitine determination** should be performed when disorders of fatty acid oxidation or carnitine metabolism are suspected, and may also be indirectly helpful in the diagnosis of organic acidemias. Carnitine exists in a free or esterified state. Several fatty acid intermediates and organic acids bind carnitine, reducing the free fraction of carnitine and elevating the esterified fraction. A secondary carnitine deficiency is noted during periods of dehydration in normal children and in the unstable child with metabolic disease. However, low carnitine may also be evident when a child affected by a disorder of fatty acid or carnitine metabolism is otherwise well.

3. **Blood acylcarnitines** are a useful diagnostic tool for identifying disorders of fatty acid oxidation and organic acidemias (see sec. **4** below).

4. **Lactate and pyruvate determinations** should be performed when a congenital lactic acidemia or mitochondrial disorder is suspected. Some metabolic disorders may show secondary increases in lactate (e.g., biotinidase deficiency). A normal lactate-pyruvate ratio is approximately 10–15 : 1 (upper limit 25 : 1). An elevated ratio may be suggestive of respiratory chain disorders or pyruvate carboxylase deficiency, particularly in a normally perfused child.

5. **Peroxisomal testing** includes measurement in the blood of a combination of very long-chain fatty acids, phytanic acid, pipecolic acid, and red blood cell plasmalogens. The particular pattern of biochemical abnormalities depends on the specific disorder being considered. With the exception of very long-chain fatty acids, peroxisomal tests may be age dependent, and false-negative results can occur. If blood testing is negative and a peroxisomal disorder is strongly suspected, evaluation using cultured skin fibroblasts is indicated.

D. **Urine tests**

1. **Amino acid quantitation** in urine (together with blood amino acids) should be done on all patients suspected of having an amino acid, organic acid, or urea cycle disorder, as well as in those suspected of having a congenital lactic acidemia or mitochondrial disease.

2. **Organic acid determination** by gas chromatography/mass spectrometry should be performed for suspected amino acid, organic acid, fatty acid oxidation, and mitochondrial disorders.

3. **Orotic acid determination** is essential in patients suspected of having a urea cycle disorder.

4. **Acylcarnitine and acylglycine determination** in urine are useful primarily for the diagnosis of defects in fatty acid oxidation and carnitine metabolism, as well as in organic acidemias. Many intermediate metabolites within these pathways conjugate with carnitine or glycine, or both, when present in excessive quantities, particularly during episodes of metabolic decompensation. However, these abnormal conjugates are also frequently detectable during healthy periods.

5. **Thin-layer chromatography** is a sensitive and specific screen for mucopolysaccharide, oligosaccharide, and sialic acid disorders.

6. **Qualitative urinary bile acid** abnormalities are detected in peroxisomal diseases and other disorders of bile acid intermediate metabolism.

E. **Cerebrospinal fluid (CSF) tests**

1. **Cerebrospinal fluid protein** is elevated in certain storage disorders (e.g., Krabbe's disease), mitochondrial disease (e.g., Kearns-Sayre syndrome), and other demyelinating processes.

2. **Amino acids** are important for the diagnosis of an infant with nonketotic hyperglycemia (severe hypotonia, seizures, developmental delay) in which a high CSF–blood glycine ratio is diagnostic. In children with mitochondrial disease, an elevated CSF alanine may reflect an elevated lactate.

3. **Lactate and pyruvate** determinations may be useful for the identification of mitochondrial disease even when blood levels are normal.

F. **When a metabolic diagnosis is being considered, it is essential that diagnostic specimens be obtained during the acute phase of illness** (see **J** below). **The greatest chance of detecting unusual intermediate metabolites occurs at these times. Even a few hours of intravenous therapy can dilute or mask a previously identifiable abnormality.** Consultation with a metabolic specialist can often help direct the workup, especially when patient specimens are limited in quantity.

G. In the event that samples cannot be obtained during the acute illness, or when an initial workup is negative, **specialized stress testing or fasting studies** can be performed in a controlled hospital setting (usually a clinical research center). Consultation with a metabolic specialist can help maximize study efficiency and safety.

H. **Diagnosis of specific enzyme deficiencies** can often be confirmed using erythrocytes, leukocytes, fibroblasts, liver, or muscle specimens. The diagnostic tissue of choice depends on the enzyme of concern.

I. **Consumers beware! Quality control standards for most complex metabolic testing do not currently exist,** and the **reporting of inaccurate results or misinterpretations, or both, can occur.** Thus, care must be taken to ensure that the laboratory used for performing these tests employs a specialist with experience in clinical metabolic disease to review all test results, that it provides a written clinical interpretation for these results, and that the metabolic specialist is available to answer questions regarding abnormal results.

J. In the case of an **emergency or imminent death,** when a metabolic disorder is suspected but there is no time to determine a workup, **serum (3–5 ml minimum), plasma (3–5 ml minimum),** and **urine (10 ml minimum)** should be collected and **promptly frozen** (in smaller aliquots if possible) for later diagnostic studies. A blood specimen on filter paper (newborn screening or PKU card) is also helpful. A **skin biopsy** should be performed and a fibroblast culture begun for future enzyme studies. The importance of a **postmortem examination** for diagnostic purposes should be discussed with the parents or family since a definitive diagnosis is necessary for accurate genetic and recurrence-risk counseling as well as prenatal diagnosis. When a complete autopsy is denied, a partial examination may be permitted. Sections of affected tissues (particularly liver, heart, kidney, brain, and skeletal muscle) should be **quick frozen at −70°C** as soon as possible after death to preserve enzyme integrity for future testing.

V. **Treatment of acutely ill patients when the possibility of a metabolic disorder cannot be ruled out** (see also Chap. 6, p. 200)

A. **General principles. Acute metabolic decompensation can be rapidly progressive and life threatening.** Prompt institution of appropriate therapy is important, even before a specific diagnosis is made, and should be implemented concurrently with other routine therapies.

1. **Discontinue all oral feedings** while the child is acutely ill until a specific diagnosis is made and a special diet prepared if necessary.

2. Provide adequate respiratory and circulatory support, **with correction of metabolic acidosis** (see p. 379) **or hyperammonemia** (see p. 380), **or both,** when present.

3. Begin the **collection of diagnostic specimens** as soon as possible (see Table 12-2).

4. Attempt to reduce the ongoing catabolic process (and subsequent endogenous production of toxic substrate) by providing **IV 10% dextrose** at a flow rate greater than maintenance.

   a. Insulin therapy promotes anabolism and may be required, especially since the renal threshold for glucose may be altered during a period of decompensation.

   b. Keep glucose levels higher than normal (>100–120 mg/dl) during the presenting phase of illness.

   c. Use intralipid with caution and only when a disorder of fatty acid oxidation is not possible.

   d. Avoid the use of any solution that contains lactate.

5. Facilitate the removal or excretion of toxic intermediate compounds. This may involve a trial of **vitamin cofactors** in organic acidemias (see p. 379), **carnitine** in organic acid disorders (see p. 379), and intravenous **urea cycle medications** for hyperammonemia of less than 500 to 600 μg/dl (see sec. **E** below). However, in cases of severe hyperammonemia (>600 μg/dl), intractable acidosis, or deteriorating mental or neurologic status in a patient with a metabolic

disorder or clear indications of a metabolic disorder, **dialysis** is indicated. **Hemodialysis** is likely superior to peritoneal dialysis; exchange transfusions are not adequate. Transfer to a more specialized center should **not be delayed** for a trial of a less effective mode of therapy.

6. Because acute metabolic crises can be precipitated by stress or infection, **evaluation and prompt treatment for sepsis or infection, or both,** should be instituted promptly.

   a. Gram-negative sepsis may develop in up to 20 to 25% of untreated neonates with **galactosemia.** Therefore, sepsis must be ruled out in any newly diagnosed infant with galactosemia who has worrisome symptoms.

   b. Some **organic acidemias** (e.g., propionic and methylmalonic acidemia) are associated with significant **neutropenia and thrombocytopenia** during acute crises or periods of inadequate metabolic control.

7. **Careful monitoring** of intake/output, electrolytes, blood pH, total carbon dioxide, ammonia, glucose, neurologic status, and other relevant clinical parameters is necessary.

B. **Metabolic acidosis** (see also Chap. 4 pp. 66ff)

1. Distinguish between a *primary metabolic acidosis* (i.e., *low* pH, *low* carbon dioxide tension [PCO_2], *low* bicarbonate) and a *primary respiratory alkalosis with compensatory metabolic acidosis* (i.e., *high* pH, *low* PCO_2, *low* bicarbonate).

   a. The first case suggests an **organic acidemia,** congenital lactic acidemia, or mitochondrial disorder and requires therapy with sodium bicarbonate or other alkali.

   b. The second scenario occurs in many individuals with **severe hyperammonemia** (ammonia is a central respiratory stimulant). Bicarbonate correction is not indicated.

2. Acidosis should be treated, particularly when the blood pH drops below 7.22 and the bicarbonate below 14 mEq/liter. Below these levels, effective physiologic compensation may not occur.

3. **Intravenous bicarbonate or acetate** solutions help to correct an acidosis. Following a bolus, continue with an infusion. In severe metabolic crises, as much as 1 mEq/kg/hr alkali may be required.

4. **Monitor acid-base status** carefully so that overcorrection does not occur. Rapid correction of blood pH can cause a paradoxical drop in central pH and worsening of CNS symptoms.

5. **As a rule, avoid solutions that contain lactate** (which can aggravate the status of a child who is already predisposed to having a high lactate).

C. **Vitamin/cofactor therapy**

1. When an organic acidemia cannot be ruled out, a trial of vitamin/cofactor therapy is indicated to potentially stimulate any residual enzyme activity and thereby enhance the degradation of the accumulated (toxic) substrate.

2. Consider the use of the following vitamins or cofactors (they can be administered simultaneously).

   a. **Biotin** when propionic acidemia, multiple carboxylase deficiency, or pyruvate carboxylase deficiency is a consideration (10 mg/day).

   b. **Vitamin B$_{12}$ (preferably hydroxocobalamin over cyanocobalamin)** when methylmalonic acidemia is a possibility (1 mg/day); **riboflavin** when glutaric acidemia is being considered (100 mg/day).

   c. **Thiamine** when a congenital lactic acidemia is contemplated (20 mg/day).

3. The patient's abnormal biochemical parameters should be monitored (urine organic acids, blood lactate, etc.) to determine whether or not cofactor therapy is effective.

D. **Carnitine therapy**

1. Any individual with a potential organic acidemia or systemic carnitine deficiency warrants a trial of carnitine PO or IV. A baseline quantitative carnitine level should be obtained with other diagnostic laboratory tests before the onset of therapy.

2. Both oral and intravenous preparations are now commercially available. The

starting oral dosage is 100 mg/kg/day in two or three divided doses. The IV dose should begin at 25 mg/kg/day and increased to 100 mg/kg/day as tolerated.

E. Hyperammonemia

1. Perhaps the most common reason for an elevated ammonia level is improper technique or handling of the specimen. A *free-flowing specimen* (especially arterial in a patient with diminished perfusion) should be obtained. Specimens should generally be kept on ice, and transported immediately to the laboratory to avoid artifactual elevations.

2. **Severe hyperammonemia** (>600 μg/dl) should be managed with dialysis, preferably hemodialysis.

3. Significant and prolonged hyperammonemia may be associated with **increased intracranial pressure.** Intervention should exclude the use of steroids because of their catabolic potential (which can aggravate the hyperammonemia).

4. When hyperammonemia is less severe (<500–600 μg/dl), **pharmacologic therapy** to facilitate waste nitrogen excretion is indicated. This includes intravenous sodium benzoate (250 mg/kg/day) and sodium phenylacetate (250 mg/kg/day) given as a bolus followed by a continuous infusion. These medications are available on an experimental protocol basis from Dr. Saul Brusilow at Johns Hopkins Hospital (410–955–0885). The oral form for these medications (marketed as Ucephan) is commercially available through Kendall-McGaw Pharmaceuticals.

5. When hyperammonemia is associated with low levels of arginine, **arginine** should be supplemented intravenously (210 mg/kg/day).

6. Once a specific urea cycle diagnosis is made, adjustments in the doses of these intravenous medications may be required.

7. **Ammonia levels must be monitored regularly,** every 4 to 6 hours, until they have normalized. Given the composition of the urea cycle medications, electrolytes and gases should be monitored closely as well.

Endocrine Disorders

Joseph I. Wolfsdorf and
Louis Muglia

I. General approach to endocrine disorders

A. The endocrine history

1. A **directed history** should include assessment of diet, sleep pattern, bowel and bladder habits, activity level, behavior, and school performance.
2. The **family history** should include growth familial patterns of pubertal development. Actual height measurements of family members should be obtained if possible.

B. The physical examination
assesses somatic growth (height or length, weight, arm span, ratio of upper-to-lower segments), sexual development, and the rate and sequence of bodily changes (Tables 13-1 and 13-2; see Figs. 3-2 through 3-5, (p. 31)).

C. Therapy

1. Because most endocrine disorders are chronic diseases, **parent and patient education** are essential. The psychosocial effects of these conditions must be addressed. It is important to relate the child to his or her chronological age, despite size or sexual development.
2. **Hormonal therapy** attempts to replace a deficiency of a specific hormone and rarely mimics the normal pattern of hormone secretion.
3. **Personality and behavior** can be directly affected by hormonal excess or deficiency. It may be difficult to determine the relative contributions of organic factors and psychological problems resulting from a chronic disease.
4. **Medic Alert bracelets** or **necklaces** should be worn by patients who have diabetes mellitus, diabetes insipidus, congenital adrenal hyperplasia, or adrenocortical insufficiency.

II. Disorders of growth

A. Short stature

1. **Etiology** (Table 13-3).
2. **Evaluation**
   a. **History.** Gestational history, birth weight and length, perinatal events, rate of growth, nutritional history, symptoms of intracranial space-occupying lesion or hypothalamic dysfunction, psychosocial adjustment, review of systems, and family history.
   b. **Physical examination.** Accurate measurements of height, weight, upper and lower segments of the body, and arm span. Staging of pubertal development, neurologic examination including visual fields, and fundoscopic examination.
   c. **Laboratory tests** (Table 13-4).
   d. **Specialized tests.** Provocative tests for growth hormone (GH) release, thyrotropin-releasing hormone (TRH) stimulation test, gonadotropin-releasing hormone (GnRH) stimulation test, and MRI of the head, particularly the hypothalamus and pituitary.
3. **Diagnosis**
   a. **Familial short stature (FSS) and constitutional growth delay (CGD)**
      (1) History and physical examination are normal. Growth velocity is normal (0–12 mo, 18–25 cm/yr; 1–2 yr, 10–13 cm/yr; 3–5 yr, 6.0–7.5 cm/yr; 5 yr–puberty, 5–6 cm/yr).

Table 13-1. Tanner stages of sexual development

Stage	Characteristics	Mean age at onset (97th–3rd percentiles)*
Testis		
1	Prepubertal (<4 ml or long axis <2.5 cm)	
2	Testes enlarge (4 ml or long axis ≥2.5 cm)	11.5 (9.5–13.5)
3	Testes 12 ml (long axis 3.6 cm)	14.0 (11.5–16.5)
Pubic hair		
1	Prepubertal; no coarse, pigmented hair	
2	Minimal coarse, pigmented hair at base of penis	12.0 (9.9–14.0)
3	Coarse, dark curly hair spread over the pubis	13.1 (11.2–15.0)
4	Hair of adult quality but not spread to junction of medial thigh with perineum	13.9 (12.0–15.8)
Penis stage		
1	Prepubertal	
2	Earliest increased length and width	11.5 (9.2–9.7)
3	Increased length and width	12.4 (10.1–14.6)
4	Continued growth in length and width	13.2 (11.2–15.3)
Peak height velocity		13.5 (11.7–15.3)
Boys who mature at an average time		9.5 (7.1–11.9) cm/yr
Boys who mature early (+2 SD)		10.3 (7.9–12.5) cm/yr
Boys who mature late (+2 SD)		8.5 (6.3–10.7) cm/yr
Breast stage		
1	Prepubertal	
2	Breast buds palpable; areolae enlarge	10.9 (8.9–12.9)
3	Elevation of breast contour; areolae enlarge	11.9 (9.9–13.9)
4	Areolae and papilla form a secondary mound on the breast	12.9 (10.5–15.3)
Pubic hair		
1	Prepubertal; no coarse, pigmented hair	
2	Minimal coarse, pigmented hair mainly on labia	11.2 (9.0–13.4)
3	Dark, coarse, curly hair spreads over mons	11.9 (9.6–14.1)
4	Hair of adult quality but not spread to junction of medial thigh with perineum	12.6 (10.4–14.8)
Menarche		12.7 (10.8–14.5)
Peak height velocity		11.5 (9.7–13.3)
Girls who mature at an average time		8.3 (6.1–10.4) cm/yr
Girls who mature early (+2 SD)		9.0 (7.0–11.0) cm/yr
Girls who mature late (+2 SD)		7.5 (5.4–9.6) cm/yr

*97th percentile refers to the earliest age and the 3rd percentile refers to the latest age at which the physical characteristic appears.
Source: Adapted from JW Tanner, PWS Davies. *J Pediatr* 107:317, 1985.

Table 13–2. Penis and testis size

Age (yr)	Penis length (cm)*	Testis length (cm)*
0.2–2.0	2.7 ± 0.5	1.4 ± 0.4
2.1–4.0	3.3 ± 0.4	1.2 ± 0.4
4.1–6.0	3.9 ± 0.9	1.5 ± 0.6
6.1–8.0	4.2 ± 0.8	1.8 ± 0.3
8.1–10.0	4.9 ± 1.0	2.0 ± 0.5
10.1–12.0	5.2 ± 1.3	2.7 ± 0.7
12.1–14.0	6.2 ± 2.0	3.4 ± 0.8
14.1–16.0	8.6 ± 2.4	4.1 ± 1.0
16.1–18.0	9.9 ± 1.7	5.0 ± 0.5
18.1–20.0	11.0 ± 1.1	5.0 ± 0.3
20.1–25.0	12.4 ± 1.6	5.2 ± 0.6

*Mean ± SD.
Source: Data from JSD Winter and C Faiman. Pituitary-gonadal relations in male children and adolescents. *Pediatr Res* 6:126,1972.

Table 13-3. Causes of short stature

Normal
Familial (genetic)
Constitutional growth delay

Pathologic

disproportionate

Long bones
  Rickets
  Hypochondroplasia
  Achondroplasia
Spine
  Vertebral anomalies
  Spinal irradiation

Proportionate

Prenatal
  Intrauterine growth retardation
  Placental dysfunction (toxemia)
  Intrauterine infections (e.g., congenital rubella)
  Teratogens (ethanol, drugs, smoking)
  Chromosomal abnormalities (e.g., trisomy 21)
Postnatal
  Malnutrition (primary, dieting, food fads, anorexia nervosa)
  Chronic disease
    Cardiac—congenital heart diseases
    Respiratory—cystic fibrosis, severe asthma
    Renal—renal tubular acidosis, chronic renal insufficiency
    Gastrointestinal—celiac disease, Crohn's disease
    Hematologic—sickle cell disease, thalassemia
    Immunologic—rheumatoid disease, connective tissue
      disorders
  Psychosocial deprivation (functional hypopituitarism)
  Drugs (glucocorticoids, cancer chemotherapy)
  Endocrinopathies
    Hypothyroidism
    Growth hormone deficiency, abnormalities of growth
      hormone action
    Glucocorticoid excess
    Inadequately treated diabetes mellitus, diabetes insipidus
    Gonadal dysgenesis (Turner's syndrome)
    Pseudohypoparathyroidism
    Late effects of precocious puberty

Table 13–4. Screening evaluation of children with growth failure

Detailed history and physical examination
Analysis of growth pattern from all available data and carefully plotted growth chart
Urinalysis including pH and specific gravity
Tests of renal function: BUN, creatinine, electrolytes, venous pH, and TCO_2
Tests for rickets: serum calcium, phosphorus, alkaline phosphatase, radiographs of hand, wrist, and knee
Assessment of nutritional status: serum albumin, carotene, CBC; antiendomysial antibodies to rule out gluten enteropathy
Thyroid function: serum thyroxine, thyroid-stimulating hormone
Erythrocyte sedimentation rate to rule out inflammatory disease
IGF-1, IGF-BP3, and postexercise measurement of growth hormone for deficiency of growth hormone
Radiograph of hand and wrist to assess skeletal maturity **(bone age)**
Cranial MRI to identify abnormalities in the area of the hypothalamus and pituitary
Karyotype to rule out abnormalities of the X chromosome in girls (Turner's syndrome)

TCO_2 = total carbon dioxide; IGF-1 = insulin-like growth factor-1; IGF-BP3 = IGF-binding protein 3.

    (2) The patient frequently has a family history of short stature or delayed puberty, or both.
    (3) Bone age corresponds with chronological age in FSS but is delayed in CGD.
    (4) The age of onset of puberty is normal in FSS, whereas it is delayed in CGD.
  b. **Hormonal disorders** that result in short stature (see under specific hormones). The patient is usually overweight for height; growth velocity is subnormal, and the bone age is retarded.
 4. **Treatment**
  a. Catch-up growth followed by a normal growth velocity occurs if the underlying cause is treated effectively.
  b. No treatment has yet proved to significantly increase the final height of children with FSS or CGD.
  c. Low doses of long-acting testosterone preparations (e.g., testosterone enanthate, 50 mg IM q1mo) can be used to induce puberty and enhance growth in boys with CGD who have severe psychological problems and social maladjustment. Final adult height is not diminished by such therapy.
III. **Disorders of sexual development**
 A. **Ambiguous genitalia. The birth of a baby with ambiguous genitalia is a psychosocial emergency. It is essential to avoid announcing the sex assignment based on the first impression of the external genitalia before a complete evaluation has been performed by the pediatrician in consultation with a pediatric endocrinologist, pediatric urologist, radiologist, and geneticist.** The parents should be told that an immediate decision cannot be made because the baby's sexual development is immature or incomplete. However, with appropriate treatment, genital appearance will ultimately be normal and adult sexual function will be possible (perhaps not reproduction).
  1. **Etiology** (Table 13-5).
  2. **Evaluation and diagnosis**
    a. The **history** should include an inquiry about maternal virilization and the possibility of maternal hormone ingestion. Family history includes infants with ambiguous genitalia, unexplained infant deaths, and relatives with disorders of puberty, amenorrhea, or infertility.
    b. Blood pressure, heart rate, and hydration must be monitored carefully. The **physical examination** should attempt to ascertain the presence of gonads in the labioscrotal folds. The phallus is examined and measured; the posi-

Table 13-5. Causes of ambiguous genital development (intersex)

Disorder	External genitalia	Phenotype Gonads	Karyotype
Disorders of gonadal differentiation			
True hermaphroditism	Ambiguous	Ovarian and testicular tissue	46,XX; 46,XY; 46,XX/46,XY chimerism or mosaic
"Pure" gonadal dysgenesis	Female	Streak gonads or hypoplastic ovaries	46,XX
	Female or ambiguous	Dysgenetic testes or dysgenetic testes and streak gonads	46,XY
Mixed gonadal dysgenesis	Ambiguous	Streak gonad and dysgenetic testis	45,X/46,XY; 46,XYp⁻
Female pseudohermaphroditism (masculinization of the genetic female)			
Congenital adrenal hyperplasia			
21α-hydroxylase deficiency	Ambiguous	Ovaries	46,XX
11β-hydroxylase deficiency	Ambiguous	Ovaries	46,XX
3β-OH steroid dehydrogenase deficiency	Ambiguous	Ovaries	46,XX
Transplacental synthetic progestogens	Ambiguous	Ovaries	46,XX
Maternal androgen excess	Ambiguous	Ovaries	46,XX
Male pseudohermaphroditism (incomplete masculinization of the genetic male)			
Testicular unresponsiveness to HCG and LH (Leydig cell hypoplasia or agenesis)	Ambiguous	Testes	46,XY
Disorders of testosterone synthesis	Ambiguous	Testes	46,XY
Side chain cleavage enzyme deficiency			
17α-hydroxylase deficiency			
3β-OH steroid dehydrogenase deficiency			
17-lyase deficiency			
17-ketosteroid reductase deficiency			
End-organ resistance to testosterone			
Complete testicular feminization	Female	Testes	46,XY
Incomplete testicular feminization	Ambiguous	Testes	46,XY
Disorder of testosterone metabolism			
5α-reductase deficiency	Ambiguous	Testes	46,XY
Vanishing testes syndrome	Variable	Absent gonads	46,XY
Lack of müllerian inhibiting substance	Male	Testes, uterus, fallopian tubes	46,XY

HCG = human chorionic gonadotropin; LH = luteinizing hormone.

tion of the urethra and the degree of pigmentation, rugation, and fusion of the labioscrotal folds are noted. A rectal examination is done to determine the presence of a uterine cervix. Somatic stigmata suggesting a chromosomal abnormality are noted.

c. **Laboratory: karyotype**, serum **electrolytes**, and, on the second or third day of life, blood for measurement of adrenocorticotropic hormone (ACTH) and **steroid metabolites:** cortisol, 17-hydroxyprogesterone, 17-hydroxypregnenolone, 11-deoxycortisol, dehydroepiandrosterone (DHEA) and its sulfate (DHEA-S), androstenedione, and testosterone.

   (1) Salt wasting is not evident for 3 to 7 days or more after birth but is preceded by an elevated plasma renin activity. In selected cases, measurements of plasma pregnenolone, progesterone, deoxycorticosterone (DOC), corticosterone, 18-hydroxylated corticosterone, and aldosterone levels are required for diagnosis.

   (2) A disorder of testosterone biosynthesis can be diagnosed from steroid hormone measurements in the basal state or after **stimulation with 3,000 units/m² human chorionic gonadotropin (HCG) IM** and sampling after 48 hours. The diagnosis of androgen unresponsiveness can be made in two ways.

   (a) Administer testosterone, 25 mg IM each month for 2 to 3 months, and observe the change in the size of the penis.

   (b) Androgen receptor activity can be determined in fibroblasts from a genital area skin biopsy.

   (3) **Pelvic ultrasonography** is used to identify the presence of a uterus and ovaries. A **urogenital sinogram, laparoscopy, surgical exploration, and histologic examination of the gonads** (and excision of discordant gonadal and ductal tissue) may be necessary.

3. **Treatment**

   a. Assignment of the sex of rearing is based on the diagnosis, the potential to achieve cosmetically and functionally normal external genitalia by surgical and hormonal therapy, and the potential for fertility. In rare cases, when either a male or female sex assignment is possible, the decision is influenced by the preference of the parents. The decision to recommend a male sex of rearing is based on the size of the phallus and its potential for growth during childhood and puberty. This can be ascertained by a 3-month trial of testosterone in consultation with an endocrinologist.

   b. A baby with **congenital adrenal hyperplasia** (see p. 397) will usually be raised concordant with the chromosomal sex, with glucocorticoid and mineralocorticoid therapy to stop further virilization. Reconstructive surgery on the genitalia of girls with congenital adrenal hyperplasia is performed early in the first year to reduce the size of an enlarged clitoris; definitive vaginoplasty is usually deferred until adolescence.

   c. Infants with severe **androgen resistance** are raised as girls. Ambiguity of the external genitalia occurs with **incomplete androgen resistance** and requires surgical reconstruction.

   d. In some instances, a **true hermaphrodite** can be raised either as a boy or girl, and the decision may be influenced by the presence of normally functioning testicular or ovarian tissue. In general, surgically creating a vagina is less difficult than constructing an adequate penis and penile urethra.

   e. A child who would be expected to be unable to function as a male because of a small, androgen-unresponsive penis should not be raised as a boy because of the high likelihood of serious psychological problems in the future.

   f. Reconstruction of the penis and correction of severe forms of hypospadias may have to be done in stages. To preserve valuable tissue for reconstruction, **circumcision is contraindicated.**

   g. If a genetic (46, XY) boy is to be raised as a girl, intraabdominal or inguinal testes are removed because of the high risk of future malignant degeneration, and the possibility of virilization during puberty.

    h. Growth and sexual development should be monitored closely and **hormone therapy** instituted as indicated (see below).

    i. The diagnosis and prognosis for sexual and reproductive function should be discussed frankly with the parents and later with the patient.

B. Delayed puberty

  1. Etiology

    a. Constitutional delay of pubertal development occurs more frequently in boys than in girls.

    b. CNS abnormalities: pituitary and hypothalamic tumors, congenital vascular anomalies, severe head trauma, birth asphyxia, psychosocial deprivation, and Kallmann's and Laurence-Moon-Biedl syndromes.

    c. Systemic conditions: anorexia nervosa; severe cardiac, pulmonary, renal, or gastrointestinal disease; malabsorption syndromes; weight loss or weight gain; sickle cell anemia; thalassemia; chronic infection; hypothyroidism; or Addison's disease.

    d. Primary gonadal insufficiency due to Turner's, Noonan's, Klinefelter's, and Sertoli-cell-only syndromes; testicular feminization; pure or mixed gonadal dysgenesis; cryptorchism and anorchism; trauma; infection; pelvic radiation; and surgical castration.

  2. Evaluation. Differential diagnosis of delayed puberty should be considered when a girl over 14 or a boy over 15 lacks any secondary sexual characteristics, or when an adolescent has not completed maturation over a period of 5 years.

    a. History. Detail chronology of sexual development, previous growth pattern, CNS symptoms including anosmia, and nutrition. **Family history** of abnormal puberty, amenorrhea, infertility, or ambiguous genitalia should be elicited.

    b. The **physical examination** should include all growth measurements, sexual staging, careful observation of the genitalia for ambiguity, palpation for inguinal masses, a pelvic examination (or at least a rectal), and a search for stigmata suggesting a syndrome.

    c. Review of past growth data. An increase in growth rate may be the first indication of impending sexual development. Conversely, deceleration may be a sign of active disease.

    d. The **laboratory evaluation** often includes a complete blood count, urinalysis, luteinizing hormone (LH), follicle-stimulating hormone (FSH), estrogen, testosterone, DHEA-S, bone age, and cranial CT or MRI scan. A karyotype is sometimes indicated, as are prolactin and thyroid hormone levels.

  3. Diagnosis

    a. The diagnosis of constitutional or hereditary delay is always tentative because it can be confirmed only after normal sexual development has occurred.

    b. Patients with hypothalamic or pituitary deficiencies have low levels of LH or FSH.

    c. In primary gonadal failure, gonadotropins are usually elevated by age 12 to 13 years.

  4. Treatment

    a. Constitutional and genetic delay. Progression of development should be monitored and emotional support offered. For certain patients, temporary hormone therapy, testosterone enanthate, 25 to 50 mg IM monthly for 3 to 4 months, may be warranted for psychological reasons, and used without compromising final stature.

    b. CNS abnormalities. Patients with hypogonadotropic hypogonadism require hormonal therapy. If the pituitary is intact, treatment with GnRH analogues makes it possible to mature completely and to reproduce.

      (1) In girls, the replacement regimen includes an oral conjugated estrogen, for example, Premarin, 0.3 mg/day, with the dosage gradually increased to 0.65 to 1.25 mg/day over 9 to 12 months; medroxyprogesterone acetate, 10 mg/day on days 12 to 25 of each month, is then added to induce cyclic bleeding. When full maturation is achieved, oral contraceptive pills can be used instead of Premarin and medroxyprogesterone.

    (2) In boys, ideal therapy consists of subcutaneous GnRH analogue infusion by minipump, or HCG, 1,000 to 2,500 IU IM q5d. Serum testosterone is helpful in monitoring dosage.

  c. Systemic conditions. Improvement of the underlying medical condition may be followed by normal puberty.

  d. Primary gonadal insufficiency

    (1) In girls, treatment consists of administering estrogens and progesterone (see sec. **b.(1)** above).

    (2) In boys, a therapeutic trial of HCG should be attempted if testicular function is possible. If no response is demonstrated, testosterone enanthate, 100 to 200 mg IM every 2 to 4 weeks, will induce virilization, normal libido, and sexual potency. The prognosis for fertility requires additional evaluation.

C. Sexual precocity

  1. Etiology (Table 13-6).

  2. Evaluation should focus on the points emphasized in sec. **B.2** above.

    a. Skin should be examined for multiple café au lait spots (neurofibromatosis) or larger irregular brown macules (McCune-Albright syndrome). Dimensions of breast areolae and glandular tissue in girls, and testes and phallus in boys, should be recorded. Presence of pubic or axillary hair and apocrine odor should be noted. Asymmetry or nodules in the testes suggest the presence of a tumor. In girls a pale-pink vaginal introitus with developed labia minora suggests active estrogenization, which can be quantitated using a vaginal smear (maturation index). A rectoabdominal examination may reveal an adnexal mass if an ovarian tumor or cyst is present.

Table 13-6. Causes of sexual precocity

True central precocious puberty (pituitary gonadotropin secretion)
Idiopathic
Russell-Silver syndrome
Neurogenic (CNS disorder)
  Hypothalamic hamartoma
  Space-occupying lesions: astrocytoma, optic glioma with neurofibromatosis, tumors associated with tuberous sclerosis, teratoma
  Cerebral damage resulting from CNS anomalies, irradiation therapy, surgery, trauma, prior inflammation (encephalitis, meningitis), hydrocephalus
Pseudoprecocious puberty (source of sex steroids independent of pituitary)
Androgen- or estrogen-secreting tumors
  Ovarian (granulosa cell, theca cell, luteomas, follicular cysts)
  Testicular (Leydig cell, adrenal rest)
Congenital adrenal hyperplasia
Adrenal adenoma or carcinoma
Exogenous sex steroids (oral contraceptives, estrogen-containing creams, consumption of estrogen-fed poultry or cattle)
Exogenous human chorionic gonadotropin (HCG) in boys
McCune-Albright (polyostotic fibrous dysplasia)
Gonadotropin or HCG-producing tumors: chorioepithelioma, teratoma, hepatoblastoma (boys)
Familial male gonadotropin-independent precocity
Severe hypothyroidism (associated with ovarian cysts)
Incomplete sexual precocity
Premature thelarche
Premature adrenarche

---

  b. Source of hormone secretion (adrenal or gonadal). One must establish whether sex steroid production is independent (usually a cyst or tumor) or the result of premature activation of the hypothalamic-pituitary-gonadal axis (central precocity). This is most reliably done by performing a GnRH stimulation test.

  c. For laboratory evaluation, see Table 13-7.

 3. Diagnosis

  a. Isosexual precocity refers to an abnormally early onset (girls <8 yr of age, boys <9 yr of age) of sexual characteristics appropriate to the child's sex. Precocious puberty is much more common in girls than in boys and is usually idiopathic. Precocity in boys is more often caused by CNS lesions, hormone-secreting tumors, congenital adrenal hyperplasia, or familial male gonadotropin-independent precocity.

  b. Precocious adrenarche refers to the early appearance of pubic hair, axillary hair, and/or apocrine odor, which are effects of adrenal androgens. Increase in growth and skeletal maturation is minimal. Some of these children have mild adrenal enzyme defects (congenital adrenal hyperplasia; see p. 397).

  c. Precocious thelarche refers to the premature development of one or both breasts in 1- to 3-year-old girls without acceleration of growth or advancement of skeletal maturation.

 4. Treatment of central precocious puberty with daily injections or depot formulations of potent analogues of GnRH can suppress LH, FSH, and gonadal steroids to prepubertal levels, resulting in cessation of menses and penile erections, slowing of accelerated growth and skeletal maturation, and partial regression of secondary sexual development. Therapy must be monitored closely

---

Table 13-7. Laboratory evaluation of precocious puberty

Isosexual
Hormonal
 Serum LH, FSH (may require GnRH stimulation test to document presence or absence of pubertal response)
 Estradiol (girls)
 Testosterone (boys)
 Dehydroepiandrosterone sulfate (DHEA-S)
 Beta HCG subunit (boys)
Radiographic
 Bone age (left hand and wrist)
 Pelvic ultrasound
 Cranial MRI scan
Premature thelarche
Hormonal
 Serum LH, FSH
 Estradiol
 Cytologic examination of vaginal smear for maturation index (bioassay of estrogen effect)
Radiographic
 Bone age
 Pelvic ultrasound
Premature adrenarche
Hormonal
 DHEA-S
 17-OH progesterone (8 AM)
 Dehydroepiandrosterone (consider ACTH stimulation test for congenital adrenal hyperplasia)
Radiologic
 Bone age

in order to maximize gains in final height. Many 6- to 8-year-old girls with precocity may attain normal adult height without intervention and do not need therapy.

IV. Disorders of the pituitary

  A. Hypopituitarism. Pituitary function depends on the integrity of the entire hypothalamic-pituitary axis.

  1. Etiology

  a. Tumors of the pituitary and suprasellar tumors can disrupt pituitary function.

  b. Tissue damage involving the hypothalamus that results from perinatal insult, trauma, hemorrhage, vascular anomaly, infectious/inflammatory disease, histiocytosis, previous irradiation, and infarction can cause isolated or multiple hormonal deficiencies.

  c. Congenital anomalies: septo-optic dysplasia, midline malformations, and syndromes of abnormal forebrain development.

  d. Psychosocial deprivation alters hypothalamopituitary function.

  e. Isolated GH deficiency is usually idiopathic but occasionally is hereditary.

  f. Isolated gonadotropin deficiency occurs in association with Kallmann's and Laurence-Moon-Biedl syndromes.

  g. Isolated deficiencies of thyroid-stimulating hormone (TSH) and ACTH are rare.

  2. Evaluation. Investigation of all anterior and posterior pituitary hormones is necessary to determine the status of current function.

  a. The **history** should review past growth, CNS symptoms, and previous head or neck illnesses or therapy, specifically radiation therapy.

  b. The **physical examination** should include growth measurements, staging of sexual development, a neurologic evaluation including visual fields and fundoscopy, and a search for the signs of hypothyroidism and hypoadrenalism.

  c. Further evaluation should include height and weight curves and bone age. If pituitary insufficiency is suggested, circulating basal and stimulated levels of GH, LH, FSH, thyroxine, ACTH, cortisol, and serum, and urine values of sodium, potassium, and osmolality, should be measured.

  d. An MRI of the brain is useful to evaluate structural lesions.

  3. Diagnosis

  a. Patients with **isolated GH deficiency** have a normal weight and length; growth velocity begins to decrease at 6 to 18 months of age. Incidence is higher in neonates who had an adverse perinatal event or breech presentation. Neonatal cholestatic jaundice, hypoglycemia, and micropenis are suggestive of the diagnosis.

  (1) Patients with GH deficiency have a subnormal rate of growth (<4.0 cm/yr after the age of 4–5 yr; see p. 381).

  (2) These patients tend to have truncal obesity and immature features. They may have craniofacial disproportion with small midface and crowded teeth. Some have a high-pitched voice. The bone age is delayed.

  (3) Growth hormone does not increase in response to pharmacologic stimuli, such as insulin-induced hypoglycemia and the administration of arginine, glucagon, clonidine, L-dopa, or propranolol.

  (4) Nocturnal and diurnal pulsations of GH are greatly diminished.

  b. Deficiencies of LH and FSH may not become apparent until puberty. A micropenis suggests hypogonadotropic hypogonadism.

  c. Deficiency of TSH may be responsible for mild to severe clinical hypothyroidism. Serum TSH levels are low in pituitary hypothyroidism and normal or slightly elevated in hypothalamic hypothyroidism. TSH does not respond to TRH administration in pituitary hypothyroidism, but hyperresponds or shows a delayed response in hypothalamic hypothyroidism.

  d. Patients with **ACTH deficiency** often have a relatively mild form of adrenal insufficiency that may go undetected until they are under stress or until later in adolescence. These patients are differentiated from those with Addison's disease by their lack of hyperpigmentation or salt craving, and their low plasma ACTH. The cortisol response to ACTH or insulin-induced hypoglycemia is inadequate.

4. Treatment

  a. Growth hormone. GH-deficient patients are treated with growth hormone, 0.025 mg/kg/day SC administered in the evening.

  b. TSH deficiency is treated with l-thyroxine (as discussed in sec. **V**, p. 393).

  c. ACTH deficiency usually requires no treatment except during the stress of surgery, trauma, or illness. Then, treatment with cortisone acetate, 50 mg/m²/day IM, or in divided doses PO, is recommended. An additional 100 mg/m² hydrocortisone sodium succinate solution is administered intravenously during surgery. When the patient is symptomatic (usually in adolescence), hydrocortisone should be replaced, 12 mg/m²/day in divided doses (see p. 396).

B. Diabetes insipidus (DI)

  1. Etiology

   a. Central DI is caused by either primary deficiency of antidiuretic hormone (ADH) or is secondary to interruption of the neurohypophyseal transport of ADH by tumors, histiocytosis, granulomatous disease, and inflammatory, vascular, or traumatic lesions. The familial form is usually inherited in an autosomal dominant fashion. It may be associated with congenital intracranial defects or result from autoimmune destruction of the supraoptic and paraventricular nuclei.

   b. Nephrogenic DI is caused by renal unresponsiveness to ADH and is inherited in an X-linked (defects in the vasopressin receptor) or autosomal recessive (water channel mutations) fashion. Female heterozygotes often have a partial concentrating defect.

  2. Evaluation. The diagnosis should be suspected in any child with persistent polydipsia and polyuria.

   a. Excess water intake and urine output must be documented. Urine volume exceeds 3 liters/m²/day, and serum osmolality exceeds urine osmolality.

   b. Evidence should be sought for CNS or pituitary disease, and the workup should include a cranial MRI study.

   c. Screening for DI is done by measuring the osmolality of a fasting second voided morning urine sample. The duration of the fast should be determined from the patient's history of usual fast duration to avoid excessive dehydration. A urine osmolality greater than 650 mOsm/kg makes the diagnosis of DI highly unlikely. Hyponatremia in a random blood sample is indicative of primary polydipsia.

   d. Primary renal disease and tubular unresponsiveness to ADH secondary to hypercalcemia, hypokalemia, pyelonephritis, and sickle cell disease should be ruled out.

   e. Primary polydipsia should be considered, especially if psychiatric illness or psychosocial problems are present.

  3. Diagnosis. The water deprivation test is used to confirm the diagnosis. Body weight, osmolality, and sodium concentration of serum and urine, and plasma ADH, are measured before, during, and at the end of the period of water deprivation. The deprivation of water should be continued either until urine osmolality does not change significantly (<30 mOsm/kg) in three consecutive hourly determinations or until body weight has decreased by 5% or more. The test is positive when serum hypertonicity develops (osmolality ≥295 mOsm/kg) and plasma ADH does not rise appropriately in the face of persistent polyuria and hyposthenuria (urine osmolality <300 mOsm/kg). An injection of ADH at the end of the test should increase urine osmolality by more than 50% in patients with central DI. In nephrogenic DI, the urine osmolality does not increase significantly.

  4. Treatment (See also Chap. 4, p. 68ff)

   a. Acute DI may occur after trauma to the hypothalamopituitary region.

    (1) Initial treatment consists of matching input and output up to a maximum of 3 liters/m^2/day, with the first 1 liter/m^2 D5 ¼ normal saline (NS) and the remainder D5W. This will produce a baseline sodium of 150 to 155 mEq/liter.

    (2) Alternatively, an ADH (Pitressin) drip can be initiated at 1.5 mU/kg/hr, with restriction of fluids to 1 liter/m^2/day.

    (3) Frequent weighing and measurements of serum osmolality and electrolytes are used to guide therapy.

  b. Chronic therapy

    (1) Desmopressin acetate (DDAVP) is the treatment of choice, and is administered intranasally as a spray (for dosage multiples of 10 μg), or as a liquid delivered via a rhinyle. The dose varies with the patient's size and renal sensitivity. Initially, a bedtime dose sufficient to eliminate nocturia should be established. If a second dose is required, it is given in the morning and should be slightly less than the evening dose. A 1- to 2-hour period of polyuria should be allowed to occur each day during which any excess fluid can be excreted. DDAVP can also be injected SC, IM, or IV. Therapy is usually started with a dose of 2.5 to 5.0 μg and increased gradually in increments of 2.5 μg until satisfactory antidiuresis is achieved.

    (2) The patient's random serum sodium should be at least 140 mEq/liter to reduce the risk of water intoxication.

    (3) Therapy in infants is more complicated because their nutrition is provided largely in liquid form, making the risk of fluid overload with DDAVP greater than in older children. It may be preferable to avoid exogenous ADH and simply provide daily fluids at 3 liters/m^2/day, divided on a 3- to 4-hour feeding schedule, to allow adequate caloric intake and reduce the risk of water intoxication.

    (4) For older infants, addition of a single dose of short-acting intranasal lysine vasopressin at bedtime reduces fluid needs and allows a brief period of uninterrupted sleep.

  c. Hormone amplifiers. Chlorpropamide, 4 mg/kg/day, can be effective in patients with residual ADH secretion. Hypoglycemia is a potential side effect. Because of its thirst-stimulating activity, chlorpropamide is the preferred treatment for patients with partial DI and for those with adipsia or hypodipsia.

  d. Nephrogenic DI. Because no treatment is able to eliminate the polyuria, **polydipsia is essential for survival.** Proprietary formulas are diluted 25 to 50% with water to reduce the solute load, and chlorothiazide, 1 g/m^2/day or 30 mg/kg/day, is given in two or three divided doses to reduce glomerular filtration rate and enhance proximal water reabsorption. These maneuvers reduce the urine volume by 50% but may not supply adequate calories for growth; therefore, the formula should be supplemented with corn syrup or other glucose polymers.

C. Inappropriate ADH secretion

  1. Etiology. This usually occurs after head trauma or intracranial surgery. Other causes include intracranial tumors, CNS infections, intrathoracic diseases, drugs that stimulate ADH secretion, and lesions of the hypothalamus that cause a state of chronic ADH excess. Ectopic ADH production is rare in childhood.

  2. Evaluation and diagnosis

    a. Urine output is decreased, there is progressive weight gain, and the patient has an altered state of consciousness if hyponatremia is severe.

    b. The laboratory findings include a decreased serum sodium, urine osmolality inappropriately high (>100 mOsm/kg) for the concurrent serum hypoosmolality, and increased urine sodium. Serum levels of urea and uric acid are usually decreased. Renal and adrenal function are normal.

  3. Treatment is with fluid restriction to about 800 ml/m^2/24 hr. Loss of body weight and a steady rise in serum sodium and osmolality are evidence of therapeutic success. More aggressive therapy is indicated if hyponatremia is acute, with serum sodium concentrations below 120 to 125 mEq/liter in association with severe CNS symptoms. Slow IV infusion of 3% saline, calculated to correct serum sodium to 125 mEq/liter, is combined with furosemide to minimize further expansion of intravascular volume. Raising the serum sodium too rapidly to levels greater than 125 mEq/liter can result in CNS damage. Treatment should aim to raise the serum sodium concentration by 1 to 2 mEq/liter/hr to 125 mEq/liter and then gradually to 135 mEq/liter over the next 24 hours, not exceeding 0.5 mEq/liter/hr.

4. **Prevention.** The effects of inappropriate ADH secretion can be prevented by carefully monitoring the patient's serum electrolytes and weight, and by restricting fluid intake to match insensible water loss plus urine output.

V. Disorders of the thyroid
 A. Hypothyroidism
  1. Etiology
   a. **Congenital** causes include ectopic or aplastic thyroid gland (60–85%), dyshormonogenesis (10–25%), and hypothalamic or pituitary hypothyroidism (4–5%); rarely, thyroid hormone resistance occurs.
   b. **Transient** causes include iodine excess or deficiency, transplacental passage of drugs (iodine, radioactive iodine [^{131}I] antithyroid medications), and maternal antithyroid antibodies.
   c. **Acquired** causes include autoimmune, irradiation, and surgery.
  2. Congenital hypothyroidism
   a. **Evaluation and diagnosis**
    (1) **Clinical manifestations.** Babies appear normal at birth. Early manifestations are nonspecific: feeding difficulties, respiratory difficulties, prolonged jaundice (unconjugated hyperbilirubinemia), hypotonia, constipation, excess sleep, weak cry, large posterior fontanel, macroglossia, umbilical hernia, dry and mottled skin, and slow relaxation of deep tendon reflexes. Only 10% of infants with congenital hypothyroidism have suggestive signs when examined at 4 to 6 weeks of age.
    (2) **Neonatal screening** is the only means of early diagnosis. Thyroxine (T_4) is measured initially. If T_4 is less than 6.5 µg/dl, TSH is measured. If TSH is 20 µU/ml or more, patients are referred for evaluation. Screening is most effective using samples obtained 3 to 5 days after birth.
     (a) Premature babies may have relatively low serum T_4, but the TSH concentration is normal.
     (b) Infants with congenital hypothyroidism may be missed by neonatal screening programs.
    (3) **Laboratory**
     (a) Repeat thyroid studies determining T_4, triiodothyronine (T_3), T_3 resin uptake (or thyroid-binding globulin index), and TSH on whole blood.
     (b) Obtain a thyroid scan and radioactive iodine (^{123}I) uptake to define the anatomy of the thyroid gland and assess its function.
     (c) If the TSH is low, a TRH stimulation test is recommended to determine whether hypothyroidism is secondary to pituitary or hypothalamic dysfunction.
     (d) Bone age determination is useful in diagnosis and for evaluating the results of therapy.
   b. **Treatment** should be begun immediately.
    (1) l-Thyroxine (10–15 µg/kg/day) is recommended. This dosage should maintain the total serum thyroxine in the upper half of the normal range (10–16 µg/dl in the first 2 yr of life). This dose will normalize serum thyroxine in less than 3 weeks. Smaller dosages (7–9 µg/kg/day) take an average of 74 days to raise T_4 levels to greater than 10 µg/dl. On 10 to 15 µg/kg, TSH levels will drop to less than 10 µU/ml in

the majority of cases. Occasionally, the serum TSH remains above 20 μU/ml for 2 to 3 months or more. This is thought to be secondary to the resetting, in utero, of the feedback threshold for T_4 suppression of TSH.

(2) Therapy should be monitored by measuring serum T_4, T_3 resin uptake or thyroid-binding globulin index and TSH 2 weeks after the initiation of therapy, and at intervals of 2 months during the first 18 to 24 months, and every 3 to 4 months thereafter, as well as 4 to 6 weeks after each change in the dose of thyroxine.

(3) Because neonatal hypothyroidism is occasionally transient, therapy can be withheld at 4 to 5 years of age for a trial period of 4 to 6 weeks to determine if the hypothyroidism is permanent.

3. Acquired hypothyroidism
    a. Etiology
        (1) Chronic lymphocytic thyroiditis (Hashimoto's disease) is the most common cause.
        (2) TSH deficiency secondary to hypopituitarism.
        (3) Exogenous causes include thyroidectomy, radioactive iodine therapy, iodine excess or deficiency, fluorine, lithium, cobalt, perchlorate, thiocyanate, para-aminosalicylic acid, propylthiouracil, and anticonvulsant therapy.
    b. Evaluation and diagnosis
        (1) Symptoms may be insidious. Linear growth is particularly vulnerable. Weight gain continues despite a poor appetite. Constipation, dry skin, fatigue, anorexia, and cold intolerance may be present. Puberty is delayed.
        (2) Signs. Short and overweight for height but rarely obese; immature facies, bradycardia, and small pulse pressure; pallor, dry skin, mottled skin, cold extremities, distended abdomen, delayed relaxation phase of deep tendon reflexes. The thyroid gland may be enlarged.
        (3) Laboratory evaluation. Serum T_4 is low. TSH is elevated in primary hypothyroidism, low in pituitary hypothyroidism, and low, normal, or occasionally slightly elevated in hypothalamic hypothyroidism. Serum T_3 is usually low. Antithyroglobulin or antiperoxidase (microsomal) antibodies are present in autoimmune thyroiditis.
    c. Treatment
        (1) Treatment with L-thyroxine is begun with 0.025 mg/day, and the dosage is gradually increased by 0.025 mg every 1 to 2 weeks until the appropriate dosage is attained. Most children require 75 to 100 μg/m²/day.
        (2) Thyroid function tests are used to monitor the appropriateness of the dosage and compliance. The serum level of TSH is the most sensitive guide to the adequacy of therapy.

B. Hyperthyroidism
  1. Neonatal hyperthyroidism
    a. Etiology. One to 10% of women with **Graves' disease** have offspring with hyperthyroidism secondary to transplacental passage of TSH receptor-stimulating immunoglobulins.
    b. Evaluation and diagnosis
        (1) Clinical manifestations: irritability, failure to gain weight, diarrhea, vomiting, diaphoresis, exophthalmos, enlarged thyroid gland. The most serious threats to life are severe tachycardia with congestive heart failure, tracheal obstruction, and associated infections. The manifestations can last from 8 weeks to 6 months.
        (2) Laboratory tests. Elevated serum T_4 and T_3, undetectable serum TSH using ultrasensitive assays, and the presence of high titers of thyrotropin-stimulating immunoglobulins (TSI) or thyrotropin-binding inhibiting immunoglobulins (TBII).

c. **Treatment** consists of propylthiouracil, 5 to 10 mg/kg/day given q8h, and iodide solution such as Lugol's (126 ng iodide/ml), one drop q8h.

    (1) The infant must be carefully monitored for signs of **heart failure** and treated with digoxin if necessary.

    (2) **Respiratory distress** from a greatly enlarged goiter is encountered infrequently and is treated with elevation and extension of the neck.

2. **Acquired hyperthyroidism**

  a. **Etiology.** Almost exclusively secondary to Graves' disease (autoimmune thyrotoxicosis). It is rarely caused by a functional adenoma, subacute thyroiditis, TSH-producing tumor of the pituitary, or pituitary resistance to thyroxine.

  b. **Evaluation and diagnosis**

    (1) Patients present with increased activity, increased appetite, weight loss, irritability, restless sleep, heat intolerance, poor coordination, increased number of bowel movements, excessive sweating, palpitations, and irregular menses.

    (2) **Physical examination** reveals a tachycardia, systolic hypertension, warm and moist skin, diffusely enlarged thyroid gland often with a bruit, fine tremors of the fingers, and hyperreflexia. The eye signs are usually mild and consist of exophthalmos, lid lag, inability to converge, and, rarely, injection of the conjunctivae, excess lacrimation, and paresis or paralysis of the extraocular muscles.

  c. **Laboratory evaluation.** Serum T_4 and T_3 are elevated (on rare occasions only T_3 is elevated). Serum TSH measured by ultrasensitive assays is undetectable, except if secondary to a pituitary tumor or partial (pituitary) resistance to T_4. Thyrotropin-stimulating antibodies (TSI or TSAb) or TBII are present.

  d. **Treatment**

    (1) **Thyrotoxicosis**

      (a) **Propylthiouracil (PTU),** 50 to 300 mg or 5 to 7 mg/kg/day, depending on the age and size of the patient, is given in three equally divided doses at 8-hour intervals. The dose is increased until the desired effect is achieved. When euthyroidism has been restored, the dose is reduced to the minimum necessary to maintain normal thyroid hormone levels. Recent recommendations include adding a replacement dose of thyroid while maintaining a full blocking dose of PTU.

      (b) **Methimazole (Tapazole)** can be used instead of PTU. The dose is one-tenth that of PTU and is given in two or three equally divided doses.

      (c) **Toxic side effects** of the thionamides, PTU and methimazole, can occur at any time during the course of therapy and include erythematous rashes, urticaria, agranulocytosis, arthritis, lymphadenopathy, a lupus-like syndrome, and hepatitis. A complete blood count must be performed whenever the patient has an infectious illness, and therapy should be stopped immediately if leukopenia or granulocytopenia is present. If the side effect is not severe, a trial of the other thionamide can be attempted, with careful monitoring for recurrence of side effects.

    (2) **Thyroid storm** is a rare medical emergency that requires immediate treatment.

      (a) Thyroid hormone synthesis and release, and the peripheral conversion of T_4 to T_3, are inhibited with large doses of **PTU,** 200 to 400 mg q6h.

      (b) **SSKI** is given orally (0.5 ml bid) or sodium iodide is given IV in a dose of 1 to 2 g to block thyroid hormone secretion.

      (c) **Dexamethasone,** 1 to 2 mg q6h, is effective in reducing the serum level of T_3.

(d) **Propranolol** should be used judiciously because tachycardia is a compensatory mechanism for the high output failure. The dosage is 2 mg/kg/day and can be increased to 4 to 6 mg/kg/day. Alternatively, **esmolol,** a short-acting, beta-1–specific antagonist administered intravenously, can be used.

(e) A cooling blanket is used to **control hyperthermia** and **fluids** are given intravenously to correct dehydration.

VI. Disorders of the adrenals

A. Adrenocortical hypofunction

1. Etiology. The causes of **primary adrenocortical insufficiency** include the following:

   a. Congenital adrenal hyperplasia.

   b. Adrenal hemorrhage.

   c. Hypoplasia or aplasia of the adrenals.

   d. Congenital unresponsiveness to ACTH.

   e. Fulminating infections, especially meningococcemia.

   f. Addison's disease, isolated or associated with polyglandular autoimmune disease.

   g. Adrenal leukodystrophy.

   h. Granulomatous infiltration (e.g., tuberculosis).

   i. Acquired immunodeficiency syndrome (AIDS).

2. Secondary adrenal insufficiency is caused by

   a. Congenital hypopituitarism.

   b. Acquired hypopituitarism, including iatrogenic adrenal suppression as a result of long-term glucocorticoid therapy.

3. Evaluation

   a. The onset is usually insidious with vague and nonspecific complaints. The major **clinical features** are weakness, personality changes, increased pigmentation (primary insufficiency only), salt craving, hypotension, hypoglycemia, anorexia, nausea, vomiting, diarrhea, weight loss, and menstrual abnormalities.

   b. **Adrenal crisis,** usually precipitated by stress, is characterized by vomiting, dehydration, fever, hypoglycemia, and hypotension, culminating in shock and coma.

   c. A short ACTH test should be performed whenever adrenocortical insufficiency is suspected by obtaining blood samples for serum cortisol immediately before and one hour after IM or IV administration of Cortrosyn, 0.25 mg.

4. Diagnosis

   a. Decreased serum sodium, increased serum potassium, hypochloremic acidosis, hypoglycemia, increased urinary sodium (>20 mmole/liter), and decreased urinary potassium. Electrolyte changes are not always present, especially in secondary insufficiency.

   b. Eosinophilia and relative neutropenia may be present depending on the severity of the illness.

   c. Serum cortisol and aldosterone may be low or within normal range, but ACTH levels are significantly elevated (>200 pg/ml) in primary adrenal insufficiency, as is plasma renin activity if associated with salt wasting. ACTH is low (<50 pg/ml) in secondary adrenal insufficiency, and plasma renin activity is usually normal.

   d. The short ACTH test will diagnose primary adrenal insufficiency and most cases of secondary insufficiency. Basal plasma ACTH distinguishes between the two. The insulin tolerance test is the definitive test to confirm secondary or tertiary adrenal insufficiency.

   e. Adrenal autoantibodies are found with autoimmune adrenalitis.

5. Therapy

   a. Addisonian crisis

      (1) Shock must be treated by rapid volume expansion (20 ml/kg normal saline IV).

(2) Hypoglycemia is treated with an IV infusion of 0.5 g/kg dextrose over 5 to 10 minutes, followed by 0.5 g/kg/hr.

(3) Hydrocortisone sodium succinate, 50 to 100 mg, should be given IV; then, hydrocortisone, 100 mg/m²/day is given as a continuous infusion, gradually reducing the dose to maintenance over 5 days and changing to oral therapy when appropriate. If the diagnosis is not certain at the time of presentation, and an ACTH test cannot be performed immediately, dexamethasone in doses of equivalent glucocorticoid potency can be administered without confounding serum cortisol measurements during a subsequent Cortrosyn test.

   b. Maintenance therapy consists of hydrocortisone, 10 to 20 mg/m²/day in divided doses tid, with a larger dose in the morning; fludrocortisone (Florinef), 0.05 to 0.3 mg/day; and table salt ad lib.

   c. During periods of stress the hydrocortisone dosage should be doubled or tripled and the frequency of administration increased to q6h. Patients or parents should know how to use cortisone acetate, 25 to 50 mg IM, in emergencies. Patients should wear a Medic Alert identification tag.

   d. For **surgery** or **severe stress,** see p. 391.

B. Congenital adrenal hyperplasia (CAH)

1. Etiology

   a. Congenital adrenal hyperplasia refers to a group of autosomal recessive enzyme defects of cortisol synthesis. The most common enzyme deficiencies and their clinical and biochemical features are shown in Table 13-8.

   b. Two enzyme deficiencies, 18-hydroxylase and 18-dehydrogenase, result only in deficiencies of aldosterone synthesis.

2. Evaluation and diagnosis (see Table 13-8 and p. 384).

3. Treatment

   a. Salt-losing crisis

   (1) Salt loss is treated with infusion of normal saline.

   (2) Hypotension is treated with a fluid bolus of 20 ml/kg followed by 1.5 times maintenance fluid requirement until the patient's condition is stable. If oral intake is compromised, 5% dextrose should be included in the intravenous fluids to prevent hypoglycemia.

   (3) Glucocorticoids are administered as described above (sec. **VI.A.5a,** p. 396).

   (4) Fludrocortisone (Florinef), 0.05 to 0.3 mg/day, is used for mineralocorticoid replacement. This is begun when the patient's condition has stabilized and (s)he is ready for oral intake. A dosage of up to 0.3 mg/day may be necessary in some infants. Salt supplementation of 2 to 4 g/day is used to replace urinary losses. This can be added to the formula or solids until the child is capable of ad lib salt supplementation.

   b. The glucocorticoid-deficient varieties of CAH (21-hydroxylase, 11-beta hydroxylase, 3-beta hydroxysteroid dehydrogenase, 17-alpha hydroxylase, and side-chain cleavage enzyme or cholesterol desmolase) require cortisol replacement.

   (1) Initial treatment of the symptomatic neonate with CAH may require three to four times the usual maintenance dose of glucocorticoids to suppress ACTH levels. Newborns are treated with 5 mg hydrocortisone q8h for the first 3 days; thereafter, the dosage is reduced to 2.5 mg q8h.

   (2) Hydrocortisone, 10 to 25 mg/m²/day in three divided doses, suppresses ACTH secretion and reduces adrenal androgen synthesis.

   c. The mineralocorticoid-deficient varieties (salt-wasting 21-hydroxylase, 3-beta hydroxysteroid dehydrogenase, side-chain cleavage enzyme or cholesterol desmolase, 18-hydroxylase, and 18-dehydrogenase deficiency) are treated with a salt-retaining hormone such as fludrocortisone (Florinef), 0.05 to 0.3 mg/day, and 2 to 4 g additional salt each day.

   d. Therapy is monitored clinically by measuring blood pressure, growth, pubertal development, and skeletal maturity.

Table 13-8. Clinical and laboratory features of congenital adrenal hyperplasia

Enzyme deficiency	Clinical features					Laboratory findings						
	Newborn with ambiguous genitalia		Postnatal virilization	Salt wasting	Hypertension	Urinary excretion		Circulating hormones				
	M	F				17KS	P'triol	17OHP	Δ4A	DHEA	Testo	PRA
21-Hydroxylase												
Salt wasting	A	P	P	P	A	+	+	+	+	+/N	+	+
Simple virilizing	A	P	P	A	A	+	+	+	+	+/N	+	N/+
Nonclassic	A	A	P	A	A	+/N	+/N	+/N	+/N	+/N	+/N	+/N
11β-Hydroxylase												
Classic	A	P	P	A	P	+	+	+/N	+	+/N	+	–[b]
Nonclassic	A	A	P	A	A[a]	+/N	+/N	+/N	+/N	+/N	+/N	–/N
3β-HSD												
Classic	P	P	P	P	A	+	N/–	–/N	–/N	+	F+/M–	+
Nonclassic	A	A	P	A	A	+/N	N/–	–/N	–/N	+/N	N or F+/M–	N/+
17α-Hydroxylase	P	A	A	A	P	–	–	–	–	–	–	–[c]
17,20-Lyase	P	A	A	A	A	–	N/+	N/+	–	–	–	N
18-Hydroxylase	A	A	A	P	A	N	N	N	N	N	N	+
18-Dehydrogenase	A	A	A	P	A	N	N	N	N	N	N	+
20,22-Desmolase	P	A	A	P	A	–	–	–	–	–	–	+

17KS = 17-ketosteroids; P'triol = pregnanetriol; 17OHP = 17-hydroxyprogesterone; Δ4A = androstenedione; DHEA = dehydroepiandrosterone; testo = testosterone; PRA = plasma renin activity; M = male; F = female; N = normal; A = absent; P = present; + = increased; – = decreased; HSD = hydroxysteroid dehydrogenase.
[a]Normal blood pressure or mild hypertension.
[b]Increased DOC and 11-deoxycortisol.
[c]Increased DOC.
Source: Adapted from MI New, LS Levine. *Congenital Adrenal Hyperplasia.* Berlin: Springer-Verlag, 1984.

    (1) Plasma androstenedione, 17-hydroxyprogesterone at 8 AM, plasma renin activity, and testosterone (in girls and prepubertal boys) are used to monitor the adequacy of replacement therapy.

    (2) 24-hour urinary excretion of 17-ketosteroids and pregnanetriol provides a measure of integrated adrenal steroid production.

  e. Disorders of sexual development are managed as described in sec. **III.A.3.**

C. Cushing's syndrome

  1. Etiology. Glucocorticoid excess can be caused by adrenal tumors, adrenal hyperplasia, an ACTH-producing tumor of the pituitary (Cushing's disease), an ectopic ACTH-producing tumor, or prolonged treatment with glucocorticoids.

  2. Evaluation and diagnosis

    a. Clinical manifestations

      (1) Evidence of glucocorticoid excess includes increased appetite, weight gain, slowing or arrest of linear growth, weakness, fatigue, and personality changes.

      (2) Fat deposition occurs in the facial, nuchal, shoulder, and abdominal areas. The extremities often appear thin as a result of muscle wasting. Hypertension, plethora, purple striae, ecchymoses, and weakness may be present.

      (3) Hirsutism as a result of excess adrenal androgens is consistent with ACTH excess, but virilization (enlarged clitoris or phallus) suggests an adrenal carcinoma.

    b. Laboratory examination

      (1) There is an increase in 24-hour urinary free cortisol. Serum cortisol may be normal. Serum androgens and urinary 17-ketosteroids may be increased in Cushing's disease, ectopic ACTH, and especially adrenal carcinoma, but tend not to be increased in adrenal adenoma. Serum ACTH should be low in primary adrenal tumors and markedly elevated (typically >200 pg/ml) with ectopic ACTH-producing tumors. Serum ACTH may be normal or elevated in Cushing's disease.

      (2) A single-dose overnight **dexamethasone suppression test** (10–20 μg/kg dexamethasone given at 11 PM, with plasma cortisol measured at 8 AM) is a useful screening test. Normally, plasma cortisol is less than 5 μg/dl; greater than 10 μg/dl is consistent with Cushing's syndrome.

      (3) Glucocorticoid excess may be accompanied by a hypokalemic alkalosis, polycythemia, eosinopenia, lymphopenia, and abnormal glucose tolerance with hyperglycemia. Bone age is delayed and osteoporosis may be present.

      (4) Evaluation of hypothalamopituitary-adrenal function (high-dose dexamethasone suppression, metyrapone, corticotropin releasing factor [CRF] stimulation tests), MRI studies of the hypothalamopituitary region, and CT scan and ultrasonography of the adrenal glands are performed to determine the cause of Cushing's syndrome.

  3. Treatment

    a. If the disorder is caused by an adrenal tumor, surgical resection is the treatment of choice. If an autonomously functioning adrenal adenoma is removed, the remaining adrenal gland and contralateral adrenal gland will be atrophic; therefore, the patient must be given supplemental glucocorticoid therapy before, during, and after surgery until normal adrenal function recovers. **Bilateral diseases** (tumors, adrenal hyperplasia, micronodular disease) require total adrenalectomy and lifelong adrenal steroid replacement.

    b. Treatment of a **nonresectable adrenal carcinoma** is unsatisfactory. Excessive glucocorticoid secretion can be diminished using the adrenolytic agent o,p′-DDD (mitotane) or agents that inhibit cortisol synthesis such as metyrapone, an 11-beta hydroxylase inhibitor, or aminoglutethimide, which blocks conversion of cholesterol to pregnenolone.

    c. Cushing's disease caused by excessive pituitary ACTH secretion is treated by surgical removal of the pituitary adenoma. Postoperative ACTH deficiency, which is usually temporary, requires glucocorticoid replacement until pituitary-adrenal function is recovered.

VII. Disorders of calcium homeostasis (See also Chap. 4, p. 65)
  A. Hypoparathyroidism
    1. Etiology
      a. Idiopathic
        (1) Early-onset hypoparathyroidism (first year)
          (a) Familial hypoparathyroidism can be autosomal dominant, recessive, or X-linked recessive.
          (b) Congenital hypoplasia or aplasia of parathyroids (Di George's syndrome).
        (2) Later onset
          (a) Associated with Addison's disease and mucocutaneous candidiasis (**type 1 autoimmune polyglandular deficiency syndrome**); the syndrome can include hypothyroidism, chronic active hepatitis, malabsorption syndrome, hypogonadism, pernicious anemia, vitiligo, and alopecia.
          (b) Idiopathic isolated hypoparathyroidism.
      b. Iatrogenic (following surgery).
      c. Functional hypoparathyroidism caused by hypomagnesemia.
      d. Neonatal hypoparathyroidism
        (1) Maternal hyperparathyroidism.
        (2) Infant of diabetic mother.
        (3) Neonatal illness.
    2. Evaluation
      a. Clinical presentation. The major clinical manifestations are due to hyperirritability of the central and peripheral nervous system caused by reduction of extracellular ionized calcium. Infants and children usually present with seizures or tetany.
      b. Laboratory evaluation should include
        (1) Serum calcium, phosphorus, magnesium, and alkaline phosphatase.
        (2) Serum parathyroid hormone (PTH) and vitamin D metabolites.
    3. Diagnosis
      a. Serum calcium can range from 5 mg/dl to low-normal values; phosphorus is high, usually in the range 7 to 12 mg/dl.
      b. Serum PTH is low despite a low calcium (normally a stimulus for PTH secretion) and there is no evidence of magnesium deficiency.
      c. Plasma $1,25\text{-}(OH)_2D$ concentration is low.
    4. Treatment
      a. Tetany is treated with IV injection of 10% **calcium gluconate** solution (9% elemental calcium), 100 to 200 mg/kg (9–18 mg elemental calcium/kg), given over 10 minutes, with continuous electrocardiographic monitoring. If the heart rate decreases, the infusion should be slowed or stopped. Avoid extravasation, which can cause local tissue necrosis. Bolus administration is followed by continuous infusion of 500 mg/kg (45 mg elemental calcium/kg) per 24 hours.
      b. After tetany has been relieved with IV calcium, normocalcemia is maintained with oral calcium gluconate or glubionate (6.4% elemental calcium; Neo-Calglucon has 115 mg calcium/5 ml), 75 mg/kg/day elemental calcium in neonates and 50 mg/kg/day in older children, divided into four to six doses. In infants, sufficient calcium is added to the formula to achieve a calcium-phosphate ratio of 4 : 1. The dose of calcium is adjusted to alleviate signs and symptoms of hypocalcemia and maintain a serum calcium concentration in the normal range.
      c. In **chronic hypoparathyroidism,** therapy is with **$1,25\text{-}(OH)_2D$ (calcitriol),** supplemented, if necessary, with oral calcium. Vitamin D therapy should be withheld in postsurgical hypoparathyroidism until a chronic deficiency is documented (parathyroid function may be transiently suppressed for up to 5 days).

The starting dosage of **calcitriol** (0.25- and 0.5-μg capsules) is 10 to 50 ng/kg/24 hr. The usual daily dose is 0.25 to 1.0 μg. Calcitriol's action begins in 1 to 2 days and ceases 3 to 5 days after it has been stopped. It should be started at a low dose and increased as necessary to maintain an adequate serum calcium concentration.

d. In addition to calcitriol, the total oral intake of elemental calcium should be at least 30 to 50 mg/kg/day including dietary sources (Neo-Calglucon in infants and small children, tablet preparations of calcium gluconate or carbonate in older children).

e. To avoid harmful effects of hypercalcemia, monitor serum calcium twice a week for 1 to 2 weeks until levels are stable; thereafter, the serum calcium and urinary calcium-creatinine ratio should be measured every 3 months. Aim to keep serum calcium at a level at which the patient is asymptomatic, usually 8 to 9 mg/dl, and the urinary calcium-creatinine ratio at less than 0.25 (normal 0.05–0.19). If the serum calcium exceeds 10.5 mg/dl or the urinary calcium-creatinine ratio is greater than 0.25, calcitriol is discontinued until these parameters have returned to normal, then restarted at a 20% lower dose.

B. **Pseudohypoparathyroidism**
 1. **Etiology.** The disorder results from PTH resistance.
 2. **Treatment** is the same as for hypoparathyroidism.
C. **Hypercalcemia** is defined as a serum calcium greater than 11 mg/dl or an ionized calcium greater than 5.5 mg/dl.
 1. **Etiology**
  a. **Idiopathic hypercalcemia of infancy.**
  b. In Williams syndrome, hypercalcemia **usually** resolves by 1 year of age.
  c. **Primary hyperparathyroidism** may be sporadic or associated with other endocrinopathies in the patient or family members as part of multiple endocrine neoplasia type 1 (**parathyroid hyperplasia or adenoma** associated with pancreatic islet cell and pituitary tumors) or type 2a (**parathyroid hyperplasia or adenoma** associated with medullary thyroid carcinoma and pheochromocytoma).
  d. **Secondary hyperparathyroidism** is caused by a compensatory increase in PTH secretion and is most common in vitamin D deficiency, chronic renal failure, and malabsorption syndromes.
  e. **Hypervitaminosis D** usually is a consequence of overtreatment with vitamin D.
  f. **Hypervitaminosis A** causes hypercalcemia by stimulating osteoclastic bone resorption.
  g. **Immobilization** hypercalcemia usually occurs in adolescents placed in extensive plaster casts for traumatic fractures.
  h. **Familial benign hypercalcemia** is an autosomal dominant disorder.
 2. **Evaluation**
  a. **Presentation.** Hypercalcemia causes anorexia, nausea, constipation, polyuria, polydipsia, weight loss, headaches, behavioral and personality changes, bone pain, hypotonia, and renal stones.
  b. **Laboratory evaluation** should include
   (1) Serum calcium, phosphorus, magnesium, and alkaline phosphatase; serum calcium in both parents if familial benign hypercalcemia is suspected.
   (2) Plasma PTH and vitamin D metabolites.
   (3) Serum vitamin A concentration.
   (4) Bone films including skull and pelvis.
   (5) 24-hour urine calcium, phosphorus, magnesium, and creatinine.
 3. **Diagnosis**
  a. **Hyperparathyroidism** is characterized by an elevated plasma PTH, decreased serum phosphorus, increased serum alkaline phosphatase; bone films show osteopenia, subperiosteal resorption of bone and osteolysis of the phalanges.

    b. Williams syndrome is diagnosed on the basis of clinical features.

    c. Vitamin A toxicity is confirmed by measurement of serum levels.

    d. Patients with **familial benign hypercalcemia** have relative hypocalciuria (familial hypocalciuric hypercalcemia). Although within the normal range, PTH levels are inappropriately high for the level of serum calcium.

4. Treatment

    a. General measures include a low-calcium diet, elimination of vitamin D, and protection from exposure to sunlight.

    b. Acute hypercalcemia is treated by infusion of 0.9% NaCl solution at 1.5 times maintenance and IV administration of furosemide, 1 mg/kg, repeated at six to eight intervals, to inhibit tubular reabsorption of calcium, sodium, and water. Prednisone, 1 to 2 mg/kg/day, is useful in lowering serum calcium due to increased intestinal absorption of calcium caused by hypervitaminosis D; however, its onset of action is delayed for several days. Hypercalcemia due to increased bone resorption is responsive to SC calcitonin, 2 units/kg q4h, and etidronate, 7.5 mg/kg/day infused over 4 hours daily for 3 to 7 days. These agents inhibit bone resorption.

    c. Primary hyperparathyroidism is treated by parathyroidectomy and heterotopic autotransplantation of glandular tissue in the forearm.

    d. Secondary hyperparathyroidism due to chronic renal failure is treated by lowering the serum phosphorus level with dietary phosphate restriction and oral calcium carbonate to bind phosphorus in the gut. Acidosis is corrected and calcitriol is given to maintain the serum calcium concentration and improve bone mineralization. (See also Chap. 9, p. 311)

    e. Immobilization hypercalcemia resolves when weight bearing resumes.

D. Rickets

1. Etiology

    a. Vitamin D deficiency can result from lack of sun exposure, dietary inadequacy, fat malabsorptive states, anticonvulsant therapy, hepatobiliary disease, renal disease, and renal 1-alpha hydroxylase deficiency resulting in deficient production of $1,25\text{-}(OH)_2D$ (vitamin D dependent type I).

    b. End-organ resistance to $1,25\text{-}(OH)_2D$ (vitamin D dependent type II).

    c. Phosphate deficiency from renal phosphorus loss is seen in X-linked hypophosphatemia (vitamin D–resistant rickets), Fanconi syndrome, and Lowe syndrome. Inadequate phosphorus intake can occur in premature infants and with use of total parenteral nutrition.

    d. Renal tubular acidosis also causes rickets.

2. Evaluation

    a. Clinical presentation

        (1) Infants with florid vitamin D–deficient rickets may present with tetany or convulsions due to hypocalcemia. Poor feeding, muscle weakness, decreased muscle tone, failure to thrive, and delayed motor development are common clinical features. Frontal bossing, craniotabes, widening of wrists, bowed legs, and a rachitic rosary (enlarged costochondral junctions) may be evident.

        (2) Patients with hypophosphatemic syndromes usually have a family history of rickets.

    b. Laboratory evaluation should include

        (1) Serum calcium, phosphorus, magnesium, alkaline phosphatase, and blood pH and TCO_2.

        (2) Plasma 25-OHD and $1,25\text{-}(OH)_2D$ levels.

        (3) Plasma PTH.

        (4) Wrist and knee films.

        (5) Urinary calcium, phosphorus, magnesium, pH, creatinine, and amino acids.

3. Diagnosis

    a. Radiologic findings of rickets include widened growth plates and widened, cupped, and frayed metaphyses.

    b. In **vitamin D–deficient rickets,** serum calcium is normal or low, phosphorus is low, and alkaline phosphatase is elevated. An elevated level of PTH and low 25-OHD level confirm the diagnosis. Plasma $1,25\text{-}(OH)_2D$ is high normal or even increased due to secondary hyperparathyroidism.

c. In **hypophosphatemic (vitamin D resistant) rickets,** renal tubular resorption of phosphorus is decreased. Serum phosphorus usually is less than 3 mg/dl. Serum calcium and plasma levels of PTH and 25-OHD are normal, and alkaline phosphatase is elevated. Plasma $1,25\text{-}(OH)_2D$ levels are normal but inappropriately low in view of hypophosphatemia.

4. **Treatment**
   a. **Vitamin D–deficiency rickets** in infants heals with 1,000 to 4,000 IU (25–100 μg) per day of oral cholecalciferol (vitamin D_3). The dose is reduced to 400 IU (10 μg) daily when the rickets has healed. To prevent tetany, the diet must provide a minimum of 30 mg/kg elemental calcium per day; an oral calcium supplement may be necessary (see **A.4.a,b** above). When rickets is due to **intestinal malabsorption,** the dosage of vitamin D necessary to promote healing may have to be 5,000 to 10,000 IU (125–250 μg) per day. A calcium supplement usually is necessary.
   b. **Rickets of prematurity** cannot be prevented by vitamin D supplements alone. In addition to vitamin D_3, 800 IU (20 μg) daily, the diet must be supplemented with calcium and phosphorus (60 mg elemental calcium/kg/day, and 30 mg elemental phosphorus/kg/day).
   c. **Vitamin D–dependent rickets (1-alpha hydroxylase deficiency)** is treated with physiologic doses of calcitriol.
   d. **Hypophosphatemic disorders** require oral phosphorus supplements to maintain serum phosphorus at greater than 3 mg/dl. Doses of neutral phosphate salts usually range from 1 to 5 g elemental phosphorus per day, and are given q4h throughout the day to provide sustained correction of hypophosphatemia. This is combined with physiologic doses of calcitriol to maintain adequate calcium absorption and avoid hypocalcemia and secondary hyperparathyroidism.
   e. To avoid the **side effects** of hypercalcemia and hypercalciuria, blood and urinary calcium concentrations must be monitored frequently.

VIII. **Disorders of glucose homeostasis**
   A. **Hypoglycemia** is defined as a plasma or serum glucose concentration less than 50 mg/dl (whole blood glucose concentration <45 mg/dl).
      1. **Etiology** (Table 13-9).
      2. **Evaluation**
         a. **Clinical manifestations** are due to increased **autonomic nervous system activity** and include trembling, nervousness, sweating, pallor, tachycardia, hunger, nausea, vomiting, and **neuroglucopenia,** which causes drowsiness, headache, weakness, inability to concentrate, bizarre behavior, confusion, coma, and seizures.
         b. **Neonatal hypoglycemia** is usually transient and does not require elaborate investigation (see Chap. 6).
         c. When **neonatal hypoglycemia is persistent or recurrent,** and when **hypoglycemia occurs in an infant or older child,** a blood sample should be obtained at the time of hypoglycemia for the following analyses: glucose, lactate, free fatty acids, beta-hydroxybutyrate and acetoacetate, total and free carnitine, alanine, insulin, glucagon, cortisol, and GH. Urine should be tested for ketones, nonglucose reducing substances, organic and amino acids, and toxins. The results may be sufficient to clarify the etiology of the hypoglycemia (Table 13-10). (See also Chap. 6, p. 201 and Chap. 12, Table 12-1, p. 374)
         d. The **response to IV glucose** provides additional information about the possible cause of the hypoglycemia. Infants with hyperinsulinism require rates of glucose administration greater than 6 to 8 mg/kg/min to maintain plasma glucose above 50 mg/dl.
         e. **If the cause of the hypoglycemia is obscure, a formal fasting study may be necessary.** Blood glucose, metabolic substrates, and hormones

Table 13–9. Classification of childhood hypoglycemia

Neonatal-transient
Inadequate substrate or enzyme function (prematurity, intrauterine growth retardation)
Hyperinsulinism (infant of diabetic mother, erythroblastosis fetalis)

Neonatal, infantile, childhood-persistent or recurrent

Disorders of hepatic glucose production
Glycogenolysis
  Glycogen storage diseases types I, III, VI, IX
  Glycogen synthetase deficiency
Gluconeogenesis
  Pyruvate carboxylase, fructose 1,6-diphosphatase, phosphoenolpyruvate carboxykinase
    (PEPCK) deficiency
  Alcohol, salicylate, valproic acid, unripe Ackee nut intoxication
  Galactosemia (galactose 1-phosphate uridyl transferase deficiency)
  Hereditary fructose intolerance (fructose 1-phosphate aldolase deficiency)
  Ketotic hypoglycemia (accelerated starvation)
  Prolonged fasting

Disorders involving production of alternative fuels
Defects in fatty acid oxidation
  Carnitine deficiency, carnitine palmitoyl transferase deficiency, medium-chain
    acyl-CoA dehydrogenase deficiency, long-chain acyl-CoA dehydrogenase
Defects in ketogenesis

Hormonal abnormalities
Hyperinsulinism
  Dysregulated insulin secretion, beta-cell hyperplasia, beta-cell adenoma, Beckwith-
    Wiedemann syndrome
Panhypopituitarism
Growth hormone deficiency
Cortisol deficiency
  Primary adrenocortical insufficiency
  Secondary to ACTH deficiency or unresponsiveness

Miscellaneous causes
Associated with propionic acidemia, methylmalonic acidemia, tyrosinosis, maple
  syrup urine disease
Severe liver disease (fulminant hepatitis, Reye's syndrome)
Sepsis in newborn
Cyanotic congenital heart disease

---

are monitored at frequent intervals, and the fast is terminated when the plasma glucose concentration falls below 50 mg/dl or after 24 hours, whichever occurs first. **Glucagon (0.03 mg/kg, 1 mg maximum)** is given IV or IM at the end of the fast, and the **glycemic response** is monitored over the next 60 minutes. Urine is collected throughout the fasting study for measurement of ketones and organic acids.

3. **Treatment.** Hypoglycemia is an important preventable cause of permanent brain damage, mental retardation, and seizures, and must be treated aggressively.
   a. **Acute.** Glucose is given intravenously at approximately 150% of the basal glucose production rate (GPR; newborns, 5–8 mg/kg/min; older infants and children, 3–5 mg/kg/min). High concentrations of glucose and boluses of concentrated glucose should be avoided because, especially in a child with hyperinsulinism, this causes "reactive hypoglycemia."

Table 13-10. Evaluation of hypoglycemia

Test	Ketotic hypoglycemia	Excess insulin	Hormone deficiency	Enzyme deficiency[a]
Glucose	Low	Low	Low	Low
Insulin	Normal	↑–↑↑↑	Normal	Normal
GH	Normal	Normal	Low/normal[b]	Normal
Cortisol	Normal	Normal	Low/normal[b]	Normal
Thyroxine/TSH	Normal	Normal	Low/normal[b]	Normal
Lactate	Normal	Normal	Normal	Normal or ↑↑↑[a]
FFA	↑↑↑	Low	↑↑–↑↑↑	↑↑↑
Ketones[c]	↑↑↑	Low	↑↑–↑↑↑	↑–↑↑↑ or low[d]
Alanine	Decreased	Normal	Normal	Normal or ↑↑↑[a]

Normal = blood level is appropriate for the blood glucose concentration and duration of fast; ↑ = mildly, ↑↑ = moderately, and ↑↑↑ = markedly elevated; FFA = free fatty acids.
[a]Deficiency of key gluconeogenic enzymes such as glucose 6-phosphatase, fructose 1,6-diphosphatase.
[b]Deficiency of GH or ACTH can be isolated or associated with deficiency of other pituitary hormones.
[c]Beta-hydroxybutyrate and acetoacetate.
[d]Ketones characteristically are low in disorders of fatty acid oxidation and ketogenesis.

    b. Hyperinsulinism. Diazoxide, 10 to 25 mg/kg/day in three equally divided doses, is used to suppress insulin secretion. If benefit is not apparent within 3 to 5 days, SC administration of a long-acting somatostatin analogue (octreotide) can be given a therapeutic trial. If normoglycemia cannot be maintained, an attempt is made to locate and excise an adenoma.

    c. Hormone deficiency is treated by replacement of the specific hormone deficiency (see above). Neonatal hypoglycemia due to GH deficiency is treated with human growth hormone (HGH), 0.05 μg/kg IM daily.

    d. The treatment of **disorders of hepatic glucose production** involves avoidance of prolonged fasting by establishing a pattern of frequent feeding. When anorexia, nausea, and vomiting occur for any reason, the urine should be tested frequently for the presence of ketones. Ketonuria signifies the need for liquid forms of concentrated carbohydrate; if oral carbohydrate cannot be retained, glucose must be given intravenously at a rate of approximately 4 to 6 mg/kg/min or 10% dextrose in water (D/W) at a rate of 1,500 to 2,000 ml/m²/24 hr to forestall symptomatic hypoglycemia.

    e. Treatment of **type I glycogen storage disease** involves providing a dietary source of continuous glucose during the day with supplements of uncooked cornstarch taken with meals and 3 hours after meals. Galactose and fructose, which cannot be readily converted to glucose, and can aggravate hyperlactatemia and hyperlipidemia, should be kept to a minimum. At night, a source of continuous glucose is provided using either intermittent uncooked cornstarch or a continuous intragastric infusion of glucose via a gastrostomy or nasogastric tube.

    f. Children with **inborn errors of fatty acid oxidation and ketogenesis** must avoid prolonged fasting. Their treatment is as outlined above for disorders of hepatic glucose production. Children with these disorders cannot produce ketones normally; during fasting ketonuria is minimal or absent despite imminent or overt hypoglycemia.

  B. Diabetes mellitus

    1. Classification, etiology, and general features

      a. Virtually all children and adolescents with diabetes have **insulin-dependent (IDDM), or type I, diabetes,** which results from an absolute deficiency of insulin. Susceptibility to IDDM is inherited; siblings of a diabetic proband have a 5% risk of developing diabetes compared to 0.4% for the population at large. The risk for an identical twin is about 33%.

  b. **Non–insulin-dependent (NIDDM), or type II, diabetes** occurs in a minority of adolescents with diabetes. Most NIDDM patients are obese and insulin resistant.

  c. **Secondary diabetes** is most often caused by cystic fibrosis, glucocorticoid excess, and subtotal pancreatectomy for hyperinsulinemic hypoglycemia.

2. **Evaluation**

  a. **Clinical course**

   (1) **Onset.** The most common complaints are polyuria, polydipsia, insatiable thirst, enuresis, weight loss, lack of energy, increased fatigability, blurred vision, and perineal candidiasis in girls. About one third of patients have diabetic ketoacidosis at the time of presentation.

   (2) **Remission.** Within a few weeks or months of starting insulin treatment, about two thirds of patients enter a phase of either partial or complete remission. Partial remission is characterized by virtually normal glycemia while receiving a relatively small dose of insulin (<0.5 units/kg/day). Partial or complete remission can last from several months to 1 to 2 years, but eventually is replaced by increasing insulin requirements.

   (3) **Intensification.** Waning of the remission usually is a gradual process characterized by increasing insulin requirements and metabolic instability over a period of several weeks or months.

  b. **Laboratory evaluation**

   (1) Fasting and random plasma glucose levels are increased with or without ketonuria.

   (2) **Transient hyperglycemia and glucosuria** occasionally occur with stress.

    (a) A **glucose tolerance test (GTT)** should be performed after the child has returned to good health. The test is done in the morning after an overnight fast and at least 3 days on a high-carbohydrate diet (200–300 g/1.73 m^2/day).

    (b) The **oral glucose tolerance test (OGTT)** is performed using 1.75 g/kg glucose (maximum 75 g). Samples are obtained fasting and then at 30-minute intervals for 2 hours for measurement of plasma glucose and insulin.

    (c) Loss of first-phase insulin secretion during an **intravenous glucose tolerance test (IVGTT) predicts imminent diabetes.**

3. **Diagnosis**

  a. The OGTT is considered diagnostic of diabetes mellitus when the fasting venous plasma glucose concentration is elevated (>140 mg/dl) and there is a sustained elevation of the plasma glucose concentration (>200 mg/dl) at 2 hours and at an intervening time point.

  b. A child has **impaired glucose tolerance (IGT) if the fasting plasma glucose concentration is less than 140 mg/dl but the 2-hour value exceeds 140 mg/dl.**

4. **Therapy**

  a. **Goals.** Treatment aims to relieve symptoms and ensure normal physical, emotional, and social growth and development.

   (1) Avoidance of episodes of severe hypoglycemia and ketoacidosis is an important short-term goal of therapy.

   (2) The long-term goal is to prevent or delay the micro- and macrovascular complications of diabetes. Long-term maintenance of near-normal blood glucose levels has been proven to prevent and/or delay the development and progression of retinopathy, nephropathy and neuropathy.

   (3) **Intensive diabetes therapy** with multiple daily injections (or contin-

uous subcutaneous infusion of insulin), strict adherence to a meal plan, frequent self-monitoring of blood glucose levels, and day-to-day self-adjustment of insulin doses using an algorithm enables the motivated patient to achieve blood glucose levels that are near normal. Intensive diabetes therapy, however, is demanding and costly, and significantly increases the risk of severe hypoglycemia.

b. The patient is considered to be in satisfactory **metabolic control** when

(1) Most fasting and premeal blood glucose levels are in the range of 70 to 150 mg/dl.

(2) Ketonuria is absent.

(3) Glycosylated hemoglobin (hemoglobin A_{1c}) is less than 1.35 times the upper limit of normal.

(4) Plasma lipids are normal.

c. **Patient education** is the foundation of successful diabetes care.

(1) The process of educating the parents and child begins soon after the diagnosis is made. Because most parents are initially too anxious to assimilate an extensive body of information, the education program should be staged; initial goals are limited to an understanding of the fundamental nature of the disease and how it is treated, and acquiring the essential "survival skills" necessary for the child to be safely cared for at home and school.

(2) During the next several weeks, the basic aspects of diabetes care are consolidated by practical experience at home and frequent telephone and direct contact with the diabetes educator or physician, or both.

(3) The intricate details of diabetes management and how to cope with intercurrent illnesses, exercise, changes in appetite, and other variations that typically occur in a child's daily routine are taught in stages.

d. Insulin

(1) **Preparations** are divided into three categories according to their time of onset, peak activity, and duration of action following subcutaneous administration (Table 13-11).

(2) During the **remission** phase the disease can be well controlled in many children with a single injection of intermediate-acting insulin alone or combined with a small amount of regular insulin given before breakfast. Increased blood glucose levels at bedtime or before breakfast, or both, signifies the need for a dose of insulin before the evening meal and/or at bedtime.

(3) **Total diabetes** can be satisfactorily controlled in most children with a twice-daily insulin regimen consisting of a mixture of rapid-acting (regular) insulin and intermediate-acting (neutral protamine Hagedorn [NPH] or lente) insulin mixed in the same syringe and injected

Table 13–11. Insulin preparations

Type	Appearance	Action	Onset of action (hr*)	Maximum effect (hr)*	End of effect (hr)*
Regular	Clear solution	Rapid	0.5	2–4	6–8
NPH (isophane)	Cloudy suspension	Intermediate	1–2	6–12	18–24
Lente	Cloudy suspension	Intermediate	1–3	6–12	18–24
Ultralente	Cloudy suspension	Prolonged	4–6	8–20	24–28

*These figures are for human insulins and are approximations from laboratory studies in test subjects. The times of onset, maximum, and duration of effect vary greatly within and between patients and are affected by many factors, including size of dose, species, site of injection, exercise of the injected area, temperature, and insulin antibodies.

subcutaneously 30 minutes before breakfast and supper. For adolescents, a modification of this regimen that involves three doses daily, with regular insulin given alone before supper and intermediate-acting insulin given at approximately 10 PM.

(4) The **dose** of insulin is determined empirically for each patient. On an average, about 60 to 75% of the total daily dose is given before breakfast and 25 to 40% before the evening meal or at bedtime, or both. Usually, about one third of each dose consists of rapid-acting insulin; however, the optimal ratio of rapid- to intermediate-acting insulin for each patient must be determined by trial and error based on the results of blood glucose monitoring before meals, at bedtime, and between 2 and 4 AM. Young children usually require a smaller fraction of rapid-acting or regular insulin, for example, on the order of 10 to 20% and 80 to 90% intermediate-acting insulin.

(5) The recommended **starting dose** of insulin in a child detected early with **moderate hyperglycemia and no ketonuria** is **0.3 to 0.5 units/kg/day SC.** A single dose of intermediate-acting insulin without any regular insulin will usually suffice to restore normoglycemia and relieve the symptoms within a few days.

    (a) When **metabolic decompensation is more severe with ketonuria but without acidosis or dehydration,** start with **0.5 to 0.7 units/kg** intermediate-acting insulin and supplement with 0.1 units/kg regular insulin SC at 4- to 6-hour intervals, aiming to achieve preprandial blood glucose levels of 70 to 150 mg/dl. The insulin dose is adjusted daily until satisfactory glycemic control is achieved.

    (b) Once metabolic control has been established, adjustments in the insulin dose should be made by approximately 10% at any one time, and a minimum of 3 to 5 days is allowed to elapse after each change before further adjustments are made. Acute metabolic derangements warrant more frequent adjustments.

(6) **Injection sites** should be rotated to avoid lipohypertrophy, which alters the pharmacokinetics of insulin absorption. Recommended sites include the posterior aspect of the upper extremities, anterior aspect of the thighs, buttocks, and anterior abdominal wall.

(7) The technique of drawing up, mixing, and injecting insulin is taught to parents and, when appropriate, to the child.

(8) **Modification of dosage**

    (a) Children's insulin requirements change during the evolution of the stages of the disease (see sec. **2.a.,** p. 406) and during normal growth and pubertal development as well as with change in activity. Therefore, each child's insulin regimen must be periodically reevaluated and adjusted if necessary.

    (b) During the **remission,** or "honeymoon," period, the insulin requirement is less than 0.5 units/kg/day.

    (c) During the intensification phase and in the stage of total diabetes, the total daily insulin dose in prepubertal children is 0.5 to 1.0 units/kg/day; in pubertal individuals it is 0.8 to 1.5 units/kg/day.

    (d) Amounts of insulin that exceed the above ranges are seldom necessary and should raise the suspicion of overinsulinization or insulin omission. Rarely, one has to consider the extremely unusual syndromes of insulin resistance due to dysfunction of the insulin receptor.

e. **Diet therapy**

    (1) **General principles**

        (a) The nutritional needs of children with diabetes do not differ from those of healthy children. However, newly diagnosed children typically present with weight loss and the initial diet prescription aims to restore appropriate body weight. Once this has been achieved, the total intake of calories and nutrients must be sufficient to balance the daily expenditure of energy and satisfy the requirements for normal growth and development. A method commonly used to estimate energy requirements is based on age and can be used as a crude approximation for children up to 12 years of age. To 1,000 kcal, add 100 times the patient's age in years. Very active children need 10 to 20% more calories.

(b) The American Diabetes Association recommends that carbohydrate provide 50 to 60% of the total calories, with protein and fat making up 15 and 30%, respectively.

(c) The **diet prescription** has to be adjusted periodically to achieve an ideal body weight and to maintain a normal rate of physical growth and maturation.

(d) The main objective of dietary therapy in obese non–insulin-dependent patients is to lose weight and then maintain a desirable body weight.

(e) **Prudent fat.** Because individuals with diabetes are predisposed to atherosclerosis, the amount of fat should not exceed 30% of the total daily calories. Dietary **cholesterol** should be reduced to no more than 300 mg/day; the amount of **polyunsaturated and monounsaturated fatty acids is increased** while the consumption of **saturated fat is reduced** to less than 10% of calories.

(f) **Fiber.** Dietary fiber can benefit the diabetic patient by blunting the rise in blood glucose after meals. Soluble fiber can also reduce serum cholesterol levels.

(g) **Fruit.** To avoid abrupt increases in blood glucose, children should eat fruit **whole** and avoid fruit juices, which should be reserved for treating episodes of hypoglycemia.

(h) Because insulin is released continuously from the injection site, **hypoglycemia,** exacerbated by exercise, can occur if snacks are not eaten between the main meals. Hence, most children who receive twice-daily injections of insulin (split-mixed insulin regimen) have a snack between each meal and at bedtime.

(i) Food consumption must be matched to the time course of action of injected insulin. Meals and snacks should be **eaten at the same times each day,** and the total consumption of calories and the proportions of carbohydrate, protein, and fat in each meal and snack must be **consistent** from day to day.

(2) **Exchange system**

(a) The **meal plan** is formulated by a registered dietitian using the system of food exchanges and is individualized to meet the ethnic, religious, and economic circumstances of each family and the food preferences of the individual child.

(b) The **exchange system** is based on six food groups: milk, fruit, vegetable, bread, meat, and fat. The individual food items included in each exchange list contain approximately the same amount of carbohydrate, fat, and protein. The portion size of each item included in the six categories is given either by weight or volume. Thus, the meal plan is prescribed in terms of the number of exchanges from each food group that should be included in each meal and snack.

f. **Exercise.** The effects of exercise on diabetes are complex.

(1) Exercise acutely lowers the blood glucose concentration, depending on the intensity and duration of the physical activity and the concurrent level of insulinemia. Consequently, bursts of increased energy expenditure should be "covered" by providing an extra snack before and, if the exercise is prolonged, during the activity. A rule of thumb is to provide 15 g carbohydrate (one bread or fruit exchange) per 30 minutes of vigorous physical activity. Strenuous exercise in the afternoon or evening should be followed by a 10 to 30% reduction in the presupper or bedtime dose of intermediate-acting insulin, and a larger bedtime snack to reduce the risk of nocturnal or early-morning hypoglycemia resulting from the lag effect of exercise.

(2) Acute vigorous exercise in the child with poorly controlled diabetes can **aggravate hyperglycemia and stimulate ketoacid production.** Therefore, **the child whose diabetes is out of control (hyperglycemia with ketonuria) should be discouraged from exercising** until satisfactory control has been restored.

(3) Exercising the limb into which insulin has been injected accelerates the rate of insulin absorption. Therefore, if exercise is planned, it is recommended that the preceding insulin injection be given in a site that is least likely to be affected by exercise.

(4) Physical training increases tissue sensitivity to insulin. Youngsters who participate in organized sports are advised to adjust their insulin dose in anticipation of sustained physical activity during a specific period of the day. The precise amounts of such reductions are determined by trial and error, but are generally in the range of 10 to 30% of the usual insulin dose.

g. **Monitoring**

(1) **Blood glucose testing**

(a) Self-monitoring of blood glucose (SMBG) is routinely taught to all patients with IDDM, and the ability of patients to obtain accurate results must be confirmed.

(b) Ideally, patients should test before each meal and at bedtime. If this is impractical or intolerable, patients should be encouraged to test before each dose of insulin, with additional tests before lunch and at bedtime at least twice each week. Alternatively, for patients who cannot tolerate such frequent monitoring, or who cannot afford the cost of the reagent strips, a period of intensive monitoring before each meal, at bedtime, and between 2 and 4 AM for several consecutive days before an office visit often provides sufficient information to confirm satisfactory control or indicate where problems lie so that appropriate adjustments in the regimen can be made.

(2) Urine should be tested for the presence of ketones whenever the child is sick, when the blood glucose level exceeds 250 mg/dl, and when blood glucose levels are high before breakfast and the possibility of unrecognized nocturnal hypoglycemia is suspected.

(3) **Glycosylated hemoglobin (hemoglobin A_1 or A_{1c}).** The level of glycosylated hemoglobin is directly proportional to the time-integrated mean blood glucose concentration over the preceding 2 to 3 months. Quarterly determinations of glycosylated hemoglobin should be used to provide an objective measure of glycemia in the intervals between office visits.

5. **Acute complications**

a. **Hypoglycemia**

(1) Occasional episodes of **hypoglycemia** are an unavoidable consequence of insulin therapy aimed at maintaining blood glucose levels near to normal.

(2) The most common reasons that **hypoglycemia** occurs are bursts of physical activity without a preceding snack; prolonged or strenuous exercise without a reduction of insulin dose; meals or snacks that are delayed, omitted, or incompletely consumed; inadvertent errors in insulin dosage; and inappropriate insulin regimens.

(3) **Patients and family members must be taught to recognize the early symptoms of hypoglycemia and treat it promptly with a**

suitable form of concentrated carbohydrate. Most episodes of hypoglycemia are satisfactorily treated with 10 to 20 g glucose; 5 g is sufficient for an infant or toddler. Suitable forms of rapidly absorbed carbohydrate for treatment of hypoglycemia are glucose tablets (each contains 5 g glucose), Lifesavers (3 g each), granulated table sugar (4 g/tsp), or orange or apple juice (10–12 g/120 ml).

(4) Family members are taught to use **glucagon** (which should be available at home) to treat an episode of **severe hypoglycemia** in which the child is unconscious or unable to swallow or retain ingested carbohydrate. Glucagon (0.02–0.03 mg/kg, maximum dose 1.0 mg) is injected IM or SC and raises the blood glucose level within 5 to 15 minutes. Nausea and vomiting may follow the administration of glucagon. Oral carbohydrate to prevent further hypoglycemia should be given when consciousness has been regained after a severe insulin reaction.

(5) If the patient cannot take or retain sugar-containing solutions orally, glucose, 0.5 g/kg, is injected IV, followed by a continuous infusion of glucose at a rate that maintains a normal blood glucose concentration.

(6) A Medic Alert bracelet or necklace should always be worn to identify the patient as having diabetes mellitus.

b. Diabetic ketoacidosis (DKA)

(1) Evaluation

(a) Rapidly perform a clinical evaluation to establish the diagnosis and determine its cause and the patient's degree of dehydration. Weigh the patient and measure height or length.

(b) Determine the blood glucose concentration at the bedside with a glucose meter.

(c) Obtain a blood sample for measurement of plasma glucose, electrolytes, total carbon dioxide, BUN, serum osmolality, arterial or venous pH, carbon dioxide tension (PCO_2), oxygen tension (PO_2), hemoglobin, hematocrit, white blood cell count and differential, calcium, magnesium, and phosphorus. Calculate the anion gap $Na^+ - [Cl^- + TCO_2]$; 12 ± 2 is normal.

(d) Perform a urinalysis and obtain appropriate specimens for culture (blood, urine, throat) even if the patient is afebrile.

(e) Perform an electrocardiogram for baseline evaluation of potassium status.

(f) Determine baseline neurologic status.

(2) Supportive measures

(a) Accurately assess urine output. Bladder catheterization or condom drainage should be used, as appropriate.

(b) A flow chart must be used to record the clinical and laboratory data, details of fluid and electrolyte therapy, administered insulin, and urine output. Successful management of diabetic ketoacidosis requires **meticulous monitoring** of the clinical and biochemical response to treatment so that timely adjustments in the treatment regimen can be made.

(c) Plasma glucose, serum electrolytes (and corrected sodium), pH, PCO_2, TCO_2, anion gap, calcium, and phosphorus should be measured every 2 hours for the first 8 hours, and then every 4 hours until they are normal.

(d) Broad-spectrum antibiotics should be given to **febrile** patients after appropriate cultures of body fluids have been obtained.

(3) Fluid and electrolyte treatment (see also Chap. 4). **All patients with DKA are dehydrated** and suffer total body depletion of sodium, potassium, chloride, phosphate, and magnesium. Patients with mild to moderate DKA are usually about 5% (50 ml/kg) dehydrated, and those with severe DKA are up to 10% (100 ml/kg) dehydrated.

(a) The first priority is to start an intravenous infusion using a large-bore cannula and to infuse **10 ml/kg isotonic saline (0.9%)** in

60 minutes. The severely dehydrated patient or patient in shock should receive 20 ml/kg. If hypotension or shock persists, an additional 10 ml/kg isotonic saline (or an equal amount of fresh-frozen plasma) is given over the next 60 minutes.

(b) Once the circulation has been stabilized, change to half-normal saline and aim to **replace the calculated fluid deficit at an even rate over 24 to 36 hours.** Aim to achieve slow correction of the serum hyperosmolality and to avoid a rapid shift of water from the extracellular to the intracellular compartment. The sodium concentration of the solution should be increased to 100 to 130 mEq/liter if the **corrected serum sodium concentration** falls or fails to rise as the plasma glucose concentration decreases. The corrected sodium is calculated: Na^+ + (1.6 × [plasma glucose mg/dl − 100]/100).

(c) **Dextrose 5%** is added to the infusion fluid when the plasma glucose concentration reaches 300 mg/dl. Attempt to maintain the plasma glucose concentration at approximately 200 mg/dl for the first 36 to 48 hours. **Dextrose 10%** may be needed to avert hypoglycemia.

(d) Early in the course of therapy, **continued osmotic diuresis contributes significantly to ongoing fluid losses,** and the rate of fluid administration may have to be temporarily increased to achieve positive fluid balance and to stabilize the circulation. When the osmotic diuresis subsides, maintenance fluid is given as half isotonic saline at a rate of 1,500 to 2,000 ml/m²/day.

(e) Intravenous fluid administration should **continue until acidosis is corrected** and the patient can eat and drink without vomiting.

(f) **Persistent tachycardia** in the absence of fever is evidence of inadequate fluid administration and should be confirmed by the record of cumulative fluid balance.

(4) **Insulin.** Several insulin therapy protocols are effective in managing DKA.

(a) The preferred method is **low-dose continuous intravenous administration** controlled by an infusion pump. Insulin is diluted in saline (50 units regular insulin in 50 ml saline) and is given IV at a rate of 0.1 units/kg/hr after an IV priming dose of 0.1 units/kg. This rate of insulin infusion is sufficient to reverse DKA in the majority of patients; however, if the response is inadequate (blood glucose levels are not falling and anion gap is not decreasing) due to severe insulin resistance, the rate of insulin infusion should be increased until a satisfactory response is achieved. **Rare patients with severe insulin resistance will not respond satisfactorily to low-dose insulin infusion and require two or three times the usual dose.** The serum half-life of insulin is approximately 5 minutes; if insulin infusion is stopped, the serum insulin concentration decreases by 50% every 5 minutes so that **insulin deficiency occurs rapidly if the infusion infiltrates or is interrupted for any reason. Therefore, low-dose insulin therapy should be closely supervised.**

(b) When DKA has resolved (venous pH >7.32, total CO_2 >18 mEq/liter) and the change to **SC** insulin is planned, the first SC injection should be given 120 minutes before stopping the infusion to allow sufficient time for the injected insulin to be absorbed.

(c) Frequent **intramuscular** insulin can also effectively lower blood glucose and reverse acidosis. However, in hypotensive patients, insulin absorption may be erratic. This has the advantage of not requiring any special equipment. Initially, 0.1 to 0.25 units/kg is

Table 13-12. Potassium replacement in diabetic ketoacidosis

Serum potassium (mEq/liter)	Infusate potassium concentration (mEq/liter)
<3	40–60
3–4	30
4–5	20
5–6	10
>6	0

given as an IV bolus; thereafter, 0.1 units/kg is administered IM hourly until the plasma glucose concentration reaches 300 mg/dl, and then the insulin is given SC.

(5) Potassium replacement

(a) All patients with DKA are potassium depleted (4–6 mEq/kg) despite the fact that the initial serum potassium concentration may be normal or increased. **With the administration of fluid and insulin, serum potassium may decrease abruptly predisposing to cardiac arrhythmias.** Patients whose serum potassium level is initially low are the most severely depleted and should receive potassium early (after urinating and after insulin has been given), and their serum potassium concentration should be measured hourly.

(b) The serum potassium level should be maintained between 3.5 and 4.5 mEq/liter. If the laboratory has not reported the pretreatment level within an hour, **potassium should not be withheld if insulin has already been given** and the patient has urinated. Table 13-12 is a guide to initial potassium administration based on the serum concentration.

(c) Half the potassium is given as **potassium acetate** and the other half as **potassium phosphate,** thus reducing the total amount of chloride administered and partially replacing the phosphate deficit.

(d) The electrocardiogram can serve as a useful guide to therapy. The configuration of the T waves in standard lead II and V_2 is followed at 30- to 60-minute intervals.

(6) Routine **bicarbonate** administration neither hastens resolution of acidosis nor improves survival and can impair tissue oxygenation and cause hypokalemia. Its routine use is not recommended; however, when acidosis is severe (arterial pH < 7.0) or hypotension, shock, or an arrhythmia is present, sodium bicarbonate, 1 to 2 mEq/kg or 40 to 80 mEq/m^2, is infused over 2 hours.

(7) Cerebral edema is an uncommon complication of DKA that can cause acute brain herniation and death. It typically develops abruptly within 2 to 12 hours of starting treatment. See Chapter 7, p. 235, for diagnosis and management.

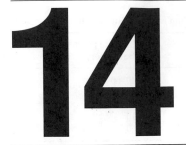

Prepubertal and Adolescent Gynecologic Disorders

Marc R. Laufer

External genital inspection should be part of the standard physical examination. Pelvic examinations should be performed routinely in sexually active adolescents by the primary care provider or closely linked referral provider.

I. **Anatomy/physiology and gynecologic examination**
   A. From **birth to 6 to 8** weeks of age
      1. **Anatomy/physiology**
         a. **Maternal estrogen and gonadotropins** (luteinizing hormone [LH] and follicle-stimulating hormone [FSH]) effects predominate.
         b. Breast tissue is engorged and breast buds are palpable.
         c. Vaginal mucosa and introitus are engorged.
         d. Genital bleeding from the uterus (endometrium) can occur as a result of the withdrawal of maternally derived estrogen.
         e. **Functional follicular ovarian cysts** may be present from the neonatal period and are generally asymptomatic. They are most commonly identified incidentally on ultrasound. The cysts are usually simple (without solid components) and may be bilateral. Since spontaneous regression is the norm, treatment is generally not warranted unless the patient is symptomatic, in which case ultrasound-guided aspiration or laparoscopy can be undertaken. Torsion is rare and laparotomy or oophorectomy should be avoided.
      2. **Gynecologic examination**
         a. A caretaker known to the child can either hold the child on his/her lap or the child can be held while lying on a table, with ankles drawn together in the frog-leg position.
         b. Grasp labia and retract forward and down to inspect hymen. The hymen can be crescentic, annular, or redundant.
         c. Visualization can be enhanced with an otoscope without the ear piece, providing light and magnification to evaluate pathology in the office setting.
   B. From **8 weeks to 2 years**
      1. **Anatomy/physiology**
         a. Maternally stimulated hormone levels (estrogen, LH, and FSH) are falling, but can do so at variable rates, resulting in **prolonged breast buds** for some girls, which may be asymmetrical. Biopsy of the area can result in amastia on the biopsied side and should be avoided.
         b. **Mastitis** is possible and should be treated aggressively, usually with intravenous antibiotics.
         c. **Functional follicular ovarian cysts:** above-mentioned neonatal ovarian simple cysts may persist as they slowly resolve. Management as listed in sec. **A.1.e** above.
      2. **Gynecologic examination as in I.A.2.**
   C. From **2 to 8 years**
      1. **Anatomy/physiology**
         a. Hypoestrogenic environment similar to menopause, readily susceptible to vaginitis if vaginal flora disrupted.
         b. Uterus involutes to 30% of adult size and is palpable on rectoabdominal examination.

   c. Ratio of the size of the cervix–uterine corpus is 2 : 1.

   d. Vagina is 5 cm long with thin, pink mucosa.

   e. Cervix is flush with the vagina.

   f. Hymen is thin and friable; hymenal opening approximately 0.5 cm in size, but dependent on examination technique.

   g. Labia minora are prominent, thin, and pink, with minimal labia majora or vulvar fat pads.

   h. Ovaries are located more cephalad than their final adult location.

2. Gynecologic examination

   a. The child is reassured that the examination is painless. Use caretaker's lap to place child in dorsal lithotomy position, with child's feet propped on knees of caretaker if child is hesitant to assume frog-leg position on examination table when so requested.

   b. Forced examinations are remembered and are **inappropriate.**

   c. As the external genitalia are inspected, the patient is asked to hold the labia apart. This allows her to participate and have a sense of control.

   d. The knee-chest position can be used for cooperative patients.

   e. Rectoabdominal examination is warranted if there is a question of a mass. The cervix feels like a small nubbin.

   f. Examination under anesthesia (EUA) is indicated when the child is unable to cooperate and there is a need for thorough gynecologic evaluation.

D. From 8 to 9 years

1. Anatomy/physiology

   a. Estrogen stimulation begins.

   b. Cervix-corpus ratio becomes 1 : 1.

   c. Vagina lengthening to 6 to 8 cm, mucosa thicker.

   d. Hymenal orifice 1 cm on average, but dependent on examination technique.

   e. Labia majora more prominent.

   f. Breast budding generally precedes onset of menstruation by about 2 years. Tanner staging is noted (see Table 13-1).

   g. Ovaries in final pelvic location.

2. Gynecologic examination

   a. Examine patient in frog-leg position to evaluate external genitalia for standard well child examination.

   b. If pathology is suspected, add the knee-chest position to visualize the vagina and in a cooperative patient to visualize the cervix. The patient is told to "lie on your tummy with your bottom in the air." As the child takes a few deep breaths and allows her spine and stomach to "sag like an old horse," the vaginal orifice falls open. An otoscope provides the necessary light and magnification needed to visualize the cervix.

   c. Rectoabdominal examination if pathology is suspected.

   d. EUA is indicated when the child is unable to cooperate and there is a need for thorough gynecologic evaluation.

E. Adolescence

1. Anatomy/physiology

   a. Adult genital anatomy; cervix-corpus ratio: 1 : 2.

   b. Vaginal length is 10 cm and vaginal fornices develop.

   c. Hymenal orifice is 1 cm but redundancy with estrogenization obscures findings.

   d. Adult-appearing vulva develops in Tanner stages.

2. Gynecologic examination/first pelvic examination

   a. Routine (at least yearly) pelvic examination including speculum examination for Papanicolaou (Pap) smear and rapid tests or cultures for gonorrhea and chlamydia should begin when the patient is sexually active or planning to be, has been sexually active in the past, or is 18 or older. (Cultures can be deferred if the patient has never had genital contact.)

   b. Explain the rationale for the examination and the information being obtained. Describe each step to the patient.

   c. Plastic models of pelvic organs will help in demonstrating the procedure.

   d. Show the instruments, beginning with a large Graves speculum and ending with a narrow Huffman, and explain your intention to use the *smallest* size appropriate for her anatomy. This helps the patient understand that you have taken particular consideration for her first examination.

   e. Whether or not a parent remains in the room depends on the parent-adolescent relationship. In general, adolescents are better examined without a parent present to provide opportunity for privileged communication.

   f. A chaperon is mandatory for a male examiner and generally preferable for all.

   g. Examination technique. Ask the patient to let her legs relax and drop apart with buttock muscles relaxed. Emphasize that the examination does not need to cause discomfort if the thigh and gluteal muscles remain relaxed. Place a hand first on the thigh or other nongenital location. Next, the examiner uses the thumb and index finger of the nondominant hand to separate the labia from above. The vulva is inspected. The forefinger of the dominant hand is then introduced through the hymenal ring; the speculum is introduced into the vagina in a posteriorly angled direction. Note the appearance of the cervix and vaginal mucosa.

   h. Obtain a Pap smear first using wooden spatula and endocervical brush. Smear onto a glass slide in a transparent layer and apply cytologic fixative immediately.

   i. Obtain gonococcal (GC) culture, with a cotton swab placed in the cervical os for 30 seconds or more, and plate *immediately* on a room-temperature Thayer-Martin plate; rapidly put in a sealed carbon dioxide environment (sealed bag and pellet; see also Chap. 5, p. 127).

   j. Take any other relevant samples (wet preps, etc.).

   k. The last specimen to be obtained should be a *Chlamydia* rapid test or culture, with a Dacron swab swirled multiple times in the endocervical canal.

   l. Next, use sterile water–soluble lubricant on one or two fingers of the dominant hand placed in the vagina; with the other hand sweep down from the umbilicus toward the vagina to palpate the uterus, and then move laterally to palpate the adnexa.

     (1) With a retroverted uterus or evidence of a posterior adnexal mass, a rectovaginal examination is then performed *after changing gloves*, with the first finger in the vagina, the second finger in the rectum, and the same motions with the abdominal hand.

     (2) In tense or obese patients, it may be difficult to identify the ovaries. An ultrasound can help define adnexal anatomy.

3. Breast examination. Although breast cancer will develop in 1 in 9 American women in a lifetime, it is extremely rare in children and adolescents. Adolescents should be taught to do breast self-examinations to promote healthy habits later in life and to become familiar with their breasts, so that when an unusual lump is noted, they will seek prompt medical attention. A family history of breast cancer, particularly if it occurred at a young age, increases future breast cancer risks and the importance of establishing good breast examination habits. The week following menses is the best time to do the examination because physiologic lumps are least prominent. If periods are irregular, an arbitrary day each month is selected.

   a. The large range of normal variation should be stressed.

   b. Benign cystic changes are found in 85% of women.

   c. Mild asymmetry is common during development. Marked asymmetry that is present after Tanner 5 breast development has been established can only be altered with plastic surgery.

   d. Accessory nipples or breasts occur in 1 to 2% of healthy patients. No therapy is indicated.

   e. The periareolar follicle may drain brownish fluid for several weeks. No treatment is needed.

f. Periareolar hair is not uncommon in healthy adolescents. No treatment is indicated. Removal of the hairs should be discouraged due to risks of infection.

II. Diagnostic studies

A. Prepubertally, a **vaginal smear for estrogen** is useful for evaluating the patient's hormonal status in the absence of infection. A calgi swab moistened with saline is twirled to scrape the side wall of the vagina, streaked on a glass slide, and sprayed with Papanicolaou fixative. The maturation index gives a scoring of basal, intermediate, and superficial cells, indicating degree of estrogenization as follows: 0 points for parabasal, ½ point intermediate, and 1 point for superficial cells. Scores indicate prepubertal (0–30), pubertal (50–60), and hypoestrogenic (31–55) levels.

B. A **Papanicolaou smear** should be done on all young woman who have a speculum examination. Those with a history of genital warts, hormonal therapy, abnormal Pap smears, or sexually transmitted disease (STD) may need Pap smears at more frequent intervals.

   1. With the speculum in place, an Ayer wooden spatula is scraped around the cervix, and the collected material is spread on a slide. A second specimen is taken from the endocervical canal with an endocervical brush, twirled once 360 degrees in the endocervical canal, and streaked on the same slide. The slide is immediately sprayed with cytologic fixative.

   2. Reporting of the results has recently been revised as follows: Specimens are designated *satisfactory* or *unsatisfactory*. Unsatisfactory smears must be repeated.

   a. No malignant cells identified (formerly class I or normal): routine yearly follow-up indicated.

   b. Atypical cells of undetermined significance (formerly class II or IIR): indication of potential abnormality, suggesting the need for, at minimum, a repeat Pap smear in 3 to 4 months. In the face of other indications of potential pathology including a prior atypical or abnormal Pap smear, history or presence of genital warts, or partner with genital warts, colposcopy is indicated. If an associated infection such as chlamydia or *Trichomonas* is present, the infection should be treated and the Pap smear repeated. *Given the high rate of false-negative Pap smears, multiple repeat Paps are often appropriate* (e.g., q3mo for 1 yr, then q6mo for 2 yr).

   c. Low-grade squamous intraepithelial lesion (formerly class III, mild to moderate dysplasia): indication for colposcopy, biopsies, and endocervical curettage.

   d. High-grade squamous intraepithelial lesion (formerly class IV or V, moderate to severe dysplasia or *carcinoma in situ*): indication for colposcopy, biopsies, and endocervical curettage.

C. **Wet preparations** are used in determining the cause of a vaginal discharge.

   1. **In the prepubertal child,** the sample is collected with a saline-moistened calgi swab or eyedropper from the introitus while the patient is supine.

   2. **In the adolescent,** the specimen is collected from the vaginal pool while the speculum is in place.

   3. The swab is mixed with one drop saline on a slide, then is mixed with one drop 10% potassium hydroxide (KOH) on a second slide.

   4. A cover slip is promptly applied and the slides are examined under the microscope (low and high dry power).

   a. In the saline specimen, *Trichomonas* infection is indicated by the presence of flagellated organisms the size of a white blood cell.

   b. In the saline specimen, *Gardnerella vaginalis* infection is indicated by leukocytes and refractile bacteria attached to large epithelial cells ("clue cells").

   c. In the KOH specimen, *Candida albicans* infection, budding pseudohyphae, and yeast forms are present.

D. **Gram's stain.** In gonorrhea the smear may reveal gram-negative intracellular diplococci. However, because *Neisseria vaginalis* organisms are normal vaginal flora, only a positive culture establishes the diagnosis.

E. Cultures. Sexually active adolescents should have a routine cervical culture or rapid test for gonorrhea and *Chlamydia* at the time of speculum examination or when indicated, such as after exposure to a new partner, or by the patient's symptoms. The sites of culture in the symptomatic patient or contact are the urethra, cervix, rectum, and pharynx.

    1. Gonorrhea. Swab the area to be cultured with a cotton swab and streak directly on a plate, using a Transgrow, modified Thayer-Martin-Jembec, or Thayer-Martin medium (Chap. 5, p. 128). All cultures from prepubertal girls should be clearly identified as "prepubertal" in the clinical information for the laboratory.

    2. *Chlamydia*
        a. In a prepubertal child, or when clinical circumstances are questionable, only **cultures** should be done because of the unacceptable consequences of a false-positive test.
        b. Microtrack screens identify inclusion bodies and are technician dependent.
        c. Enzyme immunoassay (EIA) screening tests are the most cost effective and least complicated to perform, but produce both false-positive and negative results.
        d. Polymerase chain reaction (PCR) or Ligase chain reaction (LCR) may be available in some laboratories on urine, urethral, or cervical samples. PCR and LCR are very sensitive; cross contamination is possible.

    3. *Candida.* To confirm yeast vaginitis, swab the vagina and streak on Nickerson's medium. Leave the cap of the bottle with the medium partially unscrewed and incubate the tube at room temperature. The appearance of brown colonies in 3 to 7 days confirms the diagnosis.

F. Pregnancy tests
    1. Several urine 2-minute pregnancy tests are available. They are quick and convenient, and offer a high degree of reliability. These tests detect human chorionic gonadotropin (HCG) at a level of greater than 25 mIU.
    2. The **beta subunit blood** test measures HCG in serum, is usually sensitive to a level greater than 5 mIU, and is positive within 5 to 10 days of conception. This can be used to identify and distinguish an ectopic pregnancy, missed abortion, or threatened abortion from a normal pregnancy (see sec. **VIII**, p. 429).

G. Urine dipstick should be checked for protein, blood, or glucose. In addition, if the patient has urinary symptoms, a clean-catch urine specimen should be obtained for culture.

H. Chromosomal analysis. Blood samples for chromosomal analysis are useful when evaluating patients with short stature, some cases of primary and secondary amenorrhea, and premature ovarian failure.

I. Nipple discharge. A patient can be asked to express the nipple discharge herself. A cytologic specimen of the discharge should be sprayed with fixative as with a Pap smear.

III. Common pediatric gynecologic problems
  A. Congenital abnormalities. Imperforate hymen should be corrected either at birth or before menarche. (An apparent imperforate hymen may actually be microperforate and once estrogenized may become sufficiently open that it does not require intervention.)

  B. Vaginitis
    1. Etiology. Prepubertal hypoestrogenic environment with a neutral pH is susceptible to pathogens and environmental irritants.
        a. Poor perineal hygiene is likely after the age of 3, when caretakers are not directly involved with toileting.
        b. Pinworm infestation with the subsequent anal scratching can cause vaginal irritation and discharge.
        c. Bubble bath and harsh soaps further disrupt the pH and make it easier for vulvitis and secondary vaginitis to develop.
        d. Tight-fitting or nylon underpants worn with exercise or in hot weather can cause maceration and promote yeast overgrowth.

e. Masturbation or sexual abuse can play a role. Conversely, a symptomatic vaginitis will affect behavior.

2. Evaluation

a. A careful history should be traced. Ask about the quantity, duration and type of discharge, the direction in which the child wipes the anal area, the use of bubble baths, the type of soap used, symptoms of anal pruritus, and exposure to an infected adult through sexual contact or indirectly by sharing a bed, towels, and so on.

b. Examine the child in the knee-chest position to rule out the presence of a foreign body. When indicated, obtain cultures in the frog-leg position.

c. Culture technique (see above for age-specific examination)

   (1) With a urethral swab moistened in sterile saline, take all samples with a single swipe.

   (2) The least discomfort can be obtained if the vagina can be entered without touching the hymen, but an introital specimen is also acceptable.

   (3) Aerobic sample identifies most pathology. Send the swab to the laboratory in transport media for culture on blood, MacConkey, and chocolate agar.

d. Do a wet preparation for yeast and *Trichomonas*. With a persistent or severe yeast infection, check the urine for glucose to evaluate for diabetes.

e. Persistent discharge, particularly when recurrent after a course of treatment, suggests a possible foreign body, and Examination Under Anesthesia (EUA) should be considered if an office examination does not allow adequate vaginal visualization.

f. Blood-tinged discharge is more common with *Shigella* or *Salmonella* as specific pathogens or with a foreign body, but trauma must also be excluded.

3. Diagnosis. A history of exposure to offending agents, the presence of **symptoms** (itching, discomfort, vaginal discharge), the **character of the discharge,** a positive culture, and the **physical findings** aid in establishing the diagnosis of vulvovaginitis.

4. Therapy

a. Nonspecific vaginitis (culture shows normal flora) is treated with the following measures.

   (1) Instruct the child to

      (a) Improve perineal hygiene.

      (b) Wear white cotton underpants.

      (c) Avoid bubble baths and harsh soaps.

      (d) Take sitz baths tid in plain warm water. Wash the vulvar area with mild soap (Basis) and pat dry. Allow for further drying by lying on the back with the legs spread apart for 10 minutes.

   (2) If no improvement is seen in 3 weeks, treat the child with oral antibiotics (such as amoxicillin, ampicillin, or cephalexin) for 10 to 14 days or with a topical antibacterial cream (Sultrin, AVC).

   (3) If improvement still does not occur, treat the child with an estrogen-containing cream for 2 to 3 weeks (reversible breast tenderness and vulvar pigmentation may occur) or consider EUA.

b. Acute, severe edematous vulvitis

   (1) Sitz baths should be taken q4h, with mild soap and with air drying.

   (2) Witch hazel pads (Tucks) should be used instead of toilet paper.

   (3) After 2 days, sitz baths should be alternated with painting of the vulva with a bland solution, for example, calamine lotion.

   (4) For pruritus, hydrocortisone cream 1%, Neo-Delta-Cortef Cream 1%, or Vioform-Hydrocortisone Cream should be applied to the vulva.

c. Specific vaginitis

   (1) Gonococcus (see Chap. 5, p. 127).

   (2) For **group A beta-hemolytic streptococci or pneumococci:**

  (a) Amoxicillin, 25 to 50 mg/kg/day in three divided doses for 10 days, or
  (b) Erythromycin, 30 to 50 mg/kg/day PO tid.
 (3) For *Trichomonas,* metronidazole (Flagyl), 125 mg tid PO for 5 days, or 1 to 2 g PO in one dose.
 (4) Pinworms (see Chap. 5, p. 162).
 (5) *Candida albicans.* Nystatin or other topical antifungal cream (for moist lesions) or ointment (for dry scaly lesions) should be applied to the vulva for 2 weeks. For persistent yeast infections, nystatin, 100,000 units PO qid for 2 weeks, and sitz baths in boric acid, 1 tsp per quart of warm water bid.

C. Labial adhesions
 1. Etiology. The hypoestrogenic environment of the prepubertal child makes the labia susceptible to agglutination. This may occur after minor trauma or irritation, but the etiology of labial adhesions remains unclear.
 2. Evaluation. Partial adhesions are quite common. If they extend up progressively to involve more than half the labia, urine can collect in the vagina producing odor and discharge. Complete adhesions can block urine flow.
 3. Diagnosis is made by visual inspection. The labia meet in the midline along a white line and the hymen cannot be visualized when the labia are retracted.
 4. Treatment
  a. Partial adhesions do not usually require treatment unless they block urine flow, or are symptomatic.
  b. A small amount of estrogen cream is applied only to the line of adhesion bid for 2 weeks (or until resolution) and is then continued to be applied to the area daily for at least 2 weeks after fully open. Then a bland ointment (A and D, Desitin, K-Y Jelly) is applied for several months to prevent the adhesions from reforming.
  c. If urinary retention results from the labial adhesions, surgical intervention is mandatory.

D. Genital trauma
 1. Etiology. Anatomic absence of the vulvar fat pads as well as the degree of activity make children more susceptible to genital trauma. The possibility of sexual abuse must also be considered.
 2. Evaluation
  a. The amount of bleeding correlates poorly with the degree of injury.
  b. Penetration of the hymen requires a complete EUA, as injuries can extend into the peritoneal cavity. Sexual abuse should be strongly considered when the injury is at the posterior fourchette, with hymenal transections or findings near the 6 o'clock position.
  c. Injury such as a straddle fall will usually produce anterior labial or periurethral injury, and bruising may be extensive.
  d. Critical assessment is necessary to **determine if the physical findings are consistent with the history provided** and if the child was referred promptly for evaluation, as hymenal trauma will heal rapidly and physical findings may be gone in 48 to 72 hours.
 3. Diagnosis is made by inspection. With injury that transects the hymen at 6 o'clock and is evaluated within 72 hours of occurrence, a rape kit should be collected, generally as part of an EUA. Lichen sclerosus can be diagnosed with a skin biopsy.
 4. Treatment
  a. A vulvar hematoma can usually be treated with ice packs.
  b. A Foley catheter may be necessary if urinary retention occurs. Voiding into warm water may help.
  c. Evacuation of a hematoma is necessary only if it is expanding. In that case, broad-spectrum antibiotics should be maintained intravenously for several days to prevent secondary infection.
  d. Most injuries heal well and do not need sutures unless bleeding persists,

the injury extends below the subcutaneous layer, or structures are partially avulsed and need restoration of anatomy.
E. **Foreign bodies.** The most common foreign body is a small piece of toilet paper. Foreign bodies can present with vaginal bleeding, foul-smelling vaginal discharge, or pain. Removal can be attempted in the office with the use of a plastic angiocatheter attached to a 60-ml cc syringe for irrigation of the foreign body from the vaginal vault.
F. **Sexual abuse.** Sexual abuse must be considered in all cases of vaginal bleeding, vaginal discharge, and trauma (see **D** above). Penetration injuries usually involve the lower half of the vulva and hymen while straddle injuries are associated with the anterior vulva and do not usually involve the hymen. A complete examination with documentation of forensic evidence is necessary. Photographs may be helpful. Acute management is outlined in Chap. 7, p. 242.
G. **Lichen sclerosus.** Lichen sclerosus may be mistaken for trauma or abuse because subcutaneous hemorrhages can occur with no history of trauma. However, the adjacent skin will generally be whitened, symptoms of itching are often present, and the involved skin is usually well demarcated. Diagnosis is made with biopsy and pathology. Lichen sclerosus is treated with 1% hydrocortisone ointment applied twice a day.
H. **Condyloma acuminatum**
   1. **Etiology.** Genital contact is required for transmission. Genital contact occurs in the birth canal as well as through sexual abuse. Epidemiologic evidence suggests that fomites are not a source, but this is often hypothesized.
   2. **Evaluation.** Sexual abuse should be considered, including cultures for other STDs and an age-appropriate psychosocial evaluation. A biopsy can be evaluated both histologically and for viral DNA analysis, looking specifically for a genital subtype of the human papilloma virus, which will exclude the possibility of a common wart as etiology, but does not establish the mode of transmission.
   3. **Diagnosis** is made by visual inspection and biopsy, including histology and DNA probe.
   4. **Treatment**
      a. Laser vaporization with biopsy during EUA is preferred because all lesions can be treated in one setting without conscious awareness by the child.
      b. Trichloroacetic acid and liquid nitrogen in the office setting are alternate options, but are painful and generally require multiple treatments. When sexual abuse is the etiology, this can add to the child's trauma, depending on the developmental age.
I. **Urethral prolapse.** Urethral prolapse may be mistaken for condyloma but will only involve the urethra. It can also present with vaginal bleeding. For treatment, estrogen cream is used for 2 weeks or until resolved. If the distal urethra is necrotic, surgical intervention may be required.
IV. **Common adolescent gynecologic problems**
A. **Vulvovaginitis**
   1. **Etiology.** Unlike prepubertal vaginitis, which is usually nonspecific, vaginitis in the adolescent generally has a specific cause, for example, *Neisseria gonorrhoeae*, *Trichomonas*, *Candida*, *G. vaginalis*, *Herpesvirus*, or *Chlamydia trachomatis*, and is often related to sexual contact. However, the most common cause of discharge in the adolescent is physiologic leukorrhea (normal desquamation of epithelial cells).
   2. **Evaluation and diagnosis.** A pelvic examination is required, with wet preparations, cultures, and rapid plasma reagin (RPR) if an STD is suspected.
      a. *Trichomonas.* A wet preparation (saline) reveals flagellated organisms moving under the microscope. Small punctate hemorrhagic spots may be seen on the cervical and vaginal walls.
      b. *Candida* (see pp. 417–18).
      c. **Nonspecific vaginitis.** A wet preparation reveals large epithelial cells coated with small refractile bacteria (clue cells). To identify *G. vaginalis*,

the discharge is streaked on chocolate agar and incubated under increased carbon dioxide tension.

d. Gonorrhea. A sample from the os should be cultured (see p. 416).

e. Leukorrhea. A wet preparation reveals epithelial cells only and there is no itch, burn, or smell. Most common in early puberty, and just before menarche. Cyclic variations can also occur with the menstrual cycle.

f. Condylomata acuminatum. Wart-like growths are inspected and Pap smear obtained.

g. Herpes vulvitis (see Chap. 5, p. 124). Viral cultures are obtained from a fresh vesicle and sent on ice. A culture from an ulcerated lesion may be negative even though active disease is present. If cultures are not available, the base of the lesion is scraped and stained with Wright's stain, looking for multinucleated giant cells and inclusion bodies.

h. *Chlamydia*. The endocervical canal should be cultured or detected by rapid test (see p. 418).

i. *Pediculosis pubis* (crabs). Firmly attached lice or their eggs will be seen at the base of the pubic hair.

j. Pinworms (see Chap. 5, p. 162).

k. Foreign body. Inspect the patient for the presence of a foreign body. In the adolescent, this is often a forgotten tampon.

3. Treatment. Patients and partner(s) should be treated if *Trichomonas*, gonorrhea, chlamydia, syphilis, or pelvic inflammatory disease (PID) is identified. Visible condylomata on partners should be treated.

a. For *Trichomonas* vaginitis, give metronidazole, 2 g PO, all in one dose, or 250 mg tid for 7 days. Instruct the patient not to drink alcohol while receiving metronidazole, because vomiting results.

b. For **candidal (monilial) vaginitis,** a topical or intravaginal antifungal agent for 1, 3, or 7 days depending on the product and/or sitz baths with boric acid (Borax), one tbsp per quart of warm water. Fluconazole tablets (Diflucan), 150 mg PO, for patients unable to insert applicators.

c. For *G. vaginitis* (also called nonspecific vaginitis), metronidazole, 250 mg tid PO for 7 days, or intravaginal metronidazole or clindamycin qd for 7 days.

d. Gonorrhea (see Chap. 5, p. 127).

e. Leukorrhea. Reassure the patient and recommend good perineal hygiene and the wearing of white cotton underpants.

f. Condyloma acuminatum (see Chap. 5, p. 131)

    (1) Apply trichloroacetic acid (25% or, if resistant lesions and *carefully* applied, 85%) to lesion weekly.

    (2) If lesions do not respond, cryocautery is effective.

    (3) If still resistant or increasing, laser vaporization or loop electrode excision, usually under anesthesia.

g. Herpes vulvitis. Acyclovir, 200 mg PO five doses qd for primary infections, and 400 mg bid for suppression of recurrent infections (see Chap. 5, p. 124). Valacyclovin, 500 mg bid for 5 days has been approved for recurrent infections. Symptomatic relief with lidocaine 2% jelly plus sitz baths. Urinating in the shower or tub may be necessary for patients with severe pain; occasionally, urinary catheterization is necessary for urinary retention.

h. *Chlamydia*. Doxycycline, 100 mg bid PO for 10 days, or azithromycin, 1 g PO (see Chap. 5, p. 129).

i. *Pediculosis pubis*. Permethrin (Nix) 1% once kills lice and eggs. Clothing and bedding should be washed in hot water and the partner treated simultaneously.

j. Pinworms (see Chap. 5, p. 162).

B. Genitourinary infections

    1. Gonorrhea (see Chap. 5, p. 127).

    2. Chlamydia (see Chap. 5, p. 129).

    3. Pelvic inflammatory disease (see Chap. 5, p. 129).

4. Syphilis (see Chap. 5, p. 125).
5. Chancroid.
6. Human immunodeficiency virus (HIV) (see Chap. 5, p. 151).
C. Delayed pubertal development (see Chap. 13, p. 387).
D. Secondary amenorrhea, oligomenorrhea
   1. Etiology
      a. The most common causes are pregnancy and stress, weight change, change in environment (camp, boarding school, college), or increased exercise.
      b. Also consider anorexia nervosa, obesity, polycystic ovary syndrome, thyroid disease, ovarian tumor, and diabetes.
   2. Evaluation
      a. Pregnancy. When a sexually active patient's period is late, she should have a pelvic examination and a pregnancy test.
      b. Stress. The history may elicit areas of stress in a patient's life.
      c. Anorexia nervosa. No specific laboratory test is available. Psychiatric evaluation is essential.
      d. Obesity. Determine whether or not weight gain (often rapid) is correlated with cessation of periods.
      e. Polycystic ovary syndrome, androgen excess syndromes
         (1) Hirsutism, acne, and obesity may be present.
         (2) Enlarged, cystic ovaries may be palpable on pelvic examination or identified by pelvic ultrasound but are not necessary to make the diagnosis.
         (3) Total serum or free testosterone is often elevated. There may be an increase in the LH-FSH ratio. Dehydroepiandrosterone sulfate (DHEA-S) may be elevated.
         (4) Diabetes mellitus (see Chap. 13, p. 405).
      f. Thyroid disease (see Chap. 13, p. 393).
   3. Diagnosis
      a. Pregnancy is indicated by an enlarged uterus and is confirmed by a positive pregnancy test.
      b. Stress. A stressful situation in the patient's life is identified and correlated with the onset of amenorrhea.
      c. Anorexia nervosa. The classic history of prolonged weight loss secondary to poor intake, distorted body image, excessive activity, amenorrhea, and emotional problems confirms the diagnosis of anorexia nervosa.
      d. Obesity. Documentation of excessive weight gain with resultant amenorrhea is required.
      e. Polycystic ovary syndrome. The diagnosis is considered in a patient with a history of oligomenorrhea, particularly with the physical findings of hirsutism, obesity, acne, enlarged cystic ovaries on pelvic examination, and abnormal hormonal levels.
      f. Thyroid disease (see Chap. 13, p. 393).
   4. Therapy. Identify the cause and eliminate it when possible.
      a. Stress. Medroxyprogesterone acetate (Provera), 10 mg PO for 5 days, to induce withdrawal bleeding, then initiate oral contraceptives to maintain bone mass.
      b. Anorexia nervosa. Regaining sufficient weight is critical for the individual's hypothalamic suppression to cease. A greater proportion of body weight as fat is required to restore periods than is needed to maintain them once they are reestablished. Oral contraceptives should be used to maintain bone mass until weight is restored.
      c. Obesity. Loss of excessive weight initiates spontaneous periods. Provera, 10 mg qd for 14 days a month, or oral contraceptives to maintain menses and prevent Polycystic ovaries (PCO).
      d. Polycystic ovary syndrome, androgen excess syndromes, hirsutism. Provera, 10 mg qd for 14 days a month, will prevent endometrial hyperplasia, but oral contraceptives are the treatment of choice in those who are

sexually active. For those with complaints of acne or hirsutism, a low androgenic pill is preferential, and for severe hirsutism, spironolactone, 50 to 100 mg bid, is helpful. This combination therapy can take over 3 months to have full effect.

e. Thyroid disease (see Chap. 13).

f. Diabetes mellitus (see Chap. 13).

E. Dysfunctional uterine bleeding (DUB)

   1. Etiology. One of the most common gynecologic complaints in the adolescent is irregular, prolonged menstruation.

   a. Anovulatory cycles (unopposed estrogen) with incomplete shedding of the proliferative endometrium are common for the first 2 years after menarche. A large amount of bleeding can occur without the menstrual lining being properly shed.

   b. Evaluate for pregnancy.

   c. Hematologic abnormalities, including coagulopathies, must be evaluated if bleeding is severe.

   2. Evaluation

   a. History of drug ingestion (warfarin), birth control pills.

   b. Pelvic examination with cultures for *N. gonorrhoeae* and *Chlamydia*.

   c. Pregnancy test.

   d. Complete blood count, platelet count.

   e. Prothrombin time/partial thromboplastin time (PT/PTT), bleeding time if severe bleeding.

   f. Mantoux test (in tuberculosis [TB]-prevalent areas).

   3. Diagnosis. A past history of painless bleeding with irregular intervals and particularly with irregular length suggests anovulatory bleeding. DUB is the diagnosis if an anatomic etiology for the bleeding is excluded.

   4. Treatment

   a. For irregular periods of short duration with normal hemoglobin and if the patient is not bleeding at the time of the visit, give Provera, 10 mg qd for 14 days, to bring on a proper menstrual shedding; repeat for three monthly cycles or start low-dose oral contraceptives.

   b. For **persistent vaginal bleeding** without significant anemia or no response to **a,** give Lo/Ovral, one pill q6h, until the bleeding stops, then one tid for 3 days, then bid for 2 days, then one qd to complete a 21-day course. Then, continue Lo/Ovral or another standard low-dose oral contraceptive for 3 to 6 months. Antiemetics may be needed.

   c. For **heavy vaginal bleeding** with anemia, if bleeding does not stop in 36 to 48 hours, consult a gynecologist.

F. Dysmenorrhea. Pain with menstruation is very common.

   1. Etiology. Prostaglandins released during the menstrual flow stimulate the contractility of the endometrium. Organic lesions associated with dysmenorrhea include chronic PID, vaginal agenesis, rudimentary uterine horn, and endometriosis.

   2. Evaluation. Review the menstrual history, premenstrual symptoms, timing of cramps, and how the patient deals with cramps. Patients with severe dysmenorrhea require a pelvic examination to rule out a menstrual flow obstruction.

   3. Diagnosis. Cramping lower abdominal pain usually starts 1 to 4 hours before a period and lasts for up to 24 hours. Some young women experience dysmenorrhea 2 days before the onset of menstrual flow, and the pain can last for 4 to 6 days. Nausea and vomiting may accompany the cramps.

   4. Treatment

   a. Symptomatic relief with a nonsteroidal anti-inflammatory drug

      (1) Ibuprofen (Motrin), 600 mg q6–8h.

      (2) Naproxen sodium (Anaprox), 275 to 550 mg q8–12h.

      (3) Naproxen (Naprosyn), 250 to 500 mg q8h.

      (4) Mefenamic acid (Ponstel), 250 mg q6h.

   b. Bed rest, use of a heating pad, and clear fluids can be helpful.

c. If analgesics fail, give oral contraceptives, which eliminate or substantially reduce cramps.

d. If the cramps persist or worsen despite cyclic oral contraceptives, refer the patient for a gynecologic examination to evaluate for obstructive anomalies or endometriosis.

G. Mittelschmerz is pain experienced at the time of ovulation.

1. **Etiology.** It is thought to be secondary to rupture of an ovarian follicle or irritation of the peritoneum from fluid from the rupturing follicular cyst.

2. **Evaluation.** The patient usually complains of midcycle, unilateral, dull and aching lower quadrant abdominal pain that lasts from a few minutes to 6 to 8 hours. Rarely, the pain is severe, mimicking appendicitis, ovarian torsion, or an ectopic pregnancy.

3. **Diagnosis.** The midcycle nature of the pain and absence of other significant findings establish the diagnosis.

4. **Treatment**
   a. Explain the benign nature of the pain to the patient.
   b. A heating pad and mild analgesics are helpful.
   c. If repetitive, use oral contraceptives to inhibit ovulation.

V. Breast disease

A. Breast masses

1. **Evaluation**
   a. Physical examination with routine breast examination is important.
   b. Mammography is not helpful, as an adolescent's breasts are too dense for adequate interpretation, but ultrasound is useful.

2. **Therapy**
   a. Cystic masses can be observed. If they do not resolve spontaneously, then needle aspiration is appropriate.
   b. Solid masses are most likely fibroadenomas, which are benign; removal should be considered, as they can rapidly increase in size. They may be associated with an increased risk of developing breast cancer.

B. Galactorrhea

1. **Evaluation**
   a. History of pregnancy, breast manipulation, oral contraceptive agents, chest surgery, or psychotropic medications.
   b. Physical examination to determine if bilateral or unilateral.
   c. Prolactin level.
   d. Ultrasound to evaluate for cystic masses.
   e. Unilateral discharge (see p. 418).

2. **Treatment**
   a. Conservative management with warm compresses if unilateral.
   b. For persistent or extreme symptoms that conservative management fails, surgical removal of the isolated duct is possible.

VI. Adolescent sexuality. The care of adolescents includes not only their physical and emotional well-being, but also their emerging sexuality. The spectrum of adolescent sexual concerns ranges from questions of normal secondary sexual development to sexual identity and sexual preference. To allay these concerns, the health care provider must establish a confidential, trusting relationship with the teenager, which requires time and patience. Most adolescents are reluctant to initiate discussions of sexual matters. However, sexuality introduced in the context of the system review eliminates the mutual embarrassment often felt by both provider and patient. By providing respectful, nonpatronizing information and reassurance, the health care provider can correct most sexual misconceptions.

The decision as to whether or not sex becomes a part of a teenage relationship ultimately rests with the persons involved. Young people are influenced in such a decision by family standards, religious values, society's expectations, peer pressure, internal needs, drug and alcohol usage, and partner availability. The provider's role is not to judge the patient's behavior, but to give sufficient information to permit the teenager to make a responsible decision. The issue of whose obligation it is to educate adolescents about sexuality has not been resolved. The young person has four readily available sources of information: parents, peers, educators, and health care providers. Some parents are uncomfortable discussing sexuality with their children. An equal number of children cannot tolerate discussing sex with their parents. Peers as an information source are often a cause of confusion. Children turn to their friends because they are available, approachable, and willing to listen, and they rarely make moral judgments. Their lack of expertise is rarely seen as a drawback. Schools in general cannot provide the subtle sensitivity needed to explore adolescent sexuality. Most sex education classes are limited to the mechanics of intercourse. Many states still prohibit schools from teaching family planning. Health care providers have an opportunity and the responsibility to educate and counsel their patients on sexual issues.

VII. Birth control. More than half of all first sexual encounters among teenagers are unprotected. Despite the availability of contraceptives, adolescents often refrain from using them because they are not readily offered and the individuals do not necessarily plan to have sex. If asked in a direct, nonjudgmental manner, most adolescents are willing to share information regarding their sexual activity, and to request a method of birth control that is most appropriate for them. **Remember that latex condoms are the only method of birth control that, properly used, help to prevent the spread of STDs** (see **E.2** below).

A. Oral contraceptives. The pill, taken as prescribed, will prevent pregnancy with over 99% efficiency.

   1. Side effects of oral contraceptive use may include nausea, bloating, headaches, and breakthrough bleeding. Weight gain or weight loss are statistically equally likely.

   2. Complications of oral contraceptive use may rarely include hypertension, thrombophlebitis, depression, and stroke. There is recent evidence that desogestrel and gestodene may be associated with increased risk of thromboembolic complications.

   3. Contraindications. The pill is contraindicated in patients who are pregnant, or have a hepatoma, undiagnosed genital bleeding, estrogen-dependent neoplasm, a history of thrombophlebitis, lupus erythematosus, or cholestatic jaundice of pregnancy.

   4. Prescribing the pill

   a. Patient evaluation requires the following:

   (1) A complete history and physical examination, including a pelvic examination.

   (2) Laboratory studies. Hemoglobin and Papanicolaou smear. In patients with a family history of arteriosclerotic heart disease or stroke, cholesterol and triglyceride levels should be determined. In sexually active patients, tests for syphilis and culture for gonorrhea and *Chlamydia* once to twice a year or after contact with a new partner.

   b. Choice of pill (Table 14-1)

   (1) Pills that contain 30 to 35 μg ethinyl estradiol with a low-dose progestin (desogestrel, norethindrone, or triphasic levonorgestrel) are usually prescribed for patients with regular periods and no special indication for an estrogen- or progesterone-dominant pill. Desogestrel may be associated with a two-fold increased risk of thromboembolic disease. However, the FDA does not recommend switching any patients already on and tolerating pills containing desogestrel.

   (2) A pill with high progestin efficacy (Desogen, Ortho-Cept, Lo/Ovral, Loestrin) can be given if breakthrough or dysfunctional uterine bleeding is a problem.

   (3) If **acne or hirsutism** is a problem, choosing a pill with low androgenicity (Desogen, Ortho-Cept, Ortho-Cyclen, Ovcon, Modicon) is preferable.

   (4) Patients with **glucose intolerance** should avoid a pill that contains levonorgestrel.

   (5) To avoid nausea the pill is taken at bedtime. In addition a low-

Table 14-1. Composition of oral contraceptives

Name	Progestin	mg	Estrogen	µg
Monophasics				
Demulen 1/35	ED	1.0	EE	35
Demulen 1/50	ED	1.0	EE	50
Desogen	DS	0.15	EE	30
Levlen	L-NG	0.15	EE	30
Loestrin 1/20	NEA	1.0	EE	20
Loestrin 1.5/30	NEA	1.5	EE	30
Lo/Ovral	DL-NG	0.3	EE	30
Modicon	NE	0.5	EE	35
Nordette	L-NG	0.15	EE	30
Norinyl 1/35	NE	1.0	EE	35
Ortho-Cept	DS	0.15	EE	30
Ortho-Cyclen	NO	0.25	EE	35
Ortho-Novum 1/35	NE	1.0	EE	35
Ortho-Novum 1/50	NE	1.0	EE	50
Ovcon 35	NE	0.4	EE	35
Ovcon 50	NE	1.0	EE	50
Ovral	DL-NG	0.5	EE	50
Multiphasics				
Jenest 28				
Day 1–7	NE	0.5	EE	35
Day 8–21	NE	1.0	EE	35
Ortho-Novum 7/7/7				
Day 1–7	NE	0.5	EE	35
Day 8–14	NE	0.75	EE	35
Day 15–21	NE	1.0	EE	35
Tri-Cyclen				
Day 1–7	NO	0.180	EE	35
Day 8–14	NO	0.215	EE	35
Day 15–21	NO	0.250	EE	35
Triphasil (Tri-Levlen)				
Day 1–6	L-NG	0.050	EE	30
Day 7–11	L-NG	0.075	EE	40
Day 12–21	L-NG	0.125	EE	30
Tri-Norinyl				
Day 1–6	NE	0.5	EE	35
Day 7–11	NE	1.0	EE	35
Day 12–21	NE	0.5	EE	35
Progestin only				
Micronor (Nor-Q D)	NE	0.35	None	
Ovrette	DL-NG	0.075	None	

Source: Adapted from RP Dickey. *Managing Contraceptive Pill Patients* (7th ed). Durant, OK: Essential Medical Information Systems, 1995. DL-NG = DL-norgestrel; DS = desogestrel; EE = ethinyl estradiol; ED = ethynodiol diacetate; L-NG = levonorgestrel; NE = norethindrone; NO = norgestimate; NEA = norethindrone-acetate.

estrogenic pill (Loestrin 1/20) may be better tolerated if nausea persists.

(6) Pills for 21-day and 28-day cycles are available. Since, with the latter, the teenager is taking a pill *every* day, the chances that she will forget to take it are reduced.

(7) The **minipill** is a progestogen-only pill. The pregnancy rate on this pill is higher than on combination pills (1.5–3.0 pregnancies/100 woman-years), and irregular menstrual bleeding occurs.

(8) A high-dose (50 μg) pill has no indication for use in routine family planning.

c. Follow-up. The patient should be seen in 2 to 3 months for an interval history, blood pressure, and weight check. Thereafter, she is seen every 6 months.

B. Intrauterine devices (IUDs) are available, but because infection associated with the IUD can result in permanent tubal scarring and infertility, nulliparous patients are not candidates for this method.

C. Norplant, a long-acting contraceptive, is the most effective reversible method available and does not need patient compliance for effectiveness. There are significant benefits for the adolescent who is committed to being sexually active but wants to delay childbearing for at least 5 years. Potential candidates should be extensively counseled as to side effects of headaches, breakthrough bleeding, and possible pain and scarring with removal.

D. Diaphragms. A diaphragm can only be reliably used by adolescents who are highly motivated, feel comfortable with their bodies, and are not offended by inserting a mechanical device into the vagina in anticipation of intercourse.

1. Fitting. Fitting rings of various sizes are inserted into the vagina to determine the appropriate size. A correctly fitting diaphragm covers the cervix snugly without discomfort to the patient, with the posterior lip behind the cervix and the anterior rim behind the pubic bone.

2. Instructions. The following written instructions are given to the patient on the use and care of the diaphragm.

a. Put 1 tbsp contraceptive cream in the diaphragm and on the rim.

b. Insert the diaphragm no more than ½ hour before intercourse, checking that the cervix is covered.

c. If more than ½ hour has passed since insertion, place an applicator full of contraceptive cream in the vagina while the diaphragm is undisturbed.

d. Leave the diaphragm in place at least 6 hours after intercourse.

e. After removing the diaphragm, wash it with a mild soap (cornstarch can be used after washing).

f. Check the diaphragm regularly for holes, particularly at the rim, by holding it up to the light while stretching the rubber or filling it with water to see if there are leaks.

g. The device should be replaced once a year and a weight change of 10 lbs. requires a refitting.

E. Barrier methods

1. Spermicides are a readily available form of birth control that require no prescription, but have a high failure rate if used alone. The adolescent is given the following instructions for foam/jelly/film/cream/suppositories.

a. Insert the spermicide into the vagina 1 hour or less *before* intercourse. It is not effective after intercourse.

b. Do not douche for 6 hours after intercourse; douching should be discouraged in general due to the increased incidence of PID.

c. When possible, have the partner use a latex condom to lessen the risk of pregnancy.

2. Latex condoms are the only birth control devices that lessen the risk of sexually transmitted disease transmission. Therefore, all adolescents should be strongly encouraged to use them with every act of intercourse **regardless of other contraceptive method use.** Latex condoms that contain a spermicide as lubricant are the most effective.

3. **The contraceptive sponge** is available without a prescription. It can produce a chemical vaginitis, has a 15% failure rate, and should be used with condoms.
F. **The "morning after" pill.** **High-dose estrogens/progestins** administered after unprotected intercourse are an effective means of lowering the risk of pregnancy if taken within 72 hours of intercourse. This makes it particularly useful in cases of rape or with unanticipated sex, such as after first intercourse. If there is a risk of the patient already being pregnant by previous intercourse, a pregnancy test should be performed.
   1. **Administration:** within 24 to 72 hours after intercourse.
   2. **Dosage.** **Ethinyl estradiol and norgestrel (Ovral),** two tablets PO and repeated 12 hours later. This treatment may be associated with significant nausea, requiring prochlorperazine (Compazine), 10 mg PO 1 hour before each dose, to tolerate this regimen.
VIII. **Pregnancy.** Each year, more than 1 million young women 15 to 19 years of age become pregnant. Adolescents are developmentally prone to deny the possibility of pregnancy both before and after it takes place. The majority of pregnant teenagers are neither emotionally disturbed nor promiscuous, but psychological issues may precipitate the pregnancy if the baby is seen as a love object. An adolescent may become pregnant to test her parent's love, or to achieve an adult status in an atmosphere of limited options.
A. **Diagnosis**
   1. Many girls cannot bring themselves to express concern over a missed period, and may feel immune to becoming pregnant. Every young woman should be questioned about her menstrual cycles and sexual activity.
   2. A pregnancy test is obtained to confirm the diagnosis (see p. 418).
   3. Pelvic examination and sizing of the uterus
      a. A nonpregnant uterus is firm and the size of a plum.
      b. At 12 weeks the uterus is globular and at the symphysis pubis.
      c. At 16 weeks the uterus is felt midway between the umbilicus and symphysis pubis.
      d. At 20 weeks the uterus is palpable at the umbilicus.
B. **Mortality, morbidity, and complications**
   1. The **death rate** from the complications of pregnancy, delivery, and the postpartum period is 60% higher for women who become pregnant before the age of 15 years than for those who become pregnant at a later age.
   2. The **causes of death** include preeclampsia/eclampsia, hemorrhage, and infection.
   3. Pregnancy is a common cause of school dropout; 9 of 10 girls whose first delivery occurs at age 15 or younger never complete high school.
   4. Couples who marry because of pregnancy have a higher divorce rate than that of the general population.
C. **Abortion**
   1. **Methods**
      a. **Suction curettage** is performed before 17 weeks in the outpatient setting and in many hospitals to 19 weeks. It can be done under local anesthesia, intravenous sedation, or general anesthesia. **Possible complications** include perforation of the uterus, hemorrhage (secondary to incomplete removal of the products of conception), and infection.
      b. **Saline infusion or prostaglandin therapy** is performed between 16 and 24 weeks of pregnancy. **Contraindications** to saline infusion are chronic renal disease, cardiac disease, and severe anemia. **Complications** include infection, retained products of conception, and coagulopathy.
   2. **Counseling.** Explore thoroughly with the teenager the options of abortion, adoption, or keeping the child. Once she has reached a decision, it should be supported by the health professionals caring for her. **Health professionals must not impose their own judgment on the patient.**
D. **Ectopic pregnancy** (see also Chap. 7, p. 249)
   1. **Etiology.** PID, prior abdominal surgery, congenital abnormalities, and prior ectopic pregnancy make ectopic pregnancy more likely, as adhesions or other physical factors affect tubal transport of the conceptus to the uterus.

2. **Evaluation.** Any patient with a positive pregnancy test and pain, irregular bleeding, or a uterus that does not feel pregnant on examination should receive a quantitative blood pregnancy test. If the blood value is 1,500, a vaginal probe ultrasound should confirm an intrauterine sac, or, if not available, abdominal ultrasound of the uterus should be performed to establish whether an intrauterine pregnancy is present once the level has reached 6,000. Follow the beta subunit to be sure it **increases by approximately 66% every 48 hours to confirm a normal pregnancy until it reaches the level detectable by ultrasound.** If it is not increasing appropriately, the pregnancy is abnormal and may represent a blighted ovum or an ectopic pregnancy. The uterus is then evacuated by dilatation and evacuation (D&E), and if there are no products of conception, treatment for the ectopic pregnancy must be initiated.

3. **Diagnosis.** An ectopic pregnancy is diagnosed by finding pregnancy tissue outside the uterine cavity usually by laparoscopy.

4. **Treatment**
   a. The pregnancy can be surgically removed from its location, by laparoscopy with a **linear salpingostomy with conservation of the fallopian tube.**
   b. The use of **methotrexate** to resolve an ectopic pregnancy medically is gaining in practice in the United States. This method **requires absolute patient compliance,** and may not be appropriate for noncompliant adolescents.

E. **Rape.** See Chap. 7, p. 242.

15

Hematologic Disorders

Stephan A. Grupp

I. Red blood cells

A. Normal RBC values vary with age (Table 15-1). A "physiologic nadir" occurs at 1 to 3 months in preterm and 2 to 4 months in full-term infants.

B. Anemia: initial considerations

1. **Definition:** hemoglobin (Hgb) less than 2 SD below the mean.

2. **Etiology.** There are four causes: loss, destruction, sequestration, and hypoproduction.

3. **Initial evaluation** includes patient and family history, physical examination, CBC with indices, smear, and reticulocyte count.

4. **Diagnosis** is made based on results of further investigations (see specific disorders below).

5. **Treatments** are discussed under individual disorders.

C. Anemia: specific classification. Morphologically, anemia can be classified by RBC shape, size (micro-, macro-, normocytic), and hemoglobin concentration (normochromic or hypochromic).

1. **Microcytic, hypochromic anemias** (Table 15-2)

   a. **Iron deficiency** is most prevalent.

   (1) **Etiologies** include inadequate neonatal iron stores, dietary insufficiency, impaired absorption, blood loss.

   (2) **Evaluation**

   (a) **History** should emphasize **blood loss** and **diet,** including intake of breast milk, cow's milk (see p. 362), iron-rich foods, and faddisms.

   (b) **Physical examination** should note pallor, infantile obesity ("milk baby"), and, rarely, edema, glossitis, and stomatitis.

   (c) **Laboratory evaluation** includes CBC with smear and platelet count, measurement of serum iron, ferritin, total iron-binding capacity (TIBC), zinc protoporphyrin-heme ratio (ZPP), and stool hematest.

   (3) **Diagnosis** is based on consistent laboratory findings, which may include a serum iron saturation (Fe/TIBC) less than 16%, ferritin less than 15 ng/ml, and elevated ZPP. Each of these findings is subject to confounding factors; serum Fe varies during the day and with food intake, ferritin and TIBC may be elevated as acute-phase reactants, and ZPP is elevated in other disorders as well.

   (4) **Therapy** (Table 15-3)

   (a) If iron deficiency is suspected, iron can be given for a diagnostic and **therapeutic trial.** Reticulocytosis should occur within 10 to 14 days; Hgb should rise greater than 1 g/dl by 1 month.

   (b) Therapy may be complicated by **constipation.** This can be ameliorated by decreasing the dose to 1 to 2 mg/kg qhs, or changing from iron salts to iron polysaccharide complex (Niferex). Oral supplements should **not** be given with food since this can impair absorption.

   (c) **Lack of response** to a therapeutic trial should prompt investigation into other causes of microcytic anemia.

Table 15-1. Normal RBC parameters*

Age	Hemoglobin (g/dl)	Hematocrit (%)	MCV (fl)
Birth	16.5 ± 3	51 ± 9	108 ± 10
1 mo	14 ± 4	43 ± 12	104 ± 19
2 mo	11.5 ± 2.5	35 ± 7	96 ± 19
3–6 mo	11.5 ± 2	35 ± 6	91 ± 17
1 yr	12 ± 1.5	36 ± 3	78 ± 8
2–6 yr	12.5 ± 1	37 ± 3	81 ± 6
6–12 yr	13.5 ± 2	40 ± 5	86 ± 9
12–18 yr	14 ± 2	42 ± 6	89 ± 11

MCV = mean corpuscular volume; fl = femtoliters
*Data are reported as means ± 2 standard deviations and are adapted from PR Dallman. In A Rudolph (ed.) *Pediatrics* (16th ed). New York: Appleton-Century-Crofts, 1977. P 1111.

      (d) **Severe iron deficiency** may require **transfusion therapy** or administration of **intravenous iron.** Both of these treatments should be given in consultation with a hematologist.

  b. **Lead poisoning** (see Chap. 8, p. 282).

  c. **Thalassemia syndromes**

    (1) **Etiology.** Thalassemia syndromes are genetic disorders of alpha and beta globin production that are prevalent among patients from the Mediterranean, Middle East, India, Africa, and Southeast Asia.

      (a) **Beta-thalassemia major** results from total absence of beta globin and consequently no Hgb A_1.

      (b) **Beta-thalassemia intermedia** is a less severe disorder, in which beta levels are low, but adequate to produce some functional Hgb A_1.

      (c) Patients with subclinical **thalassemia trait** have at least half normal expression of either alpha or beta globin.

      (d) **Hemoglobin H disease** is moderately severe anemia that corresponds to loss of three of four alpha genes.

      (e) **Hemoglobin Bart's disease** results from loss of all four alpha genes, leading to *hydrops fetalis* and fetal demise.

Table 15-2. Findings in microcytic anemias

	Fe deficiency	Thalassemia trait	Thalassemia major	Lead poisoning	Chronic disease
RDW	↑	N	↑	↑	N
MCV	↓	↓	↓	↓	N/↓
RBC number	↓	N	↓	↓	↓
ZPP	↑	N	N	↑	↑
Hgb A_2	N	↑ (β) N (α)	↑ (β) N (α)	N	N
Serum Fe	↓	N	↑	↓/N	↓
TIBC	↑	N	N/↓	N	↓
% Saturation	↓	N	↑	N	N/↓
Ferritin	↓	N	↑	N	N/↑

RDW = red cell distribution width; MCV = mean corpuscular volume; ZPP = zinc protoporphyrin; Hgb = hemoglobin; TIBC = total iron-binding capacity; ↑ = increased; ↓ = decreased; N = normal.

Table 15-3. Iron treatment

Preparations and dosing	Notes
Preparations*	
Ferrous sulfate (Feosol)	
Elixir	220 mg/5 ml
	44 mg elemental Fe/5 ml
	Can stain teeth, cause constipation
Tablets	200 mg each
	65 mg elemental Fe/tablet
	Can stain teeth, cause constipation
Polysaccharide-iron complex (Niferex)	
Elixir	**100 mg elemental Fe/5 ml**
	Does not stain teeth or cause GI distress
	Well absorbed
	Contains 10% alcohol
Chewable tablets	**50 mg elemental Fe/tablet**
	Does not stain teeth or cause GI distress
	Well absorbed
	Contains vitamin C
Capsules	**150 mg elemental Fe/capsule**
	Does not stain teeth or cause GI distress
	Well absorbed
Iron dextran injection	**50 mg elemental Fe/ml**
	Dosing differs from oral preparations and should be calculated on individual basis
	Anaphylaxis can occur; **hematologist should be consulted to aid in treatment**
Dosing	
Dietary supplementation	
Term infants	1 mg/kg/d elemental Fe PO starting at 4 mo
Premature infants	2 mg/kg/d elemental Fe PO starting at 2 mo
Treatment of Fe deficiency	3–6 mg/kg/d elemental Fe PO divided tid, for 3–6 mo
	A hematologist should be consulted about dosing and administration of parenteral Fe if it is indicated

*Many iron preparations are available; only a subset are listed here.
NOTE: Many foods interfere with absorption of oral iron. Iron supplementation is contraindicated in patients with hemochromatosis and in those in whom iron absorption is increased. A fatal overdose of iron is easily ingested (see p. 278). Tablets are radiopaque; elixirs are not.

(2) **Evaluation**
    (a) **Family history** is usually positive.
    (b) **Physical examination** of patients with severe thalassemia syndromes emphasizes failure to thrive, hepatosplenomegaly, bone marrow expansion, macrocephaly, and facial deformities. Patients with less severe forms may have no physical findings.
    (c) **Laboratory studies** include CBC with differential, and reticulocyte count, blood smear, and **hemoglobin electrophoresis.** Investigation of specific **molecular defects** can be undertaken for purposes of prenatal diagnosis in selected patients.
(3) **Diagnosis**
    (a) **Beta-thalassemia major** presents with severe anemia in infants between 6 and 9 months of age. Hemoglobin A_1 is absent on Hgb

electrophoresis; Hgb A_2 and Hgb F are increased. Iron saturation may be increased. Both parents have microcytic anemia and elevated Hgb A_2.

(b) **Beta-thalassemia intermedia** is similar to beta-thalassemia major but less severe, with low levels of Hgb A_1.

(c) **Beta-thalassemia trait (heterozygous condition)** is characterized by near-normal Hgb A_1 and increased Hgb A_2.

(d) **Hemoglobin H disease** presents at birth. Patients have severe anemia with Hgb Bart's (γ_4 tetramers) on neonatal electrophoresis and Hgb H (β_4 tetramers) on later electrophoreses.

(e) **Alpha-thalassemia trait.** Silent carriers with normal function of three of the four alpha genes have no hematologic findings. Those with only two normal genes display mild microcytosis and hypochromia, often without anemia. Hemoglobin electrophoresis is normal. Diagnosis is of exclusion, supported by hypochromic, microcytic anemia in one parent.

(4) **Therapy**

(a) **Thalassemia trait** disorders require no treatment, but patients should be offered genetic counseling.

(b) Severe forms of **thalassemia** are fatal if untreated. **Chronic RBC transfusions** are necessary for survival. However, iron overload eventually ensues, causing damage to liver, endocrine glands, and heart. Without chelation therapy, iron toxicity leads to death in the second or third decade of life.

(i) **Packed, leukodepleted RBC transfusions** (10–20 ml/kg) should be given every 3 to 5 weeks to maintain hematocrit (Hct) at greater than 30% and to suppress reticulocytosis. This regimen allows normal growth.

(ii) **Deferoxamine (DF) chelation** should be instituted when transferrin becomes fully saturated and a chelatable iron pool is demonstrated by DF challenge. This generally corresponds to a cumulative burden greater than 500 ml/kg of RBCs. Deferoxamine (30–50 mg/kg/day) is given daily over 10 to 12 hours by subcutaneous infusion pump. This therapy reduces iron-induced organ damage and prolongs survival **if compliance is good.**

(iii) **Splenectomy** can decrease transfusion requirements.

(iv) **Folic acid** (1 mg/day) should be prescribed to those in whom erythropoiesis is not suppressed by chronic transfusion, to prevent folate deficiency and megaloblastic crisis.

(v) **Bone marrow transplantation** is curative, though controversial due to accompanying risks.

(vi) **Prevention.** Genetic counseling and prenatal detection are effective in decreasing the incidence of severe thalassemia.

d. **Hemoglobin E** is common in Southeast Asians. Heterozygotes are not anemic, but show mild microcytosis. Homozygotes display mild anemia and extreme microcytosis. **Diagnosis** is confirmed by Hgb electrophoresis. **Treatment** is generally unnecessary. Oxidant medications should be avoided since Hgb E is unstable.

e. **Sideroblastic anemias** are extremely rare in childhood.

(1) **Etiologies** include defects in heme biosynthesis and myelodysplasia. In adults, sideroblastic anemia may herald a preleukemic state.

(2) **Evaluation** includes CBC with differential, reticulocyte count, serum iron and TIBC, ZPP, and lead screen.

(3) **Diagnosis** is suspected when hypochromia, microcytosis, and reticulocytopenia are associated with elevated iron and full transferrin saturation. It is confirmed by identification of ringed sideroblasts on bone marrow iron staining.

(4) **Treatments** include pyridoxine (some forms are responsive), transfusion, and iron chelation.

2. **Macrocytic anemias.** An elevated mean corpuscular volume (MCV) is most commonly due to an increase in the percentage of reticulocytes. Where reticulocytosis is not the cause, macrocytic anemias are classified as **megaloblastic** and **nonmegaloblastic**.

   a. **Megaloblastic anemia**

   (1) **Etiologies** include **vitamin B$_{12}$** and **folate** deficiencies, **drugs** that interfere with folate metabolism, and **metabolic disorders.**

   (2) **Evaluation**

   (a) History should emphasize nutritional deficiencies, drug intake, evidence of intestinal malabsorption (see p. 346), malaise, anorexia, constipation, sore tongue, paresthesias, and depression.

   (b) Physical examination should include a thorough evaluation for peripheral neuropathy and evidence of dorsolateral spinal degeneration.

   (c) Laboratory studies include bone marrow examination, serum lactic dehydrogenase (LDH), bilirubin, iron, vitamin B$_{12}$ level, folate level, urine methylmalonic acid, and Schilling test (see p. 345). Specialized laboratory tests may be necessary to diagnose metabolic defects.

   (3) **Diagnosis** is confirmed by identification of nuclear-cytoplasmic asynchrony in bone marrow erythroid precursors, and hypersegmentation of granulocyte nuclei ($\geq$5/cell). Etiology can be identified by specific findings, including low vitamin B$_{12}$ or folate levels or both, abnormal **Schilling test** (see p. 345), and **methylmalonic aciduria. Vitamin B$_{12}$ deficiency can cause neurologic damage as well as hematologic findings; folic acid deficiency does not affect the nervous system.** Note that multiple nutritional deficiencies can coexist, complicating diagnosis and treatment.

   (4) **Therapy. It is imperative to diagnose B$_{12}$ deficiency correctly, as treatment with folate alone can result in hematologic improvement but progressive neurologic deterioration.**

   (a) **Vitamin B$_{12}$ deficiency.** Various B$_{12}$ replacement regimens are used. A reasonable approach is to give cyanocobalamin (CN-cbl), 25 to 100 µg IM qd for 10 to 14 days, followed by maintenance therapy with 50 to 1,000 µg IM monthly to prevent recurrence. Massive doses are required for certain metabolic defects. Patients with neurologic findings are generally given more aggressive treatment. The goal is to replenish body stores (3–4 mg in adults) within the first few weeks. **Hematologic response** should be rapid, with reticulocytosis by 3 days, and resolution of anemia within 1 to 2 months. **Neurologic response** may take several months, and some neurologic damage may be irreversible. Patients should be monitored for hypokalemia and hyperuricemia early in treatment. Oral B$_{12}$ is not universally effective due to poor compliance and erratic absorption.

   (b) **Folic acid deficiency** is initially treated with folic acid, 5 to 15 mg PO qd for 10 to 14 days, followed by 1 to 5 mg PO qd for 1 to 2 months, to replenish body stores. These doses are in excess of need, but not harmful (unless the patient is vitamin B$_{12}$ deficient as well) and adequate for patients with malabsorption. If necessary, 1 mg PO qd is sufficient for chronic maintenance therapy. Rarely, IV therapy can be used in the setting of severe malabsorption. Clinical response is rapid, similar to that of B$_{12}$ deficiency.

b. **Macrocytosis** not accompanied by megaloblastic changes may be associated with liver disease, hypothyroidism, anti-epileptic drugs, oral contraceptives and bone marrow failure syndromes (see p. 444).

3. **Normocytic anemias** are caused by **hemorrhage, hemolysis,** and **hypoproduction.**
    a. Acute **hemorrhage** results in proportionate loss of plasma and red cells, with no immediate change in Hgb or Hct. Anemia ensues on reequilibration of blood volume, after hours to days.
       (1) **Evaluation** includes history, physical examination, and blood counts.
       (2) **Diagnosis** is made by identifying sites of bleeding. Initial reticulocytosis may be seen within 6 to 12 hours. Nucleated RBCs may also be seen as the marrow responds.
       (3) **Treatment** should be directed toward the underlying cause of hemorrhage. Iron replacement may be necessary in patients with chronic hemorrhage.
    b. **Hemolytic anemia**
       (1) **General features**
           (a) **Etiologies** are listed in Table 15-4. Specific disorders are discussed below.
           (b) **General evaluation.** Personal and family histories should be elicited for pallor, jaundice, gallstones, splenectomy, and exposures to precipitating agents. **General laboratory tests** include serum LDH, bilirubin, haptoglobin, reticulocyte count, and RBC morphology. **Specific laboratory tests** are listed below, under discussions of individual disorders. **Transfusion can obscure the diagnosis of intrinsic red cell disorders.** If it is necessary

Table 15-4. Causes of hemolytic anemia

Disorder	Distinctive features
Mechanical injury	Hemosiderinuria
Trauma	
Thermal injury	
Prosthetic valve	
Sequestration	(Hepato)splenomegaly
Splenic sequestration	
Erythrophagocytosis	
Vascular loss	Thrombocytopenia
Vascular malformation	
Microangiopathy	
Plasma factors	
Antibody	Coombs +
Toxin	Toxin present
Wilson's disease	↑ serum copper (Cu), ↓ ceruloplasmin
Infection	Positive culture
Infantile pyknocytosis	Treatment not necessary
Cellular factors	
Spherocytosis	Cytoskeletal abnormality; ↑ osmotic fragility
Elliptocytosis	Cytoskeletal abnormality; ± ↑ osmotic fragility
Stomatocytosis	Abnormal ion transport; ↑ osmotic fragility
Xerocytosis	Abnormal ion transport; ↓ osmotic fragility
Paroxysmal nocturnal hemoglobinuria	Abnormal Ham's and sugar water tests; bone marrow failure
Abetalipoproteinemia	Acanthocytosis
Liver disease	Acanthocytosis
Vitamin E deficiency	Prematurity, thrombocytosis
Parasites	History, organisms on thick smear
Enzymopathies	See text
Hemoglobinopathies	See text

before diagnosis, several purple top tubes of whole blood should be taken prior to transfusion and stored for later workup.

(c) **Diagnosis** is usually confirmed by findings of reticulocytosis, low haptoglobin, elevated LDH and bilirubin, and consistent red cell morphology. In **chronic** hemolytic conditions, anemia may be mild due to compensatory reticulocytosis. Such patients frequently come to medical attention during aplastic crisis (commonly due to parvovirus B19). Since reticulocytosis is absent in this situation, the underlying diagnosis of hemolysis may not be suspected.

(d) **Therapies** are discussed below for individual conditions. **General measures include**
   (i) **Folate** supplementation (1 mg/day) to prevent megaloblastic crisis in patients with chronic hemolysis.
   (ii) Treatment of **iron deficiency** (rare) if present in patients with chronic hemoglobinuria; **most patients with hemolytic anemias are not iron deficient.**
   (iii) **Transfusion** if clinically indicated for acute hemolysis or chronic hemolysis marked by severe symptomatic anemia.
   (iv) Surgical therapy may be indicated for some patients with chronic hemolysis, including **cholecystectomy** for treatment of symptomatic gallstones and **splenectomy** to prolong red cell survival. Splenectomy should be deferred until 5 to 6 years if possible.
   (v) **Steroids** or rarely **cytotoxic agents** may be of value in treating antibody-mediated hemolysis.

(2) **Hereditary spherocytosis (HS)** is the most common form of hemolytic anemia in Northern Europeans. Although spherocytes are a characteristic feature of many hemolytic states, HS represents a group of inherited (usually autosomal dominant) disorders of RBC membrane protein structure.

(a) **Evaluation** includes parental history. Splenomegaly is a prominent feature. Patients can present with neonatal jaundice or be asymptomatic until anemia is noted on a routine CBC. The mean corpuscular hemoglobin concentration (MCHC) is elevated and spherocytes are noted on blood smear.

(b) **Diagnosis** is confirmed by demonstrating increased osmotic fragility. Membrane protein analysis is occasionally useful.

(c) **Treatment** may be limited to **folate** supplementation. **Splenectomy** is performed in patients with significant anemia or increased risk of gallstones, or both. **Transfusions** are sometimes required for severe anemia secondary to intercurrent viral infections or frank aplastic crisis.

(3) **Sickle cell disorders** include homozygous Hgb SS, doubly heterozygous Hgb S/C, and Hgb S/beta-thalassemia. These genotypes are common: The incidence of sickle trait is 8% in African Americans; approximately 1 in 200 to 500 African American newborns are affected with sickle cell disease.

(a) **Etiology.** Hemoglobin S has a propensity to polymerize on deoxygenation, leading to misshapen, rigid, and adherent red cells.

(b) **Evaluation.** Newborns are asymptomatic. Vasoocclusion can begin to occur as early as 6 months of age, commonly presenting with **dactylitis** of the hands or feet, **painful crisis,** and rarely **stroke, acute chest syndrome, aplastic crisis, splenic sequestration,** or **priapism.** Late manifestations include isosthenuria, osteonecrosis, chronic pulmonary disease, cardiomegaly, and renal insufficiency. **Laboratory tests** include CBC with reticulocyte count, sickle prep, and hemoglobin electrophoresis. A room air **arterial oxygen tension (PO$_2$)** measurement is necessary to document suspected hypoxia; *cutaneous oximetry may not be reliable in patients with sickle cell disorder.* Chest x-rays and blood cultures should be obtained on febrile patients. Parvovirus polymerase chain reaction (PCR) assay or convalescent titers, or both, may be diagnostic for patients with aplastic crisis.

(c) Exposure of blood to reducing agents induces sickling ("sickle prep"). Hemoglobin electrophoresis confirms the diagnosis.

(d) Therapy

  (i) Antibiotic prophylaxis is indicated, as **functional asplenia** develops early in life. Encapsulated organisms pose the greatest threat of overwhelming sepsis. Mortality is markedly reduced by **prophylaxis** starting in the first year of life. Small children should be given **penicillin V potassium,** 125 mg PO bid; larger children should be given 250 mg PO bid. *This recommendation may change in the next few years, as the prevalence of penicillin-resistant pneumococcal strains is growing.*

  (ii) Folate should be taken daily (see above).

  (iii) Pneumococcal vaccine should be given as early as is efficacious (currently age 2 for 23-valent preparation), with boosts every 6 years. Vaccines that protect against other encapsulated organisms (*Haemophilus influenzae,* meningococcus) are also indicated.

  (iv) Fever. All fever episodes should be thoroughly evaluated. If the patient appears ill, or has a high temperature, clouded mental status, respiratory distress, lung infiltrate, or questionable compliance, **admit** and treat with **ampicillin sodium/sulbactam sodium (Unasyn),** 50 to 75 mg/kg IV q6h. Carefully selected, well-appearing, low-risk patients with good follow-up need not be admitted. They should receive **ceftriaxone,** 50 mg/kg (maximum 2 g) IV or IM immediately after cultures are drawn.

  (v) Painful crises and **dactylitis** should be treated aggressively with hydration and analgesic pain medications. **Acetaminophen** and **ibuprofen** are first-line agents. Severe episodes require hospitalization for IV fluids and **narcotics** (codeine, morphine, dilaudid, methadone). **Dosages should be tailored to individual patients and their pain;** development of tolerance to narcotics may necessitate escalating dosages if pain is persistent. Hospitalized patients should be monitored for cardiorespiratory compromise and fluid overload. **Transfusion and oxygen therapy are not indicated for uncomplicated painful crisis.** Occasionally, vasoocclusive crisis must be distinguished from cholecystitis, osteomyelitis, or acute chest syndrome.

  (vi) Acute chest syndrome is a medical emergency, characterized by fever, hypoxia, respiratory distress, chest or abdominal pain, and changes on chest x-ray (which may lag behind clinical findings). Treatment includes **oxygen, hydration, antibiotics** (Unasyn, 50–75 mg/kg IV q6hr, plus erythromycin, 10 mg/kg qid), and careful monitoring. **Exchange transfusion** may be lifesaving in severe cases.

  (vii) Aplastic crisis presents as exacerbation of anemia with reticulocytopenia, usually caused by **parvovirus B19.** **Transfusion** is frequently necessary. Spontaneous recovery is followed by lifelong immunity.

  (viii) Sequestration crisis results from sudden pooling of blood in the **spleen** or (rarely) liver, producing shock, organomegaly, and severe anemia. It is treated by **fluid resuscitation** and emergent **transfusion.**

(ix) **Stroke** requires immediate exchange transfusion followed by chronic transfusion to maintain Hgb S at less than 30%. This regimen helps prevent recurrence. **Hypertonic IV contrast** materials should be avoided in patients with sickle cell disorders.

(x) **Surgery, pregnancy, and priapism** are associated with unique problems in sickle cell patients, which should be managed in consultation with a hematologist.

(xi) **Transfusions (simple and exchange)** should be given in consultation with a hematologist and a knowledgeable blood bank, as patients with sickle cell disorders have a propensity for development of anti–red cell antibodies, which complicate future treatment. An algorithm for exchange transfusion is shown in Table 15-5. **Chronic transfusion** is indicated for a subset of patients.

(4) **Hemoglobin C disease (Hgb CC)** is a mild disorder characterized by hemolysis and splenomegaly. Abdominal pain and cholelithiasis are common. **Laboratory features** include mild anemia, prominent targets on smear, and a diagnostic Hgb electrophoretic pattern. **Treatment** is symptomatic.

(5) **Enzymopathies.** Hemolytic disorders of RBC enzymes can present at any age, though neonatal jaundice is common. **Diagnosis** is confirmed by enzyme assay, although false-negative results are frequent in the setting of hemolytic crisis due to the preponderance of young, relatively enzyme-rich cells.

(a) **Glucose 6-phosphate dehydrogenase (G6PD) deficiency,** the most common of these disorders, is inherited in an X-linked recessive pattern and occurs frequently in those of Mediterranean and African descent. Hemolysis is triggered by **oxidant stress.** Patients should avoid fava beans, sulfonamides, antimalarials, chloramphenicol, nitrofurantoin, nalidixic acid, furazolidone, acetanilid, methylene blue, phenazopyridine, aspirin, benzene, naphthalene, doxorubicin, and other oxidants.

(b) **Pyruvate kinase (PK) deficiency** is an autosomal recessive disorder associated with hemolysis, anemia, and characteristic burr cells on smear. **Folate** supplementation is recommended and **transfusions** are sometimes necessary. **Splenectomy** may be helpful in severe cases.

(6) **Autoimmune hemolytic anemia (AIHA)**

(a) **Etiologies** include infection, collagen vascular disease, malignancy, or medications.

(b) **Evaluation**

(i) **History** is often unrevealing.

(ii) **Physical examination** should note icterus, jaundice, and splenomegaly.

(iii) **Laboratory studies** include CBC, reticulocyte count, smear, serum LDH, and bilirubin.

(c) **Diagnosis** of AIHA is confirmed by Coombs' test. **"Warm" antibodies** (immunoglobin G [IgG]) display a maximal reaction at around 37°. **"Cold" antibodies** (IgM, rarely IgG) react best at low temperature, fix complement, and agglutinate red cells.

(d) **Therapy**

(i) **Secondary AIHA** often responds to treatment of the underlying condition or removal of the offending agent.

(ii) Patients with **cold** antibodies usually respond poorly to treatment and should avoid exposure to low temperatures.

Table 15-5. Exchange algorithms for sickle cell disease and polycythemia

Rapid partial volume exchange[a]

Starting Hct	Hct ≤ 15%	Hct 16–30%[e]	Hct > 30%[e]
Step 1	Exchange[b] 10 ml/kg PRBC[c] for pt's blood →	Exchange 10 ml/kg PRBC[c] for pt's blood →	Exchange 10 ml/kg saline for pt's blood →
Step 2	Exchange 20 ml/kg[d] PRBC for pt's blood	Exchange 70 ml/kg blood[c] for pt's blood	Exchange 90 ml/kg blood for pt's blood

RBC removal for polycythemia

$$\text{Volume of blood removed (ml)} = \text{volume of NS or 5\% albumin reinfused} = \frac{(\text{start Hct} - \text{desired Hct}) \times (\text{total blood volume})}{\text{start Hct}}$$

[a]Indications for rapid partial volume exchange includes severe acute chest syndrome, stroke, eye surgery, and cerebral angiography. Exchange has also been used for refractory vasoocclusive crisis. Automated erythropheresis is preferable if available and appropriate vascular access is feasible.
[b]Volume out = volume in.
[c]Packed red blood cells (PRBCs) have a hematocrit of approximately 75%; for "blood," dilute PRBC to a hematocrit of 40% with saline or plasma.
[d]Exchange in aliquots of 10–15 ml/kg; adults can usually tolerate 500-ml exchanges.
[e]Extreme caution is necessary to avoid hyperviscosity. Simple transfusion (no exchange) should not be utilized in patients with a starting Hct of >24%.
Source: Adapted from S Charache, B Lubin, CD Reid. *Management and Therapy of Sickle Cell Disease.* NIH Publication No. 92-2117, 1992.

(iii) Corticosteroids are frequently useful in **warm** antibody-mediated hemolytic anemia. **Prednisone** (or methylprednisolone) is initiated at a dosage of 4 to 6 mg/kg/day until response is seen, tapered rapidly to 1 to 2 mg/kg/day, and then tapered slowly to the minimum required to maintain an acceptable Hgb and reticulocyte count. Treatment may need to be continued for a period of months to years.

(iv) High-dose IV gamma globulin (IVGG), splenectomy, and/or immunosuppressive agents (e.g., cyclophosphamide) should be considered for patients who cannot be treated with steroids. **Plasmapheresis** may be a useful adjunct when rapid reduction of the antibody titer is desired (e.g., severe, acute AIHA).

(v) Blood transfusion may be hazardous. It must be done with extreme caution and only in the event of life-threatening anemia. High-dose IV steroids should be given before transfusion if possible. The blood bank should select the unit of blood that is least reactive on cross-match. It is infused slowly, with close monitoring. Blood should be prewarmed for patients with cold antibodies, to decrease immediate hemolysis.

c. Anemia of chronic disease is a common manifestation of numerous systemic conditions. Although usually normocytic, the MCV can be low. Characteristically both serum TIBC and Fe are diminished. Treatment is aimed at the primary condition.

D. Polycythemia (increased RBC mass), is reflected in elevations in the Hgb and Hct.

1. **Etiologies** include chronic hypoxemia from congenital heart disease and pulmonary disorders. Neonatal causes include maternal-fetal transfusion, intrauterine hypoxia, and maternal diabetes (see p. 199). **Polycythemia vera** is rare in children.

2. **Evaluation**
   a. **History** should detail headaches, dizziness, lethargy, exercise intolerance and visual disturbances, and symptoms of stroke.
   b. **Physical examination** may reveal acrocyanosis and vascular engorgement (plethora).
   c. **Laboratory** workup should be obtained by venous rather than capillary sampling. Spun Hcts are more accurate than those obtained by automated counters. Mild thrombocytopenia may be associated.

3. **Diagnosis** is confirmed by measurement of **Hct greater than 55%.**

4. **Therapy**
   a. In the absence of adequate treatment for the underlying condition, **phlebotomy** can be used to lower the Hct, alleviate symptoms of hyperviscosity, and prevent stroke. Phlebotomy is indicated for symptoms or Hct of 65% or greater.
   b. **Partial exchange transfusion** is the method of choice for newborns (Table 15-5).
   c. For older children, **automated erythropheresis** allows the Hct to be adjusted rapidly and safely without altering the total blood volume.
   d. Hematocrit should rarely be decreased by more than 10% at a time (Table 15-5).
   e. **Chronic treatment** may be necessary; it is mandatory for those with a history of stroke.

II. **Bone marrow**

A. **Primary marrow failure syndromes**

1. **Aplastic anemia (AA)** is characterized by diminished production of red cells, white cells, and platelets.
   a. **Acquired AA**
      (1) **Etiologies** include hepatitis, drugs, and radiation; often no etiology is found.

(2) Evaluation includes CBC with differential and reticulocyte count, and bone marrow examination.

(3) Diagnosis is confirmed by pancytopenia and bone marrow hypoplasia.

(4) Therapy. The prognosis in severe AA is poor, with mortality as high as 75%.

   (a) Possible **inciting factors** should be treated or removed.

   (b) Supportive care includes **transfusion** and **antibiotics.** Transfusions should be avoided unless strongly indicated; *related donor transfusions are contraindicated in any patient considered for bone marrow transplantation.* Antibiotic coverage should be instituted whenever infection is suspected.

   (c) Bone marrow transplantation offers the best chance for survival and is the treatment of choice for those with human leukocyte antigen (HLA)-matched siblings.

   (d) Immunosuppressive drugs have been used with variable success. Other agents, such as **androgens** and **hematopoietic growth factors,** may be helpful for some patients.

  b. Fanconi's anemia (FA) is characterized by bone marrow failure accompanied by an increased incidence of malignancy.

   (1) Etiology. Fanconi's anemia is an autosomal recessive condition thought to be due to DNA repair defects.

   (2) Evaluation

     (a) History should note affected siblings, growth failure dating to the prenatal period, and hearing loss.

     (b) Physical examination findings include pigmentary, skeletal, renal, and developmental abnormalities.

     (c) Laboratory tests include CBC, reticulocyte count, differential, bone marrow examination, and cytogenetic analysis in the presence of diepoxybutane.

   (3) Diagnosis. Fanconi's anemia should be suspected in patients with cytopenia(s) and phenotypic features. Diagnosis is confirmed by demonstrating increased chromosomal breakage on exposure to diepoxybutane. Prenatal diagnosis is feasible.

   (4) Therapy

     (a) Supportive care includes **transfusions** and **antibiotic** coverage for suspected infection.

     (b) Specific treatment consists of **prednisone,** 5 to 10 mg qod, and **androgens,** for example, oxymetholone, 2 to 5 mg/kg/day PO, *or* nandrolone decanoate (Deca-Durabolin), 1 to 2 mg/kg/wk IM.

     (c) Bone marrow transplantation can be curative if an appropriate donor is available.

  c. Other rare forms of **constitutional AA** include dyskeratosis congenita, Shwachman-Diamond syndrome, and other familial marrow failure syndromes.

2. Isolated cytopenias can involve any of the three cell lines.

  a. Pure red cell aplasia (PRCA) can be congenital or acquired.

   (1) Transient erythroblastopenia of childhood (TEC) is the most common form of PRCA.

     (a) Etiology is unknown.

     (b) Evaluation

       (i) History. This disorder affects healthy children from 1 month to 8 years (peak incidence, age 2). A preceding viral infection is commonly reported.

       (ii) Physical examination is remarkable for pallor of gradual onset.

       (iii) Laboratory studies include CBC with differential and reticulocyte count, and occasionally bone marrow examination.

(c) **Diagnosis** is based on a consistent clinical course. It is supported by an earlier history of normal red cell numbers, and confirmed when red cell counts recover.

(d) **Therapy.** Erythropoiesis will recover spontaneously over weeks to months. **Transfusion** may be necessary for symptomatic patients.

(2) **Acquired PRCA**

    (a) **Etiologies** include viral infection, drugs, pregnancy, anti-RBC antibodies (AIHA; see above), thymoma, end-stage renal disease (see p. 312), immunodeficiency, malignancy, and malnutrition. In patients with hemolytic or immunodeficiency disorders, **aplastic crisis** due to **parvovirus B19** can develop.

    (b) **Evaluation** should focus on a possible underlying cause. Evidence for parvovirus infection should be sought in patients with chronic hemolytic anemia or immunodeficiency. Bone marrow examination may be indicated.

    (c) **Diagnosis** is based on the findings of erythrocytopenia and reticulocytopenia in patients with conditions listed above.

    (d) **Therapy**

        (i) Red cell recovery may follow **drug removal,** nutritional repletion, **treatment of the underlying condition,** or thymectomy as indicated.

        (ii) **Splenectomy** and a variety of **immunosuppressive regimens** have been employed in persistent PRCA with occasional success.

        (iii) **Transfusion** may be necessary for symptomatic patients.

        (iv) Patients with **end-stage renal disease** can be treated with **erythropoietin** in combination with **iron.**

        (v) **Parvovirus** infection resolves spontaneously over several weeks in patients with normal immune function. Patients with immunodeficiency may develop chronic parvovirus infection, which is treated with one or more courses of **IVGG.**

(3) **Congenital PRCA or Diamond-Blackfan anemia (DBA)**

    (a) **Etiology** is unknown.

    (b) **Evaluation**

        (i) **History** is notable for pallor in the first year of life.

        (ii) **Physical examination** reveals associated congenital anomalies in 25% of patients.

        (iii) **Laboratory evaluation** includes CBC with MCV, reticulocyte count, bone marrow aspiration, and chromosome analysis.

    (c) **Diagnosis** is suggested by findings of **macrocytic anemia** with "fetal" erythropoiesis, reticulocytopenia, selective erythroid marrow hypoplasia, associated constitutional features, and normal chromosomes. DBA must be distinguished from TEC. In the absence of a prior normal CBC to confirm TEC, the diagnosis depends on the course of the illness. The absence of spontaneous improvement "confirms" DBA and warrants treatment.

    (d) **Therapy**

        (i) **Corticosteroids** are effective in up to 75% of cases. **Prednisone** is begun at a dosage of 2 mg/kg/day, with a response usually seen within 1 month. Once the Hgb and Hct have reached satisfactory levels, steroids should be tapered to the lowest possible qod dose. **Steroid dependence is the rule.** Nonresponders should be given a trial of prednisone at 4 to 6 mg/kg/day (or an alternative preparation at an equivalent dose).

        (ii) **Androgens, immunosuppressive agents,** and **hema-**

topoietic growth factors have been used with anecdotal success.

(iii) **Bone marrow transplantation** can be offered to patients with suitable donors.

(iv) **Chronic red cell transfusion** may be required; if so, patients should be monitored for development of iron overload.

b. **Neutropenia** (see p. 452).

c. **Thrombocytopenia**

(1) **Etiology** is most commonly **peripheral destruction** (see p. 450). **Decreased platelet production** may result from infection, drugs (e.g., trimethoprim, diuretics, chemotherapy), and a variety of inherited disorders.

(2) **Evaluation**

(a) **History** should probe manifestations of thrombocytopenia and their onset, drug intake, and recent infections.

(b) **Physical examination** includes a search for associated congenital abnormalities and evaluation of spleen size.

(c) **Laboratory studies** include platelet count, evaluation of platelet size and morphology, and bone marrow examination.

(3) **Diagnosis** is confirmed by paucity of megakaryocytes on bone marrow examination.

(4) **Therapy** depends on the underlying disorder.

(a) **Amegakaryocytic thrombocytopenia** is a rare congenital syndrome that invariably leads to AA. Because of the extremely poor prognosis, **bone marrow transplantation** should be considered.

(b) **Thrombocytopenia with absent radii syndrome** presents with thrombocytopenia in the first months of life. Death may occur from hemorrhage in the first year; those who survive usually demonstrate spontaneous improvement. Treatment is supportive.

(c) **Wiskott-Aldrich syndrome** is a rare, X-linked, **immunodeficiency** syndrome associated with microthrombocytopenia. **Bone marrow transplantation** can be curative.

B. **Secondary marrow failure syndromes**

1. **Leukemia** is the most common pediatric malignancy, occurring in approximately 1 in 20,000 children. All ages are affected, although the peak incidence is around age 4.

a. **Etiology** is unknown.

b. **Evaluation**

(1) **History** focuses on symptoms of anorexia, malaise, bleeding, and fever.

(2) **Physical examination** findings include adenopathy, gingival hyperplasia, hepatosplenomegaly, bone and joint pain, skin rash, papilledema, focal neurologic deficits, testicular enlargement, and respiratory compromise. Life-threatening presentations include hemorrhage, infection, and/or organ failure.

(3) **Laboratory studies** include blood smear and bone marrow examination.

c. **Diagnosis** is confirmed by the presence of increased blasts in the bone marrow. Histochemical stains, cytogenetics, and immunologic surface markers allow subtyping. **Acute lymphoblastic leukemia (ALL)** accounts for 75 to 80% of childhood leukemia, with survival rates as high as 60 to 80%. **Acute nonlymphoblastic leukemia (ANLL)** includes seven subtypes **(M1–M7)**. Survival of patients with ANLL is worse than that of ALL.

d. **Therapy**

(1) Aggressive supportive care is essential. To prevent uric acid nephropathy, **allopurinol** (50–100 mg tid), IV **hydration,** and urinary

alkalinization (5% dextrose in water [D_5W] plus 40–80 mEq/liter $NaHCO_3$ infused at 1.5–2.0 times maintenance) should be instituted immediately. Broad-spectrum **antibiotics** and **transfusions** may be indicated.

(2) **Heparin** is recommended during the initial therapy of certain forms of leukemia associated with disseminated intravascular coagulation (DIC).

(3) Hyperviscosity due to severe leukocytosis can lead to CNS or pulmonary dysfunction, requiring immediate **exchange transfusion** or **leukocytapheresis.**

(4) Patients should be referred to centers familiar with specialized **chemotherapy and radiation therapy protocols.** Outcome varies with the type of leukemia and prognostic features.

(5) **Bone marrow transplantation** is recommended for certain subtypes.

2. **Metastatic malignancies,** such as neuroblastoma, lymphoma, sarcoma, and malignant histiocytosis, may involve the marrow, resulting in cytopenias.

3. **Metabolic disorders** can lead to marrow infiltration. Examples include **Gaucher's disease** and **osteopetrosis.**

4. **Infections** involving the bone marrow include congenital **TORCH** infections, **human immunodeficiency virus (HIV), Epstein-Barr virus (EBV), cytomegalovirus (CMV),** and **tuberculosis.**

III. Coagulation

A. **Clotting factor** deficiencies are common. **Comprehensive hemophilia treatment centers are available throughout the United States for routine hemophilia management or consultation.**

1. **Hemophilia A**

a. **Etiology.** An X-linked recessive deficiency of factor VIII activity (F VIII:C) that affects 1 in 5,000 to 10,000 males.

b. **Evaluation**

(1) Family **history** is usually positive.

(2) **Physical examination** should focus on sites of past and acute bleeding.

(3) **Laboratory studies** include prothrombin time (PT), partial thromboplastin time (PTT), platelet count, and measurement of factor level.

c. **Diagnosis** is confirmed by **F VIII:C assay.** The severity of disease reflects the degree of deficiency.

(1) Mild deficiency: 5 to 30% of normal.

(2) Moderate deficiency: 1 to 5% of normal.

(3) Severe deficiency: less than 1% of normal.

d. **Therapy.** Bleeds must be treated promptly with F VIII replacement. Signs and symptoms of bleeding may be subtle. Home therapy is encouraged for all but the most severe bleeds. **Inhibitors develop in 10 to 20% of patients with severe deficiency, greatly complicating management (see p. 447).**

(1) **Factor VIII–containing products**

(a) **High-purity F VIII concentrates** are used routinely. Monoclonal and recombinant preparations are free of contaminating viruses.

(b) **Pasteurized F VIII** concentrates are less pure, but are currently considered to be safe.

(c) **Cryoprecipitate,** obtained by slow thawing of fresh-frozen plasma (FFP), contains concentrated F VIII. It is rarely used to treat hemophilia.

(d) **Deamino-D-arginine vasopressin (DDAVP)** can be used to increase F VIII levels in some patients with mild hemophilia (see p. 448).

(2) Selected patients are considered for qod factor **prophylaxis** to prevent progressive joint damage.

(3) Dose. In general, **each unit/kg** of F VIII concentrate will increase plasma levels by **2%.** Infusions are generally given bid for severe bleeds because the half-life of F VIII is 8 to 12 hours. Target levels depend on the severity of the hemorrhage. In severe bleeds, the adequacy of replacement should be assessed by measuring peak and trough F VIII levels and observing clinical response. The PTT is normal when the F VIII level is greater than 40%.

    (a) Major bleeds require correction to **100%** and maintenance of **trough levels greater than 50%.** A loading dose of 50 units/kg F VIII followed by 25 units/kg q12h usually suffices. In life-threatening situations the loading dose can be followed by continuous-infusion F VIII at 3 to 4 units/kg/hr titrated according to levels and clinical status.

    (b) Minor bleeds should be treated with **30 to 50%** correction. Factor VIII, 25 units/kg load followed by 10 to 15 units/kg q12h thereafter, should be adequate.

    (c) Joint bleeds (hemarthroses). Consultation with hematologists, orthopedic surgeons, and physical therapists who specialize in hemophilia is essential. For **early hemarthrosis** (mild trauma, normal examination) a single dose of 15 to 20 units/kg F VIII concentrate will often suffice. For **late hemarthrosis** (swollen, painful joint) levels should be maintained above 50% for several days. After the acute period, daily therapy with 25 units/kg may be necessary to prevent rebleeding during remobilization. **Elevation, ice, bed rest, and immobilization** (e.g., wraps, splints) are often helpful in controlling the acute bleed. The joint should be slowly rehabilitated with early mobilization to prevent atrophy and contractures. **Joint aspiration should be avoided.**

    (d) Forearm or calf bleeds

        (i) Factor VIII should be administered for 7 to 10 days to maintain levels between **50 and 100%.** Shorter courses may be adequate with early treatment and minimal bleeding.

        (ii) Ice and elevation are helpful.

        (iii) Close monitoring for the development of **compartment syndrome** is mandatory. Surgical fasciotomy is associated with significant risks and should be considered only as a last resort to preserve limb function.

    (e) Diagnosis of **retroperitoneal and iliopsoas bleeds** requires a high index of suspicion. Pain is referred to the **hip. Medial thigh** numbness suggests an iliopsoas bleed compressing the lateral femoral nerve.

        (i) Initially replace F VIII to 100%. Then, replace to 50% for 2 days and 30% for 1 week. A severe bleed may require 100% correction for up to 7 days.

        (ii) Close monitoring for ongoing bleeding is critical since severe anemia may develop.

        (iii) Bed rest may be helpful.

    (f) Surgery requires **100% correction** with close monitoring of levels for 10 to 14 days or as dictated by wound healing.

    (g) Dental extraction requires **100% correction** before the procedure. Follow-up therapy may be required for bleeding or hematoma formation. **Epsilon-aminocaproic acid (Amicar)** in an initial dose of 200 mg/kg PO (5 g maximum) followed by 100 mg/kg PO q6h (24 g/day maximum) should be given for 5 to 7 days following procedures associated with significant oral bleeding. **Topical thrombin** may also be of benefit.

    (h) Head trauma or severe headache requires immediate replacement to 100%, followed by thorough evaluation. Cranial CT scan should be obtained in all cases. If CNS hemorrhage is documented, treat to 50 to 100% replacement for 14 days, followed by 30 units/kg/day for 7 days. If trauma was significant but head CT was negative, factor should be given for 2 to 3 days.

(i) **Hematuria** usually resolves spontaneously with bed rest and vigorous hydration. **Prednisone** (2 mg/kg/ for 2–3 days) may be of benefit. Persistent hematuria due to kidney trauma is treated with F VIII concentrate. **Amicar is contraindicated** because of the risk of clotting and genitourinary (GU) obstruction.

e. **Complications of therapy**

(1) **Inhibitors.** Anti–factor VIII antibodies develop in 10 to 20% of patients who receive multiple concentrate infusions. **Expert advice should be sought in the management of bleeding in such patients.**

(a) The presence of inhibitors is suggested by inappropriately low F VIII levels despite replacement. **Diagnosis** is confirmed by inhibition assay. One Bethesda unit (BU) of antibody inactivates one unit of F VIII.

(b) **Patients with inhibitor levels less than 5 BU can continue to be treated with high doses of standard factor preparations.**

(c) **Patients with inhibitor levels greater than 5 BU should not receive F VIII except in the event of life- or limb-threatening hemorrhage.**

(d) **Porcine F VIII** is useful for serious bleeds in patients without **cross-reactive antibodies.**

(e) **Activated factor concentrates** that bypass F VIII (e.g., factor VIII inhibitor bypassing activity [FEIBA]) and pasteurized F IX preparations (e.g., Konyne 80) are somewhat effective.

(f) For life-threatening hemorrhage (e.g., CNS bleed, surgery), attempts can be made to overwhelm the inhibitor with large doses of F VIII. The **dose required** is roughly equal to the **(inhibitor level/ml) × (total plasma volume × 2).** This amount should be **added to the dose needed to achieve the desired correction** (i.e., 50–100% for major bleeds). This loading dose must then be followed by continuous-infusion maintenance F VIII. Massive doses may be required.

(g) **Local measures** (e.g., immobilization, ice, wraps) are the best treatment for mild bleeding.

(h) Experimental **immune tolerance** regimens are being attempted at many centers.

(2) **Infection.** Older patients with hemophilia have a high incidence of infection with HIV, HBV, and HCV viruses as a result of past treatment with contaminated F VIII concentrates.

f. **Preventative measures**

(1) **Antiplatelet medications** (e.g., aspirin) should be avoided.

(2) Hazardous activities and sports are contraindicated.

(3) **Prenatal diagnosis** is available for known carriers.

2. **Hemophilia B (Christmas disease)**

a. **Etiology.** Hemophilia B is an X-linked recessive deficiency of factor IX that is approximately one-fourth as common as hemophilia A.

b. **Evaluation** is identical to that described for factor VIII deficiency.

c. **Diagnosis** is confirmed by finding low levels of factor IX.

d. **Therapy** is similar to that of F VIII deficiency.

(1) High-purity monoclonal **F IX preparations** are now available. These do not carry a risk of thromboembolism as earlier F IX preparations did.

(2) **Dose.** In general, **for each unit/kg of factor IX administered, plasma levels will rise by 1%.** Thus, the usual dosage of factor required for minor bleeds is 30 units/kg, for major bleeds 50 units/kg,

and for severe life-threatening hemorrhage 100 units/kg. The half-life of F IX is 24 hours.

3. Inherited deficiencies of other clotting factors, including **fibrinogen, prothrombin, F V, F VII, F X, F XI, F XII, and F XIII,** are much less common than hemophilia. Bleeding tendency and laboratory features vary markedly. A **hematologist should be consulted** regarding evaluation and management.

4. **von Willebrand's disease (vWD)** is the most common inherited bleeding disorder, affecting up to 1% of the population.
   a. **Etiology.** vWD results from qualitative and/or quantitative abnormalities in von Willebrand's factor. Most subtypes are autosomal dominant.
   b. **Evaluation**
      (1) **History** should probe personal and family history of epistaxis, mucosal bleeding, excessive bruising, increased surgical bleeding, and menorrhagia.
      (2) **Physical examination** focuses on sites of bleeding and bruising.
      (3) **Laboratory evaluation** includes bleeding time (used less commonly than previously), PTT, F VIII activity, vWF antigen, ristocetin cofactor activity, and platelet count.
   c. **Diagnosis** is confirmed by finding low levels of vWF antigen and ristocetin cofactor activity. **Subtypes** can be distinguished by ristocetin titration and vWF multimer analysis.
   d. **Therapy**
      (1) **Pasteurized F VIII concentrate** (*not* recombinant or monoclonal preparations) contains high levels of vWF and carries less infectious risk than cryoprecipitate. It is first-line treatment for severe vWD or prolonged bleeding.
      (2) **Cryoprecipitate** has historically been the standard replacement product for vWD, but carries the same risks as other blood products.
      (3) **DDAVP** induces release of preformed vWF multimers, increasing circulating levels two- to threefold. This is often effective in managing bleeding in vWD in mild to moderately affected patients. Ristocetin titration testing is essential before treatment; **DDAVP is contraindicated in type IIB vWD since thrombocytopenia may be provoked.** Tachyphylaxis develops after two to three doses. Consequently, DDAVP is not useful when prolonged therapy is necessary. The major benefit is that DDAVP carries no risk of infection. A trial is required to demonstrate response **before** use in the management of bleeding. The dosage is 0.3 μg/kg (4 μg/ml in normal saline [NS]) IV over 30 minutes q12–24h for two to three doses. **Careful attention to fluid balance is vital:** with repeated administration, as symptomatic hyponatremia may develop. **Nasal DDAVP** (Stimate) is now available. This product is more convenient than IV therapy, but *extremely expensive.* It is dispensed as metered-dose sprays (0.15 mg/0.1-ml squirt); the dose is one squirt for children and two squirts for adults.

5. **Vitamin K deficiency** results in diminished production of coagulation factors II, VII, IX, and X.
   a. **Etiologies**
      (1) **Hemorrhagic disease of the newborn** (see Chap. 6, p. 199).
      (2) **Malabsorption.**
      (3) **Dietary inadequacy.**
      (4) **Vitamin K antagonism** from drugs such as warfarin (Coumarin).
   b. **Evaluation** should be tailored to the suspected etiology. Laboratory studies include PT and PTT.
   c. **Diagnosis** is suspected in patients with a prolonged **PT**. It is confirmed by response to therapeutic vitamin K administration or, if necessary, by comparing levels of vitamin K–dependent versus independent factors.
   d. **Therapy**
      (1) **Prophylaxis** with **vitamin K$_1$** (0.5–1.0 mg IM) should be given to all newborns.

(2) Treatment of older children with **vitamin K$_1$** (2.5–5.0 mg IM or slow IV) results in an increase in clotting factors and shortening of the PT within hours. Patients with normal GI absorption can be treated orally.

(3) Fresh-frozen plasma (10–20 ml/kg) can be used to treat acute hemorrhage.

6. Liver disease (see also Chap. 11)

a. Etiology. The liver is the major site of synthesis of all coagulation factors except F VIII.

b. Evaluation. The vitamin K–dependent factors, especially F VII, are most sensitive. Thus, early or mild liver disease is characterized by a prolongation of the PT. More severe dysfunction results in elevations of the PT, PTT, and thrombin time (due to diminished fibrinogen).

c. Therapy

(1) Vitamin K$_1$ (1–5 mg IM or slow IV) should be administered on a daily basis.

(2) Fresh-frozen plasma (starting at 10 ml/kg) should be given if there is active bleeding or no response to vitamin K, or both. Multiple infusions are often necessary. **Plasma or whole blood exchange** should be considered.

(3) Cryoprecipitate should be used for hypofibrinogenemia and bleeding.

(4) Platelets may be needed to treat quantitative or qualitative platelet defects.

7. Disseminated intravascular coagulation (DIC)

a. Etiologies include sepsis, shock, and acidosis.

b. Evaluation

(1) History and physical examination often reveal bleeding from the GI tract, mucosa, and/or skin.

(2) Laboratory tests include CBC, blood smear, PT, PTT, fibrinogen level, fibrin split products, and clotting factor levels.

c. Diagnosis is made by recognition of a consistent clinical picture and thrombocytopenia, microangiopathic hemolytic anemia, prolonged PT and PTT, diminished fibrinogen, low factor levels, and elevated fibrin split products.

d. Therapy

(1) Aggressive **supportive care and reversal of the underlying condition(s)** are essential.

(2) Blood product support is often required, including packed red blood cells (PRBCs), FFP, platelets, and cryoprecipitate. **Plasma or whole blood exchange** may be helpful in providing rapid, isovolemic factor replacement.

(3) Heparin has *not* been clearly demonstrated to alter the course of DIC. It is sometimes given to patients with major thrombotic complications. Heparin is also used to treat severe consumption during the initial therapy of M3 ANLL. The starting dosage is 10 to 25 units/kg/hr by continuous IV infusion. This should be used cautiously and titrated by the fibrinogen level (most sensitive), platelet count, and/or clinical response.

B. Hypercoagulable states

1. Primary or inherited prethrombotic disorders are due to abnormalities of coagulation proteins.

a. Etiologies include abnormalities of anticoagulant factors **protein C, protein S,** and **antithrombin III,** and a variant form of clotting factor V that results in **resistance to activated protein C (F V Leiden).**

b. Evaluation

(1) History of thrombosis occurring in young children, at unusual sites, in multiple family members, or recurrently is sought.

(2) Physical examination findings relate to thrombotic events.

(3) **Laboratory tests** include levels of **proteins C and S, anti-thrombin III, and resistance to activated protein C.** If available, DNA testing should be used to identify variant factor V. Measurement of anticoagulant factor levels during acute thrombosis can be misleading due to consumption; measurements of levels in parents or siblings, or both, may be more informative.

   c. **Diagnosis** is confirmed by consistently low measurements of one factor, or identification of variant factor V.

   d. **Therapy** consists primarily of anticoagulation. **A hematologist should be consulted to aid in management.**

      (1) **Coumarin** therapy can cause a decrease in the levels of protein S and C; combined initial treatment with heparin is required to prevent exacerbation of thrombosis.

      (2) **Fresh-frozen plasma** or **anti-thrombin III replacement therapy** may be required. **Protein C** concentrate is under investigation.

      (3) Female patients should avoid oral contraceptives.

2. **Secondary or acquired hypercoagulability**

   a. **Etiologies** include sickle cell disease, thrombotic thrombocytopenic purpura, DIC, collagen vascular disease, malignancy, surgery, pregnancy, immobilization, myeloproliferative disorders, autoimmune disorders, nephrotic syndrome, liver disease, paroxysmal nocturnal hemoglobinuria, metabolic disorders, vascular catheters or prosthetic devices, hyperviscosity, and medications.

   b. **Evaluation** should focus on the underlying disorder. **Laboratory tests** include PT, PTT, CBC, "lupus anticoagulant," BUN, creatinine, liver function tests (LFTs), and other studies as clinically indicated.

   c. **Diagnosis** is based on consistent clinical features.

   d. **Treatment** of the primary condition is essential; anticoagulation or thrombolysis, or both, may or may not be necessary.

C. **Platelet disorders**

1. **Thrombocytopenia** is defined as a platelet count below $150,000/mm^3$.

   a. **Etiology.** Thrombocytopenia usually results from **increased destruction** or splenic **sequestration.** Congenital hypoproduction is discussed with bone marrow failure syndromes (see p. 444).

   b. **Evaluation**

      (1) **History** should probe recent drugs and viral illnesses. Maternal history is relevant in newborns.

      (2) **Physical examination** findings include petechiae, purpura, excessive bruising, and/or mucosal bleeding.

      (3) **Laboratory tests** include CBC with smear, bone marrow examination, and antiplatelet antibodies. Mothers of thrombocytopenic newborns should have platelet counts; if normal, they should be typed for the PL^{A1} antigen.

   c. **Diagnosis** is confirmed by low platelet numbers in the absence of clumping; increased destruction is suggested by normal to increased numbers of bone marrow megakaryocytes.

   d. **Therapy**

      (1) To minimize bleeding, trauma and activities that cause increased intracranial pressure should be avoided. Antiplatelet agents should be avoided.

      (2) **Drug-induced thrombocytopenia** usually resolves with **drug withdrawal. Corticosteroids** may be helpful in the management of acute bleeding.

      (3) **Immune thrombocytopenic purpura (ITP)** is due to production of IgG platelet autoantibodies. Acute ITP may resolve without treatment, but therapy is generally recommended for patients with bleeding or platelet counts less than $20,000/mm^3$, or both. Chronic, relapsing ITP is difficult to manage.

(a) **Corticosteroids** decrease peripheral destruction of platelets and stabilize the vasculature. A pulse of **prednisone,** 2 mg/kg/ day PO for 5 to 10 days, is followed by a rapid taper over 3 to 4 days. The platelet count usually responds within 5 to 7 days. **Leukemia should be ruled out on clinical grounds or by bone marrow examination, or both, before starting steroids, as this treatment may partially treat leukemia, resulting in delayed diagnosis and impaired prognosis.** Some patients relapse after discontinuation of prednisone and can be successfully retreated. The use of high-dose steroids (30 mg/kg/day) is under investigation for multiply relapsed ITP. *Caution should be used in noninmmune patients with a history of varicella exposure,* to avoid immunocompromise and consequent overwhelming viral infection.

(b) **Intravenous gamma globulin,** 2 g/kg IV divided over 2 to 5 days, can stimulate a more rapid rise in platelet count than steroids. This treatment will not mask leukemia. Drawbacks include cost, inconvenience, risk of allergic reactions, and theoretical risk of exposure to contaminating infectious agents.

(c) **Splenectomy** is curative for many with chronic ITP, but increases the risk of overwhelming bacterial sepsis.

(d) Additional therapeutic options used for patients with chronic ITP include vincristine, cyclophosphamide, and danazol. Intravenous anti-Rh(D) globulin (WinRho) has had some effectiveness in Rh-positive patients with intact spleens.

(e) **Emergency management** of life-threatening hemorrhage should include high-dose IVGG and steroids, platelet transfusion, plasmapheresis, and, possibly, emergent splenectomy. Amicar may be useful for oral bleeding.

(f) **HIV** is commonly associated with an ITP-like disorder. First-line treatment is with zidovudine (ZDV). Steroids, IVGG, RhoGAM, and staphylococcal protein A column adsorption have also been reported to be effective in some cases. To decrease infectious complications, chronic steroids and splenectomy should be avoided if possible.

(4) **Neonatal immune thrombocytopenia** results from transplacental transfer of maternal antibodies.

(a) A low maternal platelet count is consistent with **autoimmune thrombocytopenia** in the mother. This disorder is treated as outlined above for ITP. Prenatal (maternal) treatment with IVGG or steroids may be effective in increasing fetal platelet counts.

(b) A normal maternal platelet count suggests **alloimmune platelet destruction,** often in a PL^{A1-} mother sensitized to the infant's PL^{A1+} platelets. In this situation, the standard treatment is transfusion with washed, maternal (or antigen-negative donor) platelets. While the mother is the most compatible platelet donor, her platelets should be **irradiated to prevent transfusion-associated graft-versus-host disease.** If suitable platelets are not available, steroids, IVGG, and/or random-donor platelet transfusion can be tried, with unpredictable success. Spontaneous resolution occurs by 3 to 4 months. Fetal platelet measurements, elective cesarean section, or both, may be indicated for pregnant women with a prior history of alloimmune thrombocytopenia.

(5) **Hypersplenism** from any cause can result in platelet trapping. Indications for **splenectomy** should be discussed with a hematologist.

2. **Qualitative platelet disorders** are associated with bleeding, prolonged bleeding time, and abnormal platelet aggregation studies in the absence of thrombo-

cytopenia. **Secondary dysfunction** is most common (e.g., drugs, uremia, liver disease). **Congenital disorders of platelet function** are rare. **Therapy** varies with the condition, but may include platelet transfusion (see p. 455), Amicar, DDAVP, cryoprecipitate, FFP, and avoidance of trauma and antiplatelet medications.

IV. White blood cells

A. Neutrophil counts normally range from 1,500 to 8,000/mm³. African Americans may have lower counts.

1. **Neutropenia** is defined as an absolute neutrophil count (ANC) less than 1,000/mm³, where the ANC equals the (total WBC count) × (fraction polymorphonuclear leukocytes +band forms). An ANC less than 500/mm³ represents severe neutropenia. The risk of infection increases with the degree of neutropenia.

   a. **Etiologies** include decreased marrow production and accelerated destruction (Table 15-6). Transient, self-limited neutropenia may be associated with viral infections and drugs.

   b. **Evaluation**

      (1) **History** should focus on recurrent fevers, stomatitis, adenitis, sinopulmonary disease, and other infections. Periodicity and possible exposures should be noted.

      (2) **Physical examination** is directed toward active infections.

      (3) **Laboratory studies** include CBC, evaluation of neutrophil count on multiple independent occasions, bone marrow examination, and antineutrophil antibody titers.

   c. **Diagnosis** is confirmed by repeated low ANC measurements.

   d. **Therapy** varies with the condition.

      (1) Medical evaluation and treatment are required for all **fevers** greater than 38°C.

         (a) **Empiric broad-spectrum parenteral antibiotics** should be given to patients with an ANC less than 500/mm³ (see Chap. 5), particularly when neutropenia is due to chemotherapy or bone marrow failure. Patients with uncomplicated viral suppression may have adequate marrow reserves.

         (b) Fungal, atypical, and opportunistic infections are common. Additional antimicrobial agents should be added as necessary.

         (c) **Granulocyte colony-stimulating factor (G-CSF)** may be useful; a specialist should be consulted regarding its indications.

         (d) **Granulocyte transfusion** is rarely indicated, but should be considered in cases of life-threatening or progressive infection.

      (2) **Prophylactic oral antibodies** should be given to patients with chronic neutropenia. Trimethoprim-sulfamethoxazole (TMP/SMX), 4 to 5 mg TMP/kg/day, decreases the incidence of serious infections.

2. **Disorders of neutrophil function** clinically resemble neutropenic conditions.

   a. **Etiology.** Neutrophil dysfunction can be primary or secondary (Table 15-7).

   b. **Evaluation and diagnosis.** Immunoglobulin and complement levels should be analyzed. Specific assays of phagocyte function include **prednisone stimulation** (reserve and mobilization), **opsonization and ingestion studies, Rebuck skin window** (chemotaxis), **nitroblue tetrazolium (NBT) reduction** (superoxide generation), and **flow cytometric analysis** of neutrophil receptors.

   c. **Therapy.** General principles of management of fever and infection are outlined for neutropenia (see sec. **1.d** above). Prophylactic antibiotics, IVGG, or both, are frequently beneficial. Specific treatment varies with the condition.

3. **Neutrophilia** is usually reactive in children. Etiologies include infection, inflammatory disorders, marrow invasion, exercise, and drugs (e.g., glucocorticoids, epinephrine). Rarely, neutrophilia may result from asplenia or neu-

Table 15-6. Neutropenia disorders

Etiology	Diagnosis	Treatment
Decreased production		
Infection	Usually viral, transient acquired marrow injury; occasionally severe and protracted	Supportive
Kostmann's syndrome	Severe congenital neutropenia, AR inheritance, life-threatening infections	Prophylactic antibiotics, G-CSF, marrow transplant
Benign	Mild congenital neutropenia, ANC > 500/m^3; infection is rare	Supportive
Cyclic	Oscillating neutropenia and symptoms usually q3 wk; stomatitis is frequent	Prophylactic antibiotics; G-CSF increases nadir, shortens cycle
Toxic	Drugs, radiation, chemotherapy; may be severe	Agent removal, supportive
Nutrition	Severe B$_{12}$, folate, or copper deficiency	Nutritional repletion
Shwachman-Diamond syndrome	Neutropenia, exocrine pancreatic insufficiency, AR inheritance; may evolve to AA or leukemia	Supportive, pancreatic enzymes, ? growth factors, marrow transplant
Chemotherapy induced	Expected toxicity	G-CSF, 5 µg/kg/d SQ, or GM-CSF, 250 µg/m^2/d SQ starting 24 hr post-chemotherapy and stopping when ANC > 2,000–10,000, will shorten nadir, reduce febrile neutropenia
Increased destruction		
Drug induced	Exposure history, especially antibiotics	Agent removal, supportive
Isoimmune neonatal	Severe congenital neutropenia, normal marrow, maternal anti-WBC antibodies, transient	Supportive
Autoimmune	Usually idiopathic and self-limited; may be severe; anti-WBC antibodies	Steroids, IVGG; treat underlying collagen vascular disorder

AR = autosomal recessive; G-CSF = granulocyte colony-stimulating factor; GM-CSF = granulocyte/monocytic colony-stimulating factor; AA = aplastic anemia; IVGG = intravenous gamma globulin.

Table 15-7. Disorders of neutrophil function

Etiology	Diagnosis	Treatment
Depressed chemotaxis	Seen with chronic illness (e.g., renal failure) and infection (especially skin), antibody deficiency, excess IgE and/or IgA, complement disorders, and certain drugs; Rebuck skin window test is diagnostic	Treat underlying condition, IVGG, supportive; apheresis to lower IgE sometimes helpful
Opsonization disorders	Complement and antibody deficiencies	IVGG, supportive, plasma
Chédiak-Higashi disease	Recurrent, severe infection; giant granules; neutropenia; AR inheritance; albinism	Marrow transplant, supportive
Chronic granulomatous disease	Recurrent, severe infection (especially skin, lung) with catalase + organisms; usually X linked (sometimes AR); NBT test is diagnostic	Interferon gamma, supportive prophylactic antibiotics
Neutrophil adhesion disorders	Recurrent infections, omphalitis, elevated WBC, absent receptors by cytometry, AR inheritance, abnormal Rebuck skin window test	Marrow transplant, supportive
Nutritional	Severe phosphate or zinc deficiency	Repletion

AR = autosomal recessive; NBT = nitroblue tetrazolium; IVGG = intravenous gamma-globulin.

trophil receptor defects. Normal newborns have higher neutrophil counts than older children and adults.
V. Transfusion therapy
A. All blood components have side effects; practitioners should consider indications, appropriate dose, and potential toxicities.
B. Blood products
1. **Whole blood (WB)**
   a. **Contents.** A unit of unmodified WB consists of 450 ml donor blood. The Hct is about 40%. White blood cells, platelets, and plasma proteins lose function in storage. Whole blood is an inefficient product with limited usefulness for replacement.
   b. **Indications**
      (1) **Very fresh, unrefrigerated WB** less than 6 hours old is recommended for the treatment of **neonatal sepsis with neutropenia.** Double-volume exchange q12–24h may be required to maintain a measurable neutrophil count. **Blood must be irradiated to prevent transfusion-associated graft-versus-host disease.**
      (2) **Whole blood reconstituted** from PRBCs, FFP, and platelets is employed for most other indications including acute volume loss and routine exchange transfusion.
2. **Packed red blood cells (PRBCs)**
   a. **Contents.** A unit of PRBCs consists of 200 to 250 ml with an Hct of 60 to 80% and variable amounts of WBCs and plasma.
   b. **Indications**

(1) Packed red blood cells are the standard product for treating most forms of acute and chronic anemia.

(2) **White blood cell removal** by filtration should be performed for those who require multiple transfusions, to decrease the incidence and severity of sensitization to leukocyte antigens. This also decreases the risk of CMV infection.

(3) **Packed red blood cells washed in saline** are depleted of plasma proteins.

(4) **Frozen/deglycerolized PRBCs** are depleted of WBCs and plasma. They are primarily used for those who require lifelong transfusions and/or extended RBC antigen matching (e.g., sickle cell patients).

(5) Evaluation and treatment of **transfusion reactions** are discussed in Table 15-8.

c. Dose

(1) 10–15 ml/kg results in a 7- to 10-point increase in Hct. Most patients tolerate infusion rates up to 10 ml/kg/hr.

(2) Patients with volume intolerance due to high-output heart failure should be transfused gradually with 5 to 10 ml/kg over 4 to 6 hours. Diuretics may be helpful.

(3) When rapid correction is necessary, but limited by fluid intolerance, partial exchange transfusion should be performed. Whole blood is removed in small aliquots and replaced with equal volumes of PRBCs. This can be done manually or with an automated cell separator.

3. Fresh-frozen plasma

a. Contents. Fresh-frozen plasma supplies clotting factors, albumin, and antibodies.

b. Indications. Fresh-frozen plasma should be used to replace clotting factors in bleeding patients with elevated PT or PTT. Because of potential side effects, **FFP should not be used solely for volume replacement. It is not adequate treatment for hemophiliacs.**

c. Dose

(1) 10 ml/kg increases clotting factor levels by 20%. Multiple doses may be required.

(2) Plasma exchange allows massive replacement in patients who are unable to tolerate increased volume.

(3) The rate of transfusion is limited by citrate toxicity. Close monitoring of vital signs and ionized calcium levels is essential when large or rapid infusions are used.

4. Cryoprecipitate

a. Contents. One 10-ml bag contains 200 to 300 mg fibrinogen and 80 to 100 units of F VIII.

b. Indications

(1) Bleeding associated with hypofibrinogenemia.

(2) vWD and hemophilia A (rarely used).

(3) Factor XIII deficiency.

(4) Bleeding associated with uremia.

c. Dose. 0.3 bag/kg should increase the fibrinogen by 200 mg/dl. Multiple doses may be required.

5. Platelets

a. Contents. One unit contains 5.5×10^{10} platelets with variable quantities of WBCs and plasma. Single-donor apheresis products contain 6 to 8 units per bag.

b. Indications

(1) **Thrombocytopenia with bleeding.** The aim should be to raise the platelet count to a point at which bleeding stops. Values between 50,000 and 100,000/mm³ usually suffice. Counts greater than 100,000/mm³ should be maintained for high-risk situations, such as CNS, vascular, or surgical hemorrhage.

Table 15-8. Transfusion reactions

Type	Cause	Symptoms	Treatment	Prevention
Acute hemolytic	ABO mismatch Minor mismatch with prior exposure	Fever, rigors, shock, back pain, hematuria	Stop transfusion 10–20 ml/kg saline bolus, then BP support as indicated Increase renal blood flow with furosemide, mannitol, dopamine Monitor for acute tubular necrosis Consider plasmapheresis or exchange	Cross-match
Delayed hemolytic	Minor blood group incompatibility	Develops 7–10 d after transfusion; pallor, jaundice, myalgias, arthralgias, low-grade fevers	Antipyretics Analgesics Monitor urine output	Patients with known antibodies need extended cross-matching; also consider for chronically transfused patients RhoGAM for Rh(D) mismatches
Allergic	Plasma proteins most commonly (e.g., IgA-deficient recipient)	Urticaria, pruritus, angioedema; may proceed to overt anaphylaxis	Stop transfusion Diphenhydramine, 1 mg/kg IV Methylprednisolone, 2 mg/kg IV, if no response Epinephrine and fluids for anaphylaxis	Premedication with anti-histamines, steroids, or both Rarely, washed platelets and PRBCs for patients with history of severe reactions

Febrile	Leukocyte antigens	Fever and chills	Stop transfusion only if severe antipyretics, especially prophylactically if prior history	Leukodepletion (e.g., Pall filter)
Transfusion-associated graft-vs-host disease	Engraftment of mononuclear cells from transfusion into immunodeficient recipient	Fever, rash, pancytopenia, diarrhea, hepatitis	High mortality (80%) Immunosuppressive agents, such as steroids, cyclosporin, antithymocyte globulin	Irradiation of all cellular blood products, even if leukofiltered. Irradiate if *any* suspicion of immunodeficiency: neonate, HIV, chemotherapy, transplant, etc.
Citrate toxicity	Large volumes of infused blood products, such as exchange transfusion or FFP for severe coagulopathy	Symptomatic hypocalcemia: paresthesias, diaphoresis, nausea and vomiting, abdominal pain; QT interval prolongation and hypotension follow	Hold transfusion and check ionized calcium Slow infusion rate Calcium gluconate	Prophylactic calcium administration

    (2) Prophylaxis for thrombocytopenia without bleeding. The risk of bleeding increases as the platelet count falls below 20,000/mm³. Consequently, it was once routine to transfuse platelets prophylactically in the setting of severe thrombocytopenia. Recently, many centers have relaxed prophylactic platelet transfusion guidelines, reserving transfusion for active bleeding or high-risk situations, or both. This is especially true in ITP or other antibody-mediated forms of platelet destruction. In addition, patients with chronic conditions such as aplastic anemia often develop transfusion-related complications, **making prophylactic transfusions difficult and potentially dangerous.**

    (3) Qualitative platelet disorders

        (a) In cases of acquired platelet dysfunction, platelet transfusion may be ineffective unless the underlying cause is reversed.

        (b) Bleeding patients with congenital platelet disorders usually respond to transfusion. Therapy should be determined by hemostasis and shortening of the bleeding time.

    (4) Single-donor apheresis platelets with **WBCs removed by filtration** should be given to patients who require multiple transfusions. These maneuvers decrease the incidence and severity of sensitization to leukocyte antigens.

    (5) Platelets should be **washed** in saline when it is necessary to deplete plasma proteins (e.g., maternal antibody removal).

  c. Dose

    (1) 0.1 units/kg normally increases the platelet count by 30,000 to 50,000/mm³.

    (2) Repeat or larger doses are required in the event of ongoing destruction.

    (3) Patients seem refractory to platelet transfusions if they have been allosensitized, or if they have massive ongoing bleeding. In this case, platelet counts drawn 10 to 60 minutes posttransfusion may help identify the problem (Table 15-9).

6. Albumin

  a. Contents. Standard preparations consist of 5% or 25% solutions of purified albumin.

  b. Indications

    (1) Volume restoration.

    (2) Hypoproteinemia.

  c. Dose

    (1) The usual dose is 10 ml/kg of 5% or 2.5 ml/kg of 25% albumin.

    (2) Under normal circumstances, only about 40% remains in the intravascular space. Diuretics are sometimes used in combination with 25% albumin to manage extravascular fluid overload.

Table 15-9. Causes of platelet refractoriness

Continued bleeding despite appropriate increase in count
  Systemic disorder that impairs function of transfused platelets (e.g., uremia, drugs)
  Poor platelet quality (e.g., prolonged storage)
  Other causes of bleeding (e.g., vascular lesions)
Inadequate increase in count
  Insufficient platelet dose
  Ongoing consumption (e.g., major hemorrhage, DIC, thrombus)
  Sequestration (e.g., splenomegaly)
No increase in count
  Alloimmunization to HLA antibodies
  Antiplatelet antibody (ITP)

7. Granulocytes

    a. Contents. One unit contains approximately 5×10^{10} granulocytes with variable quantities of RBCs, platelets, and plasma. Indications for granulocyte transfusion are limited, and patients may experience severe toxicity. This therapy is rarely used today, and may soon be supplanted by myeloid growth factor therapies.

    b. Indications

        (1) Severe neutropenia (ANC <500/mm³) and **life-threatening infection** without expectation of rapid marrow recovery

        (2) Sepsis neonatorum with **severe neutropenia.**

    c. Dose

        (1) Adolescents should receive 1 unit.

        (2) Children should receive 0.5 to 1.0 unit.

        (3) Neonates can be given small (e.g., 10 ml/kg) infusions or double-volume WB exchange (see p. 454).

        (4) Transfusion should be repeated q12–24h until ANC is greater than 500/mm³.

        (5) To prevent transfusion-associated graft-versus-host disease (TAGVHD), all WBC transfusions must be irradiated.

C. Side effects of transfusion. See Table 15-8.

D. Alternatives. When feasible, many donor centers offer collection of autologous blood before scheduled surgical procedures. Many parents inquire about directed donation of blood products from family members. This is usually available only for PRBCs. There are no data to support greater safety of directed donations. Additionally, family-directed donation is contraindicated for any patient in whom bone marrow transplantation is contemplated, especially patients with severe aplastic anemia. For the patient who is anemic but clinically well compensated after surgery, iron supplementation may be an alternative to transfusion. Blood substitutes are investigational. A large number of **hematopoietic growth factors** and **cytokines** have recently been cloned, offering major promise for disorders marked by diminished blood cell production. Table 15-10 lists some of these factors and their indications.

Table 15-10. Hematopoietic growth factors

Lineage	Growth factor	Indications
RBC	Erythropoietin	Anemia of renal failure
		Preoperative autologous blood donation (multiple units)
		HIV- and zidovudine-related anemia
WBC	G-CSF	Recovery from myelosuppressive chemotherapy, Kostmann's syndrome
	GM-CSF	Autologous bone marrow transplant
		Peripheral blood progenitor cell collection
Platelet	IL-11	Investigational
	Thrombopoietin	Preclinical
Progenitor cell	IL-3	Investigational
	IL-3/GM-CSF fusion protein (PIXY-321)	Investigational
	Stem cell factor	Investigational

IL = interleukin; G-CSF = granulocyte colony-stimulating factor; GM-CSF = granulocyte/monocyte colony-stimulating factor.

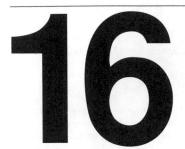

Allergic and Immunodeficiency Disorders

Lynda Schneider

I. Allergic disorders involve antigen-specific, immunoglobulin E (IgE)-mediated degranulation of mast cells.
  A. Anaphylaxis
  1. Etiology. Anaphylaxis results from an immediate IgE-mediated reaction in a sensitized individual. **Anaphylactoid** reactions are not IgE mediated, though they can result from direct mast cell activation.
  2. Evaluation. Systemic reactions occur within minutes of exposure to precipitating agents (Table 16-1).
    a. History and physical examination should probe for the following manifestations.
      (1) General. Peripheral tingling or pruritus, warm sensation, weakness.
      (2) Cutaneous. Diffuse flushing, urticaria, angioedema.
      (3) Respiratory. Range from sneezing and rhinorrhea to laryngeal or upper airway edema, or both, with stridor, bronchospasm, respiratory arrest.
      (4) Cardiovascular. Hypotension, tachycardia, shock.
      (5) Gastrointestinal. Nausea, vomiting, abdominal pain, diarrhea.
    b. Laboratory studies include the following:
      (1) Radioallergosorbent test (RAST) is a semiquantitative *in vitro* assay for allergen-specific IgE. It is less sensitive than skin testing.
      (2) Skin tests. Interpretation depends on specific allergen. If penicillin is implicated as a cause for anaphylaxis, skin testing can confirm sensitivity. RAST testing is not sufficient.
      (3) Other tests, when clinically indicated, to rule out myocardial infarction, insulin reaction, and other syndromes that can mimic anaphylaxis.
  3. Diagnosis. The diagnosis is based on the clinical syndrome and a history consistent with exposure to a precipitating agent. Evaluation for antigen-specific IgE may confirm or identify the precipitating agent.
  4. Therapy. Once anaphylaxis is recognized, therapy should be instituted immediately. Exposure to the responsible agent must be discontinued/prevented.
    a. General measures include administration of oxygen, application of a tourniquet proximal to the site of an injection or insect sting, and treatment of hypotension with isotonic fluids.
    b. Pharmacologic measures
      (1) Epinephrine, 0.01 ml/kg of 1 : 1000 solution SC, with a second dose administered at the site of a precipitating injection or insect sting.
      (2) Diphenhydramine, 1 to 2 mg/kg IV, IM, or PO q6h for at least 48 hours.
      (3) Corticosteroids, 1 to 2 mg/kg prednisone or equivalent qd for 24 to 48 hours.
      (4) See Chapter 7 for treatment of bronchospasm (p. 228), airway obstruction (p. 225), and anaphylactic shock (p. 223).
    c. Prophylaxis. To prevent recurrence, cautious avoidance of the specific allergen implicated in the original episode is mandatory.

Table 16-1. Major causes of anaphylaxis or anaphylactoid reactions

Antibiotics
  Penicillin, cephalosporins, tetracycline, streptomycin, and others
Biologicals
  Insect venoms, allergen extracts, gamma globulin, blood transfusions, antitoxins, antilymphocyte globulin, hormones, asparaginase, and others
Diagnostic agents
  Iodinated contrast media
Other drugs
  Aspirin, dextran plasma expanders
Foods
  Shellfish, peanuts, nuts, eggs, milk, fish, soy

---

(1) Epinephrine kits (e.g., EpiPen) should be given to all patients with a history of anaphylaxis. In addition, these patients should wear **Medic Alert bracelets.**

(2) Insect venom **immunotherapy** should be considered for children with anaphylaxis precipitated by stinging insect venom. Venom immunotherapy is not indicated for patients with skin manifestations only.

(3) Radiocontrast materials should be avoided in patients with documented allergy. If contrast studies are absolutely required, pretreatment with diphenhydramine and corticosteroids is mandatory.

B. Asthma (for acute asthma, see also Chap. 7, p. 228ff)

1. Etiology. Asthma is reversible obstructive lung disease characterized by hyperreactivity and inflammation of the airways in response to various stimuli, resulting in recurrent episodes of wheezing and dyspnea. Table 16-2 lists precipitating factors.

2. Evaluation

a. History should be taken for recurrent episodes of cough, dyspnea, wheezing, exercise intolerance, or "bronchitis." Inciting factors should be identified. In the acutely wheezing child, the history should include duration of wheezing, probable precipitant, past medications, and severity of previous attacks.

b. Physical examination

(1) Chronic signs of **atopic predisposition:** edema of nasal mucosa, allergic "shiners," eczema.

Table 16-2. Factors that precipitate asthma

Infections
  Viral (respiratory syncytial virus, adenovirus, influenza, parainfluenza, rhinovirus)
  Mycoplasma
  Bacteria (bronchitis, sinusitis, rarely pneumonia)
Allergens
  Seasonal pollens, animals, dust mites, molds
Irritants
  Smoke, solvents, air pollutants (ozone, sulfur dioxide, metabisulfite), cold air
Exercise
  In particular, running sports; seen less with swimming
Aspirin
  Prostaglandin-mediated, all nonsteroidal anti-inflammatory agents may have similar effect; nasal polyps may be present in aspirin triad (asthma, aspirin intolerance, and nasal polyps)

(2) If clubbing, increased anteroposterior chest diameter, recurrent sinusitis, or failure to thrive, consider underlying cystic fibrosis or immunodeficiency.

(3) Acute assessment: vital signs, breath sounds, peak flow, pulsus paradoxus, mental status (somnolence or agitation suggests hypoxia), retractions, use of accessory muscles.

  c. Laboratory data

    (1) Pulse oximetry to monitor oxygen saturation.

    (2) Arterial blood gases.

    (3) Complete blood count. Eosinophilia suggests an extrinsic precipitant.

    (4) Radiologic evaluation

      (a) Chest x-ray to rule out foreign body aspiration, congestive heart failure, pneumonia, pneumothorax.

      (b) Consider barium swallow, sinus films, and sinus CT scan if clinically indicated.

    (5) Allergy testing

      (a) Skin or RAST tests, or both, may identify precipitating allergens.

      (b) Elevated **IgE** levels suggest allergic disease.

    (6) Tuberculin skin testing if chronic cough or if steroid therapy is considered.

    (7) Pulmonary function testing in children over 5 years

      (a) To determine severity of acute exacerbations.

      (b) To assess reversible airway obstruction in patients.

      (c) To monitor patients with chronic condition and to titrate medications.

3. Diagnosis is based on the composite clinical picture and recurrent nature of symptoms.

4. Therapy. The goals of therapy are to reverse acute bronchospasm and minimize chronic symptoms. Individualized treatment has three components: avoidance of precipitants, prophylaxis against exacerbations, and titration of medications according to symptoms.

  a. Environmental control measures

    (1) Avoid nonspecific respiratory irritants: cigarette smoke, wood/coal smoke, paint, aerosolized agents, air pollution.

    (2) Control dust/mite exposure.

      (a) Encase mattress, boxspring, and pillows in airtight plastic covers.

      (b) Wash bedding in hot water weekly.

      (c) Remove dust collectors: furry toys, drapes, upholstered furniture, carpeting.

      (d) Use tannic acid solution or benzyl benzoate powder to denature mite allergens in carpeting and upholstered furniture.

      (e) Dust weekly with a damp cloth.

    (3) Remove pets from the bedroom and preferably from the house.

    (4) Use air conditioning to reduce indoor pollen.

  b. Pharmacologic agents include selective beta-2–adrenergic agents, theophylline, cromolyn, and corticosteroids. These agents are discussed individually below, and their use in acute and chronic asthma is reviewed.

    (1) Selective beta-2 agents are the mainstay of adrenergic therapy (Table 16-3). They act rapidly, have limited side effects (primarily tremor, agitation, tachycardia), have long duration of action, and can be administered orally or by inhalation. Inhaled beta agents are especially effective in exercise-induced asthma. Metered-dose inhalers used with a spacer device are suitable for children over 4 to 5 years of age (e.g., InspirEase, AeroChamber). In younger children, albuterol can be administered by nebulizer. Oral and inhaled beta agents can be

Table 16-3. Some beta-2 selective agents

Name	Forms available	Dose
Albuterol (Proventil, Ventolin)	Liquid, 2 mg/tsp Tablets, 2 or 4 mg Repetabs, 4 mg (long-acting, Proventil)	0.1 mg/kg/dose up to 4 mg tid
	Nebulizer solution, 0.5%	0.25–0.5 ml with saline or cromolyn tid–qid
	Nebulizer solution, 0.83% Metered-dose inhaler Rotohaler (Ventolin)	3 ml (one-unit dose) tid–qid 2 puffs tid–qid 1–2 capsules tid–qid
Pirbuterol (Maxair)	Metered-dose inhaler or autohaler	2 puffs tid–qid

used simultaneously for enhanced effect, although side effects are more frequent.

(2) **Cromolyn and nedocromil** sodium (Tilade) stabilize mast cells for prophylaxis of chronic asthma. They inhibit both early and late asthmatic responses. Cromolyn is available in nebulizer and inhaler forms. Nedocromil comes as an inhaler only; it has not yet been approved for children less than 12 years old. Cromolyn is a safe medication with few side effects. Nebulized cromolyn does not irritate the airway, and can be given in the face of acute wheezing. It is particularly effective in allergen-induced asthma, as well as in exercise-induced asthma.

(3) **Corticosteroids** decrease airway hyperreactivity and inflammation.

    (a) Short-term use of oral or IV steroids is indicated for severe acute exacerbations. Prednisone (or equivalent), 1 to 2 mg/kg/day divided bid–qid, is given for 3 days, followed by tapered doses over the next 3 to 4 days.

    (b) Long-term steroid therapy may be necessary; tapering to an alternate-day regimen substantially reduces side effects. Alternatively, inhaled steroids (**beclomethasone** dipropionate [Beclovent, Vanceril], **triamcinolone** acetonide [Azmacort], and **flunisolide** [Aerobid]), administered as two to four puffs bid–qid, serve as effective maintenance therapy. Side effects are minimal in recommended doses. Major complications are oral candidiasis and dysphonia, which can be prevented by the use of spacers and mouth rinse after inhalation. Rarely, beclomethasone can precipitate bronchospasm; in this case an alternate inhaled steroid should be prescribed.

(4) **Theophylline** is a bronchodilator with a narrow therapeutic window. Intravenous theophylline can be used for acute therapy; slow-release oral preparations (Table 16-4) are available for nocturnal asthma and chronic management. Dosages are given in Table 16-5.

    (a) Therapeutic blood levels range from 5 to 15 mg/ml, although significant bronchodilatation occurs at lower levels. Many factors alter metabolism (Table 16-6); serum levels should be monitored.

    (b) Dose-related side effects of theophylline include insomnia, poor concentration, agitation, abdominal pain, nausea, vomiting, headache, tremor, tachycardia, arrhythmia, and seizures. Side effects can occur at levels below the therapeutic range, especially with initial doses.

c. Treatment guidelines

Table 16-4. Some long-acting theophylline preparations

Trade name	How supplied	Dose interval
Slo-bid Gyrocaps	50-, 75-, 100-, 125-, 200-, 300-mg capsules	q8–12h
Theo-Dur	100-, 200-, 300-mg tablets	q8–12h
Slo-Phyllin Gyrocaps	60-, 125-, 250-mg capsules	q8h
Uniphyl	400-mg tablet	q24h
T-PHYL	200-mg tablet	q12h

(1) **Acute therapy**
  (a) Humidified oxygen
  (b) Adrenergic therapy
    (i) Nebulized albuterol, 0.1 to 0.15 mg/kg (maximum 5 mg) in 2 ml saline q20 min for 1 hour.
    (ii) If unable to generate peak flow or demonstrating decreased consciousness, epinephrine (1 : 1,000) 0.01 ml/kg to a maximum of 0.3 ml SC q20 min for three doses.
  (c) If symptoms improve substantially (peak expiratory flow rate >60% predicted), the patient can be discharged on oral bronchodilators with good follow-up. Patients already receiving bronchodilators should be placed on additional medications to prevent relapse. Treatment of the acute episode should continue for 5 to 7 days after symptoms have abated.
(2) **Status asthmaticus.** See Chapter 7 p. 228.
(3) **Intermittent therapy.** Beta-adrenergic agents can be used prn for infrequent, short episodes of wheezing.
  (a) Viral upper respiratory infections frequently prompt exacerbations. Wheezing can be treated prophylactically with oral or inhaled beta agents. Therapy should be continued for several days after symptoms resolve or peak flow normalizes.
  (b) Exercise-induced wheezing is minimized by inhalation of albuterol or cromolyn 10 to 20 minutes before activity.
(4) **Chronic therapy. Anti-inflammatory** therapy benefits patients with moderate to severe asthma.
  (a) Treat **moderate asthma** (>2 wheezing episodes/wk) with inhaled cromolyn or nedocromil and beta agents prn.
  (b) Treat **severe asthma** with inhaled corticosteroids +/−theophylline, long-acting beta agents, or oral prednisone. Rule out complicating factors, such as sinusitis.
    For further information on asthma management, the reader should see the National Heart, Lung, and Blood Institute (NHLBI) National Asthma Education Program's *Guidelines for the Diagnosis and Management of Asthma.*

Table 16-5. Theophylline dosing according to age

Age (yr)	Total daily dose (mg/kg/24 hr)
1–9	20
9–12	18
12–16	15
Adults	13 (or 600–900 mg/d)

Table 16-6. Factors that affect theophylline half-life

Decreased clearance
  Old age
  Very young age (<1 yr)
  Hepatic failure
  Viral illness
  Fever
  Cimetidine and ranitidine
  Erythromycin, clindamycin, clarithromycin, ciprofloxacin
Increased clearance
  Young age (toddlers, school age)
  Cigarette smoking
  IV isoproterenol
  Phenobarbital, phenytoin, carbamazepine (Tegretol)
  High-protein diet

C. Allergic rhinoconjunctivitis
  1. Etiology. Allergic rhinoconjunctivitis is a symptom complex caused by IgE-mediated reactions to environmental allergens.
  2. Evaluation
    a. History. The family history is often positive for allergies. Patients should be asked about paroxysms of sneezing, clear rhinorrhea, nasal pruritus, and improvement on antihistamines. History may correlate symptoms with allergen exposure, though reactions may occur days later.
    b. Physical examination: allergic "shiners," transverse nasal crease, Dennie's lines. Nasal polyps may be seen; if present consider cystic fibrosis.
    c. Laboratory studies include blood and nasal secretions for increased eosinophils, serum IgE, skin testing, RAST.
  3. Diagnosis is based on the clinical picture; skin and RAST testing may be confirmative.
  4. Treatment
    a. Avoidance of allergens and irritants (see p. 462).
    b. Pharmacologic agents—allergic rhinitis
      (1) Antihistamines (H_1 antagonists) are most effective for rhinorrhea and sneezing. Prophylactic use before exposure is optimal. Side effects include mild anticholinergic symptoms and somnolence (except with terfenadine [Seldane], astemizole [Hismanal], and loratidine [Claritin], which are nonsedating and approved for patients over 12 years). Multiple formulations exist, many in combination with decongestants.
      (2) Adrenergic drugs
        (a) Local vasoconstrictors (e.g., Afrin) are effective in decreasing nasal congestion. These should not be used for more than 3 days, to avoid rebound edema (rhinitis medicamentosa).
        (b) Oral adrenergic agents (e.g., pseudoephedrine) are also effective in decreasing nasal congestion and can be used alone or in combination with antihistamines.
      (3) Cromolyn is available for use as a nasal spray (Nasalcrom), two puffs tid–qid.
      (4) Topical steroid nasal sprays (e.g., beclomethasone [Beconase AQ, Vancenase AQ], flunisolide [Nasalide], triamcinolone [Nasacort], budesonide [Rhinocort], and fluticasone [Flonase]) are effective for treatment of allergic rhinitis. Side effects include transient nasal irritation and sneezing. Adrenal suppression has never been reported, even with continuous long-term use of these medications.

   c. Pharmacologic agents–allergic conjunctivitis

     (1) An ophthalmic preparation **(Naphcon-A)** with pheniramine maleate (an antihistamine) and naphazoline (a vasoconstrictor) is helpful for short-term treatment at dosages of 1 to 2 gtt q3–4hr prn. Alternatively, **levocabastine HCl (Livostin)** is a new antihistamine (1 gt bid–qid). Both agents can cause transient stinging.

     (2) Lodoxamide tromethamine ophthalmic solution (Alomide 0.1%) is a mast cell stabilizer approved for vernal conjunctivitis; dosage is 1 to 2 gtt qid for up to 3 months.

     (3) Ketorolac tromethamine (Acular) is a nonsteroidal anti-inflammatory drug (NSAID) approved for seasonal allergic conjunctivitis; dosage is 1 gt qid. Ocular irritation can occur.

   d. Immunotherapy should be considered for allergic rhinoconjunctivitis that is unresponsive to medical therapy.

D. Serum sickness is a vasculitic process that results from vascular deposition of circulating antigen-antibody complexes and secondary complement activation.

   1. Etiologies include drugs, heterologous serum proteins, viral agents.

   2. Evaluation

     a. History and physical examination. The symptom complex occurs 7 to 14 days after exposure to the offending agent and can persist for weeks. It includes fever, urticaria, angioedema, lymphadenopathy, splenomegaly, and arthralgia or arthritis. Less commonly vasculitis causes GI, CNS, pulmonary, and renal symptoms.

     b. Laboratory findings

       (1) Complete blood count may show leukocytosis, leukopenia, or eosinophilia. The erythrocyte sedimentation rate (ESR) is usually elevated.

       (2) Urinalysis rarely reveals proteinuria, microscopic hematuria, and hyaline casts.

       (3) Immune studies are notable for decreased serum complement (C3 and CH50), elevated acute-phase reactants, elevated IgG levels, and occasionally circulating immune complexes.

   3. Diagnosis. Serum sickness is a clinical diagnosis.

   4. Treatment. Most cases of serum sickness are mild and resolve spontaneously within a few days to 2 weeks after the elimination of the offending agent. Pharmacologic therapy is indicated for severe cases.

     a. Antihistamines. Diphenhydramine (Benadryl) and hydroxyzine (Atarax) are useful for symptomatic relief of urticaria and pruritus.

     b. Nonsteroidal anti-inflammatory agents such as **ibuprofen** and **aspirin** reduce fever and alleviate joint symptoms.

     c. Corticosteroid therapy should be reserved for patients with major organ system involvement. Prednisone, 1 to 2 mg/kg/day, should be initiated in divided doses, with tapering after clinical improvement and discontinuation after 10 to 14 days.

     d. Epinephrine will transiently improve acute urticaria, wheezing, and laryngeal edema.

E. Urticaria. Acute urticaria is common, with slightly higher incidence in atopic individuals. It rarely develops into **chronic urticaria** (>6 wk duration).

   1. Etiology

     a. Mechanism. Urticaria is caused by release of chemical mediators of immediate hypersensitivity. It can be mediated by IgE, complement, or direct mast cell release.

     b. Specific agents are listed in Table 16-7. Often the cause cannot be identified.

   2. Evaluation. Urticaria consists of blanchable, erythematous, pruritic papules. Urticaria and angioedema frequently coexist. Duration varies greatly; chronic urticaria should prompt investigation for underlying disorders (Table 16-8).

   3. Therapy. Known precipitants should be avoided, as should factors that non-

Table 16-7. Etiology of urticaria and angioedema

Allergic
  Ingested allergens (foods, drugs)
  Injected allergenic drugs (e.g., penicillin, biologicals)
  Inhaled allergens (e.g., cat, pollens, latex)
Complement mediated
  Serum sickness (drugs, infections)
  Vasculitis (systemic lupus erythematosus or other systemic rheumatic disease)
  Urticarial vasculitis (not associated with systemic disease)
  Infections (hepatitis B, Epstein-Barr virus, parasites)
Direct mast cell–releasing agents
  Drugs (e.g., opiates, curare, hyperosmolar solutions)
  Radiocontrast media
Agents that affect arachidonic acid metabolism
  Nonsteroidal anti-inflammatory agents (aspirin)
  Angiotensin-converting enzyme inhibitors
Exercise-induced anaphylaxis
Physical causes
  Dermatographism
  Cold
  Pressure
  Vibration
  Heat
  Solar
  Aquagenic
  Cholinergic
Neoplasms
Endocrine related (thyroid disorders with antithyroid antibodies)
Psychogenic
Idiopathic
Hereditary angioedema (urticaria does not occur)

specifically enhance urticaria and angioedema, such as NSAIDs, alcohol, heat, and tight clothing.

  a. Antihistamines. Urticaria is best controlled by round-the-clock antihistamine therapy. Dosages should be increased slowly, to tolerance or until symptoms are controlled. No agent is clearly more efficacious than the others. Hydroxyzine is used commonly; cyproheptadine (Periactin) may be better for cold-induced urticaria. Combining H_1 antihistamines can increase both therapeutic effect and side effects. Addition of an H_2 antihistamine may be beneficial.

  b. Corticosteroids. There is no role for topical steroid therapy in this condition; rarely, systemic corticosteroid treatment can be considered.

F. Atopic dermatitis (AD) is a chronic, relapsing eczematous dermatitis (see also p. 478).

  1. Etiology. Atopic dermatitis can result from type I and type IV hypersensitivity reactions, impaired IgE regulation, increased phosphodiesterase, impaired macrophage function, and increased mast cell degranulation.

  2. Evaluation

    a. The major features include (1) pruritus, (2) typical morphology and distribution, (3) chronic or chronically relapsing course, and (4) personal or family history of atopy. Acute lesions are red, edematous, and vesiculated. Chronic lesions become eczematous, lichenified, and plaque-like. Affected

Table 16-8. Urticaria and angioedema: laboratory evaluation

Suspected cause	Procedures
(General screening)	(CBC, urinalysis, chemical profile)
Vasculitis or complement related	Sedimentation rate, immunoglobulin analysis, antinuclear factor, quantitative complement (C3, C4, C1 inhibitor, CH50), skin biopsy
Infections	Culture, stool for ova and parasites, hepatitis-associated antigen, x-rays (sinuses)
Allergic	Eosinophil count, IgE, skin testing and/or RAST for suspected allergen
Physical	
Cholinergic	Mecholyl test/stress induced
Dermatographism	Firm stroking of skin
Cold	Ice-cube application, cryoglobulins, cryofibrinogens, VDRL
Solar	Light exposure
Heat	Warm-water immersion
Hereditary angioedema and acquired angioedema with lymphoma and other neoplasms	C1 inhibitor, C1, CH50, C4, C2

sites vary with age: Infants have involvement of face and extensor surfaces; older children have involvement of flexor surfaces, neck, and trunk.
  b. **Triggers** include irritants (wool, acrylic, perfume, cosmetics, soap, cleaning agents, alcohol, sand, tobacco smoke, citrus fruits), dry skin, infections, allergens, perspiration, temperature changes, illness, fatigue, and emotional stress.
  c. **Defective cell-mediated immunity** (up to 80% of patients) can result in increased susceptibility to viral and dermatophyte skin infections, and decreased responsiveness to delayed-type hypersensitivity skin testing.
  d. **Suspected food allergies should be evaluated by double-blind placebo-controlled food challenges or elimination diets;** skin testing may yield false-positive results.
3. **Diagnosis.** Atopic dermatitis is a clinical diagnosis.
4. **Treatment**
  a. **Trigger factors** should be avoided (see above).
  b. **Moisturizers** are first-line topical therapy, reducing dry itchy skin. Petroleum products are best; unscented skin creams can also be effective. Moisturizers should be applied to damp skin immediately after a tepid bath with mild soap.
  c. **Tar preparations** (in the bath or topically) may have beneficial antipruritic, disinfectant, anti-inflammatory, and/or desquamating effects.
  d. **Infections** should be treated with appropriate antibiotics or antiviral agents.
  e. **Emotional stress** can exacerbate atopic dermatitis; stress management techniques are often helpful.
  f. **Topical steroids** should be used in conjunction with other forms of therapy, especially emollients. For acute flares, potent topical steroids (e.g., difluorinated or the fluorochlorinated preparations) should be used for 7 to 10 days, followed by a midpotency topical steroid for 2 to 3 weeks until lesions have resolved. Severely affected patients may require chronic use of a low-potency topical steroid in conjunction with lubricants. Fluorinated steroids should *not* be used in infants, or chronically applied to the face, genitals, axillae, inguinal region, or skin folds. **Excessive or prolonged**

use of high-potency topical steroids can lead to local atrophy. Long-term application of steroids around the eyes or on the eyelids can lead to the development of glaucoma or cataracts. Significant systemic absorption can occur.

    g. Antihistamines (e.g., hydroxyzine or diphenhydramine) can help control itching at night. Topical antihistamines should be avoided because of low efficacy and the possibility of skin sensitization.

II. Immunodeficiency disorders

A. Etiology. The immune system can be divided into four components.

    1. Humoral system (B lymphocytes).

    2. T-lymphocyte system.

    3. Phagocytic system.

    4. Complement system. Abnormalities can involve one or more of these, resulting in a predisposition to recurrent infections.

B. Evaluation

    1. Increased frequency, duration, or severity of infection suggests underlying immunodeficiency, as does infection with unusual or opportunistic organisms.

        a. Normal children may have up to six respiratory infections per year.

        b. Chronic candidiasis, bronchiectasis, ear drainage, hearing loss, conjunctivitis, cough, or diarrhea may be a sign of immunodeficiency.

    2. Abnormal **humoral immunity** results in defective opsonization and phagocytosis of **pneumococcus** or *Haemophilus influenzae,* causing recurrent pyogenic infections (otitis, sinusitis, pneumonia, and meningitis).

        a. Early complement components (C1, C4, C2, and C3) interact with antibody-coated bacteria, promoting clearance by phagocytic cells. Absence of specific antibody markedly reduces ingestion and destruction of pathogens.

        b. Maternal IgG crosses the placenta and protects newborns for 3 to 4 months. *De novo* IgG and IgM synthesis begins as maternal IgG declines (Fig. 16-1). As a result, in children with isolated antibody deficiency infections first develop at 4 to 6 months. Adult levels of IgG, IgM, and IgA are normally present by 5 years.

    3. Abnormal **T-cell immunity** results in increased susceptibility to fungal, viral, and opportunistic infections.

    4. History will generally distinguish primary and secondary immunodeficiency disorders.

        a. Primary immunodeficiencies include

            (1) Antibody deficiency

                (a) X-linked agammaglobulinemia (XLA).

                (b) Common variable immunodeficiency.

                (c) Selective IgA deficiency.

                (d) Transient hypogammaglobulinemia of infancy.

                (e) Selective IgG subclass deficiency.

            (2) T-cell deficiency

                (a) Di George's syndrome.

                (b) Chronic mucocutaneous candidiasis.

            (3) Combined T-/B-cell deficiency

                (a) Severe combined immunodeficiency disease (SCID).

                (b) Wiskott-Aldrich syndrome.

                (c) Ataxia-telangiectasia.

                (d) Hyper-IgE syndrome.

                (e) Ommen's syndrome.

            (4) Phagocytic disorders.

            (5) Complement deficiency.

        b. Secondary immunodeficiencies may be associated with

            (1) Viral infections: human immunodeficiency virus (HIV), measles, rubeola, Epstein-Barr, cytomegalovirus (CMV).

            (2) Metabolic disorders: malnutrition, uremia, diabetes.

            (3) Protein-losing states: nephrotic syndrome, protein-losing enteropathy.

            (4) Pharmacologic immunosuppression, splenectomy.

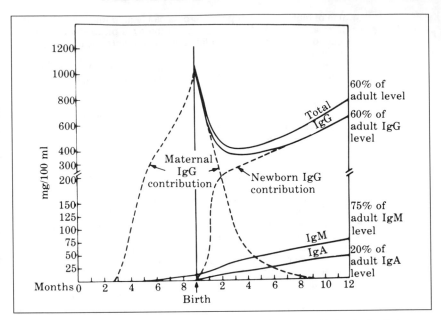

Fig. 16-1. Immunoglobulin (IgG, IgM, and IgA) levels in the fetus and infant in the first year of life. The IgG of the fetus and newborn infant is solely of maternal origin. The maternal IgG disappears by the age of 9 months, by which time the endogenous synthesis of IgG by the infant is well established. The IgM and IgA of the neonate are entirely endogenously synthesized because maternal IgM and IgA do *not* cross the placenta. (From ER Stiehm, VA Fulginiti. *Immunologic Disorders in Infants and Children.* Philadelphia: Saunders, 1973.)

> (5) Malignancy.
> (6) Prematurity.
> 5. **Physical examination** includes lymphoid tissues (tonsils, lymph nodes, spleen), skin (eczema, candidiasis, telangiectasia, or petechiae), and state of nutrition (failure to thrive, evidence of malabsorption).
> 6. **Laboratory evaluation** should be used to confirm clinical suspicion.
>> a. **Screening tests** include CBC with differential and ESR. Lymphopenia is suggestive of a T-cell disorder. Thrombocytopenia with small platelets suggests Wiskott-Aldrich syndrome. Test for cystic fibrosis and HIV infection when appropriate.
>> b. **B-cell function** varies with age, and results must be interpreted accordingly.
>>> (1) **Total immunoglobulin levels (IgG, IgM, IgA, IgE)** may be elevated in chronic granulomatous disease (CGD), immotile cilia syndrome, and HIV infection. Low IgG level accompanied by low serum albumin suggests nonspecific loss of serum proteins.
>>> (2) Normal levels of **specific antibody** to tetanus, diphtheria toxoid, measles, rubella, polio, *H. influenzae* type b, pneumococcus, and/or normal isohemagglutinins rule out severe B-cell dysfunction.
>>> (3) **Immunoglobulin G subclass levels** may be abnormal in children with recurrent sinopulmonary infections.
>>> (4) Absence of **B-cells** suggests XLA.
>> c. **Tests for T-cell function**
>>> (1) **Chest x-ray** to confirm presence of thymus.
>>> (2) **Delayed skin tests** to tetanus toxoid, diphtheria toxoid, and *Can-*

dida normally produce induration at 48 to 72 hours. Positive skin tests rule out serious T-cell deficiency. Negative tests are seen in 10 to 30% of normal individuals, and in patients receiving daily steroids. Such patients can be boosted with tetanus toxoid and retested 7 days later.

(3) **T-cell subsets** show abnormal CD4/CD8 ratios in patients with AIDS and other disorders of immunoregulation. T-cells are absent in SCID.

d. **Tests for complement** include CH50 and determination of individual components. C4 levels are invariably reduced in hereditary angioneurotic edema (HANE); C2 levels are reduced in acute attacks. The diagnosis of HANE is confirmed by determination of C1 inhibitor level.

e. **Tests for phagocytic function** include nitroblue tetrazolium test, Rebuck skin window, spleen scan, bone marrow aspiration, phenotyping for CD11, and assay for antineutrophil antibodies.

C. **Treatment of specific disorders**
  1. **General measures**
    a. **Avoid administration of live virus vaccines, especially in children with suspected T-cell deficiencies or X-linked agammaglobulinemia.**
    b. **Transfuse T-cell–deficient patients with irradiated blood products to avoid potentially lethal graft-versus-host disease.**
  2. **Antibody deficiency**
    a. **Diagnosis**
      (1) **X-linked agammaglobulinemia** presents with recurrent respiratory infections in 6- to 12-month old boys. Affected children have no peripheral B cells and make negligible amounts of immunoglobulin. The diagnosis can be made at birth by demonstrating the absence of B-cells in cord blood.
      (2) **Common variable agammaglobulinemia** affects children of both sexes. B cells are present but incapable of producing and/or secreting normal antibody.
      (3) **Immunoglobulin A deficiency** is characterized by IgA levels less than 5 mg/dl, with normal levels of IgG and IgM and normal antibody responses. Lack of secretory IgA can result in sinopulmonary infections, diarrhea, and/or malabsorption, but most IgA-deficient individuals are asymptomatic. IgG$_2$ subclass deficiency may also be present.
      (4) **Transient hypogammaglobulinemia of infancy** results from a delay in the developmental onset of immunoglobulin synthesis. Immunoglobulin G levels are low (often <200 mg/dl), and IgM and IgA may be normal or low. In the window between disappearance of maternal IgG and the onset of de novo synthesis (6–18 months), these children have little antibody protection and suffer from recurrent bacterial infections. Wheezing, cough, and diarrhea are common. Response to vaccinations is usually normal.
      (5) **Immunoglobulin G subclass deficiency** results in recurrent infections similar to those seen in individuals who lack IgG. Patients may have normal total IgG levels but marked reduction in IgG$_2$ or IgG$_3$, or both, subclasses. They respond normally to protein antigens but not to polysaccharides (e.g., pneumococcus, *H. influenzae* type b). Low IgG$_2$ subclass levels in children less than 2 years old preclude diagnosis in this age group.
    b. **Therapy**
      (1) Prophylactic antibiotics effective against probable pathogens help reduce the frequency of bacterial infections. They can be administered continuously or during periods of increased risk, in reduced or full therapeutic dosage. Side effects include allergies, diarrhea, pseudomembranous colitis, and development of bacterial resistance.
      (2) Documented infections should be treated aggressively. Bronchiectasis should be managed with physical therapy, postural drainage, and antibiotics. Malabsorption and diarrhea should be treated with di-

etary restriction and metronidazole if *Giardia* infestation is demonstrated.

(3) Children with recurrent otitis media require audiologic evaluation to identify hearing difficulties that can lead to impaired speech development.

(4) Replacement gamma globulin is highly effective in reducing the frequency of infection in antibody-deficiency states. Patients with X-linked agammaglobulinemia and common variable agammaglobulinemia require lifelong therapy with IV gamma globulin (IVGG). IVGG is occasionally required for other antibody-deficiency disorders.

(a) Intravenous gamma globulin (Iveegam, Gamimune-N, Sandoglobulin, Gammagard, Venoglobulin-S) can be used to administer large quantities of IgG (e.g., 400–500 mg/kg q3–4 wk). Trough IgG levels should be greater than 600 mg/dl. Some patients may require larger, more frequent doses of IVGG to prevent infections. Reactions (fever, chills, nausea) are managed by decreasing the infusion rate and pretreating with acetaminophen or aspirin and diphenhydramine.

(b) In patients with IgA deficiency, anaphylactic reactions to IVGG occasionally develop. Gammagard SD, which has no IgA, can be safely administered to these patients.

(c) Immune serum globulin (ISG) is administered IM, with a loading dose of 1.8 ml/kg and maintenance doses of 0.6 ml/kg every 3 to 4 weeks. Immune serum globulin is rarely given, because IVGG provides higher IgG levels and is less painful.

3. T-lymphocyte defects

a. Diagnosis

(1) Congenital thymic aplasia (Di George's syndrome) is due to an error in embryogenesis that leads to absence of thymus and parathyroids, cardiac defects, and characteristic facies. Patients have neonatal tetany (hypocalcemia), heart murmurs, and no thymic shadow on chest films. T-cell number and function are diminished.

(2) Mucocutaneous candidiasis involves recurrent *Candida albicans* infections of fingernails, toenails, mouth, and vagina. Patients may have antibody deficiency disorders or autoimmune destruction of adrenal and thyroid glands, or both, leading to Addison's disease and hypothyroidism.

(3) Miscellaneous disorders. Malnutrition, immunosuppressive drugs, and lymphocyte loss can result in T-cell dysfunction.

b. Therapy

(1) Di George's syndrome. Most children have a partial defect and gradually acquire T-cell function without treatment. Transplantation of fetal thymic tissue corrects the immune defect, although this is rarely done. Irradiate all blood products (see Chap. 15) and avoid live viral vaccines until normal T-cell function is demonstrated.

(2) Mucocutaneous candidiasis. Prophylaxis with oral antifungals such as fluconazole is the therapy of choice. Associated endocrinopathies must be treated.

4. Combined immunodeficiency

a. Diagnosis

(1) Severe combined immunodeficiency may be inherited as an X-linked or autosomal recessive disorder. Autosomal forms may be associated with deficiency of purine degradation enzymes **adenosine deaminase (ADA)** or **purine nucleoside phosphorylase (PNP)**. Affected infants lack normal lymphoid stem cells and show defects in both B-cell and T-cell immunity. A clinical triad of candidiasis, diarrhea, and pneumonitis develops after 2 to 3 months of life.

(a) Laboratory tests document low immunoglobulin levels, absent antibody responses, and few circulating T-cells. Adenosine deaminase should be assayed in red cells. Prenatal diagnosis of ADA deficiency can be made by measuring enzyme activity in cultured amniotic fibroblasts.

   (b) Bony abnormalities of the rib cage, pelvis, and spine may be seen in ADA deficiency.

   (c) Consider graft-versus-host reactions (from nonirradiated blood products and/or maternofetal transfusion) in patients with skin rash, diarrhea, hepatosplenomegaly, and failure to thrive.

(2) Wiskott-Aldrich syndrome (WAS) is an X-linked disorder characterized by eczema, thrombocytopenia, and decreased T-cell function. Bleeding and infection are potentially lethal complications.

(3) Ataxia-telangiectasia (AT) is characterized by ataxia, choreoathetosis, dysarthric speech, telangiectasias, recurrent sinopulmonary infections, IgA deficiency, and abnormal T-cell function. Alpha fetoprotein is often elevated.

(4) Hyper-IgE syndrome. These patients have elevated serum IgE and recurrent pyogenic infections, particularly *Staphylococcus aureus* skin abscesses. Antibody responses and T-cell proliferation to antigens are defective.

(5) Ommen's syndrome is a variant of SCID characterized by recurrent bacterial and fungal infections, hypereosinophilia, diffuse erythroderma, protracted diarrhea, failure to thrive, and hepatosplenomegaly. Lymphocyte populations are normal in number but oligoclonal.

b. Therapy

(1) Bone marrow transplantation is the mainstay of treatment for severe immunodeficiency syndromes (SCID, Ommen's syndrome, WAS). Bone marrow is harvested from a histocompatible donor and infused into the patient. Residual immune function in the recipient can be ablated before transplant to foster engraftment. Complications of bone marrow transplantation include **graft-versus-host disease** and infection.

(2) Complications of WAS may be diminished by splenectomy (to increase platelet survival) and prophylactic antibiotics (trimethoprim-sulfamethoxazole [Bactrim]or ampicillin). Meticulous care of eczema is mandatory.

(3) Acute infections should be treated aggressively with antibiotics. Opportunistic pathogens should be considered, in addition to standard infectious agents. *Pneumocystis carinii* pneumonia should be treated with trimethoprim-sulfamethoxazole or pentamidine (see Chap. 5).

(4) All patients with combined immunodeficiency should receive IVGG therapy antibody replacement (see p. 472).

(5) Siblings of known patients should be isolated at birth and screened for SCID.

5. Disorders of phagocytic function and complement

a. Granulocyte disorders (see Chap. 15, pp. 452–454).

b. Complement abnormalities

(1) C1 deficiency is associated with a lupus-like syndrome and susceptibility to bacterial infection.

(2) C2 deficiency is associated with anaphylactoid purpura and systemic lupus erythematosus (SLE).

(3) C3 deficiency and C3b inactivator deficiency are associated with recurrent pyogenic infections that mimic those seen in hypogammaglobulinemia. These conditions can be congenital or acquired.

(4) C4 deficiency is associated with SLE.

(5) Deficiencies of **C5, C6, C7,** and **C8** are associated with recurrent *Neisseria* infections.

(6) Therapy consists of appropriate antibiotics for infections.

c. **Splenic dysfunction.** Much of the body's phagocytic capability resides in the spleen. Splenic hypofunction increases susceptibility to bacterial infection, particularly with respiratory organisms.

    (1) Etiology

        (a) The spleen may be congenitally absent, surgically removed, or physiologically impaired (as in sickle cell disease).

        (b) Patients who undergo splenectomy before age 2 have defective processing of capsular polysaccharide antigens, predisposing to infections with pneumococcus and *H. influenzae*.

    (2) Therapy

        (a) Antibiotics are indicated for all suspected and documented infections. Because of the risk of overwhelming sepsis in asplenic patients, IV antibiotics should be started before final culture results are available.

        (b) Prevention of infections

            (i) Oral **penicillin,** 200,000 units bid, or ampicillin, 250 mg bid, should be prescribed for prophylaxis.

            (ii) Parents and patients should be educated about the risk of life-threatening sepsis and the need to seek immediate medical attention at the first sign of infection. If prompt medical attention may not be available, patients should be supplied with oral antibiotics to take if infection is suspected.

            (iii) When feasible, patients should be immunized against encapsulated pathogens before splenectomy or loss of splenic function. Conjugated vaccines are preferable.

6. Hereditary angioneurotic edema (HANE)

    a. Etiology. HANE is an autosomal dominant disorder characterized by deficiency of C1 esterase inhibitor activity. Unopposed C1 activation results in consumption of C4 and C2, and release of a vasoactive peptide that causes subcutaneous and submucosal edema.

    b. Evaluation. Intermittent episodes of nonpruritic edema of the skin, extremities, or face result from minor trauma or emotional stress. Swelling may involve mucous membranes of the upper airway, causing **laryngeal obstruction and asphyxiation.** Abdominal pain, vomiting, or diarrhea can result from edema of the intestinal wall in the absence of skin manifestations. Urticaria does not occur.

    c. Diagnosis. Most patients have decreased levels of C1 esterase inhibitor; some have a normal level of nonfunctional protein. In both groups, C4 levels are low and fall during attacks.

    d. Therapy

        (1) Laryngeal obstruction is the major complication of acute attacks; patients should be instructed to seek immediate medical attention if hoarseness, voice change, or difficulty in breathing or swallowing occurs. **Tracheotomy** may be necessary. *Epinephrine and hydrocortisone are of little benefit,* in contrast to anaphylaxis.

        (2) Administration of purified C1 esterase inhibitor is useful in acute attacks.

        (3) Androgens increase inhibitor. Routine use of danazol, 50 to 600 mg/day, or stanozolol, 2 to 24 mg/day, markedly decreases the frequency and severity of attacks.

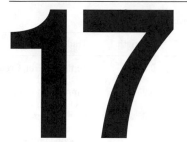

Dermatologic Disorders

Stephen Gellis and Sonja Krejci

I. General principles

A. Topical steroids of varying potencies and preparations are useful for controlling inflammation (see Table 17-1).

   1. The choice of a particular steroid is a function of the location and type of eruption, the age of the patient, and the duration of the planned treatment.

   2. Skin atrophy can occur when strong preparations are used on the face, groin, axillae, and areas of thin skin.

   3. Use of potent topical steroids over large surface areas can potentially produce adrenal suppression, particularly in small infants.

   4. An eruption that is acute and self-limited (acute contact dermatitis) can be safely treated with a potent topical steroid for 1 to 2 weeks.

   5. A chronic condition such as atopic dermatitis can be best managed by maintenance with a low- or medium-potency steroid with occasional use of a stronger preparation.

   6. Topical steroid vehicle preparations

   a. Ointments. Though greasier, ointments are more occlusive and produce greater potency that an equivalent strength in a cream form. They may be more effective in treating thick lesions.

   b. Creams and lotions may have an alcohol base, leading to irritation on application and drying.

   c. Solutions and gels are clear and nonoily, making them cosmetically acceptable when applied to the scalp.

B. Antihistamines. Systemic antihistamines are useful for control of intense pruritus.

   1. Often significant sedation is required in order to achieve the antipruritic effect.

   2. Topical antihistamines should not be utilized, as they are frequently responsible for toxic reactions.

C. Dressings

   1. Wet dressings are useful to suppress pruritus, dry moist and oozing lesions, and remove crusts. Towels, washcloths, strips of old sheets, or gauze rolls (Kerlix) can be used. These will allow evaporation and cool and soothe inflamed skin.

   a. An acceptable saline solution can be made by adding one teaspoon of salt per pint of water.

   b. Aluminum acetate (Burow's solution) can be prepared by dissolving one tablet or packet of Domeboro or Bluboro in a pint of water.

II. Specific disorders

A. Acne is a disorder of the pilosebaceous unit (follicle and associated sebaceous gland). It affects most people during their lives but is typically a disease of adolescents and young adults.

   1. Etiology. Sebum secretion by sebaceous glands is increased by androgenic hormones. Abnormal keratinization of the follicular orifice results in keratin plugs. Bacterial hydrolases (*Propionibacterium acnes*) convert triglycerides in sebum to free fatty acids, which are retained, causing distention and eventual rupture of the follicular wall with an inflammatory response.

   2. Evaluation

   a. History includes information regarding **precipitating events,** such as

Table 17-1. Commonly used topical corticosteroids

Class	Potency	Chemical name	Strength	Trade name
I	High	Clobetasol propionate	0.05%	Temovate Gel, Cream, Ointment
		Betamethasone dipropionate (augmented)	0.05%	Diprolene Cream, Ointment
II	High	Fluocinonide	0.05%	Lidex Ointment, Cream, Gel
	High	Mometasone furoate	0.1%	Elocon Ointment
III	Medium	Triamcinolone	0.1%	Aristocort Ointment
		Fluocinonide	0.05%	Lidex-E Cream
		Betamethasone dipropionate	0.05%	Diprosone Cream
		Betamethasone valerate	0.1%	Valisone Ointment
IV	Medium	Hydrocortisone valerate	0.2%	Westcort Ointment
		Fluocinolone acetonide	0.025%	Synalar Ointment
V	Medium	Hydrocortisone butyrate	0.1%	Locoid Cream
		Fluocinolone acetonide	0.025%	Synalar Cream
		Hydrocortisone valerate	0.2%	Westcort Cream
VI	Weak	Alclometasone dipropionate	0.05%	Aclovate Cream, Ointment
		Desonide	0.05%	Tridesilon Creme
VII	Weak	Hydrocortisone	1.0% & 2.5%	Hytone Cream, Ointment

menses, emotional stress, or certain **medications,** including lithium, oral contraceptives (particularly those with a high progesterone component), corticosteroids, halogens, isoniazid, and phenytoin. Careful questioning about the use of **topical products** may disclose comedogenic agents (oil-based cleansing creams, moisturizers, make-up, or cover-up; hair sprays, gels, and pomades) or potentially irritating over-the-counter acne treatments. Information about **activities** or **hobbies** may explain frictional acne from sporting gear (helmets, shoulder pads, etc.) or reveal etiologic agents such as cutting greases or chlorinated hydrocarbons.

  b. **Physical examination** should focus on areas where sebaceous glands are most active, such as the face, upper chest, shoulders, back, and scalp.
3. **Diagnosis** of acne depends on finding lesions consisting of noninflammatory open comedones ("blackheads") and closed comedones ("whiteheads") and inflammatory papules, pustules, nodules, and cysts. The underlying skin may be shiny due to increased sebum production. Sequelae of acne may include scars ("ice-pick," crateriform, hypertrophic, and keloids) and pigmentary changes.
4. **Therapy.** Most over-the-counter products produce mild peeling of the skin. They usually contain one or a combination of ingredients: salicylic acid, sulfur, and benzoyl peroxide.
  a. **Comedolytic agents.** It is important to avoid concomitant use of abrasive products, harsh soaps, scrubs, and buff puffs, as these can contribute to increased skin irritation.
    (1) **Benzoyl peroxide gel** (available in 2.5, 5, or 10%). Begin therapy nightly with the mildest agent, then increase as tolerated to bid. Advance in strength as the patient's disease activity and irritant response dictate.
    (2) **Tretinoin** (Retin-A; available in cream: 0.025%, 0.05%, 0.1%; gel: 0.01%, 0.025%, and solution: 0.05%). Cream formulations are the least irritating; gel and solutions result in a higher risk of redness, burning, and excessive peeling. Tretinoin is used qhs and a small amount ("pea-sized") is applied to a dry face. It can be used every other evening and

increased to nightly as tolerated. Note that tretinoin can increase the likelihood of sunburn in certain individuals.

(3) **Topical antibiotics** can be used in conjunction with comedolytics for mild inflammatory acne. They should be applied at an alternate time of day since simultaneous use with comedolytics can make either ineffective.

    (a) Erythromycin (1.5–2%).

    (b) Clindamycin (1%).

    (c) Tetracycline—not advised for patients under 8 years.

    (d) Oral antibiotics. For moderate and severe inflammatory acne, systemic antibiotics may be needed.

        (i) Tetracycline is very effective against *P. acnes*. It is contraindicated in children under age 8 and in pregnant or lactating women. Initial dosages may be 500 mg bid; then, once control is achieved, tetracycline can be tapered by 250-mg increments until the lowest effective dose is achieved for maintenance. Note: **Tetracycline is a photosensitizer.**

        (ii) Erythromycin at doses of 1 g/day in adolescents.

        (iii) Doxycycline and minocycline may be useful in cases that do not respond to other antibiotics. Recommended dosages are 50 to 100 mg bid.

    (e) Oral retinoids/isotretinoin (Accutane) are reserved for cases of severe nodulocystic scarring acne. Their use requires close monitoring of side effects, including hyperlipidemia, cheilitis, dry skin, musculoskeletal pain, and hair thinning. **Strict adherence to guidelines is required when prescribed in females of childbearing age due to its pronounced teratogenicity.**

    (f) Hormonal therapy. Oral contraceptives with enhanced estrogen activity may be beneficial for some female acne patients (see Chap. 14, p. 426*ff*).

B. Alopecia

  1. Etiology. Hair loss can be congenital or acquired. Organizing types of hair loss based on appearance, that is, diffuse or circumscribed, can assist in defining the cause. The most common types of hair loss in pediatrics are circumscribed and acquired (tinea capitis, traction, and alopecia areata).

  2. Evaluation

    a. History. If the alopecia is congenital, obtain information about hair, nails, teeth, and any associated factors in the patient and in family members (e.g., hair shaft abnormalities, ectodermal dysplasias, congenital syndromes). Focus on grooming methods, hairstyles, and habits (pulling, twirling, chewing) when a traumatic cause is suspected (e.g., traction, trichotillomania). Acquired diffuse hair loss should prompt investigation for systemic causes: drugs, nutritional, hormonal, or severe physical or psychological stress.

    b. Physical examination. All hair-bearing areas and nails, teeth, and skin should be examined. The pattern of loss is important to note: circumscribed versus diffuse, and localized (e.g., scalp only) versus generalized.

    c. Laboratory tests that may be of assistance in the evaluation of alopecia include

      (1) Potassium hydroxide (KOH)/Gram's stain or culture, or both, to establish infectious etiologies.

      (2) Light microscopic evaluation of plucked hairs (note cycle of hair growth [growing vs. resting]and evidence of structural abnormality of the hair shaft).

      (3) Skin biopsy may be required for diagnosis, especially in the case of scarring alopecia.

  3. Diagnosis. Associated findings, such as scale, redness, and pustules, can indicate infectious agents or associated primary skin disease. The presence of a smooth normal scalp, circumscribed alopecia, and exclamation point hairs (thick distally, tapered point) are highly suggestive of *alopecia areata*. Circumscribed areas of hair loss corresponding to areas of tension, irregular borders, and broken hairs of varying lengths may indicate *traction* or *trichotillomania*. The presence of scarring may suggest an inflammatory skin disease, infection, or trauma.

4. Therapy. Interventions are based on the etiology of the alopecia. Regrowth will occur in most acquired nonscarring alopecias.

   a. Antibiotics. Topical or systemic agents for treatment of bacterial pyodermas or folliculitis that provide coverage for *Staphylococcus*.

   b. Antifungals. Systemic griseofulvin is required for successful treatment of tinea capitis confirmed by KOH or culture. The use of topical preparations alone is not sufficient.

   c. Shampoos. Preparations that contain tar, salicylic acid, sulfur, and zinc can be beneficial for some forms of scaling scalp dermatitis (e.g., psoriasis and seborrheic dermatitis). Selenium sulfide 2.5% shampoo used twice weekly is a useful adjunct to systemic antifungals in treating tinea capitis.

   d. Corticosteroids

      (1) Topical liquids of midstrength can provide relief in inflammatory scalp dermatoses (e.g., psoriasis).

      (2) Potent topical or preferably intralesional corticosteroids can hasten hair regrowth in alopecia areata. Injections should be limited to every-6-week intervals to avoid steroid-induced atrophy.

      (3) The use of systemic corticosteroids for alopecia areata is not indicated in the majority of cases.

   e. Hair extensions, wigs, or transplantation may be required to improve appearance in refractory cases.

   f. Minoxidil (Rogaine) is available in 1% solution and is applied to the affected area 1 ml bid. This may be helpful as a topical agent to promote hair growth or diminish loss in cases of androgenetic alopecia (male- and/or female-pattern baldness). This preparation, however, does not produce appreciable effects in many cases and is expensive, and hair acquired through the use of minoxidil will be lost once application is discontinued.

C. Atopic Dermatitis (see Chap. 16, p. 467).

D. Diaper dermatitis

1. Etiology. Most cases of diaper dermatitis are due to irritation from prolonged exposure to alkaline urine and feces. In long-standing dermatitis and when systemic antibiotics are being taken, secondary invasion by *Candida albicans* can contribute. The choice of cloth versus disposable diaper has little effect on incidence of diaper dermatitis.

2. Evaluation

   a. History includes use of plastic or rubber pants, frequency of diaper changes, choice of cleansing agents, recent diarrhea, and recent administration of antibiotics.

   b. Physical examination in addition to the diaper area should include evaluation of other cutaneous surfaces. Erosions and superficial ulceration may be observed.

   c. Laboratory tests. If *C. albicans* is suspected, it can be confirmed by scraping a satellite lesion and examining for yeast or pseudohyphae with KOH.

3. Diagnosis. Involvement of scalp, retroauricular areas, and axillary folds may suggest a primary dermatitis (e.g., seborrheic dermatitis or psoriasis). When primarily convex surfaces are affected (medial thighs, waist, and perineum), chemical irritation and chafing are usually responsible. The presence of bright-red confluent erythema involving the skin folds with satellite papules and pustules is typical of *C. albicans* infection.

4. Therapy

   a. Frequent diaper changes can be beneficial.

b. Avoid occlusive plastic pants and allow the diaper area to air dry, leaving diapers off as much as is practical.

c. Irritants (soaps, bubble bath, and detergents) should be avoided.

d. In the presence of *Candida* infection, topical **nystatin** cream should be applied tid and used for 5 to 7 days following cleaning. Oral thrush should be treated simultaneously.

e. Hydrocortisone 1% cream applied bid can rapidly improve inflammation.

f. **Barrier creams** and **ointments** that contain zinc oxide can help in prevention of dermatitis by providing a protective layer against urine and feces. Cornstarch powder can reduce chafing. These products do not promote yeast infection. Oil-based emollients (Vaseline) can worsen the dermatitis by blocking pores.

E. Erythema multiforme

1. Etiology. Erythema multiforme (EM) presents in two forms: erythema multiforme minor and erythema multiforme major (Stevens-Johnson syndrome).

a. In 50% of cases **EM minor** is considered to be a specific immunologic response to herpes simplex virus (HSV) antigens manifested on keratinocytes of involved skin. This form of EM minor is often recurrent. Another identified infectious agent responsible for EM is *Mycoplasma pneumoniae*. These cases are usually not recurrent.

b. **Erythema multiforme major** appears to result from toxic injury and in most cases a specific drug (e.g., sulfonamides, anticonvulsants [diphenyl-hydantoin and carbamazepine], penicillins, barbiturates, and butazones) is implicated.

2. Evaluation and diagnosis

a. **Erythema multiforme minor** is characterized by the abrupt onset of **fixed** erythematous lesions distributed symmetrically on the skin. Over a period of days the individual lesions may acquire the typical "target" appearance of concentric color change. Lesions may be photodistributed on extensor surfaces and often are evident on the palms and soles. Usually there are no mucosal lesions, but if present only *one* mucosal surface is involved and with few lesions. Subsequent crops of new lesions may occur over a 2-week period; most cases have resolved by 3 weeks. There is usually no prodrome but history of an antecedent episode of herpes (labialis or genitalis) may be elicited. Erythema multiforms minor typically affects adolescents and young adults.

b. **Erythema multiforme major** is differentiated from EM minor by the presence of a prodrome consisting of fever, malaise, and myalgias, and sometimes associated headache, sore throat, and gastrointestinal symptoms. Initially, the skin eruption is similar to EM minor with erythematous papules and targetoid lesions but blistering and epidermal loss are more common. Additionally, at least *two* mucosal surfaces are affected, the oral mucosa, and ocular or genital mucous membranes, or both, with accompanying localizing symptoms. Significant oral erosions and crusting can lead to poor nutritional intake and dehydration. Detailed inquiry into antecedent drug ingestion should be undertaken. Often the drug history is confused by the administration of medications to treat symptoms of the prodrome. The course of EM major is more prolonged and with potential sequelae, such as visual impairment, bacterial complications (pneumonia, sepsis), cutaneous pigmentary changes, scarring, and, in rare severe cases, death.

3. Therapy

a. Prophylactic **acyclovir** can be considered in recurrent cases of EM minor and avoidance of precipitating factors of HSV activation, for example, sunlight.

b. Wet compresses with saline or aluminum acetate can help exudative skin lesions.

c. Oral antihistamines can benefit pruritus.

d. Coating and topical anesthetic agents (e.g., Kaopectate, dyphenhydramine hydrochloride [Benadryl], and lidocaine [Xylocaine]—**KBX**) applied to painful oral lesions will be useful.

  e. Hospitalization may be indicated in cases of EM major when intravenous fluids, antibiotics, and respiratory care are required.

  f. Ophthalmologic advice should be sought in instances of ocular involvement in EM major.

  g. Systemic corticosteroid use is controversial but in most cases should be **discouraged** due to potential interference with healing and increased susceptibility to infection.

F. Fungal infections (See also Chap. 5, p. 157)

  1. Etiology. Dermatophytes are a group of fungi that cause superficial infection of the skin (*tinea corporis, tinea pedis, tinea cruris*), hair (*tinea capitis*), and nails (*tinea unguium*). A lipophilic yeast-like organism, *Pityrosporum orbiculare* is responsible for *tinea versicolor.* A hypersensitivity response known as an *id reaction* can occur at sites removed from the primary infection. There should be no fungi at the *id* site and resolution is seen with treatment of the primary infectious focus.

  2. Diagnostic tests

  a. Potassium hydroxide examination. The active scaly border should be scraped with the edge of a glass slide or a No. 15 Bard-Parker blade and collected onto a second glass slide. One to two drops of KOH (10–20%) are applied to the slide, followed by a cover slip and gentle heating (not to boiling) with an alcohol flame. When scalp is examined one should evaluate broken hairs or fluorescent hairs (see **c** below). Nail and hair slides may require waiting 10 to 20 minutes before evaluation to allow the thick keratin to be degraded.

  b. Fungal culture. Scales and nail clippings or hair, or both, can be directly inoculated onto fungal culture medium. Two commonly used media are Sabouraud's and dermatophyte test medium. Incubation at room temperature is required, often for a minimum of 6 weeks.

  c. Wood's light examination is useful in tinea capitis and should be performed in a darkened room with the lamp held approximately 6 in. from the affected scalp. Dermatophtes can infect the outside of the hair shaft (ectothrix), producing bright-green fluorescence, or the inside of the hair (endothrix), yielding no fluorescence. Most cases of tinea capitis are due to *Trichophyton tonsurans*, which does not produce fluorescence.

  3. Specific fungal infections

  a. Tinea capitis. The leading dermatophytes responsible are *T. tonsurans* (acquired from a human source) and, less frequently, *Microsporum canis* (harbored by animals—dogs, cats).

  (1) Evaluation and diagnosis. Tinea capitis frequently presents without subjective complaints or perhaps only mild pruritus. Parents may report scalp dryness and hair loss.

  (a) History should include questioning about contacts with suggested symptoms and about exposure to animals, particularly new kittens.

  (b) Physical examination. One or several patches of hair loss consisting of broken hairs and thick scale suggest *M. canis.* *Trichophyton tonsurans* can produce three distinct clinical patterns: (1) fine diffuse scaling (seborrheic dermatitis–like) without obvious alopecia, (2) "black-dot" ringworm in which hairs are broken off at the follicular opening leaving small dark hairs, or (3) triangular scaly areas of alopecia with indistinct margins. Occasionally, a very inflammatory response may occur to fungal invasion of the hair shaft producing a kerion. Kerions appear as boggy plaques or masses with overlying pustules and crusting. Posterior cervical lymphadenopathy can be prominent. Without treatment there is risk of scarring and permanent hair loss.

(2) Therapy
  (a) Griseofulvin is the drug of choice since topical agents cannot penetrate the hair shaft to act on the hyphae within. Griseofulvin micronized is administered at a dosage of 10 to 20 mg/kg/day for a minimum of 6 weeks and sometimes as long as 2 to 3 months. It is available in a suspension of 125 mg/5 ml, and in 250-mg and 500-mg tablets. Ultramicrosize preparations are in tablet form only; a lower dose is effective: 3.3 mg/lb or 7.3 mg/kg/day.
  (b) Selenium sulfide 2.5% shampoo twice a week.
  (c) Family contacts with symptoms should be evaluated, cultured, and treated as well.
  (d) Prednisone at dosages of 1 to 2 mg/kg/day for 7 to 10 days is advocated by some to reduce the pronounced inflammation characteristic of kerion. This can diminish the chance of hair follicle destruction and scarring alopecia.
b. Tinea corporis
  (1) Evaluation and diagnosis. The most common complaint is pruritus. The classic presentation is of an erythematous papular lesion that progressively enlarges, becoming annular with a raised scaly border and central clearing. Occasionally, the infection extends via the follicular orifice to produce a deep, inflammatory nodular plaque known as Majocchi's granuloma.
  (2) Therapy
    (a) Topical antifungal agents are usually adequate. Numerous effective agents of various classes are available: (1) **imidazoles** (e.g., clotrimazole, miconazole, ketoconazole), (2) **allylamine** (e.g., naftifine), and (3) **nonimidazole** (ciclopirox olamine). These preparations are applied to the affected area and 1 cm beyond the lesion twice a day for 2 weeks to 1 month. Treatment should continue until 1 week after clinical resolution.
    (b) Griseofulvin is occasionally needed for treatment of tinea infection of the face and in Majocchi's granuloma.
c. Tinea cruris
  (1) Evaluation and diagnosis. Fungal infection involving the medial thighs and inguinal folds is unusual before adolescence and is often quite pruritic. Lesions are typically well demarcated areas of scaling, some with circinate elevated borders.
  (2) Therapy
    (a) Antifungal creams applied topically twice a day for at least 1 week following clearing will provide good results.
    (b) Predisposing factors, such as occlusive clothing, excess heat, and moisture, should be eliminated.
    (c) Use of an absorbent powder such as Zeasorb after showering and throughout the day is helpful.
d. Tinea pedis
  (1) Evaluation and diagnosis. Fungal infection of the feet is unusual in the preadolescent child. A KOH should be checked in any scaling or bullous plantar eruption. The clinical appearance of tinea pedis varies: (1) fissuring and erythema of the toe webs (especially between the fourth and fifth toes), (2) chronic thick scale and minimal redness in a "moccasin" pattern, and (3) a subacute type composed of blisters and pustules over the instep.
  (2) Therapy
    (a) Drying agents and absorbent powders such as aluminum chloride 20% can eliminate excess moisture from sweating and may be needed if there is prominent maceration or blistering (e.g., saline or aluminum acetate compresses).
    (b) Topical antifungals applied for 3 to 6 weeks are effective for

acute infections. Chronic infection can require 6 months of treatment.

(c) Oral antifungals are occasionally required for severely blistering tinea pedis.

(d) Attention to elimination of predisposing conditions will improve response to treatment and decrease the likelihood of recurrence. Occlusive shoes, socks, and hosiery should be eliminated. Washing and thorough drying of the feet are important.

e. Tinea unguium
   (1) Evaluation and diagnosis. Nail infection is usually acquired from adjacent infection of the skin (i.e., tinea pedis or manus). Involvement of toenails is more common since shoes often provide a warm moist environment and a potential source of trauma. Early, yellow or white discoloration of the lateral edge of the nail plate is seen. This then progresses to thickening and accumulation of debris underneath the nail plate.

   (2) Therapy. Cure of onychomycosis is difficult.
      (a) Topical agents alone are usually not successful (because of poor penetration of the nail plate) but can prevent spread to other nails if used regularly.
      (b) Daily systemic treatment with **griseofulvin** (ultramicrosize) produces response in up to one third of patients but only after 6 to 12 months of therapy, and relapse is common. With long-term treatment (6–9 mo for fingernails and 12–18 mo for toenails) laboratory monitoring for agranulocytosis, anemia, and liver function impairment is indicated.
      (c) Ketoconazole produces higher cure rates but also requires daily dosing, and close laboratory monitoring for hepatotoxicity is necessary.

f. Tinea versicolor
   (1) Evaluation and diagnosis. This eruption is asymptomatic or mildly pruritic. Patients are often most disturbed by the pigmentary changes and may complain of an inability to "tan" in certain areas. Lesions are oval macules with scale or confluent patches located over the neck, chest, upper back, shoulders, and arms. Lesions are pink to fawn colored in light-skinned individuals and appear hypopigmented in tanned or dark-skinned persons. Wood's lamp examination shows yellow-orange fluorescence due to the production of a porphyrin metabolite by *Pityrosporum*. KOH examination of the scale shows short curved hyphae and round spores ("spaghetti and meatballs").

   (2) Therapy
      (a) Selenium sulfide 2.5% suspension is applied to all affected skin for 20 minutes, then rinsed. (Overnight treatment can result in skin irritation.) It should be used daily for a month and, because tinea versicolor tends to be chronic, various maintenance regimens are advocated. One schedule is to use it once a week for a subsequent month, then once monthly indefinitely.
      (b) Topical imidazoles (clotrimazole, miconazole, ketoconazole) are very effective but may not be practical when there is extensive involvement due to their expense.
      (c) Oral ketoconazole is very effective when used in the following manner: 400 mg is ingested; after 2 hours the patient exercises to produce sweating (ketoconazole is excreted in sweat) and then showers at least 1 hour later. This process is then repeated in 1 week. It is important to remind patients that repigmentation of the hypopigmented skin will lag behind successful treatment. Sometimes 12 to 18 months are required for complete resolution of the pigmentary alterations.

G. Hemangiomas and vascular malformations. There are two major types of vascular birthmarks: hemangiomas, which are characterized by hyperplasia of endothelial cells, and malformations, which show normal division of endothelium.

1. **Hemangioma** (e.g., strawberry nevus)
   a. **Diagnosis and evaluation.** Frequently no abnormality is present at birth. In 30% there may be an initial red macule or circumscribed area of blanched skin with telangiectasias. There is a 3 : 1 female preponderance for development of these vascular tumors. The lesions grow rapidly out of proportion to the infant's growth during the first year of life. At this time they are typically red-purple plaques or nodules of variable size. (When these lesions lie deep in the dermis or subcutaneous tissue, the overlying skin may appear blue.) After a plateau in growth rate, involution begins around 15 months of age, when an early sign may be pale-gray areas developing within the hemangioma. Involution continues gradually so that 50% have returned to skin level by age 5 and 70% by age 7.
   b. **Therapy.** Since the majority of hemangiomas regress spontaneously, treatment is reserved for lesions that (1) obstruct a vital orifice (e.g., airway-subglottic hemangioma), urethra, or anus; (2) obstruct vision, causing a high risk of ambylopia; (3) cause platelet trapping (Kasabach-Merritt phenomenon—usually a single large hemangioma that collects platelets within its sluggish vascular channels, producing thrombocytopenia, disseminated intravascular coagulation [DIC], and hemorrhage); or (4) cause high-output cardiac failure (large hemangiomas or multiple cutaneous and internal organ hemangiomas).
      (1) **Systemic prednisone** is the treatment of choice at dosages of 1 to 6 mg/kg/day continued for 4 to 8 weeks. It is most effective during the growing phase, 1 to 8 months.
      (2) **Interferon-alfa-2a** is frequently used in the treatment of endangering hemangiomas that do not respond to systemic corticosteroids, though this is not an approved use. A dose of 3 to 5 million units/m^2 is given daily by subcutaneous injection for periods of 6 to 12 months. Close monitoring of neurologic examination is recommended during treatment.
      (3) **Intralesional corticosteroids** are often useful for treatment of periorbital hemangiomas.
      (4) Pulsed dye **laser** can help the superficial portion of the hemangioma or promote stabilization in growth of ulcerated hemangiomas.
      (5) **Topical or systemic antibiotics, or both,** may be needed for the management of ulcerated hemangiomas.
      (6) **Surgery** may be indicated to debulk large hemangiomas or to modify remnant fibrofatty tissue and redundant skin following involution.
      (7) Bleeding is usually controlled by applying direct pressure or use of silver nitrate sticks.
      (8) **Radiation, cryosurgery, embolization,** and **sclerosing agents** can be used but often produce less than desirable cosmetic results.

2. **Vascular malformations**
   a. **Diagnosis and evaluation.** Most malformations, in contrast to hemangiomas, are present at birth, although they may not be clinically manifest until later. Vascular malformations affect both sexes equally. These lesions grow in proportion to the growth of the child. There is no tendency for spontaneous resolution of malformations.
      (1) **Arterial malformations** are often asymptomatic until later in life when they may be revealed incidentally during evaluation for atherosclerotic disease.
      (2) **Venous malformations** are typically blue-purple in color, enlarge when in a dependent position, and diminish in size when venous outflow is enhanced (i.e., raising above the level of the heart).
      (3) **Lymphatic malformations** may present with lymphedema, usually of

the lower limbs (e.g., Milroy's disease). Lymph cysts may be single (cystic hygroma—at root of neck) or multiple ("lymphangioma"). These appear as clusters of thin-walled vesicles with clear or slightly hemorrhagic fluid ("frog spawn" appearance). Often, deeper channels are found in the subcutaneous tissue.

(4) Capillary malformations (e.g., port-wine stain) appear at birth as a pink-red-purple discoloration of skin that is sharply demarcated and usually unilateral. With age the hue deepens to dark purple and the skin becomes nodular and thickened. Port-wine stains can be associated with specific syndromes, including Sturge-Weber, Klippel-Trénaunay, and Cobb. Other common superficial capillary ectasias include nevus flammeus neonatorum—"angel's kisses," "stork bite," "salmon patch." These appear as pink macules of irregular outline on the eyelids, nuchal region, and glabella. Eyelid and glabellar stains typically fade whereas nuchal lesions may persist into adulthood.

(5) Combined malformations. Arteriovenous malformations can present with pain, pulsation, local hyperhidrosis, hypertrichosis, hyperthermia, or thrill.

b. Therapy. The exact nature of the vascular malformation and prognosis may not be evident until several evaluations over the course of time. A multidisciplinary approach will yield the best care.

H. Infestations

1. Scabies

a. Etiology. Scabies is caused by infestation with the mite, *Sarcoptes scabiei*. It is highly contagious and transmission occurs from person to person. There is little spread from fomites. The incubation period is 3 weeks before symptoms and signs appear. Patients previously infected may develop symptoms in a shorter period of time.

b. Evaluation and diagnosis

(1) The **history** of scabies includes pruritus, most notable during bedtime. The pruritus and allergic reaction leads to vesicles, papules, wheals, and eczematous plaques.

(2) On **physical examination** lesions are seen along the wrists, between the fingers, on the palms and soles, around the umbilicus and the areolae, in the axillae, along the scrotum, and over the buttocks. Attention should be paid to the presence of linear burrows, which are often seen along the fingers or wrists and are characterized by a linear papule, 5 mm in length with a thread-like scale ending in a black dot. By applying mineral oil to the burrow and gently scraping with a No. 15 blade, a specimen is obtained that may reveal a mite, eggs, or mite feces.

c. Therapy

(1) Permethrin 5% (Elimite) is the treatment of choice for all patients. However, its safety in infants under age 3 months and in pregnancy has not been established.

(a) Permethrin is applied in adults from the neck down with attention paid to the skin folds and under the fingernails. Infants may have involvement of the scalp and need the entire body surface covered.

(b) The medication is left on for 8 hours. A reapplication in one week is often recommended.

(c) All family members and close contacts should be treated even if they are asymptomatic.

(d) Pregnant patients or newborn infants can be treated with 6% precipitated sulfur in petrolatum (compounded by a pharmacist). This is applied for 3 consecutive nights.

(e) Recently worn clothing, towels, and bedding need to be either washed, placed in a hot dryer, dry cleaned, or isolated in a plastic bag for at least a week.

(f) The pruritus and rash may last for several weeks after treatment and cause additional anxiety.

(2) Antihistamines can be administered for the pruritus and emollients or anesthetic ointments for the rash.

(3) Topical steroids should be avoided since they can mask continued infection.

2. Pediculosis capitis

a. Etiology

(1) Pediculosis capitis (head lice) is caused by the insect *Pediculus humanus capitis*, a 2- to 4-mm insect.

(2) The adult female lays about six eggs (nits) per day that hatch in 8 to 10 days.

(3) Pediculosis is highly contagious and spreads through direct contact or through contact with contaminated objects, such as clothing (hats, hoods, scarves), bedding, towels, or combs and brushes.

b. Evaluation and diagnosis

(1) The nits are oval and gray, cemented to the hair shaft of the scalp, and often found along the nape of the neck. The eggs hatch before the hair has grown more than ¼ in.

(2) Nits seen beyond 1 cm of the scalp have either hatched or are dead.

(3) Live insects may be seen in a heavy infestation.

(4) Patients usually have pruritus; excoriations and erythema may be seen along the posterior hairline.

c. Treatment

(1) Permethrin (Nix) and pyrethrins (A-200, RID, R&C) are effective topical preparations that are extracts of flowers in the chrysanthemum family.

(2) Alternative therapies include lindane (Kwell) and precipitated sulfur in petrolatum.

(3) The permethrin and pyrethrins are available as shampoos that are applied for one treatment and left on for 10 minutes. Lindane also comes as a shampoo that is applied for 5 minutes on 2 consecutive nights.

(4) All family members and close contacts, even if asymptomatic, should be simultaneously treated.

(5) Clothing and bedding should be washed in hot water or placed in a hot dryer.

(6) Combs and brushes should be washed or placed in medicinal alcohol or 2% Lysol.

(7) The dead eggs can be loosened with a cream rinse, white vinegar mixed 1 : 1 with water, or formic acid (Step2), or commercially available enzyme preparations (Clear), and then removed with a fine-toothed comb.

(8) Treatment failures are usually due to reexposure.

I. Pityriasis rosea

1. Etiology. The cause of pityriasis rosea is unknown. Clusters of cases occur seasonally (spring and fall) suggesting an infectious cause.

2. Evaluation and diagnosis

a. The initial lesion (herald patch) is an oval plaque with a wet scale that appears on the trunk or the extremities. It can reach several centimeters in size, with a color ranging from pink to tan.

b. After 7 to 10 days, the herald patch is succeeded by crops of smaller oval lesions 0.5 to 1.0 cm in size that orient along the skin cleavage lines over the trunk in a Christmas tree–like pattern from the neck to the midthigh with sparing of the face. These lesions are barely raised and may show a fine collarette of scale within the border. The eruption can become confluent, lasting for 4 to 6 weeks. Considerable pruritus may be present.

c. In young children the eruption occasionally has an inverse distribution with lesions most prominent along the axillae and groin.

d. The differential diagnosis includes viral exanthems and secondary syphilis.

3. Therapy

a. Pruritus is treated with antihistamines and topical antipruritic lotions that can include Sarna or Prax.

b. In some cases, exposure to natural or artificial ultraviolet light (UVB), when initiated early, can relieve the pruritus.

c. In the inflammatory form, a trial of a topical steroid may be effective.

J. Psoriasis

1. Etiology. Psoriasis has a polygenic inheritance and is seen in 2 to 3% of the population. Its onset can occur during infancy or childhood.

a. Infections and physical trauma may predispose a susceptible individual to the appearance of lesions. In children, psoriatic lesions frequently occur following infections with streptococcus, either in the throat or the perianal area.

b. Friction and trauma (Koebner's phenomenon) also can bring out lesions seen in skin creases (inguinal, intergluteal. retroauricular), or on the elbows and knees and hands and feet.

2. Evaluation and diagnosis

a. In the infant, the initial appearance of psoriasis is characterized by well-defined bright-red plaques involving the perineum. There is involvement along the inguinal and intergluteal creases. Frequently the axillae also show erythema. The scalp may have patches with adherent heaped-up scale.

b. At times, a generalized eruption appears, consisting of well-defined red plaques with adherent white scale. If the scale is pulled off, tiny pinpoint areas of bleeding are revealed (Auspitz sign).

c. The older child will often have persistent lesions involving the scalp, retroauricular area, ear canals, genitalia, palms, and soles.

d. Involvement of the nails can occur at any age, with pitting, subungual debris, lifting of the distal nail with leakage of serum producing "oil slicks," and periungual erythema.

e. Guttate psoriasis occurs in children within one week of a streptococcal infection with sudden appearance of erythematous papules and small plaques less than a centimeter in size that are distributed over the entire body surface including the scalp.

f. Associated arthritis occurs in fewer than 5% of children.

g. Chills and loss of body heat occur with extensive involvement.

3. Therapy

a. Keep the skin well hydrated with emollients and avoid clothing or sports equipment that can traumatize the skin.

b. The first line of therapy is topical steroids of appropriate potency. Only class VII agents should be used for prolonged periods on the face, skin folds, and perineum because of the risk of thinning the skin. In sites of thick skin such as the palms, soles, knees, and elbows, a potent class I steroid may be required. The effectiveness of topical steroids can be increased by occluding with a film of plastic or the newer semi-occlusive dressings (Actiderm, Duoderm). Taper topical steroids and substitute lower-potency preparations as improvement occurs.

c. Tar preparations, available as ointments, lotion, baths, and shampoos, help maintain improvement after topical steroid use when used once or twice a day.

d. Anthralin is an effective alternative to topical steroids. Short contact treatment of up to 30 minutes is advised. Anthralin can irritate and stain the surrounding skin. It is available in a formulation for the scalp.

e. Calcipotriene, an analogue of vitamin D, has been approved recently for use in adults, and approval for use in children is pending. Irritation of skin, particularly when calcipotriene is applied to the face, can occur.

f. Exposure to natural or artificial light (UVB) may be extremely effective in treating some children, particularly in cases of guttate psoriasis.

g. In patients with severe erythrodermia, options include methotrexate, cyclosporine, psoralen and ultraviolet light (PUVA), and retinoids (Tegison, Accutane).

h. Treatment of the scalp requires initial removal of the thick scale. This can be accomplished by first applying a keratolytic gel (Keralyt) or a phenol/saline lotion (Baker's P&S) overnight. The psoriasis can then be controlled with daily application of a steroid-containing solution (Valisone, Lidex, Derma-Smoothe/FS) and a tar shampoo.

K. Seborrheic dermatitis

1. Etiology

a. There are two forms of seborrheic dermatitis: infantile and postpubertal.

(1) The infantile form may be associated with colonization of *Pityrosporum ovale*.

(2) The adult form has no known cause.

2. Evaluation and diagnosis

a. The infantile form of seborrheic dermatitis may first appear as adherent, yellowish scaling of the scalp (cradle cap) or as a sudden appearance of erythema in the skin folds of the axillae, groin, and neck. In rare instances, it may become generalized with a secondary staphylococcal infection.

b. In older patients, there is involvement of sebaceous glands with diffuse scaling of the scalp and erythema along the nasolabial folds, malar area, retroauricular folds, and over the chest.

3. Treatment

a. For the infant with scaling scalp, mineral oil can be applied overnight to gently remove the scale. Recurrence can be prevented with shampoos that contain salicylic acid, tar, zinc, or an antifungal (ketonazole).

b. In the more extensive cases in infants and children, apply topical steroids of low potency (class VII) once or twice a day. If there is evidence of infection, use a systemic antibiotic with antistaphylococcal properties.

L. Photosensitivity

1. Etiology

a. Sunlight is composed of a spectrum of wavelengths divided into

(1) UVB—290 to 320 nm.

(2) UVA—320 to 400 nm.

(3) Visible light—greater than 400 nm.

b. Sunlight between the hours of 10 AM and 3 PM is the most damaging.

c. Heightened sensitivity to sunlight can result from systemic diseases, drugs, or topical agents.

d. Photosensitizing drugs include tetracycline, minocycline, doxycycline, griseofulvin, sulfa drugs (Bactrim, Septra, diuretics), phenothiazines, psoralens, and nonsteroidal anti-inflammatory medications.

e. A localized phototoxicity can occur from contact with psoralen-containing fruits and plants (lime, lemons, celery, bergamot, parsley, parsnips).

f. Inherited conditions that predispose patients include xeroderma pigmentosum, albinism, Bloom's syndrome, Rothmund-Thomson syndrome, and Cockayne's syndrome. Acquired photosensitivity is associated with lupus, dermatomyositis, the porphyrias, vitiligo, and nutritional disorders (kwashiorkor, pellagra).

2. Evaluation and diagnosis

a. Initial asymptomatic erythema with exposure to sunlight is followed 4 to 6 hours later by a more intense erythema with stinging and burning.

b. In severe exposures, blistering and edema appear within 24 hours accompanied by fever, malaise, and chills.

3. Treatment

a. Damp compresses and cool baths with colloidal oatmeal (Aveeno) may be soothing.

b. Systemic corticosteroids, if administered early, in a dosage of 1 to 2 mg/kg/day for a total of 2 days, can relieve symptoms.

    c. Sunscreens are an effective means of protecting patients from sun sensitivity.

      (1) Para-aminobenzoic acid (PABA) and PABA esters provide partial UVB protection and no UVA protection. Benzophenone provides complete UVB and partial UVA. Cinnamates provide full UVB and partial UVA protection. Salicylates provide complete UVB and no UVA. Butylmethoxydibenzoylmethane (avobenzone or Parsol 1789) provides full UVA coverage but no UVB. Titanium dioxide and zinc oxide are physical blocks that protect against the entire spectrum of sunlight.

      (2) Any product with a sun protection factor (SPF) number equal to or greater than 15 will be adequate in screening out UVB.

      (3) Sunscreens are available in a variety of vehicles that include moisturizing creams, oil-free emulsions, and gels, any of which can produce a contact dermatitis.

      (4) Clothing specifically designed to block sunlight and broad-rimmed hats can play an important role in protection in the photosensitive patient.

M. Vitiligo

  1. Etiology. Vitiligo is an autoimmune condition in which there is a loss of melanocytes.

  2. Evaluation and diagnosis

    a. Vitiligo is often noted during the summer when lesions fail to tan and often burn.

    b. The lesions can appear on any area of the body including the scalp, where they often produce white hairs.

    c. A Wood's lamp examination will reveal lesions that are difficult to appreciate in fair skin.

  3. Therapy

    a. Early treatment rarely alters the natural history of the disease.

    b. While monitoring for the side effect of cutaneous thinning, a potent topical steroid applied daily for 1 to 2 months may be effective.

    c. Psoralen is a photosensitizing drug that can be taken orally or used topically. In combination with natural or artificial ultraviolet light, it can produce gradual repigmentation after multiple treatments.

    d. Dyes and cosmetic cover-ups are also available (Dy-o-Derm, Vitadye, Dermablend).

N. Warts

  1. Etiology. Warts are due to infection with any of 50 different types of DNA viruses known as papillomavirus. Certain types have a predilection for specific sites.

  2. Physical examination

    a. Warts on the dorsum of the extremities are skin colored to hypopigmented with a rough surface. They often form clusters around the cuticles or over joints.

    b. Plantar or palmar surface warts are raised, rough, and scaly. In some cases, the lesions are flat with a hard central core.

    c. Warts on the face can have two presentations: They can form digitate or filiform projection around the eyes and nose, or they can be light-brown, barely raised papules.

    d. Warts on the genital and rectal mucosa can appear as hypopigmented papules with pinpoint capillaries or they can form friable clusters (condyloma).

    e. Warts can exist in a subclinical state with infectious particles present but no change in the skin surface appreciated.

  3. Diagnosis is made on clinical grounds but can be confirmed by skin biopsy.

    a. The typing of lesions is done by DNA hybridization. This is important for some forms of cervical warts (types 16, 18) that have been associated with certain types of carcinoma.

   b. A useful diagnostic clue may be the presence of pinpoint hemorrhages within the wart that represent thrombosed capillaries.
  4. Therapy
   a. The treatment of warts is dependent on their location, their duration, past treatment, extent, type of lesion, and age of the patient.
   b. Most warts eventually spontaneously involute.
   c. For young children under age 4, benign neglect may be the best approach.
   d. A topical salicylic acid preparation in a collodion base (17%) or plaster (40%) applied nightly is an effective and usually painless therapy. Directions should be given to soak the affected area and to vigorously scrape off as much of the wart as possible before applying the medication. Therapy can be continued for 2 to 3 weeks. If no response is seen, a break of 1 to 2 weeks should be taken and then the treatment should be resumed for another 2- to 3-week period.
   e. Alternative treatments include continuous occlusion with tape, repetitive exposure to hot water, application of tretinoin (Retin-A is effective, particularly when applied to flat warts), and 5-fluorouracil.
   f. Liquid nitrogen freezing is helpful in older children who have had no response to topical therapy. The lesions are frozen for 20 seconds by gently applying a cotton swab immersed in liquid nitrogen. The lesion should be frozen to include a 1-mm border of normal-appearing tissue around the lesion. In resistant cases, a second freeze thaw cycle of 20 seconds can be performed. A hemorrhagic blister will appear in 24 hours and may be accompanied by considerable discomfort. Freezing is contraindicated for patients who have a history of Raynaud's phenomenon. Freezing of large lesions greater than 1 cm can produce central clearing of the wart with recurrence at the border.
 O. Molluscum contagiosum
  1. Etiology
   a. Molluscum contagiosum is caused by DNA poxvirus. It is easily spread from one child to another particularly within a family.
   b. Transmission seems to be frequently associated with public swimming pools.
   c. Lesions are easily autoinoculated by scratching.
  2. Evaluation and diagnosis
   a. Lesions present as skin-colored, shiny, 1- to 10-mm diameter papules with central white cores.
   b. The lesions can be located anywhere on the skin surface, but frequently are seen along the skin folds of the antecubital and popliteal fossae or along the flanks.
   c. Lesions may produce an eczematous area in the surrounding skin.
   d. At times, lesions may become inflamed and look infected.
  3. Treatment
   a. Lesions will spontaneously disappear over several months.
   b. If the lesions are causing pruritus or are becoming a cosmetic concern, treatment can be attempted.
   c. Lesions can be treated with cryotherapy, electrodesiccation, or curettage. These treatments are uncomfortable. A topical anesthetic (EMLA) applied before the procedures may be helpful.
   d. Retinoic acid (Retin-A) is somewhat effective when applied daily for weeks. The strongest tolerated preparation can be used.
   e. Cantharidin (Cantharone) is an excellent treatment, but is no longer for sale in the United States. It is applied to the lesions, with care taken to avoid normal skin. Wash the medication off within 6 hours of its application. It will produce blistering within 24 hours of its application.

Inflammatory Disorders

Robert Sundel

I. **Juvenile rheumatoid arthritis (JRA)** is an idiopathic chronic arthritis of children that may be associated with generalized systemic inflammation.
   A. **Etiology** is unknown.
   B. **Evaluation.** There are five modes of onset (Table 18-1). Laboratory findings in the systemic and polyarticular forms are remarkable for elevated acute-phase markers, while laboratory studies may be normal in pauciarticular disease. Joint fluid reveals low viscosity and a WBC greater than 10^3/mm with a polymorphonuclear predominance.
   C. **Diagnosis** is of exclusion: Children with at least 6 weeks of arthritis without another explanation meet criteria for JRA. Associated findings support the diagnosis.
   D. **Treatment**
      1. The **goal** is suppression of inflammation and prevention of deformity and disability.
      2. **Physical and occupational therapy** should maintain range of motion and functional joint positioning.
      3. **Anti-inflammatory drugs** provide the first line of treatment; they offer symptomatic relief but do not arrest joint damage. All medications in this category have similar efficacy; choice is based on cost, ease of administration, and toxicity.
         a. **Aspirin** (acetylsalicylic acid) is the traditional initial drug of choice in JRA. Concerns about Reye's syndrome and the need for qid dosing have led to increasing use of newer medications (see below).
            (1) A starting **dosage** of 80 mg/kg/day (maximum 3.6 g/day) is adjusted to obtain salicylate levels of 20 to 30 mg/dl. Aspirin is given with food to avoid gastrointestinal irritation. Rectal and enteric-coated aspirin are erratically absorbed. The nonacetylated salicylates choline magnesium salicylate (Trilisate) and choline salicylate (Arthropan) can reduce GI toxicity and improve compliance. These formulations do not affect platelet aggregation.
            (2) Aspirin is **metabolized** by the liver and excreted by the kidney. At high dosages, small changes in dose cause significant changes in level.
            (3) **Side effects**
               (a) **Gastrointestinal.** Nausea, abdominal pain, and diarrhea occur relatively commonly; gastric ulcers and hemorrhage rarely.
               (b) **Hepatic.** Mild liver enzyme elevations frequently occur; they tend to resolve without a change in therapy.
               (c) **Hematologic.** Platelets are irreversibly inactivated, resulting in easy bruisability and, rarely, frank bleeding for up to 14 days.
               (d) Aspirin is stopped following development of, or exposure to, chickenpox or influenza, to reduce the risk of **Reye's syndrome.** Influenza vaccination is recommended for children who are receiving chronic aspirin therapy.
               (e) Patients with nasal polyps and asthma are likely to have **aspirin sensitivity** and should avoid aspirin.
            (4) **Signs of overdosage** include tinnitus, lethargy, hyperventilation,

Table 18-1. Subgroups of juvenile rheumatoid arthritis

Subgroup	% of total	Sex ratio	Age at onset	Joints affected	Serologic and genetic tests	Extraarticular manifestations	Prognosis
Systemic onset	20	60% boys	Any age	Any joints	ANA negative, RF negative	High fever, rash, organomegaly, polyserositis, leukocytosis, growth retardation	25% severe arthritis
Rheumatoid factor Negative polyarticular	25	90% girls	Any age	Any joints	ANA 25%, RF negative	Low-grade fever, mild anemia, malaise, growth retardation	10–15% severe arthritis
Rheumatoid factor Positive polyarticular	5–10	80% girls	Late childhood	Any joints	ANA 75%, RF 100%	Low-grade fever, anemia, malaise, rheumatoid nodules	>50% severe arthritis
Pauciarticular with chronic iridocyclitis	35–40	80% girls	Early childhood	Few large joints (hips and sacroiliac joints spared)	ANA 50%, RF negative	Few constitutional complaints; chronic iridocyclitis in 50%	Severe arthritis uncommon; 10–20% ocular damage from iridocyclitis
Pauciarticular with sacroiliitis	10	90% boys	Late childhood	Few large joints (hips and sacroiliac involvement common)	ANA negative, RF negative, HLA-B27 75%	Few constitutional complaints; acute iridocyclitis in 5–10% during childhood	Clinically similar to spondyloarthrities

ANA = antinuclear antibody; RF = rheumatoid factor; HLA-B27 = histocompatibility antigen–B27.

dizziness, sweating, headaches, and nausea (see p. 279). Salicylate levels should be monitored to minimize the risk of these side effects.

b. Nonsteroidal anti-inflammatory drugs (NSAIDs). Responses to individual drugs of this class are variable; if one drug is ineffective after 1 to 2 months, another should be tried. NSAIDs are well absorbed in the GI tract and excreted by the kidney. Since all share similar toxicities, patients should receive optimal doses of a single agent, rather than different NSAIDs simultaneously.

(1) Specific agents

(a) Ibuprofen (30–40 mg/kg/day divided tid or qid) is well tolerated and approved for use in children.

(b) Tolmetin sodium (20–40 mg/kg/day divided tid or qid) is approved for children over 2 years.

(c) Naproxen (10–20 mg/kg/day divided bid) is approved for children over 2 years.

(d) Indomethacin (1.0–2.5 mg/kg/day divided tid to qid) has a higher incidence of CNS and gastric toxicity than other NSAIDs. It is approved for use in children over 14 years.

(2) Toxicity

(a) Gastric. Dyspepsia, nausea, gastritis, diarrhea, and ulceration can occur. These are seen less frequently when NSAIDs are administered with food.

(b) Hepatic. Elevation of liver enzymes is usually mild and reversible.

(c) Hematologic. Reversible platelet inactivation can lead to easy bruising and prolonged bleeding time.

(d) Renal. NSAIDs can cause fluid retention and can block the effect of some diuretics. They can precipitate acute renal shutdown in patients with decreased glomerular filtration; interstitial nephritis and nephrotic syndrome also have been reported.

(e) Dermatologic. Rashes and oral ulceration can occur at high doses. Naproxen can cause a scarring photosensitive eruption, especially in fair-skinned children.

(f) Patients with **aspirin sensitivity** should take NSAIDs with caution.

(g) Central nervous system. Headaches, drowsiness, or dysphoria occasionally limit the use of these agents.

4. Slow-acting remittive agents are drugs that affect the natural history of JRA, acting over weeks to months. Methotrexate and gold have been shown to slow or even reverse bony erosion and cartilage loss.

a. Hydroxychloroquine (Plaquenil) is an antimalarial agent with moderate anti-inflammatory activity and possibly remittive effects. It is used at 4 to 7 mg/kg/day (400 mg/day maximum) in patients whose moderate synovitis is unresponsive to NSAIDs. It is relatively contraindicated in patients with glucose 6-phosphate dehydrogenase (G6PD) deficiency. Regular ophthalmologic examinations are required to identify macular degeneration and corneal deposits, which require discontinuation of the drug. Gastric irritation and dermatitis may also occur; these are reversible with cessation of the drug.

b. Methotrexate (0.3–1.0 mg/kg once a week) is effective in treating JRA. It is generally well tolerated in children, **though the potential for severe toxicity still necessitates close monitoring. Sulfa drugs and alcohol should be avoided by patients receiving methotrexate.**

c. Gold salts at dosages of up to 1 mg/kg/wk IM are used for severe or erosive arthritis. **Dose-limiting toxicities,** including dermatitis, mucositis, vasomotor reactions, eosinophilia, blood dyscrasias, and nephrotic syndrome, are usually reversible with discontinuation of the medication.

d. Sulfasalazine (Azulfidine, 40–70 mg/kg/day divided bid or tid) has anti-inflammatory effects, especially in the spondyloarthritides. Toxicities include rash, gastritis, and bone marrow suppression; enteric-coated preparations may be better tolerated.

5. **Corticosteroids** have dramatic anti-inflammatory effects in JRA, though prolonged administration of high doses leads to unacceptable toxicity.

a. **Intra-articular steroids** are indicated for severe inflammation of a few joints; effects can persist from days to months. **Risks** include introduction of infection into the joint, and development of a transient crystal synovitis. *Repeat administrations can damage cartilage.*

b. **Oral steroids** are indicated for severe systemic manifestations of JRA or for short-term amelioration of severe polyarthritis. They are generally given in the lowest effective dose in conjunction with a slow-acting remittive agent.

6. **Topical ocular steroids** can be used for treating **chronic anterior uveitis,** the most important cause of morbidity in pauciarticular JRA. Girls with a positive antinuclear antigen (ANA) are at increased risk; all children with JRA require regular slit lamp screening.

II. **Spondyloarthritis** is chronic inflammation of the peripheral joints, axial skeleton, or both, with enthesitis (inflammation of the insertion of tendons into bone). This includes a group of related disorders: juvenile ankylosing spondylitis, psoriatic arthritis, reactive arthritis, and inflammatory bowel disease (IBD)-associated arthritis.

A. **Etiology** is unknown, though infections can trigger onset of inflammation.

B. **Evaluation**

1. **History.** Family history is frequently positive for one of the disorders listed above.

2. **Physical examination** findings include arthritis, acute iridocyclitis, mucous membrane inflammation (pyuria, oral ulceration), and skin lesions. Aortitis can occur.

3. **Laboratory tests** show association with human leukocyte antigen, (HLA)-B27 in white patients and HLA-B7 or B27 in black patients. Rheumatoid factor is negative, ANA is occasionally positive, and markers of acute inflammation are normal or elevated.

C. **Diagnosis.** The specific illnesses included in this category present with the clinical features cited above and the following associated features.

1. **Juvenile ankylosing spondylitis (JAS)** is characterized by inflammation of the spine or sacroiliac joints.

2. **IBD-associated arthritis** may precede signs or symptoms of bowel inflammation. Poor growth, fever, anemia, abdominal pain, or hematochezia associated with spondyloarthritis should prompt consideration of IBD.

3. **Reactive arthritis** is a sterile pauciarticular process that follows bacterial infections of gastrointestinal or genitourinary sites. When associated with conjunctivitis and urethritis, the triad is termed *Reiter's syndrome.* Reactive arthritis generally responds to NSAIDs in weeks to months; chronic arthritis is rare.

4. **Psoriatic arthritis** is associated with skin or nail findings of psoriasis, though arthritis can precede mucocutaneous manifestations. Presenting involvement is often pauciarticular, but the illness may progress to polyarticular arthritis, with severe destructive disease.

D. **Treatment**

1. **Supportive care** with physical and occupational therapy is crucial in maintaining mobility. Special attention should be given to the axial skeleton. Custom-made shoe orthotics are helpful for Achilles tendon and plantar enthesitis.

2. **Drugs** (see p. 492)

a. **Aspirin/NSAIDs.** Salicylates or NSAIDs are given initially. Indomethacin and tolmetin sodium seem to be more active than other NSAIDs in this form of arthritis.

b. **Intraarticular steroid injection** is used for severe inflammation of a few joints.

c. **Remittive agents,** especially sulfasalazine or methotrexate, are used for reactive arthritides that are unresponsive to NSAIDs.

III. Lyme disease
   A. Etiology. Lyme disease is caused by the spirochete *Borrelia burgdorferi*, carried by the deer tick *Ixodes dammini*.
   B. Evaluation. The initial manifestation of borrelial infection is a characteristic erythema migrans (EM) rash in about 50% of cases. This may be accompanied by flu-like symptoms, including fever, lethargy, headache, neck pain, and myalgia. Lyme arthritis occurs weeks to months after the inciting tick bite, though neither the tick bite nor the rash might be recognized. Lyme arthritis usually involves the large joints (especially the knee), and is characterized by recurrent attacks that last for weeks to months.
   C. Diagnosis is made by consistent history, physical findings, and antiborrelial antibody titers.
   D. Treatment. See Table 18-2.
IV. Acute rheumatic fever (ARF)
   A. Etiology. Acute rheumatic fever occurs following streptococcal pharyngitis and is associated with the production of antistreptococcal antibodies that cross react with tissue antigens, causing injury.
   B. Evaluation and diagnosis. Diagnosis is made using the Jones criteria (Table 18-3).
   C. Treatment
   1. **Prevention.** Acute rheumatic fever is avoided by treatment of group A streptococcal pharyngitis within 9 days of onset with benzathine penicillin (1.2 million units IM), or penicillin VK (12.5 mg/kg PO qid) for 10 days. In penicillin-allergic

Table 18-2. Complications and treatment of Lyme disease

Disease stage	Organ system	Treatment
Acute (stage 1)	General: malaise, flu-like symptoms Skin: erythema migrans	Oral regimens *Children* < 9 yr: amoxicillin, 250 mg tid, or penicillin V, 250 mg qid for 10–30 d In case of penicillin allergy: erythromycin, 250 mg tid for 10–30 d *Adults:* tetracycline, 250 mg qid; doxycycline, 100 mg bid; or amoxicillin, 500 mg qid, all for 10–30 days
Chronic (stage 2)	General: severe malaise and fatigue Skin: annular rash Neurologic: meningitis, Bell's palsy, radiculoneuritis Cardiac: first-degree atrioventricular block (P-R interval < 0.3 sec) Musculoskeletal: migratory arthralgias and arthritis	Parenteral regimens: penicillin G, 20 million units IV divided 6 × daily for 14–28 d, or ceftriaxone 2 gd for 14–28 d Oral regimens, as for early infection
Persistent (stage 3)	Skin: acrodermatitis chronica atrophicans Neurologic: chronic encephalomyelitis, spastic parapareses, ataxia Musculoskeletal: chronic arthritis, peripheral enthesopathy	Oral regimen for 1 mo usually adequate Parenteral regimen, though duration of therapy not established Parenteral regimen as for stage 2 disease

Source: Adapted from Anonymous. Treatment of lyme disease in *Med Lett Drugs Ther* 30:65–66, 1988.

Table 18-3. Jones criteria (revised)*

Major manifestations	Minor manifestations	Supportive evidence
Carditis	Fever	Recent scarlet fever
Polyarthritis	Arthralgia	Throat culture positive
Chorea	Previous rheumatic fever	for group A
Erythema marginatum	or rheumatic heart	streptococci
	condition	
Subcutaneous nodules	Elevated ESR or positive	Increased ASO or other
	CRP	streptococcal
	Prolonged P-R interval	antibodies
	on ECG	

ESR = erythrocyte sedimentation rate; CRP = C-reactive protein; ASO = antistreptolysin O.
*Two major manifestations or one major and two minor manifestations with supportive evidence of recent streptococcal infection indicate a high probability of rheumatic fever.

patients, erythromycin (7.5 mg/kg qid; maximum 1,000 mg/day) should be substituted.

2. **Acute illness.** All treatments are symptomatic; no therapy is known to alter the natural history of ARF.

   a. **General.** Benzathine penicillin, 1.2 million units IM, or procaine penicillin G, 600,000 units IV daily for 10 days, is given. When the patient is allergic to penicillin, erythromycin is used.

   b. **Carditis**

      (1) **Without cardiomegaly.** Aspirin, 80 mg/kg/day in four divided doses, is given until symptoms resolve and erythrocyte sedimentation rate (ESR) normalizes. NSAIDs may be adequate substitutes, though clinical data are lacking.

      (2) **With cardiomegaly,** prednisone is given at 1 to 2 mg/kg/day in three divided doses for 2 to 4 weeks; then aspirin therapy is begun.

   c. **Arthritis** is treated with aspirin as above.

   d. **Chorea** responds to rest and a quiet environment. Sedation with haloperidol may help in severe cases.

3. **Prophylaxis.** Penicillin is given either intramuscularly (benzathine penicillin G, 1.2 million units q3–4 wk) or orally (penicillin V, 250 mg bid). Penicillin-allergic patients are given either erythromycin, 250 mg bid, or sulfisoxazole, 0.5 to 1.0 g/day. Prophylaxis should be given for at least 5 years and continued throughout the patient's life in cases of chronic rheumatic heart disease or chorea.

V. **Systemic lupus erythematosus (SLE)** is an episodic multisystem disease characterized by circulating antibodies to nuclear and other tissue antigens (99% have a positive ANA). Autoantibodies and immune complexes mediate tissue injury. SLE is 5 to 10 times more common in females than in males.

A. **Etiology** is unknown.

B. **Evaluation and diagnosis.** SLE is diagnosed when 4 of the 11 classification criteria are present (Table 18-4) and no alternative explanation exists.

C. **Therapy** is not curative, but often will prevent incapacitating symptoms and progressive tissue damage.

   1. **Supportive measures,** including rest and avoidance of triggering factors (sun or fluorescent light exposure, fatigue, intercurrent infections), help to avoid exacerbations. Hypertension and infectious complications must be vigorously treated. Raynaud's phenomenon responds to avoidance of cold exposure, elimination of cigarettes and caffeine, and reduction of stress.

   2. **Drugs**

      a. **Aspirin/NSAIDs** (see pp. 490–491) can control fever and arthritis. The incidence of aseptic meningitis due to ibuprofen is increased in SLE.

Table 18-4. Criteria for systemic lupus erythematosus*

Criterion	Definition
Malar rash	Fixed erythema, flat or raised, over the malar eminences, tending to spare the nasolabial folds
Discoid rash	Erythematous raised patches with adherent keratotic scaling and follicular plugging; atrophic scarring may occur in older lesions
Photosensitivity	Skin rash as a result of unusual reaction to sunlight by patient history or physician observation
Oral ulcers	Oral or nasopharyngeal ulceration, usually painless, observed by a physician
Arthritis	Nonerosive arthritis involving 2 or more peripheral joints, characterized by tenderness, swelling, or effusion
Serositis	(1) Pleuritis (convincing history of pleuritic pain or rub heard by a physician or evidence of pleural effusion) *or* (2) pericarditis (documented by ECG or rub or evidence of pericardial effusion)
Renal disorder	(1) Persistent proteinuria > 0.5 g/d *or* (2) cellular casts—may be red cell, hemoglobin, granular, tubular, or mixed
Neurologic disorder	(1) Seizures (in the absence of offending drugs or known metabolic derangements, e.g., uremia, ketoacidosis, or electrolyte imbalance) *or* (2) psychosis (in the absence of offending drugs or known metabolic derangements, e.g., uremia, ketoacidosis, or electrolyte imbalance)
Hematologic disorder	(1) Hemolytic anemia with reticulocytosis, (2) leukopenia ($<4,000/mm^3$ total on 2 or more occasions), (3) lymphopenia ($<1,500/mm^3$ on 2 or more occasions), *or* (4) thrombocytopenia ($<100,000/mm^3$ in the absence of offending drugs)
Immunologic disorder	(1) Positive LE cell preparation, (2) anti-DNA (antibody to native DNA in abnormal titer), (3) anti-Sm (presence of antibody to Sm nuclear antigen), *or* (4) false-positive serologic test for syphilis known to be positive for at least 6 mo and confirmed by *Treponema pallidum* immobilization or fluorescent treponemal antibody absorption test
Antinuclear antibody	An abnormal titer of antinuclear antibody by immunofluorescence or an equivalent assay at any point in time and in the absence of drugs known to be associated with "drug-induced lupus" syndrome

*For the purpose of identifying patients, a person shall be said to have SLE if any 4 or more of the 11 criteria are present serially or simultaneously during any interval of observation
Sm = Smith antigen.
Source: Modified from EM Tan et al. The 1982 revised criteria for the classification of systemic lupus erythematosus. *Arthritis Rheum* 25:1271–1277, 1982.

    b. Hydroxychloroquine (see sec. **I.D.4.a**) can aid in controlling skin and joint manifestations, serositis, and malaise, and can prolong remissions. It is not effective for renal, CNS, or hematologic disease.
    c. Corticosteroids
        (1) Topical steroids are utilized for localized skin disease.
        (2) Oral steroids are used for life-threatening or debilitating manifestations that are unresponsive to less toxic therapies. Doses of prednisone varying from 0.5 to 2.0 mg/kg/day are generally effective for fever, dermatitis, arthritis, and serositis, as well as for severe end-organ involvement, such as cerebritis, hemolytic anemia, glomeru-

lonephritis, or vasculitis. The steroid dose is tapered when inflammation is controlled. Conversion to an alternate-day regimen can help minimize side effects.

(3) Pulse steroid therapy (methylprednisolone, 30 mg/kg IV on 1–3 consecutive days) is associated with faster clinical improvement and is used for rapidly progressive CNS or renal disease.

(4) Steroid toxicity

(a) Suppression of the hypothalamic-pituitary axis can cause hypoadrenalism as steroids are tapered. Stress doses should be provided if patients become febrile or require surgery.

(b) Immune suppression promotes susceptibility to infection (especially herpesviruses and mycobacteria) and masks signs and symptoms of infection. Clinicians must have a high level of suspicion of infection in any patient with SLE.

(c) Changes in physical appearance, such as moon facies, buffalo hump, acne, striae, weight gain, and hirsutism, are very disturbing to patients.

(d) Neurologic problems, such as euphoria, depression, psychosis, and pseudotumor cerebri, may be difficult to distinguish from neuropsychiatric manifestations of SLE, making management difficult.

(e) Metabolic effects, such as hyperglycemia, hypercholesterolemia, sodium retention, hypokalemia, and hypertension, are common.

(f) Musculoskeletal problems, including osteopenia, proximal myopathy, and aseptic necrosis, can lead to permanent disability.

(g) Ocular effects include glaucoma and cataracts.

d. Cytotoxic agents (cyclophosphamide, azathioprine, chlorambucil) are used for patients with severe prednisone toxicity or life-threatening disease uncontrolled by corticosteroids. Intravenous cyclophosphamide improves outcome in patients with diffuse proliferative glomerulonephritis. Controlled trials that demonstrate efficacy in other situations are lacking.

3. Plasmapheresis is used for rapid removal of antibodies and immune complexes, in conjunction with corticosteroid and cytotoxic therapy. Its efficacy is unproven, though anecdotal reports suggest short-term benefit in acute, life-threatening SLE.

VI. Juvenile dermatomyositis (JDMS) is characterized by diffuse microangiitis involving skeletal muscle, skin, the GI tract, and the CNS.

A. Etiology is unknown. JDMS seems to develop after an acute viral infection in many children.

B. Evaluation. Clinical features include muscle weakness and tenderness, extensor surface skin rash, and constitutional symptoms. Arthritis can occur, and GI vasculitis is a potentially fatal complication. Calcinosis and muscle atrophy may be severe long-term sequelae of muscle inflammation. JDMS is not associated with malignancy, unlike adult polymyositis.

C. Diagnosis is supported by elevated levels of muscle enzymes, rash, and typical findings on electromyography (EMG) or MRI. Muscle biopsy confirms the diagnosis.

D. Therapy

1. Supportive measures include **physical therapy** and splinting to restore muscle strength and prevent contractures. Involvement of palatal/respiratory muscles requires vigorous suctioning, postural drainage, and attention to pulmonary toilet.

2. Drugs

a. Corticosteroids (e.g., prednisone; see p. 496), 2 mg/kg/day in four divided doses, are prescribed until clinical improvement occurs, then tapered over several months to the lowest dose that maintains normal strength and muscle enzymes. Maintenance steroids may be required for years. If relapse occurs (rare after the first few years) high-dose corticosteroids are reinstituted. **Bolus intravenous methylprednisolone** may result in more rapid improvement and fewer long-term complications.

b. **Aspirin/NSAIDs** are used for arthritis (see p. 490).

c. **Cytotoxic agents** (methotrexate, cyclosporine-A) can be used in patients who are unresponsive to corticosteroids or in whom unacceptable steroid toxicity develops.

VII. **Scleroderma** is characterized by fibrosis and vascular hyperreactivity, resulting in hidebound skin, Raynaud's phenomenon, and fibrosis of internal organs (lungs, heart, GI tract, kidneys).

  A. **Etiology** is unknown.

  B. **Diagnosis** is strongly suggested by one major or two minor criteria.

    1. **The major criterion** is proximal scleroderma, that is, hidebound, thickened skin with loss of appendages proximal to the wrists.

    2. **Minor criteria** include sclerodactyly, digital pitting ulcers, and bibasilar pulmonary fibrosis.

  C. **Treatment.** There is no cure for scleroderma; therapy is aimed at treating symptomatic organ involvement. **Physical** and **occupational therapy** are used to maintain range of motion. **D-Penicillamine** slows cutaneous fibrosis and can ameliorate systemic manifestations.

VIII. **Mixed connective tissue disease (MCTD)** is a condition with overlapping features of scleroderma, dermatomyositis, rheumatoid arthritis, and SLE.

  A. **Etiology** is unknown.

  B. **Evaluation and diagnosis.** Diagnosis is based on demonstration of multiple systemic rheumatologic conditions, often meeting diagnostic criteria for more than one disease. High-titer ANA, antiribonucleoprotein (RNP), and extractable nuclear antigen (ENA) are characteristic of this disorder.

  C. **Treatment** is based on appropriate management of the patient's predominant disease manifestations (see above).

IX. **Necrotizing vasculitis** involves immune-mediated inflammation and necrosis of blood vessels.

  A. **Mucocutaneous lymph node syndrome (MLNS)** or **Kawasaki's disease**

    1. **Etiology.** MLNS appears to be caused by an as yet unidentified infectious agent.

    2. **Evaluation and diagnosis.** The diagnosis of MLNS is made in an acutely ill child with five of the following criteria in the absence of alternative diagnoses (e.g., measles or scarlet fever).

      a. **Fever** that persists for 5 or more days.

      b. **Rash** (polymorphic, not vesicular).

      c. Acute nonpurulent **cervical lymphadenopathy** (at least 1.5 cm).

      d. **Conjunctivitis** (bilateral, nonexudative).

      e. **Extremity changes** (edema of hands and feet, erythema of palms and soles, or periungual desquamation).

      f. **Mucosal changes** (erythematous and fissured lips, red oropharynx, "strawberry" tongue).

      Laboratory manifestations include elevated ESR and C-reactive protein (CRP), leukocytosis, and thrombocytosis. Untreated, there is a 15 to 25% incidence of coronary artery aneurysms and a 1 to 2% mortality.

    3. **Therapy**

      a. **Aspirin** (see p. 490), 80 to 100 mg/kg/day until afebrile for 48 hours, then 3 to 5 mg/kg/day.

      b. **Intravenous gamma globulin** (IVGG), 2 g/kg over 10 to 12 hours, dramatically reduces the incidence of coronary artery changes, the duration of acute inflammation, and the mortality. IVGG rarely causes an anaphylactoid reaction, flushing, or fever, which generally respond to slowing the infusion rate.

  B. **Polyarteritis nodosa (PAN)**

    1. **Etiology** is unknown; PAN may follow an infectious illness (especially streptococcal infection or hepatitis B).

2. **Evaluation.** Polyarteritis nodosa is characterized by systemic illness, including fever and malaise, with vasculitis involving one or more organs. Skin and renal involvement are common; liver, GI tract, cardiac, CNS, and musculoskeletal system involvement can occur.

3. **Diagnosis** is based on angiographic or biopsy evidence of vasculitis of medium-sized muscular arteries.

4. **Therapy** is similar to that of SLE (see p. 495), using steroids or cytotoxic agents to prevent organ damage.

C. **Henoch-Schönlein purpura (HSP)** is characterized by a maculopapular or purpuric rash of dependent portions of the body (typically legs and buttocks), arthritis or arthralgia, abdominal pain (possibly with GI hemorrhage or intussusception), and nephritis.

1. **Etiology** is unclear, but **HSP** often occurs after upper respiratory infection, streptococcal pharyngitis (approximately 30%), or gastroenteritis.

2. **Evaluation.** Diagnosis is made on clinical grounds; biopsy of newly affected skin often reveals perivascular deposition of immunoglobulin A (IgA). Severe renal involvement (hematuria, hypertension, and nephrotic range proteinuria) may rarely (<1%) progress to chronic renal failure. Laboratory findings include elevated serum IgA and acute-phase reactants.

3. **Treatment** is supportive.

   a. **Salicylates or NSAIDs** (see pp. 490–491) are used to treat isolated arthritis.

   b. **Corticosteroids.** Prednisone, 1 to 2 mg/kg/day, has been used for bowel involvement or severe arthritis that is unresponsive to aspirin. Nephritis is unresponsive to steroids.

X. **Sarcoidosis** is a chronic, multisystem granulomatous disease.

A. **Etiology** is unknown.

B. **Evaluation.** Manifestations include a maculopapular or nodular rash, arthritis, uveitis, fever, and malaise. Noncaseating granulomas may be found in lung, muscle, liver, skin, and nervous system. Prognosis is related to the extent of pulmonary involvement. **Laboratory manifestations** include elevated angiotensin converting enzyme (ACE) and gallium uptake in lacrimal and parotid glands. Systemic involvement is usually associated with elevated acute-phase reactants.

C. **Diagnosis** is made by biopsy of affected tissue, revealing noncaseating granulomas without an infectious cause.

D. **Treatment**

1. Skin and joint manifestations are treated with NSAIDs or hydroxychloroquine.

2. Anterior uveitis is treated with topical steroid drops.

3. **Systemic symptoms and posterior iridocyclitis** are treated with prednisone, 1 to 2 mg/kg/day.

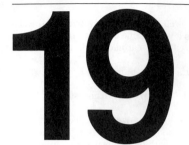

Musculoskeletal Disorders

Richard Bachur and Peter Waters

I. **Upper extremity problems**
   A. **Shoulder**
      1. **Glenohumeral joint dislocations**
         a. **Etiology:** unusual before physeal closure; anterior dislocations are most common.
         b. **Evaluation**
            (1) **History:** is usually due to a fall on the elbow or hand with the arm abducted and externally rotated.
            (2) **Physical examination.** The contour of the shoulder is altered with a prominent acromion and a depression under the acromion. Posterior dislocations are more difficult to diagnose; the anterior fullness of the shoulder is lost. Both sensory function of the axillary nerve and distal neurovascular function should be tested.
            (3) **Radiographs.** Anteroposterior (AP), lateral, and scapular "Y" views of the shoulder should be obtained before any reduction attempt.
         c. **Diagnosis:** the combination of physical examination findings and displacement of the humeral head from the glenoid fossa on radiograph.
         d. **Therapy**
            (1) Anterior dislocations are reduced by either Stimson's traction-countertraction or external rotation methods.
            (2) Reductions should be performed by experienced clinicians.
            (3) Reduction can be facilitated by narcotic analgesics or benzodiazepines.
            (4) Posterior dislocations are relocated by application of axial traction (similar to the traction-countertraction method for anterior dislocations).
            (5) Postreduction radiographs should be obtained.
            (6) Axillary nerve function should be retested after reduction.
            (7) Following reduction, the arm should be placed in a sling and swathe.
      2. **Clavicular fractures:** the most frequent bone fractured in children and the most common birth injury.
         a. **Etiology:** Clavicle fractures in newborns are caused by difficult deliveries and in older children are due to falling on an outstretched arm or directly on to the shoulder. Fractures from direct force to the clavicle may be associated with pulmonary and neurovascular injuries.
         b. **Evaluation**
            (1) **Physical examination**
               (a) **Newborns**
                  (i) Swelling at the site of the healing callus.
                  (ii) "Pseudoparalysis." This must be distinguished from other causes of weakness such as brachial plexus injury and traumatic separation of the proximal humeral epiphysis.
               (b) **Young children**
                  (i) Tenderness, swelling, and crepitus.
                  (ii) Examination of the rest of the upper extremity should be normal.

       (2) Radiographs: AP and lateral views of the shoulder.
  c. Diagnosis. The radiographs confirm the diagnosis.
  d. Therapy
     (1) Younger than 2 years of age
       (a) No treatment or a swathe to bind the arm to the trunk for a few days.
       (b) Advise the parents to be careful handling the shoulder when lifting.
     (2) Two to 12 years
       (a) The patient is usually made more comfortable if the arm is immobilized with a figure-of-eight harness or an arm sling.
       (b) Union should be present by 2 to 4 weeks and immobilization can be discontinued after 3 weeks.
     (3) Older than 12 years of age
       (a) Fractures are usually complete.
       (b) A figure-of-eight harness provides the most support and comfort; discontinue after 3 to 4 weeks.
       (c) The patient should avoid contact sports for at least 3 months.

B. Elbow injuries
  1. Radial head subluxation ("nursemaid's elbow," "pulled elbow")
    a. Etiology: excessive axial traction of an extended elbow in a child younger than 5 years of age.
    b. Evaluation
     (1) Physical examination
       (a) The affected arm is slightly flexed at the elbow and the forearm is pronated.
       (b) Decreased active motion.
       (c) The clavicle and wrist should be examined for injury as well.
     (2) Radiographs: should be obtained if the history is atypical or the examination reveals any swelling, deformity, or point tenderness.
    c. Diagnosis. Radiographs are normal. Subluxation is considered based on a consistent history and physical examination; however, the diagnosis is confirmed upon a successful reduction.
    d. Therapy. Reduction is accomplished by fully extending the elbow while firmly supinating the forearm followed by full flexion of the elbow maintaining supination. Reduction is usually palpable.
  2. Elbow fractures/dislocations: can be complicated by injury to the neurovascular structures in the forearm and hand.
    a. Etiology: result from falls on an outstretched hand and only rarely from direct blows. A nondisplaced supracondylar fracture is the most common elbow fracture.
    b. Evaluation
     (1) Physical examination. Swelling, ecchymosis, point tenderness, and pain with motion are present. Distal neurovascular function should be assessed.
     (2) Radiographs. Both AP and true lateral views of the elbow should be obtained.
    c. Diagnosis. Radiographs reveal the fracture. In the absence of an obvious fracture, the presence of a posterior fat pad also suggests an intraarticular fracture.
    d. Therapy. After assessment of the neurovascular function, the elbow should be splinted and elevated to limit swelling. *All supracondylar fractures require immediate orthopedic consultation.*

C. Fractures of the radius and ulna
  1. Etiology: falls on an outstretched hand; the type of fracture depends on the mechanism of injury and the age of the child.
  2. Evaluation
    a. Physical examination. Swelling and tenderness will invariably be present over the fracture site. Neurovascular function should be assessed especially with large deformities.

b. Radiographs. Anteroposterior and lateral views of the forearm including the elbow should be obtained.

3. Diagnosis. Radiographs demonstrate the fracture. In cases of tenderness over the physis and negative radiographs, Salter-Harris I fractures must be considered.

4. Treatment

a. A splint should be applied whenever a fracture is suspected. Elevation and splinting will reduce pain and limit swelling.

b. Displaced fractures require immediate orthopedic consultation.

c. Nondisplaced fractures can be splinted and orthopedic consultation can be delayed for up to 48 hours.

D. Injuries of the hand

1. Phalangeal fractures

a. Etiology

(1) *Distal phalangeal fractures* are usually due to a crush injury and it is common for multiple fingers to be injured simultaneously. Avulsion fractures of the distal phalanx result from forced hyperflexion (dorsal avulsion, mallet finger) or forced hyperextension (volar avulsion).

(2) *Middle phalangeal fractures* are usually secondary to crush injuries and often involve injury of the volar plate.

(3) The most common finger fracture is a Salter II *proximal phalangeal fracture* of the small finger with valgus malalignment.

b. Evaluation

(1) Physical examination. Focal tenderness, swelling, and limited range of motion will be present. Ligamentous instability and neurovascular injury may accompany phalangeal fractures. Malrotation is common with shaft fractures of the proximal and middle phalanges.

(a) Avulsion fractures of *the distal phalanx* can result in loss of function at the distal interphalangeal joint.

(b) Distal *middle phalangeal* fractures are more likely to have dorsal angulation.

(c) *Proximal phalanx* fractures tend to have volar angulation, as do proximal middle phalangeal fractures.

(2) Radiographs: AP and lateral views.

c. Diagnosis. Radiographs will confirm the fracture.

d. Therapy. Any physeal fracture requires reduction by an orthopedist.

(1) *Distal and middle phalanx* fractures are immobilized with buddy-taping to the adjacent digit. Maintaining mobility is important.

(2) All nondisplaced fractures of the *proximal phalanx* can be managed with a gutter or "trouser" splint that immobilizes the affected and the adjacent finger and holds the metacarpophalangeal joint at 70 degrees. Fractures with malrotation should be treated by an orthopedist.

2. Metacarpophalangeal (MP) and interphalangeal (IP) joint sprains and dislocations

a. Metacarpophalangeal sprains

(1) Etiology: usually involve the radial collateral ligaments of the ring and middle fingers.

(2) Evaluation

(a) Physical examination: immediately after the injury, a combination of tenderness, swelling, ecchymosis, and decreased range of motion at the affected joint. After the acute inflammation resolves, increased joint laxity may be apparent.

(b) Radiographs: AP and lateral radiographs of the joint.

(3) Diagnosis. Normal radiographs in the presence of a focal examination suggest the diagnosis.

(4) Therapy. Buddy-taping or immobilization is sufficient unless the joint is unstable, in which case orthopedic consultation is necessary.

b. Metacarpophalangeal dislocations

(1) Etiology: result from hyperextension and may have associated fractures.
(2) Evaluation
  (a) Physical examination. In simple dislocations, the proximal phalanx remains hyperextended, with the carpal head displaced volarly into the palm. In complex dislocations, the dorsal phalanx and volar metacarpal are parallel (in "bayonet" apposition). Neurovascular status should be assessed.
  (b) Radiographs. Anteroposterior and lateral views should be obtained before reduction to exclude any associated fractures.
(3) Therapy
  (a) Closed reduction is attempted with only simple dislocations.
  (b) Reduction is performed by flexion of the digit after longitudinal traction is applied.
  (c) If reduction is successful, the finger should be buddy-taped for 3 weeks.
  (d) If closed reduction of a simple dislocation fails, the finger should be immobilized, and an orthopedist consulted for possible open reduction.
  (e) *Complex dislocations involve entrapment of the volar plate within the joint and require emergency operative reduction.*
c. Interphalangeal dislocations
  (1) Etiology: result of hyperextension. Dorsal dislocations are common and volar dislocations are rare.
  (2) Evaluation
    (a) Physical examination. Most commonly, the more distal phalanx is displaced dorsally and the deformity is obvious.
    (b) Radiographs. Anteroposterior and lateral views should be obtained before the reduction.
  (3) Therapy
    (a) After digital block anesthesia, the dislocation can be reduced by applying longitudinal traction and then flexing the joint to bring the distal segment into position.
    (b) Postreduction films should be obtained.
    (c) After reduction, the joint should be tested for lateral stability. If lateral instability exists, the finger should be splinted for 3 weeks and referral for rehabilitation is necessary to prevent stiffness. If stable, the finger should be buddy-taped for 7 to 10 days.
    (d) Volar dislocations should be referred to an orthopedist because of presumed tendon and ligamentous injury.

II. Lower extremity problems
  A. Hip and thigh
    1. Toxic synovitis: the most common cause of hip pain in toddlers and young children aged 18 months to 7 years (peak incidence at age 2 yr).
      a. Evaluation
        (1) Physical examination
          (a) Unilateral hip pain with limited range of motion and antalgic gait.
          (b) The child may prefer to hold the leg externally rotated and slightly flexed at the hip.
          (c) Resistance to extension, adduction, or internal rotation of the hip may be noted.
          (d) Fever, if present, is usually low grade.
          (e) Patients with toxic synovitis appear well.
        (2) Laboratories: complete blood count and erythrocyte sedimentation rate (ESR).
        (3) Radiographs
          (a) Anteroposterior and frog-leg lateral views to determine if an effusion is present (increased distance between acetabulum and femoral head).

    (b) Ultrasound can better estimate the presence or size of a hip effusion.
  b. Diagnosis
    (1) Unlike patients with septic hips, these individuals usually have a normal peripheral white blood cell count and erythrocyte sedimentation rate.
    (2) Absence of an effusion on radiograph or ultrasound can be reassuring in the well-appearing child with hip pain.
    (3) If septic arthritis cannot be excluded clinically, joint aspiration for cell count, Gram's stain, and culture should be performed.
  c. Therapy
    (1) Toxic synovitis resolves with rest and nonsteroidal anti-inflammatory agents.
    (2) Crutches (if age appropriate) should be used until the child can painlessly bear weight.
    (3) Although most heal completely, in a small percentage Legg-Calvé-Perthes disease eventually develops.
2. Legg-Calvé-Perthes disease
  a. Etiology: avascular necrosis of the femoral head. It occurs predominantly in males (4 : 1) between the ages of 4 and 8 years.
  b. Evaluation
    (1) Physical examination
      (a) Groin or buttock pain and limp are common complaints.
      (b) *Knee pain*, referred from the affected hip, may also be the presenting complaint. An antalgic gait is present.
      (c) Internal rotation and abduction are limited and the thigh may be slightly flexed at the hip.
    (2) Radiographs: AP and frog-leg lateral views.
  c. Diagnosis. Radiographs are abnormal. Early changes consist of widening of the joint space and epiphyseal line. Late changes include flattening of the femoral head, sclerosis, and widening of the femoral neck.
  d. Therapy. All patients should be referred to an orthopedist for care.
3. Slipped capital femoral epiphysis (SCFE)
  a. Etiology
    (1) Displacement of the femoral head relative to the femoral neck at the epiphyseal plate.
    (2) Acute SCFE results from a shear force during trauma; 80% of cases are chronic.
    (3) SCFE tends to occur in the peripubertal period during accelerated growth.
    (4) Risk factors include gender (males 2–4 : 1), race (black), and obesity (80%).
    (5) Of patients who present with unilateral SCFE, 30 to 40% will progress to bilateral involvement.
    (6) SCFE may be associated with endocrinologic disorders, specifically hypopituitarism, renal rickets, and growth hormone therapy.
  b. Evaluation
    (1) Physical examination
      (a) Groin, lateral hip, buttock, or knee pain (referred from the hip) is a common complaint.
      (b) Chronic SCFE may present as a painless limp.
      (c) Pain is never severe except in acute SCFE.
      (d) Limp is present and the affected limb is externally rotated.
      (e) Hip motion, especially internal rotation abduction, and flexion will be decreased.
      (f) With flexion of the hip, there is obligate external rotation and abduction.
    (2) Radiographs: AP and frog-leg lateral.

   c. Diagnosis: demonstrates the femoral head displaced posteriorly and me-
      dially. A line drawn along the superior edge of the neck that normally inter-
      sects the femoral head will not do so in SCFE.
   d. Therapy
      (1) The patient should not bear weight.
      (2) Immediate orthopedic consultation is necessary.
      (3) The only effective treatment is operative repair.
B. Knee and lower leg problems
   1. Osgood-Schlatter disease (apophysitis of the tibial tuberosity)
      a. Etiology: commonly seen in athletic males as an "overuse syndrome."
      b. Evaluation
         (1) History. Children 10 to 15 years of age present with knee pain that
            worsens with activity, especially running. The patient may complain
            of focal pain and intermittent swelling.
         (2) Physical examination: pain to palpation or percussion over the tib-
            ial tuberorsity. Swelling may be present.
         (3) Radiographs: AP and lateral views.
      c. Diagnosis
         (1) Radiographs often demonstrate soft tissue swelling over the tuberos-
            ity and increased density of the patellar tendon at the insertion.
         (2) Radiographs in older children may demonstrate a small density sepa-
            rate from the apophysis.
      d. Therapy
         (1) Rest and nonsteroidal anti-inflammatory agents.
         (2) Immobilization can relieve severe symptoms.
         (3) Reevaluation by an orthopedist is recommended after 3 weeks.
   2. Chondromalacia patellae
      a. Etiology: an "overuse" syndrome.
      b. Evaluation
         (1) History: poorly localized pain over the patella that worsens while
            climbing stairs or prolonged sitting ("theater sign").
         (2) Physical examination: pain with compression of the patella, espe-
            cially with the quadriceps contracted. There may be crepitus when
            compressing the patella and tenderness on the undersurface of the
            patella as it is displaced laterally.
         (3) Radiographs: AP, lateral, and tunnel ("sunrise") views.
      c. Diagnosis: radiographs are usually normal but may show defects on the
         posterior surface of the patella. If the radiographs are normal, the diagno-
         sis is based on the typical history and examination.
      d. Treatment. The patient should decrease activity, avoid strenuous exer-
         cises, and perform quadriceps-strengthening exercises including straight
         leg raises.
   3. Ligamentous injuries of the knee
      a. Etiology
         (1) Medial collateral ligament (MCL). The mechanism of injury is a
            twisting motion or a blow to the lateral knee causing valgus stress.
         (2) Anterior cruciate ligament (ACL). Typically, the ACL is injured
            secondary to hyperextension or sudden deceleration with the foot
            planted, causing abduction and external rotation of the leg.
         (3) Posterior cruciate ligament. This ligament is injured by a direct
            blow to the tibia while the knee is flexed, thereby forcing the proxi-
            mal tibia posteriorly.
      b. Evaluation
         (1) Physical examination. With severe or acute injuries, pain and limita-
            tion of motion prevent a thorough examination.
            (a) MCL. Pain is elicited by palpation over the MCL. Laxity can be
               demonstrated by applying valgus stress. A joint effusion and lim-
               itation of motion often coexist.

(b) ACL. A large hemarthrosis is present, and Lachman and anterior drawer tests are positive.

(c) Posterior cruciate ligament. Posterior knee tenderness and a small effusion are present.

(2) Radiographs: AP and lateral views.

c. Diagnosis

(1) The diagnosis is made based on the examination, which often has to be delayed until swelling and tenderness subside.

(2) Radiographs should exclude any concomitant fractures.

(3) ACL injuries can be associated with an avulsion fracture of the tibial spine.

d. Treatment

(1) ACL injuries with avulsion fractures require urgent orthopedic consultation.

(2) For all other suspected ligamentous injuries, the initial management should include ice, elevation, compression, nonsteroidal anti-inflammatory agents, and rest (no weight bearing).

(3) The patient should be referred to an orthopedist once the swelling has subsided (after several days).

(4) In the case of large hemarthroses, aspiration of the joint can relieve excessive pain.

4. Meniscal injury

a. Etiology

(1) Usually results from a twisting or bending force with the knee in flexion and the foot planted.

(2) Meniscal injuries are more common in adolescents than in younger children, and the medial meniscus is injured five times as often as the lateral meniscus.

b. Evaluation

(1) History

(a) The patient may report an audible "snap" or "pop" coincident with a buckling of the knee.

(b) The injury is followed by painful motion and a limp.

(c) Swelling is acute, but symptoms subside within a few days.

(d) After the acute episode, the patient presents with symptoms of impingement: a sensation of snapping or popping in the joint, "giving out," "locking," or recurrent swelling especially after activity.

(2) Physical examination

(a) The knee is tender along the medial or lateral joint line that corresponds to the meniscus that was injured.

(b) The knee may lock in flexion or prevent full extension, which is very sensitive for internal derangement of the knee.

(c) The McMurray maneuver and the Appley's test are positive.

(3) Radiographs: AP and lateral views of the knee.

c. Diagnosis. The diagnosis is based on a typical history and examination.

d. Therapy

(1) Referral to an orthopedist after several days rest.

(2) Immobilization and compression of the knee, crutches, elevation, and compression.

5. Toddler's fracture: classically refers to an oblique nondisplaced fracture of the distal tibia without a fibular fracture.

a. Evaluation

(1) History. The child usually presents with an acute antalgic gait or refusal to bear weight, classically after a seemingly minor fall.

(2) Physical examination. Often there is minimal swelling and a careful examination is necessary to localize tenderness.

(3) Radiographs

    (a) If focal tenderness or swelling is not apparent, AP and lateral radiographs of the entire leg should be obtained.

    (b) With focal tenderness of the tibia, an oblique view can also be obtained if the other views do not delineate a fracture.

  b. Diagnosis. Radiographic findings are subtle and can only be seen on an internal oblique view.

  c. Therapy

    (1) Immobilization with a long leg cast will promote healing and provide comfort.

    (2) *In the presence of a spiral fracture, child abuse should be considered, especially if the child is not yet old enough to ambulate* (see p. 240).

    (3) In general, fractures of the tibia from child abuse are midshaft, whereas the majority of toddler's fractures are distal.

C. Ankle and foot problems

  1. Ankle sprains

    a. Evaluation

      (1) History. Inversion injury, especially during plantar flexion, is the most common mechanism of injury.

      (2) Physical examination

        (a) Swelling, ecchymosis, and tenderness may be present. Tenderness over growth plates should be noted.

        (b) The talofibular ligaments are most commonly disrupted, which leads to tenderness just anterior to the lateral malleolus.

      (3) Radiographs: AP and lateral views of the ankle.

    b. Diagnosis

      (1) Acute injuries that lead to swelling or tenderness without radiographic abnormalities are considered sprains.

      (2) However, as with other joints, physeal injuries are more common than ligamentous injuries and therefore it is impossible to exclude Salter I fractures in a young child.

    c. Therapy

      (1) Tenderness or swelling over a growth plate should be treated as a presumed Salter I fracture with casting or splinting, elevation, crutches, and orthopedic follow-up in one week.

      (2) Grade I sprains are immobilized with an elastic wrap or air splint and treated with ice, elevation, nonsteroidal anti-inflammatory agents, and crutches for 3 days or until weight bearing is possible without pain.

      (3) Grade II and III sprains require immobilization with a cast or posterior splint and crutches for 3 weeks, and then slow introduction of activity.

      (4) Rehabilitation of the ankle must be carefully planned to avoid recurrent sprains.

  2. In-toeing can be divided into three conditions (or combination of conditions).

    a. Metatarsus adductus

      (1) Evaluation

        (a) History: a strong familial tendency, usually a diagnosis in the newborn. Unilateral metatarsus adductus has a 100% association with ipsilateral hip dysplasia.

        (b) Physical examination. The forefoot is in varus and may look clinically similar to a clubfoot (fixed varus deformity of both the forefoot and hindfoot) but the hindfoot is normal. Both the lateral margin and the plantar surface of the foot are shaped like a "C."

      (2) Therapy. The foot will correct itself with time if it straightens with stroking the lateral margin. If not, the parents can perform stretching exercises to correct the problem, but orthopedic referral for serial casting may be necessary.

b. Internal tibial torsion: usually diagnosed in the early walking child
   (1) Evaluation
   (a) The degree of torsion is measured with the patient prone and the knees flexed to 90 degrees, palpating both malleoli.
   (b) Normally the medial malleolus should be anterior (15 degrees) to the transcondylar axis of the knee.
   (2) Therapy
   (a) Most resolve by 2 to 3 years of life.
   (b) Rarely, nighttime braces are indicated.
   (c) If the condition does not improve over the first year of walking, the patient should be referred to an orthopedist.

c. Femoral anteversion (medial femoral torsion)
   (1) Evaluation
   (a) History
      (i) Usually diagnosed in the older child, typically age 4 or 5 years.
      (ii) The child is often female, and commonly has a history of sitting in the reverse "W" position with the hips flexed to 90 degrees and the knees flexed to 130 degrees such that the feet are behind the child and pointing outward.
   (b) Physical examination. External rotation is limited as detected by
      (i) "Log-rolling" the legs with the patient supine and the hips and knees fully extended.
      (ii) With the patient prone and the knees at 90 degrees, allowing the legs to fall outward by gravity (internal rotation) and crossing the legs (external rotation).
      (iii) Normally, 40 to 50 degrees of internal and external rotation can be achieved.
      (iv) With femoral anteversion, the femur can be internally rotated up to 90 degrees, whereas external rotation is limited.
   (2) Therapy
   (a) The child should be discouraged from sitting in the reverse "W" position and should be encouraged to sit with legs crossed anterior to the hip.
   (b) Femoral anteversion usually resolves by age 10 to 12 years of age and rarely requires orthopedic treatment.
   (c) Treatment is only indicated when the child does not improve spontaneously and has repeated falls or severe gait disturbances.

III. Problems in the spine
   A. Cervical spine
      1. Congenital torticollis
         a. Etiology. The majority of cases are associated with difficult deliveries especially breech presentations and may be related to intrauterine malposition or muscle injury during delivery.
         b. Evaluation
            (1) The torticollis is seldom visible at birth.
            (2) After one week, a lump (pseudotumor) appears in the lower one-third of the sternocleidomastoid (SCM) coincident with an ipsilateral head tilt.
            (3) Motion of the neck is limited and plagiocephaly may be present.
            (4) Historically, the infant may always rest on the same part of the head, causing a bald spot on the ipsilateral occiput.
         c. Therapy
            (1) Stretching exercises should be instituted immediately.
            (2) Parents should be advised to position the child during sleep to facilitate stretching of the SCM.
            (3) If the torticollis is not corrected early in life, permanent facial asym-

metry can develop and persist even after surgical lengthening of the SCM.

(4) Radiographs should be obtained in resistant cases to exclude congenital cervical anomalies.

2. Acquired torticollis

a. Etiology

(1) *Atlantoaxial rotatory subluxation* following an uncomplicated upper respiratory infection or trauma results in muscular spasm of the "long" SCM in response to fixation of C1 on C2.

(2) Local reactive muscular inflammation concomitant with cervical adenitis, discitis, and vertebral osteomyelitis results in ipsilateral SCM spasm.

b. Evaluation

(1) Physical examination. Pain to palpation and decreased motion are present. The patient is unable to return the head to midline.

(2) Radiographs: demonstrate rotatory displacement of C1. Associated etiologies should be sought.

c. Therapy

(1) Patients without a history of trauma are managed with a soft cervical collar and nonsteroidal anti-inflammatory medications.

(2) Patients with known trauma, anterior displacement of C1, or any neurologic complaints or findings require immobilization, CT evaluation, and a neurosurgical consultation.

(3) Traction and muscle relaxants may be necessary.

B. Scoliosis: lateral deviation of the spine

1. Congenital scoliosis

a. Etiology: occurs from failure of formation of vertebra (e.g., hemivertebra) or failure of segmentation of the bony elements (congenital bar or block vertebra).

b. Evaluation. Congenital scoliosis should be considered when any asymmetry of the shoulders, ribs, or trunk is found or if midline defects of the back (dimples, sinus tracts, hairy patches) are present.

c. Treatment

(1) The patient should be referred to an orthopedist.

(2) As many as 50% of patients require spinal fusion to stop progressive deformity.

2. Idiopathic scoliosis. Minor degrees of scoliosis are functionally and cosmetically insignificant. Infantile (onset younger than 3 yr) form of idiopathic scoliosis resolves spontaneously in 75% of cases. Juvenile (onset between 3 and 10 yr of age) and adolescent (onset after 10 yr of age) idiopathic scoliosis more commonly require intervention. Girls are eight times more likely than boys to require treatment for scoliosis.

a. Etiology: unknown but believed to be a combination of growth asymmetry and postural imbalance.

b. Evaluation

(1) Physical examination. The following signs are associated with scoliosis.

(a) Positive bend test: asymmetrical prominence of the thoracic or lumbar region when the patient bends forward (with the arms and head fully relaxed and hanging toward the floor); reflects the rotational component of the spinal deformity. A "hump" will be noted on the convex side of the curve.

(b) Asymmetrical shoulder height, scapula asymmetry, asymmetry of the waistline or flank contour, asymmetrical distances from the arms to the trunk, a palpable curve as the hand follows the spinous processes.

(c) Pain is not typical in idiopathic scoliosis.

(2) Radiographs: standing posteroanterior x-ray of the spine.

   c. Therapy. Using the radiographs, measure the curve using the Cobb method. Consultation with an orthopedist is necessary.

     (1) Spinal curvatures less than 25 degrees require careful follow-up.

     (2) Curves between 25 and 40 degrees in skeletally immature patients can be treated with a brace and close follow-up (80–90% effective in compliant patients).

     (3) The goal of bracing is prevention of curve progression, not correction of the deformity.

     (4) Curves greater than 40 degrees usually need surgical intervention.

Neurologic Disorders

Karl Kuban and
Catherine Chapman

I. Disorders of mental status: intracranial hypertension
A. Coma and acute increased intracranial pressure (ICP) (see Chap. 7, p. 235)
B. Reye's syndrome
  1. **Etiology.** The cause is not understood, although it is probably a mitochondrial disease associated with influenza and varicella, and possibly aspirin use, that primarily involves the liver and brain.
  2. **Evaluation and diagnosis**
    a. Characteristically, an antecedent viral illness is followed by vomiting and progressive lethargy.
    b. **Examination.** Tachypnea, fever, lethargy, and stupor or coma are typical. Signs of elevated ICP and, more rarely, seizures may also be noted.
    c. **Laboratory findings**
      (1) Elevated serum **hepatocellular enzyme assays** (SGOT, SGPT, LDH) and serum arterial ammonia are the laboratory hallmarks; one may also see metabolic acidosis and respiratory alkalosis as well as hypoglycemia and prolongation of the prothrombin time (PT) and partial thromboplastin time (PTT).
      (2) **A CT scan** or **MRI scan** may be necessary to rule out an intracranial mass.
      (3) Lumbar puncture is relatively contraindicated in patients with Reye's syndrome because of the high risk of cerebral herniation.
      (4) **Liver biopsy** is generally performed when the diagnosis is in question. Questionable features include an unusual age (<1 yr old or >16 yr old) and recurrent episodes, such as are seen with disorders of carnitine metabolism.
  3. **Treatment**
    a. The primary goals are to maintain **cerebral perfusion pressure** (mean arterial pressure minus ICP) above 50 mm Hg and to avoid the complications of hepatic dysfunction. Both are directly related to the severity of the disease. Severity is indicated by a number of prognostic variables. These include serum ammonia greater than 300 μg/dl, rapid clinical evolution through the stages of coma, posturing (decortication or decerebration), and an EEG indicative of deeper stages of coma.
    b. **Clinical staging and EEG grading of Reye's syndrome.** See Table 20-1.
    c. **For the management of acute hepatic necrosis,** see Chap. 11, p. 367.
    d. **Cerebral support**
      (1) **Stage I or II**
        (a) An EEG is obtained q12h until clinical stabilization or improved grading is achieved. Progression to higher grades requires additional intervention, (see **(2)** below).
        (b) Initially, unless the patient is volume depleted, limit fluid to one-half maintenance; prevent hypoglycemia and elevate serum osmolarity to 290 to 310 mOsm.
        (c) Seizures should be treated with IV phenytoin (Dilantin) to avoid

Table 20-1. Clinical staging and EEG grading in Reye's syndrome

Grade	Clinical description	EEG characteristics by age in yr		
		<5	5–10	>10
1	Lethargic	Predominantly delta	Theta-delta	Predominantly theta
2	Agitated	Predominantly delta	Predominantly delta	Theta-delta
3	Decorticate	High-voltage delta	High-voltage delta	High-voltage delta
4	Decerebrate	Burst suppression and low voltage,		
5	Flaccid	(nearly) isoelectric		

losing the ability to monitor the patient's level of consciousness (see Chap. 7, p. 235).

  (d) Electrolytes, osmolarity, blood sugar, and BUN should be monitored q6–12h, and an arterial ammonia q12–24h. PT and PTT should also be repeated q12–24h.

  (e) The head should be placed in the midline and elevated to 30 degrees to reduce the venous component of ICP.

  (2) Stage III, IV, or V. In addition to the treatment outlines for stages I and II, the patient will require intracranial monitoring and possible additional therapy, including intubation, hyperventilation, osmotic agents, and barbiturates (see Chap. 7, p. 237).

C. Chronic increased ICP

  1. Etiology. The causes include hydrocephalus, brain tumors, brain abscess, arteriovenous malformations, and chronic subdural hematomas.

  2. Evaluation and diagnosis

  a. Examination. A lateralized examination suggests hemispheric brain tumor, subdural hematoma, abscess, or arteriovenous malformation. Asymmetrical nystagmus, truncal or appendicular ataxia, and brainstem signs suggest a similar posterior fossa process. Nonlateralized and nonfocal signs suggest hydrocephalus and pseudotumor cerebri (see **D**, p. 513).

  b. Tests

  (1) Cranial MRI scan or cranial CT scan.

  (2) Lumbar puncture is contraindicated except in pseudotumor cerebri and simple communicating hydrocephalus.

  (3) Cranial sector scanning ultrasound can be used to evaluate the ventricular system and the cerebral hemispheres when the anterior fontanel is patent.

  3. Treatment

  a. Treat as in acute increased ICP.

  b. Posthemorrhagic hydrocephalus in premature newborns can be treated medically by daily lumbar puncture and removal of at least 10 ml cerebrospinal fluid (CSF). Serial lumbar punctures do **not** prevent the development of hydrocephalus.

  c. Most patients with progressive hydrocephalus will require a shunting procedure.

  d. When surgery is contraindicated, temporization can be achieved with furosemide (0.1–0.5 mg/kg q4–6h), glycerol or mannitol (0.25 g/kg q6h), or acetazolamide (10 mg/kg q8–12h).

  e. Radiation in combination with chemotherapy or surgery is used as indicated for tumors or abscess.

D. Increased ICP without alteration of mental status: pseudotumor cerebri (benign intracranial hypertension)
   1. **Etiology.** The cause is unknown.
   2. **Evaluation and diagnosis**
      a. **History.** Headache is the rule. The patient may complain of visual loss or diplopia and, occasionally, nausea and vomiting.
      b. **Examination.** Papilledema, enlarged blind spot, visual scotoma, and sixth cranial nerve palsy may be seen. Other focal or lateralized neurologic signs, such as other cranial nerve palsies, hemiparesis, ataxia, and sensory deficits, diminish pseudotumor as a diagnostic consideration.
      c. **Tests**
         (1) A **cranial CT or MRI scan** must be performed to exclude hydrocephalus or a space-occupying lesion; the ventricles appear either normal in size or slit-like.
         (2) A **lumbar puncture** can be done if there are no localizing signs and if the CT or MRI scan is normal.
         (3) Baseline ophthalmologic evaluation and periodic reassessments of visual fields are advised.
   3. **Therapy.** Untreated, persistent ICP can lead to permanent loss of vision.
      a. A single **lumbar puncture,** with removal of enough fluid to drop the pressure to approximately 150 mm water or to 50% of the opening pressure, is frequently adequate. Symptoms (headache) are often dramatically alleviated following the lumbar puncture.
      b. Initially, some patients will require a series of lumbar punctures, daily at first, adjusting the interval according to exacerbation of symptoms (headache) and rate of reaccumulation of CSF.
      c. When repeated lumbar punctures are not successful, **acetazolamide** (Diamox) can be initiated (10–25 mg/kg in 2–3 divided doses/day).
      d. **Furosemide (Lasix),** 0.1 to 0.5 mg/kg q4–6h, can be used if acetazolamide is not successful.
      e. If previous interventions are unsuccessful, a course of **dexamethasone** at 0.2 to 0.5 mg/kg/day is recommended. Corticosteroid dependency can result, however. A response to dexamethasone generally occurs within days to a few weeks. Improvement can be evaluated by the resolution of headache and normalization of eye grounds (usually slower to resolve), as well as by lower opening pressure on lumbar puncture. With normalization of opening pressure, dexamethasone can be given every other day and then tapered over 2 to 3 months.
      f. When all other modalities to control increased ICP fail, or when vision is acutely threatened, an optic nerve fenestration procedure will alleviate optic nerve pressure and avert impending visual compromise. Some advocate the fenestration procedure in lieu of corticosteroid treatment. Alternatively, a **lumboperitoneal or ventriculoperitoneal** shunt can also save vision and alleviate symptoms associated with elevated intracranial pressure.

II. Paroxysmal disorders
   A. **Seizures** represent a symptom complex and not a disease state. The tendency to have recurrent seizures in the absence of acute metabolic alterations or CNS infection loosely defines epilepsy.
      1. **Etiology.** In the emergency room setting, the most important etiologic considerations include trauma, physical abuse, meningitis and encephalitis, fever, space-occupying lesions, metabolic causes, cerebrovascular accidents, and toxic encephalopathies. In patients with epilepsy, poor drug compliance or altered drug metabolism because of intercurrent illness is the most common cause of seizures.
      2. **Evaluation**
         a. The **history** should include questions about previous static or progressive neurologic or developmental dysfunction, symptoms of infection, or a history of headaches, early-morning vomiting, or visual alterations.

(1) Precise details of the seizure, particularly observing the initial components of the seizure and deviations of the eyes and head, are important. The postictal assessment for eye position or weakness is also useful. The duration of the postictal state should be noted.

(2) Absence of a return to baseline within one hour suggests either ongoing seizures or a response to administered medications, or it is due to the underlying disease or a supervening problem.

(3) A **family history** of febrile and nonfebrile seizures should be noted.

b. **Physical examination.** A thorough neurologic examination should be performed, with particular attention to evaluation of mental status and the fundi and a search for focal or lateralized signs. The general examination should include attention to meningeal signs, trauma, and diseases of other body systems.

c. **Specific laboratory tests** will depend on the clues provided by the history and physical findings.

(1) An **awake and asleep EEG** should be done in all patients with afebrile seizures. An EEG is particularly useful for confirming the presence of paroxysmal discharges, identifying the focus of a discharge and space-occupying lesions, choosing appropriate anticonvulsant medication, and determining when anticonvulsants should be discontinued. On occasion an EEG performed soon after a seizure will show only background slowing, which, if repeated after 7 to 10 days, will then demonstrate epileptiform activity.

(2) A **cranial MRI scan** should be performed in patients with partial seizures, with otherwise unexplained loss of seizure control, with focal or lateralized abnormalities found on the neurologic examination, with focally abnormal EEGs, or with known or suspected specific white or gray matter neurologic diseases. **A cranial CT scan** is useful as a screen to identify cerebral calcifications associated with tuberous sclerosis, congenital infections, arteriovenous malformations, or cysticercosis. A CT scan is generally not indicated for patients with well-controlled primary generalized (grand mal) or pure absence (petit mal) seizures in whom the neurologic findings are normal.

d. The **differential diagnoses** include syncope, breath-holding spells (both may be followed by a brief, clonic seizure), decerebration, narcolepsy, complicated migraine, benign paroxysmal vertigo, and hysteria (pseudoseizures).

3. **Diagnosis of seizure types**

a. **Grand mal (primary generalized, tonic-clonic)** seizures usually start without an aura or focal features. Characteristically, there is a tonic phase, usually lasting less than a minute, often associated with rolling up of the eyes. During this phase there may be tonic contraction of the respiratory musculature, resulting in cyanosis. The tonic phase is followed by clonic jerking of the extremities, usually lasting 1 to 5 minutes, with associated improved air exchange. Hypersalivation, tachycardia, and metabolic and respiratory acidosis may be present. There is usually a postictal state lasting less than 1 hour.

b. **Focal motor seizures (partial seizures with elementary symptomatology).** Characteristically, focal motor seizures start in the hand or face and are associated with head and eye deviation toward the hemisphere opposite the seizure focus. They can restricted to that area, without loss of consciousness, or they can generalize and quickly and phenotypically resemble grand mal seizures (secondary generalized, tonic-clonic seizures). Following the seizures, a Todd's paralysis or eye and head deviation **toward** the previously discharging hemisphere may be a clue to the focality.

c. **Temporal lobe or psychomotor seizures (partial seizures with complex symptomatology)** are preceded by an aura (e.g., emotional feelings, abdominal or head pain, feeling in the throat) about 50% of the time. These seizures can mimic other seizure types during various ictal episodes. Focal, motor, grand mal, or staring seizures may be present; at other times the seizures will appear more complex, with stereotyped, automatic behaviors, including running, lip smacking, laughing, and unusual movements of the face or hand. In general, there is a postictal state with full or partial amnesia for the seizure.

d. **Petit mal (primary generalized, absence seizures)** begin in childhood, usually occur after 3 years of age, and are characterized by staring with or without eyelid fluttering or head-nodding movements. The seizures are not preceded by an aura or followed by a postictal state and usually last for less than 30 seconds. They can occur many times a day and can be provoked by hyperventilation or stroboscopic lights. The associated EEG is specifically a three-per-second spike-and-wave abnormality. It is important to differentiate these seizures from partial complex seizures because of implications of anticonvulsant treatment, causation, and prognosis. Occasional grand mal seizures occur in 10 to 20% of patients with typical petit mal seizures. By puberty, the majority (75%) of patients no longer have seizures and have a normal EEG.

e. **Infantile spasms with hypsarrhythmic EEG.** Infantile spasms begin most often in the first year of life and are characterized by large myoclonic (salaam) spasms. This syndrome can occur as a consequence of various neurologic diseases or can arise without known antecedent problems. Development usually slows with the onset of spasms, and there is a high incidence of subsequent retardation, particularly among patients with antecedent neurologic disease.

f. **Mixed generalized seizures (atypical petit mal, petit mal variant, minor motor seizures).** This group of seizure disorders is typified by patients with Lennox-Gastaut syndrome, which is characterized by frequent, hard-to-control seizures, including atonic, myoclonic (sudden muscle jerks), tonic, and clonic seizures associated with an EEG pattern of atypical spike and waves (<3/sec spike and waves), multifocal spikes, and polyspikes. The age of onset is usually between 18 months and 5 years, and often follows infantile spasms. Patients frequently have developmental delay.

g. **Benign childhood epilepsy** with centrotemporal spikes (**benign rolandic epilepsy**). This is a common syndrome, thought to represent a form of idiopathic epilepsy, with an excellent prognosis. Onset is between 3 and 13. Most children have normal intelligence and neurologic examinations. Seizures are often nocturnal, although they can occur in wakefulness. Onset frequently is simple partial, involving the face and producing speech arrest. Often there is associated drooling, dysarthria, or perioral or intraoral parasthesias. EEG findings are diagnostic and consist of midtemporal central spike foci. Recurrent seizures are usually controlled with carbamazepine or phenytoin. As with most of the other idiopathic epileptic disorders, most children lose their propensity to have seizures without sequelae by mid teenage years.

h. **Juvenile myoclonic epilepsy (JME).** This seizure disorder begins in childhood with onset in the second decade. The neurologic examination is normal. JME is a familial disorder characterized by mild myoclonic seizures, generalized and tonic-clonic seizures, or clonic-tonic-clonic seizures and occasional absence seizures. Myoclonic seizures usually occur in the morning and involve the upper extremities, often presenting as a tendency to drop or throw objects that are held in the hands. Valproate is the most efficacious treatment, but clonazepam can also be used.

i. **Febrile seizures** occur between 6 months and 5 years of age in the context of fever, usually above 38.5°(101.5°F), and most often as the temperature rises or is at its peak. The seizures are usually grand mal, although they can be tonic, atonic (limp), or clonic.

(1) They are considered to be simple if they are single and last less than 15 minutes, and if no focal features are present during or following an

episode. Implicit to the definition is an absence both of metabolic disarray and of nervous system infection. An EEG is unnecessary unless seizures are recurrent with atypical features (low-grade fever, complex seizure, abnormal examination).

(2) Complex febrile seizures are multiple, prolonged, or focal.

(3) All febrile patients *under 18 months* or *over 3 years* of age with a first seizure require **lumbar puncture** and a **metabolic screen,** as does any patient with complex febrile seizures, altered mental status, neurologic signs, meningeal signs, or uncertain follow-up.

(4) Risk factors for subsequent development of epilepsy include

  (a) Antecedent abnormal neurologic or developmental status.

  (b) A family history of afebrile seizures.

  (c) Complex febrile seizures.

(5) The presence of a single risk factor is associated with a less than 2% chance of the development of afebrile seizures. This contrasts with an approximately 6 to 10% occurrence with two or three risk factors. Further, each feature of seizure complexity (length >15 min, multiple or focal) increases the risk of developing subsequent epilepsy. The presence of all three complex features is associated with near 50% risk of subsequent epilepsy.

(6) Prophylaxis for febrile seizures. Medications proven to be effective prophylactically include phenobarbital, diazepam, and valproate. Carbamazepine and phenytoin are not effective.

  (a) Patients with febrile seizures generally do not require prophylactic treatment unless seizures occur frequently or are recurrently life threatening (status epilepticus). When phenobarbital is used, it should be continued for 1 year or until 3 years of age, after which the incidence of febrile seizures declines. Serum levels of at least 15 μg/ml are required for effective prophylaxis.

  (b) Oral diazepam at the onset of illness or fever, or both, at a dosage of 0.33 mg/kg q8h until the child is afebrile for 24 hours, has been shown to prevent recurrent febrile seizures in some children. Its efficacy has been questioned, and side effects can complicate the physician's ability to evaluate the child for symptoms of meningitis. If used, we recommend a maximum of 2.5 mg per dose after the initial dose.

  (c) Although valproate is effective in preventing recurrent febrile seizures, **the potential for life-threatening liver toxicity** (particularly in children <2 yr of age) **excludes this drug as a reasonable prophylactic alternative.**

4. Therapy. See also Table 20-2.

  a. General principles

  (1) Acute seizure management. For management of status epilepticus, see Chap. 7.

  (2) Chronic management

    (a) The choice of anticonvulsant should be based on clinical and EEG assessment of the seizure type, with consideration of benefit-risk ratio of the drug (Table 20-3).

    (b) A single drug at a therapeutic level is more likely to be effective and causes fewer adverse reactions than multiple drugs at subtherapeutic levels.

    (c) The most effective level of the appropriate drug is established by increasing the dose until seizures are controlled, side effects are sustained, or the maximum therapeutic level is exceeded.

    (d) It is often helpful to obtain peak (2–3 hr postdose) and trough (predose) blood levels in order to ascertain adequacy of levels throughout the day, establish frequency of dosing, and help determine the utility of giving larger doses at certain times (such as hour of sleep to cover early-morning hours better).

Table 20-2. Drugs used for treatment of seizure disorders

Anticonvulsant	Half-life (hr)	Dosage (mg/kg/day)	Time/day	Approx. therapeutic range (µg/ml)	Common side effects
Phenytoin (Dilantin)	24–50	5 (5–12)[a]	bid	10–20 (5–10)[b]	Rash, hirsutism, gingival hyperplasia, hypertrichosis
Phenobarbital or mephobarbital (Mebaral)	60–92	3–5 (5–18)	qd	10–45	Lethargy, hyperactivity
Primidone (Mysoline)	6–14	5–25	tid	5–10	Lethargy, irritability
Carbamazepine (Tegretol)[c]	9–15	15–30	bid–tid	3–11	Lethargy, blurry vision, granulocytopenia
Ethosuximide (Zarontin)	20–60	20–30	bid	40–120	Nausea, hiccups
Valproic acid[c] (Depakene)	8–15	25–60	bid–tid	50–120	GI discomfort, tremor, alopecia
Clonazepam (Klonopin)	24–48	0.02–0.2	bid–tid	10–60	Lethargy, ataxia, hypersalivation
Lamotrigine[d] (Lamictil)	15–24	150–500 in adults (see text)	qd–bid	—	Rash, diplopia, lethargy, ataxia, and headache
Gabapentin (Neurontin)	4–6	600–1200 in adults; 20 in children	tid	—	Mild fatigue, dizziness, nystagmus, hypotension

[a]Phenytoin is very poorly absorbed and/or has a very short half-life in the neonatal period; this problem gradually improves through the first years of life.

[b]Depakene has interactions with phenytoin and phenobarbital. Total phenytoin will be reduced by approximately one-half and free phenytoin will be doubled. Thus, dosages of phenytoin should not be altered, and the therapeutic range should be considered to be between 5 and 10 µg/ml. Free Dilantin level (therapeutic: 1–2 µg/ml). Depakene also tends to increase phenobarbital levels.

[c]Requires weekly CBC and liver functions for 2 wk, then monthly for 3 mo, then q3–6 mo.

[d]Lamotrigine is not recommended for children under 16 years of age.

(e) To alter anticonvulsant regimens, modify one drug at a time, allowing for reequilibration to the new level, which will depend on the drug's half-life. Reequilibration will usually require approximately five half-lives. Giving loading doses will substantially reduce the time to equilibration, but can cause a greater number and degree of side effects.

(f) When substituting a new anticonvulsant for another, it is prudent to add the new anticonvulsant first and attain therapeutic levels before tapering away the previous medication.

(g) Discontinuation of an anticonvulsant, especially phenobarbital, carbamazepine (Tegretol), and the diazepines, should be done slowly, usually over a period of 1 to 6 months.

(h) When possible, tablets or capsules should be used in preference

Table 20-3. Anticonvulsant choice by seizure type

Seizure type	Principal drug of choice	Second-line or adjunctive drugs
Primary generalized (grand mal) seizures	Phenobarbital, mephobarbital (Mebaral) Phenytoin (Dilantin) Carbamazepine (Tegretol)	Valproic acid Acetazolamide (Diamox)
Partial elementary seizures (focal)	Phenobarbital Phenytoin Carbamazepine Primidone (Mysoline)	Valproic acid Methsuximide
Partial complex seizures (temporal lobe epilepsy)	Carbamazepine Phenytoin Primidone	Phenobarbital Valproic acid Acetazolamide Methsuximide Gabapentin Lamotrigine
Primary generalized (petit mal, absence) seizures	Ethosuximide (Zarontin) Valproic acid (Depakene) Methsuximide (Celontin)	Acetazolamide Clonazepam (Klonopin) Phenobarbital
Infantile spasms	ACTH Valproic acid Clonazepam	Phenytoin Phenobarbital Acetazolamide
Febrile seizures	Phenobarbital	Valproic acid
Mixed generalized seizures	Phenobarbital Valproic acid Clonazepam	Acetazolamide Diazepam Ethosuximide Phenytoin ACTH Clorazepate (Tranxene) Lorazepam Methsuximide Carbamazepine Triple bromides Ketogenic diet
Neonatal seizures	Phenobarbital Phenytoin	Paraldehyde Valproic acid

ACTH = Adrenocorticotropic hormone.

to liquid formulations. This is more likely to ensure uniformity of dosage. Most tablets can be crushed and mixed with food if necessary.

   (i) In general, anticonvulsants can be discontinued when the patient has had no seizures for 2 years and has nonparoxysmal waking and sleeping EEGs. After 2 years of complete seizure control, a paroxysmal or epileptiform EEG predicts a recurrence incidence of approximately 50%; a nonparoxysmal/nonepileptiform EEG is associated with a 5 to 10% recurrence rate, usually within 6 months of discontinuation of medication.

b. Specific anticonvulsant therapy (see Table 20-2)
   (1) Phenobarbital
      (a) The long half-life permits once-a-day dosing, usually best given at hour of sleep.

(b) It can promote hyperactivity/attention deficit disorder (ADD) in some children.

(c) Drug interactions

(i) Predictably reduces the *Tegretol* level when given concomitantly.

(ii) Level will increase when *valproate* is added as a second drug.

(d) Data related to reduced (3–6 pts) IQ scores in children treated with phenobarbital are controversial and inconclusive. Any decision to use pharmacologic interventions must always be based on an analysis of benefit-risk ratio.

(2) Valproate (VPA; Depakene)

(a) The relatively short half-life requires tid dosing.

(b) Valproate has been associated with liver necrosis and death in over 100 instances; the risk for this is enhanced under the age of 2, in the setting of multiple anticonvulsant medication use, and possibly by deficient baseline serum carnitine values. **Bone marrow suppression can also occur.**

(c) Baseline alanine aminotransferase (ALT), ammonia, and CBC values should be obtained and repeated frequently initially (weekly for the first 4 wk; monthly for the next 3 mo; then q3 mo).

(d) Drug interactions

(i) Serum *phenobarbital level* will increase 10 to 25%.

(ii) *Valproate* will double the *free Dilantin* (usually 10% of total Dilantin), but reduce the *total Dilantin* value by half.

(iii) Use with clonazepam will occasionally provoke an episode of status epilepticus.

(3) Carbamazepine (Tegretol)

(a) The relatively short half-life requires bid/tid/qid dosing.

(b) The risk of irreversible hepatic necrosis or bone marrow suppression is minimal (on the order of 1/100,000); reversible dose-responsive or transient granulocytopenia is more common.

(c) Drug interaction

(i) *Carbamazepine* levels tend to drop in the face of most other anticonvulsants.

(ii) Concomitant use of *erythromycin* will markedly increase the serum *carbamazepine* value, often prompting symptoms of toxicity.

(d) Nongeneric formulary is preferred.

(4) Diphenylhydantoin (Dilantin, phenytoin)

(a) The half-life requires bid/tid dosing.

(b) Use of Dilantin in the first few years of life leads to erratic and low serum levels at usual maintenance doses (see **B** below).

(c) Drug interactions

(i) Valproate (see above).

(ii) Tegretol (see above).

(d) Nongeneric formulary is preferred.

(5) Ethosuximide (Zarontin)

(a) The half-life allows bid dosing.

(b) The most common side effects are gastrointestinal disturbances (nausea, emesis, loss of appetite). Rarely, ethosuximide causes hiccups, alopecia, psychosis, or a lupus-like reaction.

(c) Drug interactions are not consistent. Carbamazepine, phenobarbital, and phenytoin can decrease ethosuximide levels.

(d) Monitoring of levels is needed along with a liver enzyme profile.

(6) Gabapentin (Neurontin)

(a) The half-life requires tid/qid dosing.

(b) Gabapentin is a gamma aminobutyric acid (GABA)-related amino acid that is effective in treatment of partial and complex partial seizures. It is approved as adjunctive therapy to treat patients older than 12.

   (c) So far, according to the manufacturer, gabapentin is reported to have no antiepileptic drug interactions and has low toxicity although experience is limited.

   (d) Side effects include somnolence, dizziness, fatigue, and headaches.

   (7) Felbamate (Felbatol) is *not* indicated as a first-line antiepileptic drug. It is recommended for use only in those who have intractable seizures that are unresponsive to alternative treatment and whose seizures are so severe that the substantial risk of aplastic anemia is deemed acceptable in light of the benefits conferred by its use.

B. Neonatal seizures (see also Chap. 6, p. 214)

   1. Etiology. The causes can be categorized in the following manner.

   a. Metabolic. Hypoglycemia, hypocalcemia, hypomagnesemia, hyponatremia, and hypoxemia.

   b. Toxic. Maternal drug ingestion (withdrawal), inadvertent local anesthetic poisoning.

   c. Hemorrhagic. Intraventricular, subdural, and subarachnoid hemorrhage.

   d. Infectious. Bacterial, viral (TORCH).

   e. Effects resulting from inborn errors of metabolism. Organic acidemias, errors of amino acid metabolism, pyridoxine dependency, and so forth.

   f. Effects of asphyxia (hypoxia, ischemia). We specifically avoid the term *hypoxic-ischemic encephalopathy,* preferring to use the term *neonatal encephalopathy,* unless there is very clear and direct evidence of prenatal ischemia or postnatal hypoxia or ischemia, or both.

   g. Cerebral dysgenesis.

   h. Benign familial seizures.

   2. Evaluation

   a. A full **perinatal history** and **neonatal examination** will help differentiate the causes.

   b. Laboratory assessments of blood sugar (Dextrostix), calcium, magnesium, sodium, CBC and cultures, and a toxic screen. A CSF examination, EEG with pyridoxine infusion, cranial ultrasound, and/or cranial CT scan are frequently important for diagnostic, therapeutic, or prognostic purposes.

   3. Diagnosis. Seizures can be tonic, focal clonic, multifocal clonic, myoclonic, or, most commonly, subtle, which includes eye deviation, nystagmus, apnea, sucking movements, tongue thrusting, and bicycling and swimming movements.

   4. Therapy

   a. Attention must first be directed at **vital signs.**

   b. Therapy should subsequently be directed at the underlying cause.

   c. Anticonvulsant therapy is required when glucose and pyridoxine administration (50–100 mg IV) is unsuccessful, or when the possibility of such a deficiency has been excluded.

   d. The cornerstone of therapy is **phenobarbital;** a loading dose of phenobarbital at 10 to 20 mg/kg can be administered over 5 to 10 minutes. **Phenytoin** can be used as a second drug at a loading dose of 20 mg/kg, and phenobarbital can be readministered at 10 mg/kg at hourly intervals for two further doses, if necessary. For ongoing seizures, careful monitoring of blood pressure and heart rate is required with anticonvulsant loads. After loading with phenobarbital and phenytoin, rectal **paraldehyde** is the next drug of choice. Rectal **valproate** is used on rare occasions.

   e. See Formulary for maintenance anticonvulsant doses. Phenobarbital is well absorbed orally. Phenytoin is very poorly absorbed orally or has an exceedingly short half-life in the first months of life, or both, and should generally be avoided if possible.

f. Anticonvulsants can be discontinued at the time of discharge or at 3 months if the patient is no longer having clinical seizures, the EEG is not paroxysmal, and the neurologic findings are normal. Anticonvulsant levels should be monitored at the time of recurrent seizures, when side effects develop, and 2 to 3 weeks subsequent to an alteration of the maintenance dosage.

C. Migraine headache. The majority of childhood headaches not associated with acute illness are migrainous. Migraine occurs in 5% of children.

1. Etiology. The neurologic symptoms associated with migraine are considered to be a function of cerebrovascular constriction, leading to diminished cerebral blood flow to specific brain areas. The pain is thought to occur because of vasodilation, leading to stretching of intramural nerves.

2. Evaluation and diagnosis. Migraine headaches are typically periodic. They can be conveniently divided into classic (hemicranial, throbbing, and preceded by an aura), complicated (classic and a neurologic deficit), or common (no aura, generalized or bilateral head pain). Rarely, vomiting alone or abdominal pain alone is the only symptom of a migraine attack. Cyclic vomiting can be viewed as a form of migraine equivalent.

a. History and physical examination

(1) The diagnosis of migraine rests on identifying the *intermittency* and the nature of the headache. The majority of children have associated nausea and vomiting, photophobia, and sonophobia.

(2) Auras, identified in 10 to 25% of patients, can include visual scotoma or scintillations, vertigo, malaise with associated pallor, perioral numbness, or alterations of perception.

(3) Neurologic findings can include confusional state, aphasia, brainstem signs, ataxia, hemiparesis, hemisensory loss, and loss of consciousness. In 90% of children, a family member has migraines, and many children suffer from motion sickness.

(4) A diary can help to identify provoking factors, such as certain foods, activities, or environmental variables.

b. Laboratory evaluation. The history and physical findings will determine which tests are necessary. The aim of the tests is to rule out other causes of headache, which will depend on the clinical setting.

3. Therapy. The approach to treatment of migraine headache depends on headache frequency, the degree of disability, and age.

a. Migraine-provoking agents, such as chocolates, cheeses, nitrite-containing foods (processed meats), and monosodium glutamate–containing foods, should be eliminated if they appear to be associated with headaches.

b. Other complicating factors, such as emotional stress and withdrawal from chronic intake of caffeinated beverages, should also be evaluated.

c. Pharmacologic treatment can be either symptomatic (Table 20-4) or prophylactic (Table 20-5).

(1) Symptomatic treatment of headache

(a) Common analgesics such as acetaminophen and the nonsteroidal anti-inflammatory agents (NSAIDs), ibuprofen, and naproxen are commonly used for headache.

(b) Mixed barbiturate analgesics (butalbital/caffeine/acetaminophen) are useful in older children. These potent analgesics pose a habit risk.

(c) Narcotics are not recommended for the pediatric population.

(d) If acetaminophen and ibuprofen are ineffective, **abortive therapy** can be considered. **Ergotamine** derivatives may be effective in decreasing the headache pain; however, associated nausea and emesis are often worse than the headache itself. Rebound headache can also occur with these agents. An antiemetic can be used 30 minutes before the use of the ergot preparation in order to avoid excessive emesis.

Table 20-4. Symptomatic treatment of migraine headache

Drug	Dosage and route of administration	Age 3–10 yr	Age 11 yr and older
Aspirin	Usual analgesic dosages PO or PR	Preferred	Preferred
Acetaminophen	Usual and analgesic dosages PO or PR	Preferred	Preferred
Butalbital, 50 mg; caffeine, 40 mg; aspirin, 325 mg/acetaminophen, 300 mg (Fiorinal, Fioricet, Esgic)	Under 5 yr, ½ tablet; over 5, 1 tablet; age 11 yr and older, 1–2 tablets	Not preferred	
Ergotamine tartrate,* 1.8 mg; caffeine, 100 mg (Cafergot)	PO: 1–2 tablets at onset of headache; 1 tablet q½h to maximum of 4	Not preferred	Preferred
Ibuprofen (Motrin, Advil)	Usual analgesic dosage PO	Preferred	Preferred
Isometheptene, 65 mg; acetaminophen, 325 mg/dichloralphenazone, 100 mg (Midrin)	1–2 capsules immediately if needed, then repeat 1/hr to a maximum of 3/d (or 5/wk)	Not preferred	Preferred
Sumatriptan (Imitrix)	Subcutaneous injection, 6 mg	Not preferred	Preferred

*Not to be taken with complicated migraine. Give no more than 6 PO tablets or 2 PR tablets in 24 hr. Limit to 8 PO tablets or 4 suppositories/wk.

(2) **Prophylaxis** is considered when the frequency is greater than once a week, leading to school absence or major changes in lifestyle or quality of life; when headaches are unresponsive to symptomatic treatment; or when side effects of the acutely administered medications lead to a similar or worse disability. Cyproheptadine, propranolol, phenobarbital, and amitriptyline are the more commonly used prophylactic agents. Calcium-channel blockers have been used successfully as prophylaxis in adults and may be useful in children as well. Occasionally, prophylaxis with propranolol or ibuprofen can be used just before specific times when such activities are known to provoke migraine attacks (e.g., just before strenuous activity such as a soccer match).

    d. **Nonpharmacologic treatment.** Biofeedback and relaxation techniques have been useful in patients with common migraine or muscle tension–based headaches, and in those in whom emotional issues and anxiety provoke migraine attacks.

III. Cranial nerve disorders

  A. Optic neuritis

    1. **Etiology.** Optic neuritis can occur during or following an infection or can arise separately, as with immune-mediated disorders or the first signs of a recurrent demyelinating disorder. It involves demyelination of the optic nerve head (papillitis) or the area behind the nerve head (retrobulbar neuritis).

    2. **Evaluation and diagnosis**

      a. **History.** The clinical history is that of lost vision; this may be unilateral or bilateral, and visual acuity may be reduced considerably. Associated ocular pain may be present.

      b. **Examination.** Visual acuity is reduced. With papillitis, papilledema is seen; with retrobulbar neuritis, the fundoscopic findings are essentially normal.

Table 20-5. Prophylactic treatment of migraine headache

Drug	Dosage and route of administration	Age 3–10 yr	Age 11 yr and older
Phenobarbital	3–5 mg/kg/day qhs PO	Preferred	Not preferred
Phenytoin (Dilantin)	5 mg/kg/day bid PO	Preferred	Less commonly used or less effective than others
Propranolol[a] (Inderal)	(1) 0.5–3.0 mg/kg/day tid or qid (or bid for LA preparation)	Less commonly used or less effective than others	Preferred
Amitriptyline	0.2–0.5 mg/kg/day (in qhs dosages) PO	Not preferred	Preferred
Cyproheptadine	0.25 mg/kg/day bid/tid PO	Preferred	Preferred
Verapamil	40–80 mg PO bid/tid	Not preferred	Preferred
Methysergide[b] (Sansert)	2 mg qd PO	Not preferred	Less commonly used or less effective than others
Biofeedback behavioral modification		Preferred	Preferred

[a]Not to be given to patients with asthma, sinus bradycardia with first-degree block, or congestive heart failure.
[b]Can cause retroperitoneal fibrosis and vascular insufficiency. It is to be given only for brief periods (<5 mo) in adolescence.

A careful neurologic examination may reveal other neurologic deficits to suggest a more disseminated disease.

  c. **Laboratory tests**
    (1) A **cranial CT or, preferably, an MRI scan** may be necessary to rule out raised ICP, disseminated white matter disease, or chiasmatic region mass, which can lead to acute visual loss.
    (2) A **lumbar puncture** is necessary for similar reasons; CSF can be assessed for a more generalized involvement of the nervous system to include basic myelin protein and gamma globulins. (There may be a mild pleocytosis with optic neuritis.)
    (3) Somatosensory, brainstem, visual, and auditory evoked responses may identify more extensive white matter disease.
 3. **Therapy**
    a. Optic neuritis is often self-limited. When the disease progresses, particularly to both eyes, acute disseminated encephalomyelitis can be assumed and treated aggressively with high-dose IV **methylprednisolone** for 5 to 7 days with a rapid taper.
    b. Alternatively, adrenocorticotropic hormone (ACTH), 60 to 80 units IV, given in two divided doses over 4 to 8 hours each, should be used; this is changed to IM ACTH gel after 3 to 7 days and then is slowly tapered over 1 to 3 months.
    c. Patients must be carefully monitored for complications associated with the use of high-dose corticosteroids. Concurrent antacid or H_2 blocker therapy is recommended.
 B. **Facial (Bell's) palsy**
    1. **Etiology.** Facial nerve palsy can occur as a result of head injury, demyelina-

tion, tumor, hypertension, infection (including Lyme disease), or infarction. Idiopathic cases are termed **Bell's palsy.**

2. **Evaluation and diagnosis** of Bell's palsy
   a. **History.** Unilateral facial paralysis is preceded by an upper respiratory infection in approximately 75% of cases. Patients frequently complain of pain behind or in front of the ear for 1 or 2 days before or concurrent with the development of the facial weakness, which evolves over a few hours. Rarely, it can recur one or several times.
   b. **Examination.** Mandatory findings in patients with Bell's palsy include weakness of both the lower and upper face, absence of other cranial nerve dysfunction, and normal blood pressure. Findings consistent with the diagnosis of Bell's palsy include hyperacusis of one ear, loss of taste on one side of the tongue, and unilateral overflow of tears or a dry eye.
   c. **Tests**
      (1) **Skull x-rays,** with attention to mastoid and petrous bones, are required to rule out infection or tumor.
      (2) A **CBC, heterophil antibodies,** and Lyme disease antibody titers may also be useful.
3. **Treatment**
   a. **Supportive.** Protection of the involved eye should include the use of a protective eye glass, and a methylcellulose eye lubricant is suggested if the eye is dry.
   b. **Specific.** If begun within 72 hours, a 10-day course of prednisone, starting with 0.75 mg/kg/day and reducing the dosage by 0.25 mg/kg/day every third day, can alleviate the pain associated with Bell's palsy, shorten recovery, and reduce instances of complete, permanent paralysis.

IV. **Peripheral nerve disorder: acute inflammatory demyelinating polyradiculoneuropathy/Guillain-Barré syndrome (AIDP/GBS)**
   A. **Etiology.** This acute or subacute symmetrical ascending disease of predominantly motor nerves is thought to be immune mediated.
   B. **Evaluation and diagnosis**
      1. **History.** There is usually an antecedent viral illness or surgical procedure. Frequently, the patient complains of paresthesia or weakness of the lower extremities, or both.
      2. **Physical examination**
         a. The cranial nerves are usually normal; bifacial weakness often appears later in the course.
         b. The Fisher variant (descending weakness with ataxia) may present with ophthalmoplegia or facial palsy early in the course of the disease.
         c. Distal hypotonia, symmetrical weakness, and reduced deep tendon reflexes are most often noted.
         d. There should be absent extensor plantars, no sensory levels, and no perianal sensory loss.
      3. **Laboratory tests.** Cerebrospinal fluid protein will usually be elevated **following** the first 48 hours of symptoms. Mild pleocytosis (up to 50–100 cells) does not exclude GBS.
   C. **Treatment.** The therapy is largely symptomatic. There are, however, special considerations.
      1. **Monitoring of respiratory status.** Compromise of the nerve roots innervating the phrenic nerve, C3, C4, and C5 can cause rapid respiratory embarrassment. Vital capacity must be monitored frequently, and a fall below 15 ml/kg warrants artificial ventilatory support. Compromise of C3, C4, and C5 is usually preceded by weakness of the upper extremities and occurs within the first 2 weeks of the onset of symptoms.
      2. **Preparing patient and family.** It is critical that the patient and family be counseled that intubation may be necessary as routine support for the disease before urgent measures are required.
      3. Substantial data in adults affirm the benefit of **plasmapheresis** in AIDP as measured by rapidity of acute and long-term improvement, and it can reduce

the risk for required ventilation support. There are more limited data from studies involving children, but similar benefits have been reported. Since plasmapheresis has inherent potential morbidity, we recommend its use in children when need for intubation, a procedure that also has potential inherent morbidity, appears likely by virtue of rapidity of evolution of symptoms or signs and/or involvement of lumbar and thoracic spinal segments. **Plasmapheresis** is generally also only used in the first 2 weeks of the disease. Treatments are given every other day for four to eight sessions. Each exchange involves the removal of 25 to 40 ml/kg plasma and replacement with Plasmanate, immunoglobulins, or an equivalent solution.

4. **Intravenous immunoglobulin** (IVIG) can also be used for the acute treatment of AIDP. It can be administered in most hospital settings, making it more practical than plasmapheresis. However, the data substantiating benefit with IVIG in children are still very limited and in our experience it may not be efficacious in some children. The recommended dosage of IVIG is 400 mg/kg/day for 5 days. Further courses can then be determined every 3 weeks dependent on the clinical profile.

5. **Corticosteroids.** The efficacy of corticosteroids in this disease is controversial and considered by some to lead to an increased incidence of relapse. On the other hand, corticosteroids are extremely effective for the *relapsing* or chronic form of polyneuritis.

6. Hypertension can occur. Propranolol and, if needed, an alpha-adrenergic blocker are recommended (see Chap. 9).

7. **Physical therapy** to prevent contractures is important during the recovery phase.

V. **Neuromuscular junction disorders: myasthenia gravis**
   A. **Etiology and evaluation.** Myasthenia gravis is usually an immune-mediated disease involving the neuromuscular junction. It can occur as three clinical syndromes.

   1. **Transient neonatal myasthenia gravis** is thought to occur because of passively transferred immunoglobulin G (IgG) antibodies. The signs and symptoms of weakness can be severe.

   2. **Congenital myasthenia gravis** can present before birth with reduced fetal movements, postnatally, or up to several years after birth. The mother does not have myasthenia gravis. The symptoms are milder, though more persistent, than the transient disease.

   3. **Juvenile myasthenia gravis** can occur any time during childhood and usually presents with ptosis, diplopia or other bulbar symptoms and signs, and weakness.

   B. **Evaluation.** The response to **edrophonium** (Tensilon), 0.2 mg/kg with a maximum of 10 mg, is transient, lasting less than 5 minutes, and can provoke profound cholinergic side effects. Therefore, neostigmine (Prostigmin) is used intramuscularly in neonates and occasionally in older children; 0.04 mg/kg neostigmine will elicit a response within 10 minutes and peak at 30 minutes. With either edrophonium or neostigmine, cardiac rhythm and blood pressure must be monitored, and atropine at 0.01 mg/kg/dose, with a maximum of 0.4 mg, must be available for intravenous injection.

   C. **Diagnosis.** The response to anticholinesterase administration is the cornerstone of diagnosis. Repetitive nerve stimulation seeking a decremental response is confirmatory.

   D. **Therapy**
   1. **Transient neonatal myasthenia gravis**
      a. **Supportive therapy** alone will be adequate only in a minority of patients.
      b. With feeding or respiratory difficulty, IM and oral neostigmine are helpful. The IM dosage range is 0.05 to 0.3 mg/kg; with oral doses it is 10 times higher. The frequency of administration can be ascertained clinically by respiratory function and force of the cry and may be necessary q1–12h. Intramuscular doses can be given 20 minutes before feedings.
      c. **Plasmapheresis** or **exchange transfusion** can be used for symptoms

that are unresponsive to anticholinesterase therapy. Gamma globulin infusion has been reported to be effective as well.

2. **Congenital myasthenia gravis** can be managed as transient myasthenia in the neonatal period, although serious problems are not as evident. Plasmapheresis or exchange transfusion is not likely to be helpful. Chronic anticholinesterase treatment is often disappointing at any age.

3. **Juvenile myasthenia gravis**
    a. **Anticholinesterase drugs** are the basis of management, both chronically, for cranial nerve dysfunction and weakness, and for acute respiratory embarrassment.
        (1) Neostigmine or pyridostigmine (Mestinon) is used, starting at 0.3 to 0.5 mg/kg and 1 mg/kg tid, respectively, with increasing dosage and adjustment of frequency of administration according to the response and its duration. Treatment frequency should be loaded toward the early times of the day.
        (2) Time span (sustained release) 180-mg tablets are available when dosing amounts permit their use.
    b. When anticholinesterase medications at higher doses are not effective, **prednisone** is used, starting at 0.5 to 1.0 mg/kg and increasing by 0.2 mg/kg up to 60 mg/day every other day until an optimal effect is achieved. The prednisone should subsequently be slowly tapered. **The risk of steroid dependency is substantial.**
    c. **Thymectomy** may be effective therapy when other means of treatment have failed or when requirements for corticosteroids are prolonged, daily, and at high doses. Thymoma rarely occurs in childhood.
    d. **Plasmapheresis** has shown promise as a means of *transiently* improving severe symptoms and signs.

4. When using anticholinesterase medications, **overmedication can result in weakness, leading to the so-called cholinergic crisis.** Systemic cholinergic symptoms and signs suggest the proper diagnosis, and a Tensilon test distinguishes *cholinergic crisis* from *myasthenic crisis.* **Atropine,** 0.4 mg IV, is the treatment of choice for cholinergic crisis.

VI. Movement disorders

A. **Gilles de la Tourette syndrome** is characterized by multiple, complex tics occasionally associated with unusual vocalizations.

1. **Etiology.** This disease is thought to be caused by an alteration of dopaminergic neurotransmitter systems.

2. **Evaluation and diagnosis.** The diagnosis rests on the clinical identification of multiple, complex tics that continue for at least 6 months. Occasionally, this picture can be provoked by stimulant therapy. Children often have an associated ADD, learning disabilities, behavioral difficulties, obsessive-compulsive symptoms, or emotional problems as well.

3. **Therapy**
    a. Discontinuation of stimulant drugs.
    b. **Pimozide** (Orap) or **haloperidol** (Haldol) is indicated when the frequency of movements has a negative impact on the child's physical, educational, social, or psychological well-being. Both medications are major tranquilizers and can produce side effects associated with phenothiazine at therapeutically effective doses.
        (1) Pimozide (Orap) produces sedation and lethargy, although less frequently than haloperidol. Generally, use of the smallest dosage that produces the desired effect is appropriate and the long half-life allows qhs administration. Dosing should be incremented slowly with changes instituted at weekly, every-other-weekly, or greater intervals depending on side effects. The starting dose is 1 mg.
            (a) **Major side effects** include dry mouth or sedation, or both, either of which may dissipate with time. Acute dystonic reactions occur 5 to 9% of the time and an initial dose of 0.5 mg benztropine at bedtime will prevent this side effect. After several

weeks the benztropine can be discontinued. Doses should not exceed 20 mg/day or 0.3 mg/kg/day and most children require less than 8 mg/day.

(b) A baseline **ECG** should be performed and a QTc greater than 0.44 seconds should prompt a cardiologic evaluation. Electrocardiography should also be performed during therapy and an increase of the QTc 25% above baseline, development of T waves, a QTc value of 0.47 seconds or greater, or a heart rate of less than 50 per minute should prompt a reduction in the pimozide dosage.

(2) Haloperidol (Haldol) dosages will range from 0.25 mg bid to as high as 4 mg tid. Initial dosages should be small, 0.25 mg bid, and increased at weekly or greater intervals until satisfactory control is achieved or sedative side effects necessitate discontinuation or reduction of the drug.

(3) Clonidine is effective in tic reduction especially in the setting of comorbid ADHD.

(a) Starting dosage is 0.05 mg PO bid and can be increased to 0.2 mg/day in 0.05 increments. The side effect most commonly cited is sedation. Mild sedation usually subsides after 6 weeks of therapy.

   c. Psychological counseling and modification of the educational program are often indicated.

B. Sydenham's chorea

   1. The **etiology** is unknown.

   2. Evaluation is that of acute rheumatic fever (see Chap. 5, p. 111).

   3. The **diagnosis** rests on noting choreiform movements of the arms and fingers, unusual postures of the outstretched arm, facial grimacing, darting of the tongue, and an explosive speech pattern. The patients are frequently restless and emotionally labile. Hypotonia is present and deep tendon reflexes are pendular and may be "hung up" on repetitive tapping. Signs can be asymmetrical or unilateral.

   4. Therapy

     a. Prednisone therapy (1–2 mg/kg/day) reportedly leads to improvement within a week.

     b. Haloperidol (0.02–0.1 mg/kg/day in 2 divided doses) is reputed to be effective within 2 weeks.

     c. Phenobarbital (3–5 mg/kg/day) or chlorpromazine (50–100 mg tid) can be used as a sedative for symptomatic relief from the movements.

     d. Valproate has been reported to offer benefit.

     e. A restful environment will help reduce external stimulation.

C. The **syndrome of opsoclonus-myoclonus (SOMy)** is also known as myoclonic encephalopathy of infancy.

   1. Etiology. This syndrome is associated with neuroblastoma and encephalitis, or can be idiopathic. It is thought to occur because of inflammation of the brainstem or cerebellum, or both.

   2. Evaluation and diagnosis

     a. Evaluated in the same manner as occult neuroblastoma.

     b. Physical examination. The patients are most often irritable and photophobic. They usually have conjugate, chaotic, quick movements of the eyes in any direction of gaze, often aggravated when they are tired and noted during sleep. Jerking movements of the legs, particularly when attempts are made to place the child on his or her feet, are present. The child may appear markedly ataxic; similar movements may be noted in the patient's upper extremities when reaching.

     c. Laboratory evaluation. These patients should first have a head CT or MRI scan to rule out a posterior fossa mass and then a lumbar puncture to rule out enteroviral or arboviral infection. To evaluate for neuroblastoma, chest and abdominal MRI as well as urinary excretion of homovanillic acid and vanillylmandelic acid are recommended.

3. Therapy

    a. Treatment of the underlying neuroblastoma or waiting for a few weeks following a clear infectious cause may be all that is necessary.

    b. When SOMy persists, ACTH, given IM, is advocated (60–80 units/m², rapidly tapering to every other day and, subsequently, as clinically indicated, over 1–3 mo). Some patients become ACTH dependent.

D. Wilson's disease (see Chap. 11).

VII. Human immunodeficiency virus (see p. 369) **(HIV)-associated neurologic disease** (see Chap. 5, p. 151).

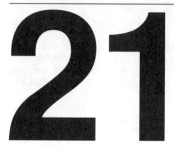

Management of the Child with Developmental Disabilities and Specialized Health Care Needs

Thomas J. Silva and
Marilynn Haynie

I. Introduction and definitions

A. Optimal care of children with developmental disabilities should combine a careful systems-based approach to medical care, a careful analysis of a child's abilities in major developmental fields, and a thorough assessment of a family's hopes and goals for their child.

B. The World Health Organization (WHO) Classification System (1980): separation of a child's particular "condition" from the child's abilities and ultimate role in life.

1. An **impairment** or **disease** is any loss or abnormality of physiologic function or anatomic structure. Impairments pertain to *biologic* anomalies and may or may not significantly affect the function (activities/employment) of an individual.
2. A **disability** is a restriction or lack of function due to an impairment.
3. A **handicap** is a social or vocational disadvantage imposed by impairment or disability environmental factors.
4. A **developmental disability** has been defined by the Developmental Disabilities Assistance and Bill of Rights Act Amendment of 1987 as an impairment in physical or mental ability that is manifested before 22 years of age, causes functional limitations of major life activities, and is likely to persist indefinitely.
5. A **chronic medical condition** or illness is one that lasts longer than 3 months and is expected to last for at least one year. Many children have chronic medical conditions that overlap with developmental disabilities.
6. **Technology-assisted children** rely on the daily use of a device to replace or enhance essential bodily function or require daily skilled nursing to prevent further disability or death.
7. **Family-centered care** recognizes the family as the only constant factor in the child's life, facilitates family and professional collaboration, honors cultural diversity in families, and ensures flexible, accessible, and comprehensive supports for families.

II. General principles and goals of family-centered care

A. Parent-physician collaboration

1. **Parents' role.** From the earliest point, parents should be encouraged to take charge of their children's medical and (re)habilitation plans. Physicians should review families' short- and long-term goals for their children and help to incorporate them into safe medical care plans.
2. **Parental education.** Pediatric providers should educate their patient's parents about
   a. Health and educational choices.
   b. The justification, target effects, and untoward effects of medications and procedures.
   c. Their children's rights as pertain to education and educational mediation.
3. **Plan for smooth transitions in health care.** Many children with specialized health care and developmental needs experience acute exacerbations of chronic health problems, and some shuttle almost continuously between acute hospitalizations, step-down units, and home care. These acute episodes can interrupt a child's developmental or educational progress. The primary provider

and family must organize the child's care and ensure that overriding goals are continued.
4. **Making difficult decisions.** Providers should anticipate and help families through times of crisis. Issues such as level of care decisions, "do not resuscitate" status, redirection of care, placement, and guardianship may need to be addressed, and these issues should be openly discussed well before a crisis occurs.

B. **Medical management**
1. **Establish primary diagnosis.** The root cause of a child's developmental impairments must be identified if at all possible. Accurate primary diagnosis allows for
   a. Identification of related medical problems.
   b. Anticipation of educational/functional difficulties.
   c. Genetic counseling.
2. **Identify and treat existing medical problems.** See Table 21-1.
3. **Screen for associated medical conditions.** Some primary diagnoses carry an increased risk of particular medical conditions, for example, Down's syndrome and hypothyroidism and Hirschprung's disease, as well as William's syndrome and subaortic stenosis.
4. **Routine health maintenance** (see Chap. 3, p. 25)
   a. **Immunizations.** Children with developmental impairments historically have had decreased immunization rates. They should have the same immu-

Table 21-1. Commonly Encountered Medical Problems in Children with Developmental Disabilities

Respiratory: microaspiration of saliva, frank aspiration, reactive airway disease, functional upper airway obstruction, recurrent pneumonia, obstructive sleep apnea, chronic or recurrent hypoxemia secondary to obstruction or aspiration
Cardiovascular: primary malformation, hypertension secondary to renal disease, Raynaud's phenomenon, poor perfusion to anesthetic extremities, autonomic dysreflexia
Gastrointestinal: dysphagia, gastroesophageal reflux, peptic ulcer disease, intestinal dysmotility, bacterial overgrowth, lactose intolerance, constipation, dumping syndrome
Endocrine: hypothyroidism, precocious/delayed puberty, temperature instability, amenorrhea/dysmenorrhea
Immunologic/infectious: recurrent otitis/sinusitis, recurrent pneumonia, increased hepatitis B/C risk, increased tuberculosis exposure
Renal/urologic: hypertension/chronic renal failure mainly secondary to neurogenic bladder dysfunction in spinal dysraphism, infection
Hematologic: nutritional anemias, leukopenia secondary to medication effect (anticonvulsants)
Dermatologic: eczema, maceration, contact dermatitis abrasion (adaptive equipment), pressure necrosis (from braces), sun sensitivity (medication effects), fungal infection (nails, skin)
Orthopedic: joint contractures due to abnormal tone, degenerative joint disease due to abnormal mechanics, scoliosis, osteopenia secondary to immobility and antiepileptic medication
Dental: gingival hyperplasia, caries, malocclusion
Ophthalmologic: refractive errors, strabismus and amblyopia, visual field cuts
Otolaryngologic: conductive and sensorineural hearing impairments, otitis media, otitis externa secondary to auricular aids, tonsillar/adenoidal hypertrophy, obstructive apnea, laryngotracheal malacia, vocal abuse, intubation injuries
Neurologic: seizures, motor impairment, inattention, mental retardation, communication disorders, sensory impairments
Psychiatric/psychological: depression, parental depression, chronic stress on family function, self-injurious behaviors, behavior/adjustment disorders, inattention, possible early-onset dementia

nization schedule as other children, **including** pertussis unless there are specific contraindications (see Chap. 3, p. 25).

b. Anticipatory guidance. Accidental injury, malnutrition, lead poisoning, and untreated dental caries can have important additive consequences.

5. Maximize growth and nutrition.

C. Functional management deals with a child's physical, cognitive, and interpersonal abilities regardless of diagnosis. This should include assessment of a child's ability to eat, move, perform self-care activities, communicate, think, learn, play, and relate to peers.

1. Delineate functional abilities. Pediatricians should describe accurately a child's abilities in the following areas in order to decrease the disabilities imposed by the child's biologic impairments and design an effective rehabilitation plan.

a. Gross motor—mobility.

b. Fine motor—dexterity.

c. Vision.

d. Hearing.

e. Cognition.

f. Communication.

g. Social interaction.

h. Mental health (especially adolescents).

Medical management should aim toward increasing or enhancing function in these areas.

2. Multidisciplinary assessment should be a cornerstone of care. The team, which might include physicians, nurses, social workers, psychologists, physical therapists, occupational therapists, speech/language therapists, and nutritionists, must

a. Monitor achievement of milestones.

b. Document the rate of acquisition of new skills.

c. Provide ongoing therapies as indicated with clearly documented goals.

d. "Augment" existing skills with equipment as indicated.

e. Maintain equipment.

f. Provide family-centered mental health services.

g. Monitor school function.

3. Cognitive assessment can be done as part of local early intervention services or as part of an evaluation for school placement. At times structured nonverbal assessment or adapted testing conditions are necessary. Self-care and social abilities must be taken into account.

4. Maximize inclusion and recreational opportunities. Children with disabilities need the same experiences and opportunities that their siblings and peers have. Opportunities to observe and model normal behavior and communication patterns are very important to development. At the same time recreational activities that have been "adapted" to match certain impairments may allow children to be more active and successful in play (challenger baseball and adaptive horseback riding are two examples).

III. Common medical management problems. Certain disorders and problems occur commonly in children with disabilities regardless of their individual diagnoses. The presentation of these problems as well as typical childhood health problems may differ from their presentation in otherwise healthy children. A list of disorders that commonly affect these children is given in Table 21-1.

A. Nutritional disorders (see also Chap. 11, p. 337). Both malnutrition and obesity are commonly seen in these children.

1. Severe protein calorie malnutrition can adversely affect attention, cognition, development, immune function, and exercise tolerance. Prolonged malnutrition impairs wound healing and skin care, and can lead to postoperative complications. Inadequate caloric intake, particularly in the context of altered energy expenditures is most common. Disorders of digestion and absorption are discussed in Chap. 11, p. 346.

a. Etiologies of inadequate caloric intake can be detected by history.

(1) Children with limited physical or cognitive abilities may have **limited access** to food and fluids throughout the day.

(2) **Oral motor impairments** can make ingestion of certain textures laborious. Mealtimes in excess of 30 minutes, coughing, sweating, or irritation during meals can signify critical oral motor difficulties.

(3) **Fine motor impairments** can make self-feeding difficult. A history of uncomfortable oral procedures or prevention of feeding during early infancy can create **oral aversion.**

(4) **Pain** from gastroesophageal reflux, ulcers, or extreme constipation can decrease appetite.

b. **Evaluation and diagnosis**

(1) **Physical examination** should include careful measurement of height (length), weight, and head circumference to determine the degree and duration of malnutrition. A *functional* neurologic examination, including **cranial nerves, gross motor control, and fine motor assessments,** will help determine safe swallowing abilities and the need for adaptive positioning or tableware equipment.

(2) **Laboratory assessment** can include

(a) A complete blood count to screen for anemia and iron deficiency, total protein and albumin, thyroid function tests, and fecal occult blood testing.

(b) A modified barium swallow to assess swallowing function as well as an upper GI series and pH probe if significant gastroesophageal reflux is suspected.

(3) Other evaluations: **consultation** with the following:

(a) A **clinical nutritionist** in conjunction with a 3-day intake diary can determine caloric intake and screen for trace element and vitamin deficiency.

(b) A **speech pathologist** can identify dysfunctional chewing and swallowing, and can assist in finding safe textures for use in increasing caloric intake.

(c) A **dentist** is often indicated to treat caries or malalignment, which can further impact on feeding abilities.

(d) A **gastroenterologist** for further evaluation may be necessary.

c. **Treatment**

(1) The first step in **treatment** is to supplement calories orally with appropriate textures and caloric density using appropriate positioning equipment. Once calories have been supplemented, subsequent growth should be monitored every 2 or 3 months (or more frequently for an infant). If predicted growth does not occur, a more thorough investigation for disorders of digestion or absorption should be considered.

(2) If oral supplementation cannot be accomplished, temporary nasogastric (NG) or permanent gastrostomy feeding should be considered.

(a) Indications for temporary nasogastric feedings include

(i) Temporary alterations in caloric requirements coupled with temporary alterations in feeding abilities (nutritional stress of hip or spine surgery in a child with spastic quadriplegia who will not be able to sit postoperatively).

(ii) Inability to ingest sufficient calories for growth in an otherwise intact patient (nighttime NG feeds in an adolescent with chronic respiratory symptoms of cystic fibrosis).

(iii) Temporary nasogastric feeding in infancy before sufficient feeding skills develop (prematurity or cleft lip and/or palate).

(iv) As a therapeutic trial to determine whether gastrostomy will be effective.

(v) Airway-protective responses are a prerequisite for nasogastric feeding.

(b) Indications for gastrostomy feedings can include

    (i) Congenital malformations of the craniofacial structures, upper airway, or GI tract that preclude successful swallowing.

    (ii) Severe physiologic oral motor dysphagia.

    (iii) Absent airway-protective responses.

    (iv) An underlying irreversible process affecting intake.

2. Obesity exacerbates immobility, isolation, chronic respiratory failure, scoliosis, and decubitus ulcers. It contributes to lifelong problems of diabetes, hypertension, and acquired heart disease.

  a. The **etiology** is usually an excess of caloric intake over energy expenditure. Abnormal body composition (increased fat in denervated extremities) also plays a role. Many disabling conditions of childhood carry an increased risk of hypothyroidism, which can add to this problem.

  b. Evaluation and diagnosis

    (1) The **history** should include

      (a) Careful analysis of intake, with emphasis on the use of food for behavioral reinforcement at home and school.

      (b) Family eating and exercise habits.

      (c) Activity and opportunities for supervised exercise and wheelchair use.

      (d) Obsessive mealtime behavior and compulsive eating habits.

    (2) Physical examination should include anthropometric measurements and comparison to National Center for Health Statistics (NCHS) growth charts.

  c. The **treatment** of obesity includes a combination of caloric restriction, altering the percentage of calories taken as fat, and increasing activity. The use of food as a positive reinforcer should be stopped. Obese children who are inactive or isolated should be enrolled in a supervised, ability-matched exercise program.

B. Disorders of **posture, mobility,** and **dexterity** are common to most disabling conditions. Addressing a child's ability to hold still, move, and manipulate allows for problem solving and better inclusion in age-appropriate activities.

  1. Evaluation

  a. The **assessment of gross motor function** should include a developmentally based line of questioning, starting with head control, still sitting abilities, rolling/standing abilities, and ambulation.

  b. Fine motor function, such as self-feeding, dressing, grooming, drawing, and writing, should be assessed. Exercise or normal activity tolerance should be clearly determined.

  c. The **physical examination** should include assessment of resting tone and strength. Persistent primitive reflexes should be sought, as these play an important role in prescription of adaptive positioning devices. Description of a child's effective movements allows the physician/therapist to capitalize on these movements and "augment" abilities with equipment.

  2. Treatment

  a. The **treatment** plan can include orthopedic, psychiatric, occupational, or physical therapy consultation/treatment and use of orthoses and adaptive positioning and mobility devices.

  b. Adaptive equipment should be used to prevent deformity or to simplify complex movement patterns.

  c. Children with physical impairments (spastic diplegia, lumbar meningomyelocele) often require tremendous energy expenditure (60–75% maximal oxygen consumption (VO_2)) for ambulation. A balance must be found between maximizing unaided physical activity and augmenting mobility at an unreasonable energy cost.

C. Disorders of communication frequently add to the disability imposed by developmental impairment. Proper communication assessment and treatment are part of every child's rehabilitation program.

1. **Evaluation**
   a. The **assessment** should be done by a certified speech/language patholo-gist and occupational therapist. All children with communication impair-ments must have
      (1) Formal hearing assessment.
      (2) A functional visual assessment.
      (3) Assessment of cognitive skills, attention, oral motor skills, and fine motor skills.
      These skills all play a role in receptive and expressive language.
   b. Phonation, airway anatomy, and swallowing abilities are also important and may require additional referral (otolaryngology) or testing.
   c. The ability to produce clear speech should be separated from language or overall cognitive abilities in order to help parents recognize the often hid-den communication abilities of their children.
2. **Treatment** should be multimodal and will depend on the child's inherent skills, personal interests, situational communication requirements, and physical abili-ties. **Augmentive communication** involves the use of nonverbal communica-tion to convey a child's thoughts. This may include visual pointing, gestures, signing, picture boards, icon pointing, or computer programs. Even severely physically impaired children may be able to operate sophisticated computer programs with switches controlled only by head movements or limb thrusts.

D. **Acute and chronic respiratory** disorders can affect development both by making cooperation with therapeutic and educational programs difficult and by the direct effects of hypoxia on brain function.
1. **Upper airway obstruction and hypoxia** is common in children with upper airway and jaw anomalies, bulbar palsies, and neuromuscular disorders.
   a. **Evaluation** should include
      (1) **History**
         (a) Situations/positions that produce stridor.
         (b) Mental state or color during maximal symptoms.
         (c) History of foreign body aspiration.
         (d) Sleep history, including snoring, respiratory pauses, or excessive daytime somnolence.
         (e) History of prolonged intubation, repeated episodes of "croup," or vocal abuse.
      (2) **Physical examination** should include
         (a) Assessment of extraneous respiratory noise in different head and trunk positions.
         (b) Inspection for digital clubbing.
         (c) Inspection of pharyngeal tonsil size.
      (3) **Laboratory testing** can include
         (a) Fluoroscopy.
         (b) Referral for direct laryngoscopy/tracheoscopy.
         (c) Overnight oximetry or multichannel polysomnography (gold standard for obstructive sleep apnea).
   b. The goal of **management** should be to protect normal lung function. This can include
      (1) Tonsillectomy and adenoidectomy,
      (2) Improvement in adaptive seating (including head supports),
      (3) Nighttime oxygen or continuous positive airway pressure, or
      (4) Tracheostomy.
2. Signs of **lower airway disease,** including coughing, wheezing, cyanosis, exer-cise intolerance, or exposure-related bronchospasm, are seen in a variety of disabling conditions.
   a. **Evaluation** should include
      (1) **History**
         (a) Exacerbation with exposures and feeding.
         (b) Seasonal exacerbation.
         (c) Recurrent pneumonia.

(d) Choking/foreign body aspiration.
(2) **Physical examination** should include
(a) Respiratory rate.
(b) Inspiratory/expiratory ratio.
(c) Distribution of breath sounds.
(d) Inspection for rib anomalies, kyphosis, scoliosis, and proximal muscle weakness that could alter chest compliance or vital capacity.
(3) **Laboratory testing** could include
(a) Oximetry.
(b) Arterial blood gas analysis.
(c) Pulmonary function tests.
(d) pH probe.
(e) Allergy testing, sweat testing, or immunologic evaluation.
b. **Management** can include
(1) Removal of allergens/exacerbants.
(2) Adaptive seating, bracing, or orthopedic surgery to preserve chest compliance.
(3) Beta agonists, inhaled steroids, or inhaled mast cell stabilizers.
(4) Chest physical therapy and postural drainage.
3. **Chronic unrecognized hypoxia is a significant cause of added morbidity in children with disabling conditions, including congenital malformations** (Pierre Robin sequence), **pharyngeal hypotonia** (Down's syndrome), and **neuromuscular diseases** (fascioscapulohumeral muscular dystrophy).
IV. **Management of children assisted by medical technology** requires parental training, provider training, maintenance care, and troubleshooting.
A. **Tracheostomy** is used when a variety of congenital and acquired structural and neuromuscular diseases complicate breathing.
1. **Equipment** needed includes two tracheostomy tubes (use and spare), gauze and ties, portable and stationary suction device, suction catheters, resuscitation bag, saline dosettes, oxygen/compressed air, humidifying device, gloves, and artificial "nose" (protects trachea from dry air and particles). Children with tracheostomies commonly require a home oximeter and cardiac/apnea monitor for use during sleep.
2. **Training** includes the biologic basis for therapy, recognizing early clinical signs of airway compromise, and mastering technical skills needed in care and accessing care when needed. Caregivers must be trained in CPR, including the ability to ventilate via tracheostomy and bag. Children with tracheostomies who attend school should travel with a nurse.
3. **Maintenance care** is dependent on age of the patient, age of the tracheostomy, size, anatomy, and neuromuscular condition. Many children do not require routine tracheostomy changes, but this should be dictated by the attending otolaryngologist. Most children will require routine suctioning (up to once an hour). At times this requires substantial home nursing support. Tracheostomy ties are changed at least daily. Skin care usually includes washing the site and neck with a peroxide/water mixture once or twice a day. Powder should never be used around a tracheostomy.
4. **Troubleshooting** includes recognizing signs of respiratory distress, responding to a change in secretions, and maintaining skin integrity around the stoma.
a. Frequently, a **change in tracheal secretions** signifies dehydration or excessive cooling of tracheal mucosa. Color change from white to yellow or green that is not associated with fever or respiratory distress can be treated with increasing oral hydration or increasing inhaled humidity.
b. **Fever or persistent thick discolored secretions** could signify bacterial tracheitis. At this time tracheal aspirate for Gram's stain and culture can help dictate antibiotic choice. Excessive oral antibiotic use can breed highly resistant organisms and should be avoided as much as possible.
c. **Frequent episodes of tracheitis or bloody secretions** could signify poor suctioning technique and this should be reviewed. Intratracheal com-

plications such as granuloma formation should be considered with episodes of tracheal bleeding and increasing respiratory distress.

d. **Site complications** usually are caused by excessive tube motion, excessive secretions, and irritation caused by friction or prolonged contact with dressings. These can be resolved by more frequent local hygiene, topical antibiotics and antifungals, barrier creams, and topical steroids as indicated. These creams and ointments should never contain a petroleum base.

B. **Gastrostomy** (see also Chap. 11, p. 338) devices are used when oral feeding is insufficient to meet caloric or hydration requirements.

1. **Equipment** for gastrostomy feedings includes two gastrostomy devices (use and spare), formula, syringes, or feeding bags and a pump.

2. **Training** for gastrostomy feeding should include monitoring for feeding intolerance (vomiting, retching, pain, or dyspnea), bolus and continuous feeding, and skin care.

3. **Maintenance** includes providing nutrition, replacing devices when necessary, and assessing skin condition. Both age-appropriate formulas and pureed food can be given via gastrostomy. If physiologically possible bolus feeding is preferred in order to preserve a hunger/satiety cycle. This may facilitate a return to oral feeding. Gastroesophageal reflux is common after gastrostomy regardless of its preoperative presence. A history of reflux should be explored at each visit. Skin care should be as simple as washing with soap and water. However, at times leakage, granuloma formation, and infection affect the gastrostomy site.

4. **Troubleshooting** can include formula or dietary changes, responding to redness or bleeding, or changing/replacing devices.

   a. **Formula or dietary changes** may be necessary when lactose intolerance or specific allergy is suspected.

   b. **Redness at the site** can be a sign of leakage, infection, or contact dermatitis.

      (1) **Acid leakage** is irritating. At times leakage can be decreased by changing to a different variety of tube or by increasing the inflation of the anchoring balloon. Leakage is a consequence of poor wound healing and tract formation. Increasing the gauge of feeding tube rarely if ever solves this problem. Painting the skin with liquid antacids around the gastrostomy site helps neutralize the acid leakage and can allow the skin to heal.

      (2) If superficial swelling, streaking, or pain accompanies redness, **infection** with staphylococcus or streptococcus should be suspected and topical or systemic antibiotics instituted.

      (3) **Granuloma** formation, minor bleeding from trauma, or small areas of recalcitrant maceration can be treated with topical cauterization with silver nitrate.

   c. When a gastrostomy device is pulled out, it must be **replaced** within a few hours to prevent tract occlusion. If a particular type of device is not immediately available, a Foley catheter of the same gauge should be inserted temporarily.

C. **Ventriculoperitoneal** and other types of **extracranial** shunts are surgically implanted catheters that reroute cerebrospinal fluid (CSF) to prevent accumulation of fluid and increased intracranial pressure.

1. Equipment: Most children with hydrocephalus are treated with extracranial shunts, where a catheter is surgically implanted in the skull, and sufficient tubing is attached to the valve to reach a compartment of the body where the CSF can drain freely. The reservoir is usually placed to permit access to CSF in the shunt, and can be tapped under aseptic conditions. Many valves can be "pumped" to ascertain flow. Both tapping the reservoir and pumping the valve should be performed only by physicians or neurosurgeons with expertise in shunts. Occasionally valveless shunts are used.

   a. Ventriculoperitoneal shunts: Tubing is placed subcutaneously running

from the scalp down to the abdomen, and enters the peritoneum. In small children, extra tubing is provided to accommodate linear growth.
  b. Ventriculoatrial shunts are used less frequently, and deliver CSF to the right atrium.
  c. Ventriculopleural shunts are infrequently used, due to accumulation of pleural effusions in children.
2. Training: Minimal parent training needed.
3. Maintenance: No specific maintenance needed.
4. Troubleshooting: All shunts are at risk for shunt malfunction due to obstruction, infection, and disconnection. A shunt malfunction is a potentially life-threatening emergency. Nonemergent revision of a shunt may be necessary with linear growth of the child.
  a. **Shunt infection** is the most common complication of ventricular shunts and occurs most commonly in younger children.
    (1) **Etiology.** The most common **organism** causing shunt infection is *Staphylococcus epidermidis*, usually from the patient's own skin flora. Streptococci, yeast, and gram-negative enteric bacteria are other organisms that cause internal shunt infections, while *Staphylococcus aureus* and gram-negative bacteria can cause internal shunt infection through infection of the wound.
    (2) **Evaluation.** Manifestations of shunt infections include fever, headache, meningeal signs, and occasionally vomiting and lethargy, as well as erythema and tenderness overlying the tract. Children with ventriculoperitoneal shunts may complain of abdominal pain.
    (3) **Diagnosis** of shunt infection relies on examination and culture of CSF from the shunt.
    (4) **Treatment** of shunt infections includes the use of appropriate intravenous and intraventricular antibiotics to cover the specific organism. In many cases the ventricular catheter may need to be removed, and an external drainage system used until the infection is cleared. In other cases, the catheter is left, but connected to a temporary external drain. Antibiotics should be continued for 10 to 14 days after cultures of CSF are sterile.
V. **School attendance for children with disabilities and special health care needs.** In the United States, all children are entitled under the Individuals with Disabilities Education Act (IDEA) to a free, appropriate public education in the least restrictive environment from age 3 through 22. "Least restrictive environment" means as much as possible in the regular classroom setting. The same law provides for early intervention services for infants and toddlers aged birth to 3 years.
A. **Early intervention.** The purpose of these services is to identify, evaluate, and provide necessary services to a child with a disability early, in order to prevent or ameliorate subsequent developmental delays. In order to be eligible, a child must be under the age of 3 and have a diagnosed condition (such as cerebral palsy or Down's syndrome) or have developmental delays or be at risk for having delays due to low birth weight or "environmental" factors such as abuse.

Each child enrolled in early intervention is entitled to a range of developmental services, including physical, occupational, and speech therapy, as well as case management, medical diagnostic services, family counseling, and transportation. These services are documented in the **Individualized Family Service Plan (IFSP),** which is developed with the family based on the evaluation of the child, and outlines the plan of intervention for the child.
B. **Services for children aged 3 to 5.** Children with disabilities, such as mental retardation; speech, hearing and visual impairments; emotional disturbance; and physical and other health impairments, are entitled to services through the public school system that assist the child in benefiting from special education. These **related services** include early identification and assessment of the child's disabilities, diagnostic medical services, nursing services, counseling, and therapies, such as physical, occupational, and speech. In order to qualify for these services, the

child must meet the definition of disability as specified by law, and must have an **Individualized Education Plan (IEP),** which, like the IFSP, documents the child's needs and the plan for intervention. Some school systems provide these services in the child's home, while others provide preschool programs at school for the child to attend.

C. **Children aged 5 to 22.** If the school-aged child meets the criteria for disability specified by law, that child is entitled to an IEP and necessary related services provided by the public school in school. **Inclusion** means having children with disabilities and other special health needs attending regular classrooms instead of being segregated into substantially separate classrooms. Full inclusion means adaptation of the complete classroom environment to accommodate a student's needs, including communication, special education, and physical access.

22

Behavioral Disorders

John R. Knight, Barbara Burr,
and Carolyn Frazer

I. Evaluation of behavioral disorders. (See Table 22-1 for suggested readings.)

A. Interview. Project an attitude of unconditional acceptance and empathy. Always protect confidentiality unless safety is in jeopardy.

1. **Family.** Obtain a full pediatric history by interview, supplemented by questionnaires, from the parents or caretakers. Include early temperament, school experience, functioning at home and in the neighborhood, medical problems, attentional difficulties, and specific character strengths and weaknesses. Obtain a detailed description of problem behavior, including onset, frequency, context in which it occurs, the meaning to the parents, and effect on the family structure.

2. **Child**
   a. Observe all children *under 6 years* of age while in the office for unusual behaviors, quality of play, and interaction with parents.
   b. Conduct a supplemental interview with *school-aged children* (without parents present).

3. **Adolescents.** Ask about
   a. Problems with *parents* and *peers*.
   b. Use of *tobacco, alcohol,* and *other drugs*.
   c. *Sexual history* (including history of sexual abuse or assault).
   d. *Emotional state* (including suicidal ideation).

4. **Other.** Obtain from the school, day care, or other care providers descriptions of current placement and functioning, any special assistance program, and the results of prior evaluations.

B. Physical examination

1. Perform a complete examination, including vision and hearing screens, complete neurologic exam, height, and weight.
2. Check face, hands, and feet for presence of congenital anomalies.
3. Examine the skin for evidence of past or present trauma and neurocutaneous markings.
4. Plot a growth curve.

C. Educational and psychological testing. Some of the following **evaluations** will require a consultant.

1. **Neurodevelopmental examination.**
2. **Educational evaluation,** including achievement tests.
3. **Psychological testing,** including
   a. **Cognitive** (IQ) testing (e.g., Wechsler Intelligence Scale for Children III (WISC-III), Wechsler Adult Intelligence Scale (WAIS), McCarthy).
   b. **Projective** testing

D. Laboratory and other diagnostic examinations

1. Based on findings from the history or physical, consider analysis of chromosomes, amino acids, organic acids, and toxins in blood or urine.
2. Incontinence may require urinalysis or abdominal x-ray.
3. Children with eating disorders may need evaluation for electrolyte disturbances, anemia, and endocrine abnormalities.
4. Obtain an EEG when staring spells are present.
5. In the absence of seizures or neurologic deficits, head imaging (CT or MRI) *is not often helpful.*

Table 22-1. Suggested readings on behavioral issues

Diagnostic and Statistical Manual of Mental Disorders (4th ed). Washington DC: American Psychiatric Association, 1994.
Ferber R. *Solve Your Child's Sleep Problems.* New York: Simon and Schuster, 1985.
Harper G. Eating disorders in adolescence. *Pediatr Rev* 15:72, 1994.
Levine MD, Carey WB, Crocker AC (eds). *Developmental Behavioral Pediatrics* (2nd ed). Philadelphia: Saunders, 1992.
Lewis M (ed). *Child and Adolescent Psychiatry.* Baltimore: Williams & Wilkins, 1991.
Miller WR, Zweben A, DiClemente CC, Rychtarik RG. *Motivational Enhancement Therapy Manual.* NIAA Project MATCH Monograph Series, Vol 2. NIH Publication No. 94-3723, 1994.
Parker S, Zuckerman B (eds). *Behavioral and Developmental Pediatrics: A Handbook for Primary Care.* Boston: Little, Brown, 1995.
Prochaska JO, DiClemente CC. Transtheoretical therapy: Toward a more integrative model of change. *Psychotherapy: Theory, Research and Practice* 19:276, 1982.
Schmitt BD. *Your Child's Health* (2nd ed). New York: Bantam, 1991.
Wiener JM (ed). *Textbook of Child and Adolescent Psychiatry.* Washington, DC: American Psychiatric Press, 1991.

II. Treatment modalities

A. Behavioral interventions. Behavioral management techniques are based on observation that when a behavior is followed by a rewarding event (**positive reinforcer**), it tends to occur more frequently. If the behavior is followed by no event (**extinction**) or by an aversive event (**negative reinforcer**), it tends to be weakened and occurs less frequently. Over time, **punishment is not an effective intervention.** Unless parents are motivated and willing to model appropriate behavior, **no** program will be effective. Behavioral interventions should be targeted to the child's **developmental level** and not chronological age.

  1. Effective use of "Time Out." Time Out is most useful in toddlers and preschoolers, and presents an alternative for parents to making empty threats, scolding, or spanking. Once a problem behavior has been identified, parents must offer praise to their child when not engaged in that target behavior. However, when the problem behavior is manifested, Time Out combines extinction and negative reinforcement in a safe and effective manner.

    a. Select a boring place, usually a chair in a room that has no TV, books, games, or other people (not the child's bedroom, bathroom, attic, or cellar).

    b. Explain Time Out to the child.

    c. Send child to Time Out immediately after problem behavior.

    d. Use active ignoring during the Time Out period. Discussions and apologies are better processed afterwards.

    e. One minute of Time Out for each year of age. Use of a portable timer is recommended. Consistency is essential.

  2. Behavioral plans. More substantive behavioral plans, often called "sticker plans," are appropriate for older, school-aged children.

    a. Specify the target behavior.

    b. Measure the target behavior (baseline). Have the family record the frequency, time, and duration of the behavior.

    c. Choose the reinforcer(s). Together with the child and family, search for an appropriate reward or reinforcer. Do not forget praise and affection.

    d. Arrange the contingency

      (1) Apply reinforcers immediately and consistently.

      (2) In the beginning make them easily obtainable. Increase requirements as progress is made.

      (3) Stickers, stars, or points can be posted on a chart or pasted in a book, and later turned in for a prize. In cases in which parent-child conflict

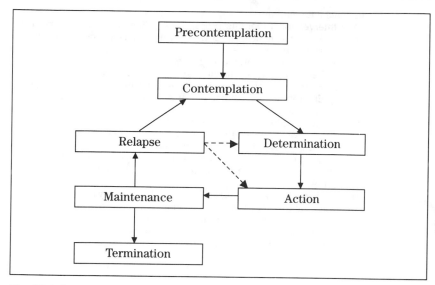

Fig. 22-1. Stages of change. Based on data from Prochaska JO, DiClemente CC: *Psychother Theor Res Pract* 1982;19(3):276.

is a major factor (often seen in enuresis/encopresis), encourage the child to keep his or her own sticker chart and bring it to you for review.
  e. Monitor the progress.
3. **Motivational enhancement.** For adolescents, **motivational enhancement** is a promising new therapeutic approach based on the premise that ambivalence to change in behavior is normal and acceptable, and change is a process rather than an event.
  a. Avoid pressuring an adolescent (which only leads to increased resistance to change).
  b. Ask questions that elicit self-motivational statements from the adolescent. ("How might you imagine your life could improve if you gave up using drugs?")
  c. *Summarize* and *support* those statements that favor change.
  d. Identify the adolescent's **stage of change** regarding the problem behavior (Fig. 22-1). In any single encounter, try to move him or her to the next stage.
  e. Brief intervention. Use the strategies that are summarized in the **FRAMES** mnemonic:

F	Give **F**eedback on personal risk or impairment.
R	**R**esponsibility for change rests with the adolescent.
A	Give Clear **A**dvice to change.
M	Present a **M**enu of options for change.
E	Develop **E**mpathy as a counseling style.
S	Support **S**elf-efficacy (optimism).

B. Educational interventions

1. **Early Intervention Programs (EIPs).** All children aged 0 to 3 years in the United States who are defined "at risk" for developmental delays are eligible for early intervention services.

   a. There are three categories of eligibility.
      (1) **Established risk:** a medical condition such as Down syndrome.
      (2) **Biologic risk:** a medical history of prematurity or low birth weight.
      (3) **Environmental risk:** factors such as poor nutrition, teen parent, or drug abuse.

   b. **Services include** monitoring of growth, development, and health status; general developmental stimulation; physical therapy; occupational therapy; and speech and language therapy. Services are provided through home visitation or at the EIP, or both, and can vary in each community.

   c. **Role of health care provider:** *document* areas of risk and *advocate* for services.

2. **Individualized Educational Plans (IEPs).** In the US, every child is guaranteed by law the right to an **appropriate** education, which can include an IEP. Be familiar with available structures in your local area.

   a. Accommodation within the mainstream classroom.
   b. Majority of time within the mainstream classroom.
   c. Majority of time in a special setting.
   d. A totally separate classroom within the public school.
   e. Special schools.
   f. Residential programs.
   g. Specialized hospitals.

   The **content** of educational programs can be tailored for any of the following: *language disorders, behavioral problems, attentional issues, psychiatric illness, cognitive disability,* or other specific *learning disabilities.* Special services, such as *physical therapy, occupational therapy, speech and language therapy,* or *vocational training,* can be included. *Recommend remediation in areas of significant lag.* Advise parents and educators to strongly encourage an area of success (i.e., athletics, music, art, a collection, etc.).

C. Psychotherapy

1. **Individual psychotherapy.** Recommend therapists who are well versed in child development and use both **play therapy** (younger children) and **conversation** (older children and adolescents). The goals for therapy include improvement in self-esteem, facilitation of age-appropriate coping skills, lessening of depression and anxiety, and better peer relationships.

2. **Family therapy** regards the **family unit** rather than the "identified patient" as the focus for intervention. Chronic family conflict, poor communication, and ineffective problem-solving skills can be improved by family therapy treatment. Young children can be included in family therapy with some modification of communication style and activities.

3. **Group psychotherapy** for children and adolescents promotes therapeutic and educational goals in a safe and supportive setting, with rules and boundaries established by the group therapist.

   a. **Support groups** can be helpful for difficulties in interpersonal relationships, behavioral problems, poor social skills, learning difficulties, and so forth.

   b. **Special groups** for divorce, abuse, chronic illness, substance abuse (AA), parental substance abuse (ALANON), and so forth, can facilitate improved adaptation.

   c. **Parent groups** can be effective means of teaching improved parenting skills, and dealing with severe stressors, such as the death of a child, chronic illness, or handicapping conditions.

D. Psychopharmacologic intervention. Pharmacotherapy should be used as an adjunct in treatment (see **Table 22-2**). Consult a psychiatrist if at all possible.

Table 22-2. Commonly used psychopharmacologic agents*

Drug class	Generic name	Proprietary name
Stimulants	Methylphenidate	Ritalin
	Dextroamphetamine	Dexedrine
	Pemoline	Cylert
Antidepressants	Imipramine	Tofranil
	Nortryptyline	Pamelor
	Desipramine	Norpramin
Selective serotonin reuptake	Fluoxetine	Prozac
inhibitors (SSRIs)	Sertraline	Zoloft
	Paroxetine	Paxil
Sedatives	Clonidine	Catapres
	Diphenhydramine	Benadryl
	Hydroxyzine	Vistaril
Benzodiazepines	Diazepam	Valium
	Clonazepam	Klonopin
	Lorazepam	Ativan
Mood stabilizers	Lithium Carbonate	—
	Valproic acid	Depakene, Depakote
	Carbamazepine	Tegretol
Neuroleptics	Haloperidol	Haldol
(antipsychotics)	Thioridazine	Mellaril
	Perphenazine	Trilafon

*See Formulary for complete prescribing information.

III. Management of neurodevelopmental disorders*

A. Language disorders include any impairment in speech or language, including comprehension, production, articulation, and social pragmatics. They are the most common developmental problems found in preschoolers (5–10% prevalence).

1. Evaluation and diagnosis

a. History. Ask about prematurity, perinatal infection, CNS infections, toxins, recurrent otitis media with conductive hearing loss, or general developmental delay. Problems with early feeding and persistent drooling may indicate oral motor dysfunction.

b. Physical examination. Perform a careful head, eyes, ears, nose, and throat (HEENT) (including head circumference) and neurologic examination, and check for dysmorphic features.

c. Other examinations. Obtain formal **audiologic testing.** Perform an initial language screening and then refer for formal **speech and language evaluation** when a problem is identified.

2. Treatment

a. Speech and language therapy. Base the type and degree of therapy on individual ability and age.

b. Amplification may be indicated for permanent hearing loss.

c. Tympanostomy tubes may be indicated for persistent middle ear effusion with conductive hearing loss.

*Sections III through VIII deal with defining (within categories) specific developmental, behavioral, and psychiatric disorders. All definitions are adapted from the *Diagnostic and Statistical Manual of Mental Disorders* (4th ed) (*DSM IV*) when applicable. As the etiology of these disorders is multifactorial (genetic, medical, psychological, social-environmental, characterologic) and often poorly understood, sections include descriptions of evaluation, diagnosis, and treatment only.

   d. Recommend **educational remediation** in the areas of reading and writing for the school-aged child.
   e. **Behavioral therapy** can help with behavioral problems due to frustration with inability to communicate.
   f. **Counseling** may be indicated for emotional distress.
B. **Pervasive developmental disorder (PDD) and autism** are developmental disorders with impairments in social interaction, communication, and imaginative activity, with a **preference for repetitive and stereotyped activities.** Onset is before age 30 months, and the degree of impairment varies. Associated features include **mental retardation, stereotyped movements** (spinning, rocking, flapping, toe walking), **tantrums, overactivity,** and **extreme fears.** PDD has been associated with organic diseases, including phenylketonuria, congenital rubella, tuberous sclerosis, hypsarrhythmia, and Fragile X syndrome.
   1. **Evaluation and diagnosis**
      a. **History.** Ask about early temperament and development, onset of symptoms, any loss of skills, social functioning, and behavior.
      b. **Physical examination**
         (1) Observe for **atypical language** (echolalia, poor use of pronouns, screeching), **stereotypic behaviors, repetitive behaviors** (opening and shutting doors, turning lights on and off), and **decreased social relatedness** (poor eye gaze, lack of response to others).
         (2) Assess head circumference (increased in Fragile X syndrome), presence of dysmorphic features, neurocutaneous findings, overall tone (often decreased), coordination (often awkward), and reflexes.
      c. **Other**
         (1) Recommend formal audiologic examination (most children with PDD have language delays) and a formal developmental-educational-psychological assessment.
         (2) Consider chromosome and Fragile X syndrome testing, amino acids, organic acids, and EEG (if evidence of seizures).
   2. **Treatment.** Early intervention for language and social impairments has been shown to correlate highly with improved prognosis.
      a. **Skilled special education** in a structured and supportive environment. Recommend a *full-day, year-round* program.
      b. Recommend **behavioral treatment** for improving social responses and communication, and decreasing inappropriate behaviors.
      c. Assist with **parent training.**
      d. Prescribe **medications** for **associated** problems (seizures, hyperactivity, inattention, compulsive behaviors, affective disorders, and sleep disorders).
      e. Treatments such as auditory training, facilitated communication, yeast, and magnesium have shown only limited **anecdotal** success.
C. **Mental retardation** (see Chap. 21, p. 530).
D. **Attention deficit (with hyperactivity) disorder (ADHD)** is a disorder with developmentally inappropriate **inattention, impulsivity,** and **distractibility** with or without **hyperactivity** that occurs in 3 to 10% of the population. The predominant symptoms vary with age: hyperactivity in the preschooler, distractibility and impulsivity in the older child and adolescent. ADHD is often associated with other learning disabilities (particularly language based), low self-esteem, mood lability, low frustration tolerance, and temper tantrums.
   1. **Evaluation and diagnosis.** Distinguish from inattention secondary to sensory deficits (vision or hearing), language disorders, learning disability, mental retardation, PDD emotional stress (i.e., depression, anxiety, neglect), petit mal seizures, sleep disorders, illicit drug use, and age-appropriate overactivity (i.e., active, but not haphazard or poorly organized, behavior). However, **ADHD can coexist** with any of these problems.
      a. **History**
         (1) Obtain a full developmental and school history with parent and teacher questionnaires (such as Conner's, Achenbach). **Symptoms**

may be less prominent in a novel and structured environment such as the physician's office.

(2) Ask about lead exposure or prior lead testing, or both (see also Chap. 8, p. 283).

b. **Physical examination.** Check for "soft neurologic signs" (synkinesia, stress gait posturing, choreiform movement, incoordination, motor overflow); screen vision and hearing. Tics or tremors can indicate ADHD associated with Tourette's syndrome.

c. **Other examinations.** Consider CBC, lead level, and thyroid function tests. EEG and MRI are indicated in cases of neurologic abnormality. Educational and neurodevelopmental testing, and psychiatric assessment, may be indicated.

2. **Treatment** must be a combination of educational remediation, counseling, and medication. Clarification regarding the underlying neurologic problem is essential, as much of the child's behavior may be wrongly attributed to laziness or willfulness by parents and teachers.

a. **Educational remediation** (academic underachievement is common).

b. **Counseling:** cognitive therapy to help the child increase attention span and decrease distractibility and impulsivity (i.e., "think first").

c. **Medication** (see Formulary for dosage information)

(1) **Stimulant medications** (methylphenidate, dextroamphetamine, and pemoline) are the first-line drugs for attentional disorders and are effective in 75% of children.

(a) Individual children may respond differently to the three stimulants. Try all three **before declaring treatment failure.** Long-acting preparations (Dexedrine, Ritalin-SR, Cylert) are associated with improved compliance. Dosages for children 6 years or older are

(i) Methylphenidate: 0.6 to 2.1 mg/kg/day divided into two to three doses. Usual starting dose is 5 or 10 mg bid. Available in 5-mg, 10-mg, and 20-mg tablets, and in 20-mg sustained release.

(ii) Dextroamphetamine: 0.30 to 1.5 mg/kg/day divided into two to three doses. Usual starting dose is 5 mg bid. Available in 5-mg tablets, and sustained release 5 mg, 10 mg, and 15 mg, providing the greatest flexibility in SR dosing of all three stimulant medications.

(iii) Pemoline: Maximum daily dose is 112.5 mg. Usual starting dose is 37.5 mg/day. Available in tablets of 18.75 mg, 37.5 mg, and 75 mg.

(b) Teachers are usually the best source of information concerning medication response (i.e., questionnaires, telephone contact).

(c) *Maximal learning may occur at a lower dosage than that which provides the most improvement in behavior.*

(d) **Reversible side effects** include insomnia, decreased appetite (usually transient), slowed growth (monitor growth curves), abdominal pain, and (rarely) psychosis.

(e) **Tics may not disappear** or improve once developed. **Stimulants can exacerbate Tourette's syndrome or other tic disorders.** Use cautiously when a child has multiple or complex (movement plus verbal) tics or a family history of the same.

(2) Use **tricyclic antidepressant** such as **imipramine** when stimulants are not tolerated. Monitor for side effects (tachycardia, dry mouth); follow serum levels and conduction intervals (PR, QRS, QTc) on ECG. Psychopharmacology consultation is recommended.

(a) Imipramine dosage

(i) 0.5 mg/kg/day divided into one to two doses.

(ii) Usual starting dose for child older than 6 years is 25 mg/day.

(3) Consider **clonidine** when impulsivity is a major symptom or tics are present. Monitor for sedation or hypotension, or both. Psychopharmacology consultation is recommended.

    (a) Clonidine dosage

        (i) 4 to 5 μg/kg/day divided into two to three doses.

        (ii) Usual starting dose for child older than 6 years is 0.025 mg bid, with dosing gradually increased every other day until therapeutic range is achieved.

E. Learning disabilities are characterized by difficulty in acquiring specific academic skills in listening, speaking, reading, writing, reasoning, or mathematics due to underlying central nervous system dysfunction. There may be a discrepancy between academic performance and general intellectual function (underachievement), and associated attentional and sensory deficits.

  1. Diagnosis. Distinguish from ADHD, mental retardation, sensory deficits, language disorder, emotional stress, petit mal seizures, sleep disorder, and illicit drug use. The diagnosis is confirmed on **neurodevelopmental and educational testing.**

  2. Treatment. Educational remediation is indicated for areas of weakness. Modifications in the educational program may be necessary depending on individual needs (see p. 542).

IV. Management of nutritional disorders

  A. Nonorganic failure to thrive (FTT) is a feeding disturbance manifested by failure to gain weight or loss of weight over at least one month that is not due to an associated GI disturbance, other general medical condition, other mental disorder, or lack of available food.

    1. Evaluation and diagnosis are confirmed by evidence that parent-child interactional problems interfere with feeding. Improvement in feeding and weight gain when caregivers are changed (e.g., during hospitalization) confirms the diagnosis.

      a. History. Ask about economic stress, disorganized families, social isolation, parental depression, and history of loss.

      b. Physical examination. There is frequently a mixed organic and nonorganic cause. Look for minor congenital anomalies, prenatal malnutrition, prematurity, and ongoing medical illness. Observe feeding and nonfeeding situations between parent(s) and child, looking for decreased, inconsistent, or nonmutual interactions. Assess the child's **development,** including social responsiveness.

      c. Laboratory examination. Obtain hemogram (CBC), serum albumin, and total protein. These may indicate problems *secondary* to poor nutrition. Consider analysis of chromosomes, amino acids, organic acids, or perinatal infection (TORCH screen). Structural abnormalities of the GI tract can be excluded with abdominal CT, ultrasound, or contrast studies (upper GI, barium enema, etc.). Bone age may be helpful in ascertaining potential for catchup growth.

    2. Treatment

      a. Nutritional rehabilitation and treatment of any associated medical problems.

      b. Interactional difficulties must be directly addressed with parents. Psychiatric or social service consultation, or both; behavioral therapy; and counseling are often needed.

      c. Developmental stimulation of the child through community infant-stimulation programs can be helpful.

      d. Pediatric follow-up is indicated, given the risk for subsequent behavior problems, cognitive delays, school difficulties, and slow growth.

  B. Anorexia nervosa is a symptom complex that includes a weight greater than 15% *below* expected for height, intense fear of gaining weight, distorted body image, and amenorrhea for more than three cycles. Female-male preponderance is about 20 : 1.

1. **Evaluation and diagnosis.** Exclude any physical illness that would account for the weight loss (inflammatory bowel or renal disease, endocrine disorder, neoplasm) and major thought or mood disorder. *Superior mesenteric artery syndrome* (postprandial vomiting secondary to intermittent gastric outlet obstruction) should be distinguished from anorexia nervosa, but can occur as a complication of emaciation.

   a. **History.** Findings include a self-imposed diet that gradually leads to drastic caloric reduction (restricting), marked weight loss, preoccupation with food, an intense fear of gaining weight, distorted body image, and sometimes purging (self-induced vomiting, laxative or diuretic abuse, and/or excessive exercising).

   b. **Physical findings** include hypothermia; bradycardia or hypotension, or both; lanugo hair; dry skin; muscle wasting; and dependent edema. Both primary and secondary amenorrhea and growth retardation occur.

   c. **Laboratory findings**

   (1) Anemia, leukopenia, lymphocytosis, low erythrocyte sedimentation rate, hypercholesterolemia, and low fibrinogen levels can occur.

   (2) Electrolyte disturbances are most common with purging, and can be life threatening.

   (3) Calcium and magnesium can be affected, and sudden drops in phosphorus during the first 1 or 2 weeks of refeeding are common. Osteoporosis may be irreversible.

2. **Treatment**

   a. Nutritional education, counseling, encouragement, and support, along with **firm and unchanging weight gain expectations,** are indicated. **Target weight** is calculated using the Frisch tables for the 10th to 25th percentile or 10th percentile plus 10 lb (see RE Frisch et al. *Hum Biol* 45:469–483, 1973) as a weight at which menses are likely to reoccur, growth will resume, and the patient is usually physiologically stable. Target weight may need to be adjusted 5 to 10 lb higher if menses do not return in 6 to 12 months, the patient has a large frame, or instability continues.

   b. **Outpatients** should be seen medically at least once a week for **weight monitoring. Postural vital signs** should be checked, along with urine specific gravity (to exclude water loading).

   c. **Hospitalization** is often necessary. Indications include severe malnutrition, vital sign instability, acute dehydration, electrolyte imbalance (e.g., hypokalemic alkalosis), and/or inability to eat. Management requires a collaboration between pediatrics and psychiatry. **Care during hospitalization** includes the following:

   (1) **Baseline weight** is set after rehydration (about 24 hr) and the patient is measured in a gown each morning after voiding. Activity is increased with improvements in vital signs and weight gain.

   (2) A nutritional consultant determines intake necessary to gain 1.4 kg/week. Daily caloric totals are quite small at first (1,500 kcal/day), and are increased by 250 kcal every 2 days. The nutritionist divides the daily totals into planned meals and snacks.

   (3) Meals and snacks must be eaten in the presence of a nurse or assistant within 30 minutes. If the patient is unable to comply, 500 kcal (2 cans) of a liquid supplement is ingested (e.g., Ensure, Sustacal) over the next 30 minutes. Patients who are unable to finish this supplementation by mouth must be tube fed (rarely required).

   (4) Restrictions must be **gently,** but **firmly** and **consistently** applied in order to be effective. Observation for 30 minutes following meals (including bathroom observation) is essential to prevent purging.

   (5) Constipation is relieved by eating nutritional or supplementary fiber, or stool softeners (Ducosate). **Stimulant and cathartic laxatives are to be avoided.**

   (6) A multivitamin and phosphorus supplement (e.g., Neutra-Phos, 500

mg 2–4×/day) should be given during initial refeeding. A single IM dose of thiamine, 100 mg, is indicated for patients with prolonged periods of malnutrition.

   (7) Neuroleptics, sedatives, and antidepressants have been used with limited success.

   d. Individual **psychotherapy** or family therapy, or both, are indicated during hospitalization and after discharge. Self-help groups (Anorectic-Bulimics Anonymous, Overeaters Anonymous) can be very useful.

C. Bulimia nervosa is a disorder characterized by recurrent episodes of binge eating (>1,500 kcal in one sitting), a sense of lack of control over eating, and recurrent inappropriate compensatory behavior to prevent weight gain (fasting, exercising); misuse of laxatives, diuretics, or enemas; or self-induced vomiting. Most patients weigh within the normal range, yet exhibit persistent overconcern about body shape and weight.

   1. Evaluation and diagnosis. Exclude epileptic equivalent seizures, CNS tumors, and abdominal pathology.

   a. History. Obtain a careful weight history, plus onset, frequency, and duration of binge eating. Specifically ask about vomiting, and use of emetics, diuretics, and laxatives.

   b. Physical findings can include erosion of dentition; abrasions over the knuckles or dorsum of the hand; exercise injuries and stress fractures; tender, swollen parotids; or facial petichiae.

   c. Laboratory findings include electrolyte imbalance and elevated serum amylase (with normal serum lipase). Normal chemistries do not exclude purging.

   d. Complications include Mallory-Weiss tears, esophagitis, aspiration pneumonia, gastric rupture, mediastinal dissection, bloody diarrhea, and congestive heart failure.

   2. Treatment

   a. Outpatient **behavioral treatment** can be used with some success in mild cases. Twelve-step support group programs are often effective.

   b. Psychiatric consultation and treatment plan (as above for anorexia nervosa) is recommended.

   c. Dehydration and **electrolyte imbalance** (hypokalemia) secondary to the vomiting, cathartics, or diuretics may need correction with intravenous fluids.

   d. Hospitalization is often required, and treatment is similar to that of anorexia nervosa. Bathroom observation is always required.

D. Obesity is a marked increase in body fat, resulting in a weight that is more than 20% above the mean. Obesity **need not** denote a behavioral or psychiatric disturbance, but is often associated with emotional disorders (and distortions in body image). Obesity can result from **binge eating** in the **absence** of the compensatory behaviors seen in bulimia. Social, emotional, learning, genetic, and physical activity factors, and/or fat cell size and number have also been implicated as causes. Favorable outcomes are entirely dependent on the ability of both child and family to make significant, permanent changes in food selection and exercise patterns.

   1. Evaluation and diagnosis. Exclude weight gain secondary to craniopharyngioma, pituitary tumor, Prader-Willi syndrome, ovarian dysfunction, or Cushing's syndrome.

   a. History

   (1) Historical data should be gathered and plotted on a growth chart. **Normal height effectively excludes primary endocrine disorders.**

   (2) Food diaries can be useful, although this information is often unreliable. Obese individuals often consume larger amounts during evening (inactive) hours.

   b. Physical examination may reveal striae secondary to weight gain (rather than Cushing's syndrome). Distribution of fat (centripetal, generalized subcutaneous, omental) should be noted. Blood pressure should be recorded with an appropriately sized cuff.

    c. Laboratory tests (rarely indicated)
- **(1)** Mild abnormalities in thyroid, adrenal, or gonadotropic function are often secondary to morbid obesity.
- **(2)** Analysis of serum lipoproteins is indicated when the patient has a family history of early-onset coronary artery disease and once after puberty for all children.
- **(3)** Chromosome analysis if suggested by physical examination.

2. Treatment. Successful treatment requires high motivation and **family involvement.**
- **a.** Important components include a *balanced low-calorie diet* and *increased physical activity.*
- **b.** Though not ideal, behavioral treatment programs involving positive reinforcement for stepwise weight reduction have been effective.
- **c.** Adolescents may respond to **motivational enhancement and group support** (Weight Watchers, Overeaters Anonymous, etc.).
- **d.** Obesity is a chronic disorder; therefore, the prognosis for sustained weight loss is poor and relapse is common. This should never lead to provider abandonment or hopelessness.
- **e.** Prevention via early recognition and nutritional advice is important.
- **f.** Inappropriate use of food to calm a child's discomfort should be discouraged.

V. Management of psychiatric disorders

  A. Conduct disorders are conditions in which **repetitive, persistent** behaviors violate either the basic rights of others or major age-appropriate societal rules (lasting at least 6 mo). Behaviors include serious aggression, coercion, cruelty, theft, destruction of property, running away, and so forth.

    1. Evaluation and diagnosis. Exclude oppositional defiant disorder, a pattern of negativistic, hostile, and defiant behavior (although usually not including sociopathy).
- **a. Interview** with the family reveals a history of persistent and severe behavior problems, such as lying, fighting, bullying, truancy, and/or criminal acts.
- **b. Problematic parent-child relationships,** abuse, difficult temperament, poor supervision, and lack of or excessively harsh discipline can predispose to conduct disorder.
- **c. Comorbid problems,** such as ADHD, learning disabilities (LD), depression, or substance abuse, may be present.

    2. Treatment
- **a. Prevention** is important: counseling about discipline, management of difficult temperament, or referral to parent effectiveness training groups.
- **b.** Assist family in identifying **structured recreational experiences** or individuals who can provide a **supportive relationship** for the child, or both.
- **c. Refer to a child psychiatrist** if symptoms are persistent or escalating.
- **d.** In extreme cases, refer to the **Juvenile Court** for **residential placement** or **inpatient psychiatric hospitalization.**

  B. Anxiety disorders are characterized by *excessive worry and fear,* symptoms of *autonomic hyperarousal, increased vigilance,* and *anticipatory dread.*

    1. Specific types
- **a. Generalized anxiety disorder** is defined by excessive anxiety and worry almost daily.
- **b. Separation anxiety disorder** is developmentally excessive anxiety concerning separation from home or familiar caretakers.
- **c. Specific phobia** includes marked and unreasonable fear cued by the presence or anticipation of a specific object or situation.
- **d. Panic disorders** are discrete attacks with intense fear accompanied by somatic or cognitive symptoms, followed by persistent worry about recurrence or the implications of the attack.
- **e.** In **posttraumatic stress disorder** the individual is a victim of or exposed to an extreme traumatic stressor and experiences intrusive recollections, nightmares, hyperarousal, and numbing of responsiveness.

  f. Obsessive-compulsive disorder (OCD) includes persistent obsessions or compulsions, or both, such as hand washing or checking, which are time consuming and disrupt normal routines.

 2. Evaluation and diagnosis

  a. History includes excessive worrying, crying, tantrums, unreasonable fears, excessive rituals, school refusal, clinginess, multiple somatic complaints, sleep disturbance, and exposure to traumatic experience.

  b. Family history of anxiety is common.

  c. High performance pressure on the child may be present.

  d. Panic attacks can **mimic** cardiac or neurologic problems.

  e. Transitory fears are usually normal in younger children.

 3. Treatment

  a. Support and reassurance for child and family.

  b. Psychiatric consultation if symptoms are debilitating or persistent. Traumatized children and their families should always be referred.

  c. Medications for acute anxiety may be helpful (benzodiazepines or other sedatives; see **Table 22-2**).

  d. Obsessive-compulsive disorder and **panic disorder** can be helped by selective serotonin reuptake inhibitors (SSRIs), benzodiazepines, or antidepressants (see **Table 22-2**). Psychopharmacological consultation is recommended.

  e. Relaxation techniques to reduce stress and somatic complaints, and to improve sleep.

  f. Behavioral therapy can be helpful in treating phobias, panic attacks, and OCD symptoms.

C. Depression. A **major depression** is characterized by a period of at least 2 weeks during which the child exhibits depressed mood and loss of interest or pleasure in most activities. In children, the mood may seem more irritable than sad. Additional features can include appetite and sleep disturbance, loss of energy, poor concentration, feelings of worthlessness, or suicidal thoughts.

Bipolar disorder, which is less common in children, is characterized by manic episodes (abnormally and persistently elevated mood), often alternating with periods of depression.

 1. Evaluation and diagnosis

  a. Interview for history of sudden loss, parental rejection, physical illness, school problems, behavioral problems or sleep disturbance.

  b. The **child** should be asked directly about the severity and frequency of sad feelings. Inquiring about suicide (e.g., "Do you ever think about hurting yourself?") will not precipitate the event, and will often provide relief as well as facilitate intervention.

  c. Family history often includes relatives with depression or substance abuse.

  d. Transitory depressed moods in children that are not disabling are common.

  e. Medical causes for depression (e.g., hypothyroidism) should be excluded.

 2. Treatment

  a. The pediatrician should establish a **supportive relationship** with the child, and assist with identification of positive coping mechanisms. Additionally, environmental interventions, such as school changes, parent education, and so forth, are helpful.

  b. Psychiatric consultation is recommended for evaluation and treatment of persistent depression and bipolar disorder.

  c. Psychopharmacologic treatment (tricyclic antidepressants and SSRIs, see **Table 22-2**) may be helpful, but close monitoring is required.

  d. Suicidal behavior (see Chap. 7, p. 245) requires emergency evaluation.

D. Acute psychosis (see Chap. 7, 245).

VI. Management of other behavioral disturbances

 A. Tantrums are **out-of-control behaviors,** such as crying, screaming, kicking, or head banging, caused by frustration or anger centered around power struggles and issues of autonomy. Although "normal" in toddlers, tantrums can be a sign of emotional immaturity or distress in the older child. Tantrums are a problem if the behavior is impacting the child's functioning at school, or if the child is aggressive or destructive.

1. **Evaluation and diagnosis**
   a. **History.** Evaluate onset, context in which it occurs, and previous treatments the family has tried. Assess problems such as temperament, emotional stress, sleep difficulties, developmental delay, language delay, PDD, or mental retardation.
   b. **Examination.** Observe child's play, behavior, and parent-child interaction for social-emotional and cognitive functioning.
2. **Treatment.** Decrease situational triggers, decrease the attention the child gains during the tantrum, and set firm limits. See p. 540 for details of **behavioral management.**
   a. **Decrease frustrating situations.** Offer choices for the toddler to avoid autonomy struggles; provide warnings before any change in activity or routine for the child; develop appropriate expectations for the child's behavior and temperament.
   b. **Ignore the tantrum behavior** while assuring the child's safety.
   c. **Set firm limits** and consistent rules.
   d. **Counseling** with a behavioral specialist may be indicated.

B. **Sleep disorders**
1. **Delayed sleep initiation and maintenance** are characterized by difficulty in falling asleep or frequent wakening, or both. These problems are more common in younger children and are typically behaviorally based.
   a. Specific causes include the following:
      (1) **Inappropriate sleep associations** occur when a child learns to fall asleep only when certain conditions, such as rocking, feeding, or pacifiers, are present.
      (2) **Feedings** during the night can cause increased wakening due to learned hunger and increased wetting.
      (3) **Erratic scheduling** results in difficulty in establishing a regular sleep pattern.
      (4) **Ineffective limit setting** can also contribute to the problem.
   b. **Evaluation and diagnosis.** Obtain a complete sleep history, including sleep schedules, sleep environment, and bedtime routines. Look for contributing problems such as parental stress. Ask parents to keep a sleep diary.
   c. **Treatment**
      (1) **Explain** the problem in a nonjudgmental manner.
      (2) **Discuss strategies** for dealing with inappropriate sleep associations. For example, put the child into the crib while still awake to avoid a learned association with rocking.
      (3) **Reduce nighttime feeding** by decreasing the amount of fluid given or the amount of time spent nursing over successive nights.
      (4) **Establish a regular routine** during the night and day.
      (5) Discuss consistent **limit setting** (see p. 540).
      (6) **Close follow-up** by phone or office visit to implement the changes.
2. **Disorders of arousal.** Non–rapid eye movement (NREM) parasomnias occur in the first third of the night during a transition from deep NREM sleep to another sleep stage. The child is often confused and unresponsive to the environment, may have autonomic symptoms (tachycardia, sweating, pupillary dilatation), and has retrograde amnesia for the event.
   a. Specific types include the following:
      (1) **Confusional arousals** are identified when the child looks confused and agitated, and there may be verbal (talking, crying, or screaming), motor (thrashing in bed or walking around the room), or autonomic features (most common in the first 3 yr of life).
      (2) In **sleepwalking** the sleeping child walks calmly around the house.

Occasionally, unusual behavior such as urinating on the floor is seen (most common between 6 and 12 yr).

   (3) Sleep terrors are brief (up to 45 min) episodes, which begin with a terrified scream, an intense autonomic response, and fearful behaviors such as running away. Night terrors are distinguished from nightmares in that they occur early in the night during NREM sleep, and the child is not arousable, has no memory of the episode, and returns to sleep easily following the episode (most common between 4 and 7 yr old).

   b. Evaluation and diagnosis. Exclude seizure disorders.

   (1) History. Obtain frequency, time of onset, time during sleep cycle, and history of child's typical sleep schedule. A sleep diary kept by the parents is helpful.

   (2) Physical examination. Check for neurologic abnormalities.

   (3) Other examination: EEG if seizures are suspected (early morning episodes, history of tonic-clonic movements).

   c. Treatment

   (1) Explain that episodes are self-limited and not medically dangerous. Parents should minimize physical contact during the episode, intervening only to prevent injury. For night terrors, efforts to **console the child make the episode worse.**

   (2) Regularize the sleep schedule.

   (3) Safety proof the house to avoid any injuries during the episodes.

   (4) Pharmacologic therapy with benzodiazepines or tricyclic antidepressants may be indicated if arousals are disruptive or dangerous.

   (5) Scheduled awakening before the time that the event typically occurs is occasionally helpful.

3. Obstructive sleep apnea syndrome is a *potentially lethal condition* characterized by multiple episodes of obstructive or mixed apneas during sleep, repetitive episodes of loud snoring, and excessive daytime somnolence. It is caused by anatomic factors (e.g., large tonsils or adenoids, small posterior oropharynx) and possible CNS dysfunction.

   a. Evaluation and diagnosis. Differentiate from benign snoring.

   (1) History. Identify excessive daytime sleepiness, loud intermittent snoring at night, frequent nocturnal apnea, poor school performance, headaches, and enuresis. Ask for tape recording of sleep. Frequent upper respiratory infections and mouth breathing may indicate tonsillar and adenoidal hypertrophy.

   (2) Physical examination. Look for enlarged tonsils, mouth breathing, and nasal voice. Assess growth, as sleep apnea is more common to the obese.

   (3) Other examinations

   (a) X-ray the upper airway to evaluate obstruction.

   (b) Obtain an **ECG** to detect right ventricular hypertrophy, cor pulmonale, and arrhythmias.

   (c) A **sleep study** confirms the diagnosis.

   b. Treatment

   (1) Avoid all forms of sedation, as they can exacerbate the apnea.

   (2) Time can relieve symptoms in some younger children as the airway grows and the relative size of the tonsils and adenoids decreases.

   (3) Surgery to remove obstruction (e.g., adenoids, tonsils) has varying success.

   (4) Tracheostomy cures the problem but the cost-benefit ratio must be considered.

   (5) Weight loss is beneficial in obese patients.

C. Incontinence

1. Encopresis relates to the deposition of stools in the child's underwear on a regular basis after age 4 years (due to *chronic constipation, loss of internal* *sphincter competence,* and *resultant leakage of stool).* Primary encopresis indicates that bowel continence has never been achieved; secondary encopresis indicates incontinence after being fully trained for at least 6 months.

  a. Evaluation and diagnosis. Exclude pathologic causes including spinal cord lesions, autonomic dysfunction, seizures, cerebral palsy, muscular disorders, hypothyroidism, and Hirschsprung's disease (aganglionic megacolon). Identify psychosocial stresses.

    (1) History

      (a) Determine onset, frequency, the time that accidents usually occur, caliber and bulk of stools, history of previous constipation, prior treatment regimen, and family's perception of the problem.

      (b) Nighttime accidents are rare and suggest emotional or neurologic etiologies.

      (c) Constipation since birth with small-caliber (pencil-like) stools suggests Hirschsprung's disease.

    (2) Physical examination

      (a) Include growth parameters.

      (b) Check anal wink and cremasteric reflex (in boys) to assess lower spinal cord function.

      (c) Assess stool retention by abdominal and rectal examination.

    (3) Other examinations

      (a) Abdominal x-ray helps to assess the degree of stool retention and patient education.

      (b) Obtain **urinalysis and urine culture** in girls with encopresis due to increased incidence of urinary tract infections.

      (c) Anal manometry and rectal biopsy may be indicated in rare cases (if Hirschsprung's is suspected).

  b. Treatment

    (1) Education. Explain that the distended colon has lost sensation and muscle tone, and thus lack of control is not the child's fault. Involve the child directly in the treatment plan.

    (2) Establish regular bowel habits

      (a) Ensure access to a private bathroom at school.

      (b) Use a foot support for younger children (to assist in Valsalva maneuver).

    (3) Initial catharsis to disimpact the bowel. A regimen that combines oral and suppository cathartics with enemas is recommended for the average 7-year-old child (appropriate adjustments should be made for larger and smaller children).

      (a) Home treatment. For moderate to severe retention (majority of patients), go through three to four cycles (9–12 days total).

        (i) Day 1: hypophosphate enema (Fleet, adult size).

        (ii) Day 2: bisacodyl (Dulcolax) suppository.

        (iii) Day 3: bisacodyl tablet.

        (iv) More recently, **polyethylene glycol** electrolyte solution (GoLYTELY), given orally at a starting dose of 40 ml/kg over 6 hours, has been used.

      (b) Inpatient treatment is reserved for severe retention or when home compliance is poor. Order daily enemas and suppositories along with regular use of the toilet after meals.

    (4) Maintenance therapy after initial catharsis is complete will minimize relapse (common).

      (a) Use **mineral oil** (at least 2 tbsp) or other stool softener (ducosate sodium) bid for at least 4 to 6 months. Due to the risk of aspiration, mineral oil should not be used in children less than 2 years old unless it is mixed with food such as yogurt.

      (b) Oral laxatives (senna or danthron) can be used for severe cases or during relapse. Use daily for 2 to 3 weeks, then on alternate days for one month.

(c) Reinforce **regular daily toilet sitting** for 5 minutes, twice a day, after meals.

(d) **High-roughage diet.**

(e) Vitamin supplements since mineral oil can decrease vitamin absorption.

(5) Warn children and parents about the **possibility of relapse.** Signs of relapse include large-caliber stools, increased mineral oil leakage, abdominal pain, decreased frequency of defecation, and soiling. Advise parents not to punish or blame the child.

(6) **Biofeedback** may be useful in refractory cases.

(7) **Psychiatric referral** may be indicated in cases in which the child's self-esteem has been damaged or when significant parent-child conflict impairs treatment.

D. Enuresis is urinary incontinence after the age of 4 years for daytime wetting and after the age of 6 years for nighttime wetting. There is a large variation in children developmentally and across cultures. By age 5, 92% of children have attained daytime continence and 80% have achieved nighttime continence. By age 12, 95% of children have attained nighttime continence.

1. **Evaluation and diagnosis.** Exclude **organic causes,** including structural anomalies of the genitourinary tract (i.e., ectopic ureter), urinary tract infections, diabetes mellitus, neurologic abnormalities including seizures, and diabetes insipidus. Constipation and psychological stress can exacerbate enuresis.

   a. **History.** Obtain urinary and toileting history, including patterns of wetting (time of day, number of times per night and per week, number of daytime voidings, periods of dryness), sleep abnormalities, dysuria, polyuria, description of urinary stream, family history, toilet training efforts, parent and child perceptions, stresses, and medications.

      (1) **Diurnal enuresis** can be due to bladder spasms or vaginal reflux (usually in overweight girls).

      (2) **Nocturnal enuresis** can be due to small functional bladder capacity.

   b. **Physical examination.** Perform a genital examination (including location of the urethral meatus), and neurologic and spine examinations. Palpate the abdomen for an enlarged bladder or fecal impaction.

   c. **Other examinations**

      (1) Obtain a **urinalysis in all cases.** Urine culture may be indicated, particularly in girls.

      (2) Measure **bladder capacity.**

      (3) Radiologic studies may be indicated in cases of suspected anatomic abnormality.

      (4) Obtain BUN and creatinine if renal disease is suspected, and an EEG if seizures are suspected.

2. **Treatment.** Organic causes for enuresis should be treated appropriately. In all cases, try to decrease the blame and guilt feelings of the child, and discourage struggles between the parents and child.

   a. **Reassurance** is sufficient in some cases, such as with younger children, since a large proportion will have spontaneous resolution.

   b. **Awakening exercises** or having the parents teach the child to wake at night may be successful in some cases.

   c. Emphasize **proper voiding** to decrease vaginal reflux. Instruct girls to sit on the toilet with legs as wide open as possible, or to sit facing backward on the toilet and wait briefly after voiding.

   d. **Bladder training exercises** to stretch the bladder and increase its capacity may be helpful. Once a day the child is asked to hold onto his or her urine for as long as possible.

   e. **Enuresis alarms** are the therapy of choice, with 70% efficacy and a low relapse rate. The small alarms attach to the underwear and are commercially available; they should be used with a **positive motivational (e.g., sticker chart) program.** It can take 4 to 6 months for the enuresis to be fully resolved.

  f. **Medications** (imipramine and intranasal desmopressin) have 50% efficacy. However, the relapse rate is much higher than for alarms (up to 90% on discontinuation). Medications have a more immediate effect than alarms and are therefore indicated when symptoms may prevent the child from having visiting friends overnight or from going to camp, and in adolescent patients. Medications can be used in conjunction with an alarm to accelerate time to dryness and thus increase motivation.

   (1) **Imipramine** is given nightly at 1 mg/kg 1 hour before bedtime. If no effect is seen after 10 to 14 days, the dosage can be increased to a maximum of 50 mg for younger children and 75 mg for older children. Medication should be given for a maximum of 4 months and should be tapered over 4 to 6 weeks. **Life-threatening cardiac arrhythmias can occur with overdosage and thus supervised administration is mandatory.**

   (2) **Desmopressin** (DDAVP) is a synthetic analogue of the antidiuretic hormone vasopressin that increases water reabsorption in the distal tubules. Intranasal administration starts at a dose of 20 μg (one spray in each nostril), with a maximum dose of 40 μg. Dose should be administered at bedtime, with **no subsequent fluid intake. It is contraindicated in patients with hypertension or cardiac disease.**

E. **School avoidance** (school refusal, school phobia) refers to repeated absences or dismissals from school due to physical symptoms that are emotionally based. Often symptoms occur on Monday mornings and resolve by midmorning. The etiology may be **separation anxiety** (symptoms often most prominent at the beginning of the school year or following a vacation), **fear of school** (class bully, difficulty with teacher, learning problems), or **secondary gain** from staying home.

  1. **Evaluation and diagnosis.** Exclude medical illness (e.g., strep throat, mononucleosis, etc.), depression, truancy (child is neither at school nor at home), and illicit drug use.

   a. **History.** Suspect the problem when a child has vague physical complaints with normal physical and laboratory findings. Ask about earlier separation problems, previous undefined illness with prolonged school absence, temporal pattern of symptoms (absence of symptoms on weekends or holidays), and stresses at school and home.

   b. **Physical and other examination** is indicated by the symptoms. Emphasize the normal findings to reassure the parents.

  2. **Treatment.** The **goal is regular school attendance.** The longer the sustained absence and the older the child, the more serious and urgent the problem.

   a. **Reassure** the parents and the child after the physical examination and necessary laboratory tests that the symptoms do not represent serious disease.

   b. **Acknowledge** that the child is experiencing the symptom and explain that anxiety can cause physical discomfort. The child and family should not feel that the symptoms are being dismissed or attributed to "faking."

   c. **Insist that school is the child's job** and that there are few acceptable excuses for absence.

   d. **Insist that the child be seen that morning** for examination by the physician if allowed to stay home from school. If the examination is normal, the child must return to school.

   e. **Help the family organize a specific plan** for getting the child to school. Arrange for adjustments in workload to help the child catch up in school. Work with the school nurse to support the child at school.

   f. **Prepare the parents for an initial escalation** of symptoms when attendance is enforced.

   g. **Psychiatric referral** is indicated for persistent problems, for more general social withdrawal, and for all adolescents.

F. **Somatization and conversion disorders** are characterized by many physical complaints, treatment seeking, and significant impairment in functioning. Symptoms usually involve pain, gastrointestinal distress, or pseudoneurologic symptoms that cannot be fully explained or that exceed those expected by medical causes. **The symptoms are not feigned** (as in factitious illness).

1. **Evaluation and diagnosis.** The differential diagnosis includes systemic lupus erythematosus, multiple sclerosis, and inflammatory bowel disease, all of which can present with vague, recurrent symptoms.

   a. **History.** Ask about previous history of undiagnosable physical symptoms and multiple health care providers. A **coexisting organic illness** does not rule out the diagnosis. **Emotional stress** before the symptom or exposure to a person with similar physical symptoms is frequent.

   b. **Physical examination.** Frequent physical assessments may be required to allay anxiety, establish a working relationship with the patient and family members, and exclude comorbid or previously undiagnosable physical pathology.

   c. Keep **laboratory** and other diagnostic tests to a minimum.

2. **Treatment**

   a. **Psychiatric consultation** is indicated. Tell the child that this support is needed to help him/her **deal with the distress caused by the symptom** and resultant life disruption. Attributions such as "it's all in your head" will only increase anxiety and resistance to treatment.

   b. **Support of the family.** Offer reassurance about symptoms that are not medically serious. Ask parents to minimize secondary gain.

   c. **Organic illness** is eventually discovered in 10 to 30% of patients with a diagnosis of conversion disorder. Provide continuing medical care during psychiatric investigation and treatment.

VII. **Management of special adolescent issues**

A. **Adolescent adjustment** is a term that describes difficulties that often accompany the profound, and sometimes turbulent, changes of adolescence (not DSM IV).

1. **Evaluation and diagnosis. Puberty** refers to the physiologic changes that occur during this period (growth spurt and emergence of secondary sexual characteristics). **Adolescence** refers to psychosocial changes that accompany puberty, including the following:

   a. **Cognitive.** Formal operations are developed, leading to propositional, (abstract) as opposed to syllogistic (concrete), thinking. Abstract concepts, such as "the future," are not well developed until late in adolescence.

   b. **Characterologic**

      (1) Adolescents believe that they are the center of attention ("imagined audience"), and as a result somehow superior to others and invulnerable to harm ("personal fable").

      (2) Adolescent developmental norms also include questioning of rules and authority, limit testing, risk taking (see f below), and experimentation.

   c. **Social.** Parental influence diminishes in favor of peer relationships. Do not underestimate the importance of conformity to peer group dress and behavior.

   d. **Sexual**

      (1) *Early adolescence* is a time of bonding to same-sex peers.

      (2) *Middle adolescence* involves viewing the opposite sex with interest largely as objects of experimentation and potential gratification.

      (3) *Late adolescence* contains the potential for mutually satisfying emotional-sexual relationships with members of the opposite sex.

      (4) Homosexual and bisexual youth may experience significant, potentially life-threatening, isolation and stress during this time.

   e. **Emotional**

      (1) Adolescence is a time of emotional lability and wide mood swings. Rapid physical changes can lead to dissatisfaction with body image and sexuality.

(2) Difficulties in relationships with parents, peers, and love interests may be viewed catastrophically, without the adult perspective that such difficulties are transient and normal.

f. **Risk taking.** The three leading causes of mortality in adolescents are accidents (particularly motor vehicle), homicides, and suicides. These can result from a tragic combination of risk taking, experimentation (with alcohol and other drugs), a feeling of invulnerability, emotional lability, and the need for peer acceptance. In addition, adolescents place themselves at risk for pregnancy, sexually transmitted diseases, and human immunodeficiency virus (HIV) infection.

2. **Treatment.** Provide education regarding "normal" adolescent development and behavior, and offer guidance and support both to adolescents and their families.

a. **Parental guidance.** Remind parents that their goal is to "put oneself out of business." They must simultaneously relax "rules" while encouraging self-responsibility. Unusual dress, hairstyle, taste in music, and so forth, should be tolerated. The only "battles" worth fighting are those that risk the adolescent's life, health, or future.

b. **Support.** Provide the adolescent with education regarding normal pubertal and emotional changes. Anxieties over emerging sexuality require nonjudgmental listening and continuity of care, even if referral for therapy is necessary.

c. **Risk assessment.** As part of routine health assessment, ask each adolescent

(1) When was the last time you rode in a car whose driver (including you) had been using alcohol or another drug?

(2) Whether you are sexually active. If sexually active, when was the last time you didn't use a barrier method of contraception (condom) during sexual intercourse?

(a) Are you having sex with anyone?

(b) What kind of protection (if any) are you using?

(3) When was the last time you thought that your life was no longer worth living, or thought of hurting yourself or someone else?

Positive answers call for an immediate brief intervention (see Motivational Interviewing, p. 541).

B. **Alcohol and other drug (AOD) abuse** (see also Chap. 8, p. 272) is the maladaptive pattern of substance use that causes impairment in social or school functioning, physical risk, or legal problems and continued use despite that harm. Dependence is manifested by tolerance or withdrawal symptoms, or both. Try to place each patient on the continuum of use (see **Table 22-3**).

1. **Evaluation and diagnosis**

a. **History.** Ask about family history of alcoholism or drug abuse, or both; decline in school performance; legal problems; risky behavior; and other dys-

Table 22-3. The spectrum of adolescent substance use and abuse

Experimental-regular use	Occasional use of AOD			
Problematic use	Regular use of AOD	Negative consequences		
Substance abuse	Increased frequency, amount, variety	Major life disruptions	Continued use despite harm	
Chemical dependency	Constant use when available	Physical and mental deterioration	Complete loss of control over use	Tolerance and/or withdrawal

function. Answers to questions regarding frequency and amount can be misleading. Use the CAGE questionnaire:

C	Have you ever felt a need to **C**ut down on your AOD use?
A	Do you get **A**nnoyed when people comment on your AOD use?
G	Do you sometimes feel **G**uilty (or bad) about your AOD use?
E	Do you sometimes use AOD **E**arly in the day (before school)?

Two or more "yes" answers indicate a significant problem.
   b. **Physical findings** (see also Chap. 8, p. 273). Check vital signs and pupillary size for indications of intoxication or withdrawal. Dilated pupils, yawning, tachycardia, hypertension, and hyperactive bowel sounds may indicate opiate withdrawal. Examine nasal mucosa for inflammation or erosion from "snorting" cocaine or heroin, or both. Examine skin for needle marks (rare in adolescents).
   c. **Laboratory.** Urine or serum screens, or both, for toxicologic examination should be performed only with the knowledge (and consent, unless life-threatening circumstances exist) of the adolescent.
2. **Treatment.** Establish a *supportive relationship* with the adolescent that is also firm, consistent, and nonrejecting. The substance abuser may be difficult to engage in formal treatment programs, but **motivational interviewing** (see p. 541) is an effective tool. Offer a menu of choices, which can include the following:
   a. **Abstinence challenge.** Present this as a diagnostic test ("If AOD use isn't a problem for you, you shouldn't have any trouble **not** using them for ____ days. Why don't you give it a try and we'll meet again and talk about how it went."). Typical time periods are 30 to 90 days.
   b. **Controlled use trial (CUT).** If the adolescent refuses an abstinence challenge, ask for a contract requiring *risk elimination* (AOD use while driving), *pattern normalization* (no AOD use on school days/nights), and *reduction in harm* (no fights, arrests, suspensions, failures, tardiness, etc.). Tell the adolescent that failure to complete either the abstinence challenge or CUT indicates a need for more intensive treatment.
   c. **Twelve-step support groups** such as Alcoholics Anonymous or Narcotics Anonymous are helpful. Meeting lists, which include specific designations for young people's meetings, are obtained by calling the number in your local telephone directory. Make referrals to specific meetings (recommendations can be obtained from recovering patients).
   d. **Other**
      (1) Outpatient counseling referrals may be offered. Make psychiatric referral for psychopharmacologic assessment and management when dual diagnosis is suspected.
      (2) Refer adolescents with total loss of control (or where tolerance or withdrawal is present) to **inpatient detoxification.** This can then be followed by a **residential treatment center, therapeutic community, halfway house,** or **day hospital program.**
      (3) Stay involved in the patient's aftercare.
VIII. **Management of psychosocial problems**
   A. **Chronic illness** in a child constitutes a major stress for the entire family. The reactions of the family may pass through a number of phases, including shock and disbelief, protest and anger, and restitution (positive adaptation).
      1. **Evaluation and diagnosis.** Maladaptive responses of the child include *overdependence, noncompliance, aggressiveness,* and/or *withdrawal.*

2. **Treatment**
   a. Establish a long-term, **supportive relationship** with the family and child.
   b. Give **clear and accurate explanations** regarding medical issues, taking into account the child's cognitive development.
   c. **Siblings** often feel guilt or resentment. Keep them informed.
   d. Encourage parents to minimize the "sick child" role.
   e. Offer referral to **support groups.**

B. **Hospitalization** is most emotionally stressful for children between the ages of 6 months and 4 years due to separation anxiety and fear of the strange environment.
   1. **Evaluation and diagnosis.** Focus on maladaptive responses. Beginning around age 4, children have increasing worries about illness and bodily harm. Around the age of 10 years, they begin to fear death.
   2. **Treatment**
      a. Provide **support** and clear explanations to both parents and child.
      b. Allow parents to **room in** for younger children, and allow frequent visitation for older children.
      c. Encourage **activity** and **familiar routines.**
      d. Obtain **psychiatric consultation** if behavior is problematic or the child is withdrawn.
      e. Prepare children in advance for elective hospitalizations.

C. **Family disruption**
   1. **Substance abuse and mental illness** in parents increase the risk of disturbed child development.
      a. **Evaluation and diagnosis.** Screen for lack of sensitivity to children's needs, parental unavailability, poor parenting skills, excessive conflict or violence within the family, and abuse or neglect.
      b. **Treatment**
         (1) **Set clear limits** regarding the child's basic health care and developmental needs.
         (2) **Refer the family** to the appropriate social service or mental health agency.
         (3) Encourage **parents** to obtain individual psychiatric care and to participate in recovery programs such as Alcoholics Anonymous.
         (4) Refer **children** to counseling and support groups such as Alateen.
         (5) In cases of grossly inappropriate care or neglect, file a report with the state **Social Services Department.**
   2. **Divorce** affects children of all ages.
      a. **Evaluation and diagnosis** of the specific impact differs at developmental stages, but all children are adversely affected by ongoing marital conflict and will wonder if they caused the divorce.
      b. **Treatment**
         (1) Encourage **parents** to relate specific and honest facts about the divorce to their children. **Reassure children that they are not to blame.**
         (2) The **child should be protected** from ongoing disputes. Visitation should not be used by one parent against another.
         (3) **Refer for counseling** if children and family are highly distressed.
   3. **Domestic violence.** Ask questions regarding domestic violence when interviewing parents of behaviorally disturbed children.

D. **Coping with loss**
   1. **Death of a family member.** A child's grief usually goes through phases, as in chronic illness. The child's coping ability is related to developmental stage and to parents' capacity to cope. Before age 10, the child may view death as reversible.
      a. **Diagnosis and evaluation.** During the grieving process, many behavioral and psychosomatic symptoms may be observed.
      b. **Treatment**
         (1) Counsel parents to **reassure the child,** and at the same time avoid evasive explanations of what happened.

(2) Warn children of an impending death and allow visitation.

(3) Tell the child explicitly that he or she is **not to blame** for the loss.

(4) Allow the child to attend all or part of the **funeral in the presence of a supportive adult.** Parents should share their genuine beliefs regarding death, and include the child in some memorial activities.

(5) Refer for counseling if the grieving process is protracted or significant behavior or emotional problems emerge.

2. **Death of a child.** There is probably nothing more painful to parents than the death of their child.

   a. **Diagnosis and evaluation.** Severe distress and prolonged mourning are common. Reactions generally pass through stages of denial and shock, guilt and anger, grieving, and acceptance or resignation.

   b. **Treatment**

      (1) Communicate **bad news** in an unhurried, private setting and as honestly as possible. Parents should be given time to express shock and grief.

      (2) Reassure **parents** and siblings about their own handling of the situation.

      (3) Parents and pediatrician should agree on what to **tell the dying child,** and who will provide the information.

      (4) Offer a **follow-up interview** to the family a few months after the death.

      (5) The **pediatrician** may find it helpful to process his or her own reactions with supportive peers.

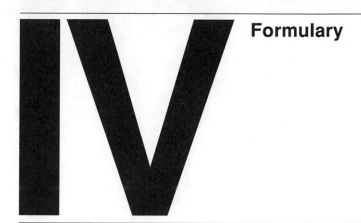

Formulary

Formulary

Gregory J. Young and
Cedric J. Priebe

I. **Acetaminophen**
   A. Available preparations: Drops: 100 mg/ml—15-ml btl
   Solution: 160 mg/5 ml—4-oz btl
   Suppository: 125, 650 mg
   Tablet: 80 mg (chewable), 325 mg
   B. Dosage: 65 mg/kg/day in 4–6 divided doses
II. **Acetazolamide**
   A. Available preparations: Capsule: 500 mg
   Injection: 500-mg vial
   Tablet: 125, 250 mg
   B. Dosage
   1. **Diuretic:** Parenteral or oral: 5 mg/kg/24 hr daily or every other day
   2. **Epilepsy, glaucoma:** Oral: 8–30 mg/kg/24 hr in 3–4 divided doses
   3. **Neonatal hydrocephalus: Oral: 50–100 mg/kg/day**
III. **Acetylcysteine sodium (Mucomyst)**
   A. Available in solution: 20%—10-ml vial, and 10%—10-ml vial
   B. Dosage
   1. Pulmonary mucolytic: 3–5 ml by nebulization tid–qid
   2. Acetaminophen ingestion: Oral: 140 mg/kg once; then 70 mg/kg/dose q4h
   for 17 doses; repeat dose if emesis occurs within 1 hr of dose
IV. **Actifed***
   A. Available preparations: Solution: 2.5, 5 ml units/day†, and 120-ml btl
   Tablet: Combination product
   B. Dosage: Children, 4 mo–2 yr: 1.25 ml tid–qid
   2–4 yr: 2.5 ml tid–qid
   4–6 yr: 3.75 ml tid–qid
   6–12 yr: 5 ml or ½ tablet tid–qid
   12 yr: 1 tablet tid–qid
   C. Contains: Triprolidine HCl, 1.25 mg/5 ml, 2.5 mg/tablet
   Pseudoephedrine HCl, 30 mg/5 ml, 60 mg/tablet
V. **Acyclovir**
   A. Available preparations: Capsule: 200 mg
   Injection: 500 mg—1-g vial
   Ointment: 5%—15-g tube
   B. Dosage
   1. Mucosal and cutaneous herpes simplex or varicella zoster in immuno-
   compromised patients: Infants: See Chapter 6.
   2. Herpes simplex encephalitis and varicella zoster: 30 mg/kg/24 hr (1,500
   mg/m^2/24 hr) in 3 divided doses given over 30–60 min for 7–14 days
   C. Caution: Do not exceed 4 doses in 24 hr

*Trade name.
†Unit dose.

VI. Adenosine
A. Available in solution: 6 mg—2-ml vial
B. Dosage: 0.1 mg/kg; can repeat after 5 min at twice the dose (must be rapid IV push)
C. Caution: Dosage and frequency should be adjusted in patients with acute or chronic renal impairment

VII. Albuterol
A. Available preparations: Metered dose inhaler (MDI): 90 μg/dose—17-g aerosol container
Syrup: 0.4 mg/ml
Tablet: 2, 4 mg
Tablet, extended release: 4 mg
Solution for inhalation 0.5%: 0.25–0.5 mL
Dry powder inhaler: 200 μg/dose
B. Dosage
  1. Oral
    a. 2–6 yr: 0.1–0.2 mg/kg/dose tid; maximum dose not to exceed 4 mg 3 times/day
    b. 6–12 yr: 2 mg tid–qid; maximum dose not to exceed 16 mg/day (divided doses)
    c. >12 yr: 2–4 mg tid–qid; maximum dose not to exceed 8 mg 4 times/day
  2. Inhalation MDI: Albuterol, 90 μg/spray, 17 g (Proventil, Ventolin)
    a. <12 yr: 1–2 inhalators qid using a tube spacer
    b. >12 yr: 1–2 inhalations q4–6h
  3. Inhalation
    a. Neonatal ICU patients: 5–20 breaths of ½ or full-strength 0.083% albuterol q4–6 h (can be given more frequently according to need)
    b. ≤12 yr: 0.02–0.03 ml/kg to a maximum of 1 ml 0.5% albuterol diluted in 2–3 ml normal saline until nebulized q4–6h (can be given more frequently according to need)
    c. >12 yr: 0.5–1.0 ml 0.5% albuterol diluted in 2–3 ml normal saline until nebulized q4–6h (can be given more frequently according to need)

VIII. Alcohol, dehydrated (ethanol 100%)
A. Available by injection: 2-ml ampul
B. Dosage
  1. As a metabolic blocking agent in an ethylene glycol or methanol ingestion
  2. Parenteral, IV
    a. Loading dose: 0.6 mg/kg either as a 10% IV or a 20–50% oral solution
    b. Maintenance dose: 110–130 mg/kg/hr adjusted as needed to provide a serum concentration ≥ 100 mg/dl

IX. Allopurinol
A. Available preparations: Injection: 500-mg vial (investigational)
Tablet: 100, 300 mg
B. Dosage: Hyperuricemia: Oral: 10 mg/kg/24 hr in 3–4 divided doses; after 48 hr of treatment, titrate dose according to serum uric acid levels
C. Caution
  1. Do not exceed 600 mg/24 hr
  2. Inhibits inactivation of 6-mercaptopurine and azathioprine (requires that doses of these agents be reduced by 60–75%)
  3. Avoid use with iron supplements
  4. Reduce dose in renal impairment

X. Aluminum carbonate
A. Available preparations: Capsule: 600 mg
Suspension: 400 mg/5 ml—360-ml btl
Tablet: 500 mg
B. Caution
  1. 2.8 mg sodium per capsule
  2. 2.1 mg sodium per tablet
  3. 2.4 mg sodium per 5 ml

4. Avoid prolonged use of aluminum-containing antacids in dialysis patients
XI. Aluminum hydroxide
  A. Available preparations: Capsule: 500 mg
                             Suspension: 600 mg/5 ml—30 ml units/day, 150 ml
                             Tablet: 300, 600 mg
  B. Caution
    1. <2.5 mg sodium per 5 ml
    2. 1.8 mg sodium per 300-mg tablet
XII. Aluminum phosphate
  A. Available preparation: Suspension: 4%—120-ml btl
  B. Caution: 12.5 mg sodium per 5 ml
XIII. Amantadine hydrochloride
  A. Available preparations: Capsule: 100 mg
                             Solution: 50 mg/5 ml—16-oz btl
  B. Dosage
    1. 1–9 yr: 4–8 mg/kg/24 hr in 2–3 divided doses to a maximum of 150 mg/24 hr
    2. 9–12 yr: 100 mg—200 mg/day in 2 divided doses
  C. Special considerations
    1. Useful for prophylaxis of influenza A in an epidemic setting when it is too late to immunize; continue for at least 10 days following a known exposure
    2. Useful therapeutically to reduce duration of symptoms and to decrease small airway disease
XIV. Amikacin
  A. Available as injection: 250 mg/ml—4-ml vial
  B. Dosage
    1. Newborn: 15 mg/kg/24 hr in 2 divided doses
    2. Children: 22.5 mg/kg/24 hr or 750 mg/m^2/24 hr in 3 divided doses to a maximum of 1.5 g/24 hr
  C. Special considerations
    1. Allowable predose level; <10 µg/ml
    2. Allowable 1-hr postdose range: 15–35 µg/ml
XV. Aminocaproic acid
  A. Available preparations: Injection: 250 g/ml—20-ml vial
                             Solution: 1.25 g/5 ml—16-oz btl
                             Tablet: 500 mg
  B. Dosage: See text
  C. Caution: See text; contraindicated in disseminated intravascular coagulation and hematuria.
XVI. Aminophylline
  A. Available preparations: Injection: 25 mg/ml—10-ml vial
                             Solution: 105 g/5 ml—8-oz btl
                             Tablet: 100 g, 200 mg
                             Tablet: prolonged release, 225 mg
  B. Dosage
    1. Neonates
      a. Apnea (aminophylline concentration 2 mg/ml, pharmacy prepared)
        (1) Loading dose: 5 mg/kg; each 1 mg/kg raises the blood level - 2 µg/ml
        (2) Maintenance 1–3 mg/kg/dose q8–12h; administer IV push 1 ml/min (2 mg/min)
      b. Wheezing: 4–6 mg/kg q6h
      c. Theophylline levels should be drawn q4–6h initially (longer intervals are OK when infant's condition is stable)
    2. Treatment of acute bronchospasm; >6 mo of age
      a. Loading dose (in patients not currently receiving theophylline)
        (1) Based on aminophylline: 6 mg/kg over 20–30 min
        (2) Based on theophylline: 4.7 mg/kg
      b. Maintenance dosage, by infusion (first 12 hr)
    3. 6 mo–9 yr: Aminophylline: 1.2 mg/kg/hr; theophylline: 0.95 mg/kg/hr

    4. 9–16 yr and young adult smokers: Aminophylline: 1 mg/kg/hr; theophylline: 0.79 mg/kg/hr

    5. Older patients and patients with cor pulmonale: Aminophylline: 0.6 mg/kg/hr; theophylline: 0.47 mg/kg/hr

    6. Patients with CHF or liver failure: Aminophylline: 0.5 mg/kg/hr; theophylline: 0.39 mg/kg/hr. Second 12-hr period: Dosage should be adjusted according to serum level

  C. Caution

    1. Approximately 85% of the aminophylline dose is anhydrous theophylline

      a. Therapeutic level: Asthma: 5–15 µg/ml

                  Neonatal apnea: 6–13 µg/ml

    2. Toxicity is common at >20 µg/ml

XVII. Amiodarone

  A. Available as tablet: 200 mg

  B. Dosage: 10 mg/kg/day for 10 days or until arrhythmia is adequately controlled. Dose is then reduced to 5 mg/kg/day

  C. Caution: Pulmonary, hepatic, and neurologic toxicity is common

XVIII. Amitriptyline

  A. Available as tablet: 10, 25, 50, 75, 100, 150 mg

  B. Dosage

    1. Depression, daily dose range: 0.5–5.0 mg/kg/24 hr (older adolescents 3.5 mg/kg/24 hr); increase by 0.5 mg/kg/24 hr q3 days

    2. Attention deficit disorder, daily dose range: 0.2–0.5 mg/kg/24 hr in 1 or 2 divided doses

  C. Caution

    1. Not recommended in children <6 yr old

    2. In many patients the long half-life permits single daily dosing at bedtime, thereby utilizing the sedative effect

    3. Reference range: 125–250 ng/ml

XIX. Ammonium chloride

  A. Available as tablet: 500 mg

  B. Dosage

    1. Urinary acidification: 75 mg/kg/dose qid to a total of 2–6 g/24 hr

    2. Refractory hypochloremic metabolic alkalosis: Calculate the dose from the following formula: Ammonium chloride (mEq) = chloride deficit (mEq/liter) $\times$ (0.3 $\times$ wt in kg). Administer ½ to ⅔ of the calculated dose, then reevaluate

  C. Caution

    1. Use with caution in infants

    2. Do not use in patients with liver disease

XX. Amoxicillin

  A. Available preparations: Capsule: 250, 500 mg

                          Suspension, oral: 25 mg/ml (150 ml); 50 mg/ml (150 ml)

  B. Dosage

    1. Oral

      a. Children: 20–40 mg/kg/day in 3 divided doses

      b. Adults: 250–500 mg 3 times/day; maximum dose: 2–3 g/day

XXI. Amoxicillin and clavulanate

  A. Available preparations: All preparations have half as many milligrams of clavulanic acid as amoxicillin. Doses expressed as amoxicillin

    1. Suspension, oral: Amoxicillin: 50 mg, 25 mg/ml

    2. Tablet: Amoxicillin: 250, 125 mg

    3. Chewable tablets: 125, 250 mg

  B. Dosage: Oral: Calculate and prescribe based on the amoxicillin component

    1. Children <40 kg: 20–40 mg/kg/day in 3 divided doses

    2. Adults: 250–500 mg q8h

  C. Caution: Contraindications: Known hypersensitivity to amoxicillin or clavulanic acid (penicillins), infectious mononucleosis, concomitant use of disulfiram

XXII. **Amphotericin B**
  A. Available as injection: 50 mg/vial
  B. Dosage: The dilution for amphotericin B infusions is 0.1 mg/ml in 5% dextrose in water (D5W)
    1. Test dose: 0.1 mg/kg/dose to maximum of 1 mg, infuse over 30–60 min; if test dose tolerated, give therapeutic dose
    2. Initial therapeutic dose: 0.25 mg/kg; daily dose can then be increased to 0.5–0.6 mg/kg the next day
    3. Severely ill patients: The full dose can be given after the test dose. Maintenance dose: 0.5–1.0 mg/kg/day given once a day; infuse over 2–6 hr; once therapy established, amphotericin B can be administered on an every-other-day basis at 1.0–1.2 mg/kg/dose; maximum dose: 1.5 mg/kg in children
    4. Adults: IV: 1 mg/kg/day **or** 1.5 mg/kg every other day
  C. Caution
    1. Do not administer through filters smaller than 1 μ
    2. Premedication with acetaminophen, meperidine, and/or antihistamines can reduce side effects. Side effects can include fever, chills, hypotension, nausea, vomiting, or headache. Dose-related side effects include renal failure, hypomagnesemia, and hypokalemia

XXIII. **Ampicillin**
  A. Available as injection: 1-gm vial
  B. Dosage
    1. **Infection:** Neonates: Premature, <1 wk: 50–100 mg/kg/24 hr in 2 divided doses
       Premature, >1 wk: 100 mg/kg/24 hr in 3 divided doses
       Term infants, <1 wk: 150–250 mg/kg/24 hr in 3–4 divided doses
       Infants and children: 100–400 mg/kg/24 hr in 4–6 divided doses
    2. **Meningitis:** Neonates, <1 week: 100–200 mg/kg/24 hr in 2 divided doses
       >1 wk: 200–400 mg/kg/24 hr in 3–4 divided doses
       Infants and children: 300–400 mg/kg/24 hr in 4–6 divided doses
  C. Contains: 3 mEq sodium per gram

XXIV. **Ampicillin and sulbactam**
  A. Available in powder for injection
    1. 1.5 g = ampicillin sodium, 1 g, and sulbactam sodium, 0.5 g
    2. 3 g = ampicillin sodium, 2 g, and sulbactam sodium, 1 g
  B. Dosage should be calculated and prescribed as the ampicillin dosage
    1. Uncomplicated urinary tract infection: 100 mg/kg/day (ampicillin) in 4 divided doses
    2. Cellulitis, skeletal and abdominal infection, and to rule out sepsis: 200 mg/kg/day (ampicillin) in 4 divided doses; maximum dosage: 2 g (ampicillin) q6h
  C. Caution: Should not be used to treat meningitis; once culture results are available, other antibiotics may be more appropriate

XXV. **Amrinone**
  A. Available in solution: 20-mg ampul
  B. Dosage: Load 1–3 mg/kg over 15 min; infusion of 5–20 μg/kg/min
  C. Caution: Reduce dose in renal failure

XXVI. **Amyl nitrite vaporol**
  A. Available as ampul: 12/box
  B. Dosage: **Cyanide poisoning:** Inhale contents of vaporol 30 sec out of every minute; use a new vaporol q3 min
  C. Caution: Consult with the Poison Control Center for management of cyanide poisoning

XXVII. Ascorbic acid
  A. Available preparations: Injection: 500 mg/ml—1-ml ampul
                          Drops: 35 mg/0.6 ml
                          Tablet: 100, 250, 500 mg
  B. Dosage
    1. Urine acidification: 2–8 g/m^2 in 6 divided doses
    2. Dietary supplement: 50–60 mg/day
XXVIII. Aspirin
  A. Available preparations: Chewable tablet: 81 mg
                          Suppository: 125, 300, 600 mg
                          Tablet: 325, 500, 600 mg
  B. Dosage
    1. Analgesic and antipyretic: Oral, rectal: 10–15 mg/kg/dose q4–6h
    2. Anti-inflammatory: Oral: 80–100 mg/kg/day in 3–4 divided doses
    3. Kawasaki disease: Oral: 100 mg/kg/day in 4 divided doses; after fever re-
       solves: 3–5 mg/kg/day once a day
  C. Special considerations
    1. Reference range: Salicylate blood levels for anti-inflammatory effect:
       150–300 µg/ml; analgesic and antipyretic effect: 30–50 µg/ml
    2. Strong association with Reye's syndrome
XXIX. Atenolol
  A. Available in tablets: 25, 50, 100 mg
  B. Dosage: 1–2 mg/kg/day
  C. Caution: Reduce dose in renal failure. Avoid abrupt discontinuation
XXX. Azathioprine
  A. Available preparations: Capsule: 10 mg (special prep)
                          Injection: 5 mg/ml (20 ml)
                          Tablet: 50 mg
  B. Dosage
    1. Initial: renal transplant, parenteral or oral: 3–5 mg/kg/24 hr
    2. Maintenance, oral: 1–3 mg/kg/24 hr
    3. Rheumatoid arthritis: Oral: 1 mg/kg/day for 6–8 wk; increase by 0.5
       mg/day q4 wk until response, or up to 2.5 mg/kg/day
  C. Caution: Reduce dose to ¼–⅓ of usual dose if allopurinol is given concur-
       rently
XXXI. Aztreonam
  A. Available as injection: 2 g
  B. Dosage: IV
    1. Postnatal 0–7 days: <2 kg: 60 mg/kg/day in 2 divided doses
                            >2 kg: 90 mg/kg/day in 3 divided doses
    2. Postnatal 7–30 days: <2 kg: 90 mg/kg/day in 3 divided doses
                             >2 kg: 120 mg/kg/day in 4 divided doses
    3. >1 mo and children: 90–120 mg/kg/day in 3–4 divided doses
    4. Cystic fibrosis: 150–200 mg/kg/day; maximum 6–8 g/day
  C. Caution: Reduce dose in renal failure
XXXII. Beclomethasone dipropionate
  A. Available preparations: Nasal inhaler: 42 µg/inhalation—16.8-g aerosol
                          Aqueous nasal solution: 42 µg/spray—25-g btl
                          Oral inhaler: 42 mg/inhalation—17-g aerosol con-
                          tainer
  B. Dosage
    1. 6–12 yr: 1–2 inhalations tid–qid
    2. >12 yr: 2 inhalations tid–qid
  C. Caution: Do not exceed 10 inhalations/24 hr
XXXIII. Bisacodyl
  A. Available preparations: Tablet: 5 mg
                          Suppository: 10 mg
  B. Dosage
    1. Oral: 3–12 yr: 5 mg/dose

≥12 yr: 5–15 mg/day as a single dose
2. Rectal suppository: 2–11 yr: 5–10 mg/day as a single dose
≥12 yr: 10 mg/day as a single dose
C. Caution
1. Swallow tablet whole; do not crush or chew
2. Do not administer milk or antacids within 1 hr of receiving tablet
3. **Do not use for children <2 yr old**
XXXIV. **Bretylium tosylate**
    A. Available as injection: 50 mg/ml—10-ml ampul
    B. Dosage: 5 mg/kg bolus IV followed by additional doses of 5 mg/kg q6h for up
        to 48 hr
    C. Caution: Can cause hypotension. Increases sensitivity to catecholamines
XXXV. **Brompheniramine maleate and phenylpropanolamine hydrochloride**
    A. Available preparations: Elixir: 0.4 mg brompheniramine and 2.5 mg phenyl-
                        propanolamine/ml
                        Tablet, sustained release: 12 mg brompheniramine
                        and 75 mg phenylpropanolamine
    B. Dosage
      1. 1–6 mo: 1.25 ml tid–qid
      2. 7–24 mo: 2.5 ml tid–qid
      3. 2–4 yr: 3.75 ml tid–qid
      4. 4–12 yr: 5 ml tid–qid
      5. Adults: 1 tablet bid
XXXVI. **Calcifediol**
    A. Available in capsule: 20, 50 μg
    B. Dosage
      1. Chronic renal failure—dialysis patients: Initial: 300–350 μg/wk (given
          daily or on alternate days)
      2. Patients with normal calcium: 20–100 μg/day or 50–200 μg on alternate
          days
    C. Caution: Titrate by adjusting dose at 4-wk intervals
XXXVII. **Calcitonin**
    A. Available as injection: 400-units vial
    B. Dosage
      1. Paget's disease: IM or SC: Initial: 100 units/day
          Maintenance: 50 units/day or 50–100 units q1–3 days
      2. Hypercalcemia: 4 units/kg q12h; after 1–2 days may increase to 8
          units/kg q12h until more specific treatment is established
XXXVIII. **Calcitrol**
    A. Available in capsule: 0.25, 0.5 μg
    B. Dosage: Oral: individualized dosage to maintain Ca^{++} levels of 9–10 mg/dl;
        adjust dose at 4- to 8-wk intervals
      1. Renal failure
        a. Children: Initial: 15 ng/kg/day
              Maintenance: 5–40 ng/kg/day; 0.25–2.0 μg/day has been used
              (with hemodialysis); 0.014–0.041 μg/kg/day (not receiving
              hemodialysis)
        b. Adults: 0.25 μg/day or every other day; may require 0.5–1.0 μg/day
      2. Hypoparathyroidism/pseudohypoparathyroidism
        a. <1 yr: 0.04–0.08 μg/kg/day
        b. >1 yr and adults: 0.25 μg/day
        c. Most children 1–5 yr require 0.25–0.75 μg/day
        d. Most children > 6 yr and adults require 0.5–2.0 μg/day
      3. Hypocalcemia in premature infants: 1 μg/day for 5 days
      4. Vitamin D–dependent rickets: 1 μg/day
      5. Vitamin D–resistant rickets (familial hypophosphatemia): 2 μg/day; ini-
          tial: 15–20 ng/kg/day; maintenance: 30–60 ng/kg/day
XXXIX. **Calcium chloride**
    A. Available as injection: 100 mg/ml—10-ml vial (27 mg/ml elemental calcium)

    B. Cardiac arrest: Infants and children: 20 mg/kg/dose or 0.2 ml/kg/dose IV; can repeat in 10 min if necessary

    C. Caution: Do not administer IM or SC

XL. Calcium glubionate

    A. Available in solution: 1.8 g/5 ml—16-oz btl

    B. Dosage

      1. Neonatal hypocalcemia: 1,200 mg/kg/24 hr in 4–6 divided doses

      2. Maintenance: 600–2,000 mg/kg/24 hr in 4 divided doses to maximum of 9 g/24 hr

    C. Contains: 115 mg elemental calcium per 5 ml

XLI. Calcium gluconate

    A. Available as injection: 100 mg/ml—10-ml vial (9 mg/ml elemental calcium)

    B. Dosage

      1. Cardiac arrest: Infants and children: 100–200 mg/kg/dose

      2. Hypocalcemic tetany: Infants and children: 100–200 mg/kg/dose IV for 1 dose, then an infusion of 500 mg/kg/24 hr

XLII. Calcium lactate

    A. Available in tablet: 300 mg

    B. Dosage: **Maintenance** (or **mild hypocalcemia**): Infants: 400–500 mg/kg/24 hr in 3–4 divided doses

    C. Contains: 42 mg elemental calcium (18%) per tablet

XLIII. Captopril

    A. Available in tablet: 12.5, 25, 50, 100 mg

    B. Dosage

      1. <2 mo: Initial starting dose: 0.1–0.25 mg/kg/dose q8–24h. Titrate dose up to 0.8 mg/kg/dose q6–24h

      2. >2 mo: Initial starting dose: 0.5 mg/kg/dose. Titrate to a maximum of 6 mg/kg/day in 1–4 doses or 75 mg/day

XLIV. Carbamazepine

    A. Available preparations: Suspension: 20 mg/ml

                             Chewable tablet: 100 mg

                             Tablet: 200 mg

    B. Dosage: See text

    C. Caution: **Discontinue if evidence of significant bone marrow depression**

XLV. Cefazolin

    A. Available as injection: 250 mg and 500 mg, and 1-, 10-, and 20-g vial

    B. Dosage: Infants > 1 mo and children: 50–100 mg/kg/24 hr in 3 divided doses. **Prophylaxis:** 40 mg/kg/24 hr in 3 divided doses for 1 day

    C. Contains: 2 mEq sodium per gram

XLVI. Cefixime

    A. Available preparations: Suspension: 20 mg/ml

                             Tablet: 200 mg

    B. Dosage: Children: 8 mg/kg/day as a single dose

                   Adults: 400 mg daily

XLVII. Cefotaxime

    A. Available in powder: 1, 2, 10 mg

    B. Dosage

      1. Neonates: <7 days: 100 mg/kg/day ÷ bid; >7 days: 150 mg/kg/day ÷ tid

      2. Infants: ≥1 mo and <12 yr: <50 kg: 100–200 mg/kg/day ÷ tid; >50 kg: 1–2 g tid

XLVIII. Cefoxitin

    A. Available as injection: 1-g vial

    B. Dosage: Neonates <1 wk: 40 mg/kg/24 hr in 2 divided doses

                   Children: 80–160 mg/kg/24 hr in 4 divided doses

    C. Contains: 2.3 mEq sodium per gram

XLIX. Cefprozil

   A. Available preparations: Suspension: 125, 250 mg/5 ml
                                Tablets: 250, 500 mg
   B. Dosage
      1. Children: 30 mg/kg/day ÷ bid
      2. Adults: 500 mg–1 g/day ÷ bid
L. Ceftazidime
   A. Available as injection: 1-g vial
   B. Dosage
      1. Neonates: 60 mg/kg/24 hr in 2 divided doses
      2. Infants and children: 100–150 mg/kg/24 hr in 3 divided doses
      3. Cystic fibrosis: 200 mg/kg/24 hr; maximum: 6 g/day
   C. Contains: 2.3 mEq sodium per gram
LI. Ceftriaxone
   A. Available as injection: 1-g vial
   B. Dosage: 50–100 mg/kg/24 hr in 1 or 2 doses to a maximum of 4 g/24 hr
   C. Contains: 3.6 mEq sodium per gram
      1. Can be given IM or IV, qd or q12h
      2. No dosage adjustment is necessary for patients with impaired renal or hepatic function
LII. Cephalexin
   A. Available preparations: Capsule: 250 mg
                                 Suspension: 125 mg/5 ml—100-, and 200-ml btl
                                   250 mg/5 ml—100-, 200-ml btl
   B. 25–50 mg/kg/24 hr in 4 divided doses
LIII. Chloral hydrate
   A. Available preparations: Capsule: 250, 500 mg
                                   Solution: 500 mg/5 ml—16-oz btl
   B. Dosage: Oral or rectal, **sedative:** 15–25 mg/kg/dose to a maximum of 2 g/dose; **hypnotic:** 50 mg/kg/dose
   C. Caution
      1. When given orally, the solution should be well diluted with water or milk
      2. Can increase warfarin effect
LIV. Chloramphenicol
   A. Available preparations: Capsule: 250 mg
                                   Injection: 1-g vial
                                   Ophthalmic ointment: 1%—3.5-g tube
                                   Ophthalmic solution: 0.5%—7.5-ml drop btl
                                   Suspension: 150 mg/5 ml—60-ml btl
   B. Dosage
      1. Premature infants, <4 wk: 25 mg/kg/24 hr in 2 divided doses
      2. Term infants, <1 wk: 25 mg/kg/24 hr in 2 divided doses
      3. Infants, 1–4 wk: 50 mg/kg/24 hr in 4 divided doses
   C. Caution
      1. Draw drug level at 1 hr postdose and adjust dosage as necessary
      2. Therapeutic range: 15–25 µg/ml
      3. Can cause aplastic anemia
LV. Chloroquine phosphate
   A. Available in tablet: 250 mg (= 150-mg base)
                         500 mg (= 300-mg base)
   B. Dosage calculated using base
      1. Amebiasis: 10 mg/kg/24 hr qd to a maximum of 300 mg/24 hr for 21 days
      2. Malaria, treatment: 10 mg/kg once, to a maximum of 600 mg/dose, then 5 mg/kg qd for 2 days
      3. Malaria, prophylaxis: 5 mg/kg once a week to a maximum of 300 mg/dose; begin 1 wk before and for the duration of exposure and continue for the following 6 wk
   C. Caution
      1. Parenteral form not recommended

2. Administer with food

LVI. Chlorothiazide
  A. Available preparations: Injection: 500 mg—20-ml vial
  Suspension: 250 mg/5 ml—8-oz btl
  Tablet: 250, 500 mg
  B. Dosage
  1. <6 mo, oral: 30 mg/kg/24 hr in 2 divided doses
  2. >6 mo: 20 mg/kg/24 hr in 2 divided doses
  C. Caution
  1. Can cause hypokalemia
  2. Monitor potassium, especially in patients receiving digitalis

LVII. Chlorpheniramine
  A. Available preparations: Capsule: 8, 12 mg
  Solution: 2 mg/5 ml—230-ml btl
  Tablet: 4 mg
  B. Dosage: Solution or tablet: 0.35 mg/kg/24 hr in 4–6 divided doses
  Capsule: 0.2 mg/kg/24 hr bid–tid

LVIII. Chlorpromazine
  A. Available preparations: Concentrated solution: 30 mg/ml—120-ml btl
  Injection: 25 mg/ml—1-ml ampul
  Solution: 10 mg/5 ml—120-ml btl
  Suppository: 25 mg
  Tablet: 10, 25, 50 mg
  B. Dosage
  1. Parenteral, IM: 1.5–2.0 mg/kg/24 hr in 4–6 divided doses
  2. Oral: 2 mg/kg/24 hr in 4–6 divided doses
  3. Rectal: 2–4 mg/kg/24 hr in 3–4 divided doses
  C. Caution: SC injection is not advised. The IV route is only for severe hiccups and surgery

LIX. Cholestyramine
  A. Available preparations: Powder: 9-g units/day pkt (440 mg resin/g powder),
  378-g cans
  Powder with aspartame: 5-g units/day packets, 210-g cans
  (4 g resin/5 g powder)
  B. Dosage
  1. <6 yr: Initiate therapy with small doses and adjust as needed; no dose has been established
  2. >6 yr: 240 mg/kg/24 hr in 3–4 divided doses
  C. Caution
  1. Do not take in dry form. Mix with water or other fluids
  2. Can bind with other drugs given concurrently.

LX. Cimetidine
  A. Available preparations: Injection: 150 mg/ml—2-ml vial
  Solution: 300 mg/5 ml—237-ml btl
  Tablet: 200, 300 mg
  B. Dosage
  1. Neonates: 10–20 mg/kg/24 hr in 4–6 doses
  2. Children: 20–40 mg/kg/24 hr in 4 divided doses
  C. Caution
  1. Administer one hour apart from antacid
  2. Lower dose in renal insufficiency

LXI. Ciprofloxacin hydrochloride
  A. Available preparations: Tablet: 250 mg
  Injection: 2 mg/ml (20 ml)
  B. Dosage: 20–30 mg/kg/24 hr in 2 divided doses
  C. Caution
  1. Dilute to 1–2 mg/ml; infuse over 60 min

2. Not recommended in prepubertal children; modify dosage in patients with renal impairment

LXII. Cisapride

  A. Available preparations: Tablet: 10 mg

  Oral solution concentration: 1 mg/ml

  B. Dosage: 0.6–0.9 mg/kg/24 hr PO in 3 divided doses before meals (maximum dose 20 mg)

  C. Caution: Should not be used in combination with clarithromycin, erythromycin, fluconazole, itraconazole, ketoconazole, and miconazole due to reports of serious cardiac arrythmias

LXIII. Clarithromycin

  A. Available preparations: Suspension: 125, 250 mg/5 ml

  Tablet: 250, 500 mg

  B. Dosage

   1. Children: 15 mg/kg/day ÷ bid

   2. Adults: 250–500 mg/dose bid

LXIV. Clindamycin

  A. Available preparations: Capsule: 75, 150, 300 mg

  Oral suspension: 15 mg/ml

  Injection: 150 mg/ml—6-ml vial

  Topical solution: 1%—60-ml btl

  B. Dosage

   1. Parenteral, IM or IV: Neonates, <1 mo: 15–20 mg/kg/24 hr in 3 divided doses

   Children, >1 mo: 15–40 mg/kg/24 hr in 3–4 divided doses

   2. Topical solution is applied bid

LXV. Clonazepam

  A. Available in tablet: 500 µg, 1 mg, 2 mg

  B. Dosage: 10–30 µg/kg/24 hr in 2–3 divided doses to a maximum of 50 µg/kg/24 hr

LXVI. Clotrimazole

  A. Available preparations: Topical cream: 1%—30-g tube

  Vaginal cream: 1%—45-g tube

  Topical solution: 1%—30-ml squeeze btl

  Vaginal suppository: 100, 500 mg

  B. Dosage

   1. Vaginal cream: 1 applicatorful at bedtime for 7–14 days

   2. Vaginal suppository: one 100-mg suppository intravaginally at bedtime for 7 days or two 100-mg suppositories at bedtime for 3 days (only if not pregnant) or one 500-mg suppository once

LXVII. Codeine

  A. Available preparations: Injection: 30 mg/ml—1-ml vial

  Solution: 15 mg/5 ml—500-ml btl

  Tablet: 15, 30 mg

  B. Dosage

   1. Analgesic: 0.5–1.0 mg/kg PO or IM q3–4h

   2. Antitussive: 1.0–1.5 mg/kg/day in 4–6 divided doses

LXVIII. Cosyntropin

  A. Available preparation as injection: 250-µg vial

  B. Dosage: <2 yr: 125 µg; >2 yr: 250 µg

  C. Caution: Administered as single dose over 2 min; may need retest

LXIX. Cromolyn sodium

  A. Available preparations: Inhalant solution: 20 mg/2 ml—60/box

  Inhaler, oral: 800 µg/spray (8.1 g)

  B. Dosage: >2 yr: Solution: 20 mg by nebulizer qid; >5 yr: 2 sprays qid

LXX. Cyanocobalamin

  A. Available as injection: 100, 1,000 µg/ml in 1-, 10-ml vials

B. Dosage: **Vitamin B$_{12}$ deficiency:** 100 µg qd for 10 days followed by 100 µg monthly maintenance

LXXI. Cyproheptadine

A. Available preparations: Solution: 2 mg/5 ml—16-oz btl
   Tablet: 4 mg

B. Dosage: 2–14 yr: 0.25 mg/kg/24 hr in 2–3 divided doses; do not exceed 16 mg/24 hr

C. Caution: **Concurrent use of monoamine oxidase (MAO) inhibitors contraindicated**

LXXII. Dantrolene

A. Available preparations: Capsule: 25, 50 mg
   Injection: 20-mg vial
   Suspension: 25 mg/5 ml—120-ml btl

B. Dosage
   1. **Chronic spasticity:** Oral: Initiate 0.5 mg/kg bid, increase by 0.5 mg/kg up to as high as 3 mg/kg 3–4 times a day
   2. **Malignant hyperthermia:** IV: Rapid IV push of 2 mg/kg and continuing until symptoms subside or the maximum cumulative dose of 10 mg/kg has been reached

C. Caution
   1. Monitor liver function including frequent aspartate aminotransferase (AST) or alanine aminotransferase (ALT)
   2. Safety of dantrolene has not been established in children <5 yr

LXXIII. Dapsone

A. Available in tablet: 25, 100 mg

B. Dosage
   1. Primary *pneumocystis carinii* (PCP) prophylaxis in human immunodeficiency virus (HIV)-positive patients with CD4 counts <200 cells/mm (can be used as an alternative to cotrimoxazole for prophylaxis of PCP). Adults: 100 mg/day PO in 1–2 divided doses
   2. Primary toxoplasmosis prophylaxis in HIV-infected patients with fewer than 100 CD4-positive cells in combination with pyrimethamine. Adults: 50 mg PO once a day in combination with pyrimethamine. The dosage of 100 mg PO bid (in combination with pyrimethamine) has been shown to be effective for primary prophylaxis of both PCP and *Toxoplasma* infection
   3. Secondary toxoplasmosis prophylaxis
      a. >1 mo: 1 mg/kg PO once a day up to a maximum of 100 mg/day
      b. Adult: 100 mg PO twice a week
      c. Special consideration: Can be administered without regard to meals

LXXIV. Deferoxamine

A. Available as injection: 500-mg vial

B. Dosage
   1. Acute iron intoxication: IV: 15 mg/kg/hr continuous infusion; maximum: 6 g/24 hr
   2. Chronic iron overload
      a. IM: 20–25 mg/kg/day
      b. IV: 500 mg–2 g with each unit of blood transfused
      c. SC: 20–40 mg/kg/day over 8–12 hr

C. Caution: Contraindicated in anuria

LXXV. Desmopressin (DDAVP)

A. Available preparations: Solution: 100 µg/ml—2.5-ml drop btl
   Injection: 4 µg/ml—10-ml vial

B. Dosage
   1. Diabetes insipidus: 3 mo–12 yr: Intranasal: 2.5–3.0 µg/day in 1 or 2 divided doses; allow diuretic phase between doses to avoid water intoxication
   2. Hemophilia: >3 months: IV: 0.3 µg/kg by slow infusion 30 min preoperatively

Nocturnal enuresis: ≥6 yr: Intranasal: Initial: 20 µg at bedtime; range 10–40 µg

C. Caution: Titrate dose to achieve control of excessive thirst and urination

LXXVI. **Dexamethasone**

   A. Available preparations: Injection: 4 mg/ml

   Solution: 0.5 mg/5 ml—10-ml units/day and 120-ml btl

   Tablet: 0.5, 1.5, 4 mg

   B. Dosage

   1. Anti-inflammatory or immunosuppressive: 0.03–0.2 mg/kg/24 hr in 2–4 divided doses

   2. Cerebral edema: Initial: 1.5 mg/kg/dose

   Maintenance: 1.5 mg/kg/24 hr in 4 divided doses for 5 days; taper slowly over the next 5 days and discontinue

   3. Airway edema: 0.25–0.5 mg/kg/dose qid as needed for croup or beginning 24 hr before planned extubation; then continue for 4–6 doses

   4. Shock: 3–6 mg/kg/dose q4–6h for a maximum of 48–72 hr

LXXVII. **Dextroamphetamine sulfate**

   A. Available preparations: Capsule: 10, 15 mg

   Tablet: 5 mg

   Sustained release capsule: 5, 10, 15 mg

   B. Dosage: Hyperkinesis, attention deficit

   1. >6 yr: 5 mg in morning for 2 days; then 5 mg in morning and at noon for 2 days; increase by 5 mg/day at 2 to 4-day intervals to gain optimal response. Dose range: 5–80 mg/24 hr

   2. 3–6 yr: Use ½ of the above dose

   C. Caution: Not recommended for treatment of hyperkinesis, attention deficit in children < 3 yr

LXXVIII. **Diazepam**

   A. Available preparations: Injection: 5 mg/ml—2-ml syringe

   Tablet: 2, 5 mg

   B. Dosage

   1. Sedation or muscle relaxation

   a. Oral: 0.12–0.8 mg/kg/day in divided doses q6–8h

   b. IM, IV: 0.04–0.3 mg/kg/dose q2–4h; maximum: 0.6 mg/kg within an 8-hr period if needed

   2. Status epilepticus: IV

   a. ≥1 mo and ≤5 yr: 0.05–0.5 mg/kg/dose q15–30 min to a maximum total dose of 5 mg; repeat in 2–4 hr as needed

   b. >5 yr: 0.05–0.3 mg/kg/dose q15–30 min to a maximum total dose of 10 mg; repeat in 2–4 hr as needed **or** 1 mg q2–5 min to a maximum of 10 mg

   C. Caution

   1. Rapid IV injection can cause apnea. IV rate should not exceed 5 mg/min. Do not mix diazepam with other drugs or IV solutions

   2. Diazepam injection is not approved for use in infants < 30 days of age

LXXIX. **Diazoxide**

   A. Available preparations: Injection: 15 mg/ml—20-ml ampul

   Suspension: 50 mg/ml—30-ml btl

   B. Dosage

   1. Hypertensive crisis: Parenteral: 3–5 mg/kg dose IV push within 30 sec; repeat in 20 min if no effect observed; then q3–10h as needed

   2. Hyperinsulinemic hypoglycemia: Oral

   a. Infants and newborns: 8–15 mg/kg/24 hr in 2–3 divided doses

   b. Children: 3–8 mg/kg/24 hr in 2–3 divided doses

   c. Caution: Can cause hyperglycemia

LXXX. **Dicloxacillin**

   A. Available preparations: Capsule: 125, 250, 500 mg

   Suspension: 62.5 mg/5 ml—100-ml, 200-ml btl

B. Dosage: 25–50 mg/kg/24 hr in 4 divided doses
Osteomyelitis: Up to 100 mg/kg/24 hr in 4 divided doses
C. Caution: Disagreeable taste limits use of suspension

LXXXI. Digoxin
    A. Available preparations: Injection: 100 µg/ml—1-ml ampul; 250 µg/ml—2-ml
                       ampul
                       Solution: 50 µg/ml—2-oz drop btl
                       Tablet: 125 µg, 250 mg
    B. Dosage
       1. Digitalization is accomplished by giving 50, 25, and 25% of total digitalizing dose at 8- to 12-hr intervals
       2. Maintenance doses are divided in 2 doses approximately 12 hr apart
       3. See Chap. 10 (Cardiac Disorders).
    C. Caution
       1. Maximum dose in children: 0.25 mg/24 hr
       2. Digitalization loading dose not essential in small infants
       3. Digoxin should be ordered in "mg" doses carried to not more than 2 decimal places
       4. The oral solution should be ordered in "ml" followed by "mg" in parentheses

LXXXII. Dimenhydrinate (Dramamine)
    A. Available preparations: Injection: 50 mg/ml—1-ml cart
                       Tablet: 50 mg
    B. Dosage: Oral, parenteral, IM: 5 mg/kg/24 hr in 4 divided doses

LXXXIII. Dimercaprol
    A. Available as injection: 100 mg/ml—3-ml ampul
    B. Dosage: Chap. 8 (Poisoning).

LXXXIV. Dimercaptosuccinic acid
    A. Available in capsules: 100 mg
    B. Dosage: Lead poisoning (≥45 µg/dl): 30 µg/kg/day ÷ tid for 5 days followed by 20 µg/kg/day ÷ bid for 14 days

LXXXV. Dimetapp*
    A. Available preparations: Tablet: combination product
                       Solution: 4-oz btl
    B. Dosage
       1. Solution: 1–6 mo: 1.25 ml tid–qid
                 2–4 yr: 3.75 ml tid–qid
                 4–12 yr: 5 ml tid–qid
                 >12 yr: 5–10 ml tid–qid
       2. Tablet: >12 yr: 1 tablet bid
    C. Contains: Brompheniramine, 12 mg/sustained-release tablet, 2 mg/5 ml
                Phenylpropanolamine, 75 mg/sustained-release tablet, 12.5/5 ml

LXXXVI. Diphenhydramine
    A. Available preparations: Capsule: 25, 50 mg
                       Injection: 50 mg/ml—1-ml syringe
                       Solution: 12.5 mg/5 ml—4-oz btl
    B. Dosage: 5 mg/kg/24 hr in 4 divided doses; do not exceed 300 mg/24 hr
    C. Caution: Concurrent use of MAO inhibitors is contraindicated

LXXXVII. Disopyramide
    A. Available in capsule: 100, 150 mg
    B. Dosage: Infants: 10–20 mg/kg/day ÷ qid
               Children: 5–15 mg/kg/day ÷ qid
    C. Caution: Reduce dose in renal failure

LXXXVIII. Dobutamine
    A. Available as injection: 250-mg vial
    B. 2.5–15.0 µg/kg/min based on patient's response

*Trade name.

LXXXIX. Docusate sodium (Colace)
  A. Available preparations: Capsule: 50, 100 mg
  Concentrated solution: 10 mg/ml—30-ml drop btl
  Syrup: 4 mg/ml
  B. Dosage
  1. <3 yr: 10–40 mg/24 hr in 1–4 divided doses
  2. 3–6 yr: 20–60 mg/24 hr in 1–4 divided doses
  3. 6–12 yr: 40–120 mg/24 hr in 1–4 divided doses
  4. Adolescents: 50–200 mg/24 hr in 1–4 divided doses
  C. Caution: Concurrent administration with mineral oil is contraindicated
XC. Docusate and casanthranol (Peri-Colace)
  A. Available preparations: Capsule: combination product
  Solution: 16-oz btl
  B. Dosage: Syrup: 5–10 ml at bedtime
  Capsule: 1 at bedtime
  C. Caution: Contains: Docusate, 100 mg/capsule, 20 mg/5 ml
  Casanthranol, 30 mg/capsule, 10 mg/5 ml
XCI. Dopamine
  A. Available as parenteral solution: 40 mg/ml
  B. Dosage: 3–20 µg/kg/min IV; titrate to desired response
  C. Caution: Inactivated by alkaline (e.g., sodium bicarbonate) solutions
XCII. Doxycycline
  A. Available preparations: Capsule: 50, 100, 300 mg
  Tablet: 100 mg
  Oral solution: 50 mg/5 ml
  Parenteral: 100, 200 mg/ml
  B. Dosage: ≥8 yr: 2–4 mg/kg/day in 1–2 divided doses to a maximum of 200 mg/day
XCIII. Droperidol
  A. Available as injection: 2.5 mg/ml
  B. Dosage: Premedication or induction of anesthesia: 2–12 yr: IM or IV: 0.09–0.165 mg/kg
XCIV. Edetate calcium disodium (EDTA)
  A. Available as injection: 200 mg/ml
  B. Dosage: See Chap. 8 (Poisoning)
XCV. Edrophonium (Tensilon)
  A. Available as injection: 10 mg/ml
  B. Dosage: Myasthenia gravis test: 0.2 mg/kg as a single dose IV
  1. Infants: Initial: 0.1 mg; if no response follow with an additional 0.4 mg for a maximum total dose of 0.5 mg
  2. Children: Diagnosis: Initial: 0.04 mg/kg followed by 0.16 mg/kg if no response; maximum total dose: 10 mg
  3. Titration of therapy: 0.04 mg/kg one time; if strength improves, an increase in neostigmine or pyridostigmine dose is indicated
  4. Reversal of nondepolarizing neuromuscular blocking agents: 1 mg/kg/dose
  C. Caution: Can precipitate cholinergic crisis
XCVI. Enalapril
  A. Available preparations: Tablet: 2.5, 5, 10, 20 mg
  Injection (enalaprilat): 1.25 mg/ml in 1- and 2-ml vials
  B. Dosage: Congestive heart failure or hypertension
  1. Adults: 5 mg PO once a day initially, increased gradually as necessary; the usual dosage required is 10–40 mg PO per day, given as a single dose or in 2 divided doses. Maximum daily dose is 40 mg/day *Note:* In patients receiving diuretics, the initial dose should be 2.5 mg. Patients unable to tolerate oral enalapril can be given enalaprilat injections of 0.625–1.25 mg IV q6h.
  2. Patients with renal impairment: CrCl <30 ml/min: Reduce PO dose to 2.5 mg/day PO initially, then gradually titrate dosage as needed or reduce IV

dose to 0.625 mg; can be repeated after 1 hr if clinical response is adequate

C. Special considerations
1. Oral administration: can be administered without regard to meals
2. Intravenous administration
   a. Can be administered undiluted or in up to 50 ml of a compatible IV infusion solution
   b. Administer by slow, direct IV infusion over a period of at least 5 min

XCVII. **Epinephrine**
A. Available preparations: 1 : 1,000 (aqueous): 1 mg/ml
   1 : 200 (Sus-Phrine*): 5 mg/ml
   2.25% (racemic)
   1 : 10,000 (aqueous): 100 µg/ml
B. Dosage
1. 1 : 1,000 (aqueous): 0.01 ml/kg/dose SC (maximum single dose 0.3 ml)
2. 1 : 200 (Sus-Phrine): 0.005 ml/kg/dose SC (maximum single dose 0.15 ml)
3. 2.25% (racemic): 0.05 ml/kg to maximum of 0.5 ml; 1 dose diluted to 3 ml with 0.9% NaCl via nebulizer
4. 1 : 10,000: 0.1 ml/kg; 1 dose; can be given via endotracheal tube

XCVIII. **Erythromycin**
A. Available preparations
1. Erythromycin ethylsuccinate: Suspension: 200, 400 mg/5 ml
   Drops: 100 mg/2.5 ml
   Tablet: 200, 400 mg
2. Erythromycin lactobionate: Vial: 500, 1,000 mg
3. Erythromycin estolate: Tablet: 250, 500 mg
   Capsule: 125, 250 mg
   Suspension: 125, 250 mg/5 ml
4. Erythromycin stearate: Tablet: 250, 500 mg
B. Dosage: Parenteral, IV: 20–40 mg/kg/24 hr in 4 divided doses
   Oral: 30–50 mg/kg/24 hr in 4 divided doses
C. Caution
1. GI side effects common
2. Can cause elevated digoxin, theophylline, and carbamazepine levels
3. Estolate causes hepatotoxicity in adults but rarely in children

IC. **Esmolol**
A. Available in solution: 100 mg/vial
B. Dosage: 0.5 mg/kg bolus; infusion of 50–200 mg/kg/min
C. Caution: Limited experience in children

C. **Ethambutol**
A. Available in tablet: 100 mg, 400 mg
B. Dosage: > 12 yr: 15–25 mg/kg/24 hr as a single daily dose
C. Caution: Not recommended in children <12 yr

CI. **Ethosuximide**
A. Available preparations: Capsule: 250 mg
   Solution: 250 mg/5 ml
B. Dosage
1. <6 yr: 15 mg/kg/day ÷ bid
2. >6 yr, initial: 250 mg/24 hr in 2 divided doses
3. Maintenance: Increase dose by 250 mg q4–7 days to maximum of 1.5 g/24 hr
C. Caution: Collect blood sample at steady state (6–24 hr after dose). The ideal serum concentration is 40–100 µg/ml

CII. **Fentanyl**
A. Dosage
1. Sedation for minor procedures/analgesic

---

*Trade name.

a. 1–3 yr: IM: 2–3 µg/kg/dose; can repeat after 30 min–1 hr; IV: 0.5–2.0 µg/kg/dose

b. 3–12 yr: IM: 1–2 µg/kg/dose; repeat after 30 min–1 hr; IV: 0.5–1.0 µg/kg/dose

2. Continuous analgesic: 1–3 µg/kg/hr

CIII. Ferrous gluconate (11.6% Fe)
  A. Available preparations: Solution: 300 mg (35 mg Fe)/5 ml
  Tablet: 320 mg (37 mg Fe)
  B. Dosage: See Ferrous sulfate

CIV. Ferrous sulfate (20% Fe)
  A. Available preparations: Drops: 75 mg (15 mg Fe)/0.6 ml
  Syrup: 90 mg (18 mg Fe)/5 ml
  Elixir: 220 mg (44 mg Fe)/5 ml
  Tablet: 200 mg (40 mg elemental Fe)
  B. Dosage
  1. Therapeutic: 6 mg/kg/24 hr (elemental iron) in divided doses tid
  2. Prophylactic: Preterm infant: 2 mg/kg/24 hr (elemental iron) in divided doses q8–12h
  Term infant: 1 mg/kg/24 hr (elemental iron) in divided doses q8–12h

CV. Flumazenil
  A. Available preparation: 0.1 mg/ml
  B. Dosage: See Chap. 8 (Poisoning)

CVI. Flunisolide
  A. Available preparations: Metered-dose inhaler: 250 µg/puff
  Nasal spray
  B. Dosage: Inhaler: 2–4 puffs bid
  Nasal spray: 2 sprays bid

CVII. Folic acid
  A. Available preparations: Injection: 5 mg/ml
  Tablet: 1 mg
  B. Dosage: 1 mg daily regardless of age

CVIII. Furosemide
  A. Available preparations: Injection: 10 mg/ml
  Oral solution: 10 mg/ml
  Tablet: 20, 40, 80 mg
  B. Dosage
  1. Premature newborns: Parenteral, IM or IV: 1–2 mg/kg/dose q12–24h
  Oral: not recommended
  2. Infants and children: Parenteral, IM or IV: 1 mg/kg/dose q12h; can increase by 1–2 mg/kg/dose after 2 hr to a maximum of 6 mg/kg/dose qd–bid
  Oral: 2 mg/kg/dose of q6–8h; increase by 1–2 mg/kg/dose after 6–8 hr to a maximum of 6 mg/kg/dose qd–bid
  C. Caution
  1. Can cause hypokalemic metabolic alkalosis and volume depletion
  2. Prolonged use in premature infants can result in nephrocalcinosis
  3. Avoid use with aminoglycosides when possible

CIX. Gentamicin
  A. Available preparations: Injection: 10 mg/ml, 40 mg/ml
  Intrathecal: 2 mg/ml
  Ophthalmic ointment: 0.3%
  Ophthalmic solution: 0.3%
  B. Dosage
  1. Neonates, <1 wk: 5 mg/kg/24 hr in 2 divided doses
  2. For older children, divide tid: >1 wk: 7.5 mg/kg/24 hr
  <5 yr: 7.5 mg/kg/24 hr
  5–10 yr: 6 mg/kg/24 hr
  >10 yr: 4.5 mg/kg/24 hr
  3. Ophthalmic ointment: Apply bid–tid

    4. Ophthalmic solution: **Severe infection:** up to 2 drops every hr
                   Mild infection: 1–2 drops 6 times a day
  C. Caution: Allowable predose level: <2 µg/ml
              Allowable 1-hr postdose range: 4–10 µg/ml

CX. Glucagon
  A. Available as injection: 1 mg/ml
  B. Dosage: Neonates: 0.03 mg/kg/dose q4h as needed
             Children: 0.03–0.1 mg/kg/dose, repeated in 20 min as needed

CXI. Griseofulvin, microsize
  A. Available preparations: Suspension: 125 mg/5 ml
                    Tablet: 125, 250, 500 mg
  B. Dosage: 10–20 mg/kg/24 hr in 1–4 divided doses for 2–3 mo
  C. Caution: Best absorbed when given with a fat-containing meal (e.g., milk or
      ice cream)

CXII. Guaifenesin (Robitussin)
  A. Available in solution: 100 mg/5 ml—8-oz btl
  B. Dosage: 2–5 yr: 2.5–5.0 ml 6 times a day
             >5 yr: 5–10 ml 6 times a day

CXIII. Haloperidol
  A. Available preparations: Concentrated solution: 2 mg/ml
                    Injection: 5 mg/ml
                    Tablet: 1, 2, 5, 10 mg
  B. Dosage
    1. Oral: 3–12 yr
      a. Agitation or hyperkinesia: 0.01–0.03 mg/kg/day once a day
      b. Tourette's disorder: 0.05–0.75 mg/kg/day in 2–3 divided doses
      c. Psychotic disorders: 0.05–0.15 mg/kg/day in 2–3 divided doses
    2. IM: 1–3 mg/dose q4–8h; maximum 0.1 mg/kg/day
  C. Caution
    1. Not recommended for children <3 yr of age
    2. Oral dosage range is 2–20 mg/24 hr

CXIV. Heparin sodium
  A. Available as injection: 10, 100, 1,000 units/ml
  B. Dosage: Initial: 50 units/kg IV bolus
             Maintenance: 15–25 units/kg/hr as continuous infusion

CXV. Hydralazine
  A. Available preparations: Injection: 20 mg/ml
                    Tablet: 10, 25, 50 mg
  B. Dosage
    1. Hypertensive crisis: Parenteral, IM, or IV: 0.1–0.2 mg/kg/dose 4–6 times
      a day
    2. Chronic hypertension: Oral: 0.25–1.0 mg/kg/dose hr bid–qid
  C. Caution: See Chap. 9 (Renal Disorders)

CXVI. Hydrochlorothiazide
  A. Available preparations: Tablet: 25, 50, 100 mg
                    Solution: 10 mg/ml
  B. Dosage: <6 mo: 2–3 mg/kg/24 hr in 2 divided doses
             >6 mo: 2 mg/kg/24 hr in 2 divided doses

CXVII. Hydrocortisone
  A. Available preparations: Cream: 0.5, 1, 2.5%
                    Injection: 50 mg/ml
                    Ointment: 1%
                    Oral suspension: 10 mg/5 ml
                    Tablet: 5, 10, 20 mg
  B. Dosage
    1. Physiologic replacement: 10–20 mg/m^2/day ÷ tid
    2. Anti-inflammatory or immunosuppressive
      a. IV: 0.8–4.0 mg/kg/day ÷ qid
      b. Oral: 2.5–10.0 mg/kg/day ÷ tid–qid

C. Caution: See text

CXVIII. Hydromorphone hydrochloride

    A. Available preparations: Tablet: 1, 2, 3, 4 mg

                                        Injection: 1, 2, 4 mg/ml, in 1-ml ampul

                                        Solution: 5 mg/5 ml

                                        Suppository: 3 mg

    B. Dosage

        1. Oral: Adults: 1–6 mg PO q4–6h, prn or around the clock

        2. SC, IM, or IV dosage: Adults: 1–2 mg SC, IM q4–6h, prn or around the clock. Severe pain may require 3–4 mg SC or IM q4–6h. (Dosage can be administered by slow IV over 3–5 min)

        3. Rectal dosage: Adults: 3 mg suppository PR q6–8h, prn or around the clock.

        4. Children: Safety and efficacy have not been established

    C. Special considerations

        1. Oral administration: Can be administered with food or milk to minimize GI irritation

        2. Parenteral administration: Hydromorphone is administered SC, IM, or IV

CXIX. Hydroxychloroquine

    A. Available in tablet: 200 mg

    B. Dosage

        1. Juvenile rheumatoid arthritis (JRA) or systemic lupus erythematosus (SLE): 3–5 mg/kg/24 hr in 1–2 divided doses to a maximum of 7 mg/kg/24 hr

        2. Malaria treatment

            a. Prophylaxis: 5 mg/kg weekly (not to exceed 400 mg)

            b. Acute attack: 10 mg/kg initially, then 5 mg/kg 6 hr later and once a day on days 2 and 3.

CXX. Hydroxyzine

    A. Available preparations: Tablet: 10, 25, 50, 100 mg

                                          Capsule: 25, 50, 100 mg

                                        Syrup: 10 mg/5 ml

                                        Suspension: 25 mg/5 ml

                                        Injection: 25, 50 mg/ml

    B. Dosage: Oral: 2–4 mg/kg/24 hr in divided doses q6h

                      Parenteral: 0.5–1.0 mg/kg/dose q4–6h IM as needed

CXXI. Ibuprofen

    A. Available preparations: Tablet: 200, 400, 600, 800 mg

                                          Chewable tablet: 50, 100 mg

                                          Suspension: 100 mg/5 ml

    B. Dosage: Oral: Fever: 5–10 mg/kg/dose q6–8h

                         Oral: JRA: 35 mg/kg/24 hr in 4 divided doses

CXXII. Imipenem-cilastatin (Primaxin)

    A. Available as injection: 500 mg (as imipenem)

    B. Dosage: IV infusion: based on imipenem component

            a. <12 yr: 60–100 mg/kg/day in 4 divided doses

            b. Adults: 45–60 mg/kg/day to a maximum of 4 g/day ÷ qid

    C. Caution

        1. Contains 3.2 mEq sodium per gram

        2. Adjust dose in renal failure

CXXIII. Imipramine

    A. Available in tablet: 10, 25, 50 mg

    B. Dosage

        1. Depression: *Initial:* 0.5 mg/kg/24 hr for 2–3 days; increase by 0.5 mg/kg/24 hr q1–2 wk to a maximum of 5 mg/kg/day

        2. Enuresis: 0.5–2.0 mg/kg qhs

    C. Caution: Not recommended for children <6 yr; except for enuresis

CXXIV. Immune globulin IM (gamma globulin)

    A. Available as injection: 2-ml vial

B. Dosage
1. **Hepatitis A case contacts:** 0.02 ml/kg/dose
2. **Travelers:** 0.02–0.05 ml/kg/dose (dependent on length of stay)
3. **Immunoglobulin deficiency:** 0.6 ml/kg/dose given q3–4 wk; double dose at onset of therapy; some patients require more frequent injections
C. Caution: Administer by deep IM injection only

CXXV. **Immune globulin IV**
A. Available as injection: 3-g vial; 6-g vial
B. Dosage
1. **Immunodeficiency syndrome:** 0.4 g/kg/dose by IV infusion q3–4 wk
2. **Idiopathic thrombocytopenic purpura (ITP):** 2 g/kg ÷ over 2–5 days
3. Kawasaki's disease: 2 g/kg once
C. Caution: See text

CXXVI. **Indomethacin**
A. Available preparations: Capsule: 25, 50 mg
Injection: 1-mg vial
B. Dosage: Closure of ductus arteriosus: IV only: A course of therapy is 3 IV doses given at 12- to 24-hr intervals; dosage according to age is as follows:
1. <48 hr: 1st dose: 0.2 mg/kg; 2nd and 3rd dose: 0.1 mg/kg
2. 2–7 days: 1st dose: 0.2 mg/kg; 2nd and 3rd dose: 0.2 mg/kg
3. >7 days: 1st dose: 0.2 mg/kg; 2nd and 3rd dose: 0.25 mg/kg

CXXVII. **Ipecac syrup**
A. Available in solution: 1.4 mg/ml
B. Dosage
1. <1 yr: 10 ml followed by 200 ml water
2. >1 yr: 15 ml followed by 200 ml water; repeat once in 20 min *only* if no emesis occurs
C. Caution: See text

CXXVIII. **Ipratropium**
A. Available in metered-dose inhaler: 18 µg/dose—14-g aerosol canister
B. Dosage: Bronchospasm: oral inhalation dosage (aerosol inhaler)
1. Adults: 36 µg (2 inhalations) tid–qid taken not more often than q4h. Initial doses of 72 µg (4 inhalations) may be required by some patients for maximum effect. Maximum adult dose is 216 µg (12 inhalations) per 24-hr period
2. Children under <12 yr: Dosage has not been established
C. Special considerations: aerosol inhalation
1. If the patient is using other inhalers, give instructions to use ipratropium first and to wait 5 min, then to use other inhalers as directed
2. A tube spacer extension may be beneficial in children
3. Following administration, instruct patient to rinse mouth with water to minimize dry mouth

CXXIX. **Isoniazid**
A. Available preparations: Injection: 100 mg/ml—10-ml vial
Tablet: 100, 300 mg
B. Dosage: **Active tuberculosis:** 10–20 mg/kg once a day
Prophylaxis: 10 mg/kg/24 hr given daily
C. Caution: Follow liver function tests (LFTs); supplemental pyridoxine (1–2 mg/kg/day) is recommended for children with low milk and meat intake.

CXXX. **Kanamycin sulfate**
A. Available preparations: Capsule: 500 mg
Injection: 37.5, 250 mg/ml
B. Dosage: Parenteral: IM or IV
1. <1 wk and <2 kg: 15 mg/kg/24 hr in 2 divided doses
2. <1 wk and >2 kg: 20 mg/kg/24 hr in 2 divided doses
3. >1 wk and <2 kg: 20 mg/kg/24 hr in 2 divided doses
4. >1 wk and >2 kg: 30 mg/kg/24 hr in 3 divided doses
5. Children: 30 mg/kg/24 hr in 3 divided doses to a maximum of 1.5 g/24 hr
C. Caution: Follow serum levels

CXXXI. Ketoconazole
  A. Available in tablet: 200 mg
  B. Dosage: <20 kg: 50 mg/day
    20–40 kg: 100 mg/day
    >40 kg: 200 mg/day
  C. Caution: Closely monitor patients for liver toxicity
CXXXII. Ketorolac
  A. Available preparations: Solution: 15, 30 mg/ml
    Tablet: 10 mg
  B. Dosage: Adults, IM: 15 or 30 mg q6h
    PO: 10 mg q4–6h
  C. Caution: Reduce dose in renal failure
CXXXIII. Labetalol
  A. Available preparations: Tablet: 100, 200, or 300 mg
    Injection: 100 mg/20 ml
  B. Dosage
    1. Hypertension: oral dosage
      a. Adults: 100 mg PO bid initially. If necessary, increase in increments of 100 mg bid q2–3 days until desired response is achieved. The usual maintenance dosage is 200–400 mg PO bid. Some patients require the total daily dose divided in 3 doses because of side effects. In severe hypertension, the maximum recommended dosage is 2,400 mg/day in 2 or 3 divided doses
      b. Children: Dosage has not been established
    2. Hypertensive emergency: intravenous dosage
      a. Adults: Initially, 20–80 mg by slow IV injection. If necessary, repeat q10 min up to total dose of 300 mg. Alternatively, can administer as an IV infusion at a rate of 2 mg/min. Adjust rate to patient response. The maximum total dose is 300 mg
      b. Children: dosage not established
  C. Special considerations
    1. Oral administration: Food delays GI absorption but increases absolute bioavailability
    2. Direct IV injection
      a. No dilution necessary
      b. Inject slowly over a 2-min period at intervals of 10 min. Monitor blood pressure before and at 5-min intervals after each injection
    3. IV infusion: Dilute in a compatible IV infusion solution
    4. Abrupt discontinuation can result in the development of myocardial ischemia, infarction, ventricular arrhythmias, or severe hypertension, particularly in patients with preexisting cardiac disease
CXXXIV. Lactase
  A. Available in solution: 16,000-units/ml drop btl
  B. Dosage: Add 5–15 drops per quart of milk, depending on level of lactose conversion desired.
  C. Caution: 4–5 drops hydrolyzes approximately 70% of the lactose in 1 qt of milk at refrigerator temperature, at 42°F (6°C) in 24 hr, or will do the same in 2 hr at 85°F (30°C); additional time and/or enzyme required for 100% lactose conversion. One quart of milk contains approximately 50 g lactose
CXXXV. Lactulose
  A. Available in solution: 3.3 g/5 ml—30 ml units/day and 64-oz btl
  B. Dosage
    1. Infants: 2.5–10.0 ml/24 hr in 3–4 divided doses
    2. Children and adolescents: 40–90 ml/24 hr in 3–4 divided doses
    3. Chronic therapy: 30–45 ml tid–qid
  C. Caution: Titrate dose to produce 2–3 soft stools per day
CXXXVI. Levothyroxine sodium
  A. Available preparations: Injection: 200-μg vial
    Tablet: 25, 50, 100, 150, 200 μg

B. Dosage
  1. Oral: 0–12 mo: 10–15 μg/kg/day
        >12 mo: 75–100 μg/m^2/day
  2. IV, IM: 75% of the oral dose
C. Caution: Dose is adjusted according to individual response

CXXXVII. Lidocaine
  A. Available preparations: Injection: 0.5%, 1%
                                Jelly: 2%
                                Ointment: 5%
                                Topical solution: 4%
                                Oral viscous solution: 2%
  B. Dosage
    1. Parenteral, **antiarrhythmic**
      a. *Loading dose:* 1 mg/kg/dose IV push; can repeat in 10 min to desired effect or for total of 3 doses
      b. *Maintenance:* 10–50 μg/kg/min infusion
    2. Oral solution: <3 yr: 2.5 mg 6–8 times a day
                      >3 yr: 5 ml 6–8 times a day
  C. Caution: Maximum local anesthetic dose is 5 mg/kg

CXXXVIII. Lindane
  A. Available preparations: Cream: 1%—60-g tube
                                Lotion: 1%—60-ml btl
                                Shampoo: 1%—60-ml btl
  B. Dosage
    1. Cream and lotion: Apply and leave on for 8–12 hr, then wash off thoroughly; can repeat in 1 wk if necessary
    2. Shampoo: Use 15–30 ml and lather for 4–5 min, then rinse thoroughly; can repeat in 1 wk if necessary

CXXXIX. Lithium carbonate
  A. Available in capsule: 300 mg
  B. Dosage should be individualized to the patient's response and serum levels.
    1. *Initial:* 300 mg bid; increase by 300 mg at 5- to 7-day intervals with serum levels 4–5 days after dose change
    2. *Maintenance:* 300 mg tid or qid; adjust dose to achieve therapeutic levels; most clinicians recommend a steady-state level between 0.5 and 1.5 mEq/liter
  C. Caution: Doses for children <12 yr of age have not been established; however, clinicians at Children's Hospital, Boston, use 15–60 mg/kg/day in 3 to 4 divided doses

CXL. Lomotil * (diphenoxylate with atropine)
  A. Available preparations: Solution: 2.5 mg/5 ml
                                  Tablet: 2.5 mg
  B. Dosage
    1. 2–5 yr: 2.5 mg tid
    2. 5–8 yr: 2.5 mg qid
    3. 8–12 yr: 2.5 mg 5 times a day
  C. Caution
    1. Contraindicated for children <2 yr of age due to decreased margin safety
    2. Reduce dose as soon as initial control of symptoms is achieved
    3. Combination product: Contains: diphenoxylate, 2.5 mg; atropine sulfate, 0.025 mg

CXLI. Loperamide
  A. Available in capsule: 2 mg
  B. Dosage
    1. Acute diarrhea: 0.04–0.8 mg/kg/day in 2–4 divided doses
    2. Chronic diarrhea: 0.08–0.24 mg/kg/day in 2–3 divided doses
  C. Caution: Discontinue if no improvement seen in 48 hr. Maximum dose = 2 mg

*Trade name.

CXLII. Lorazepam
   A. Available preparations: Injection: 2, 4 mg/ml
                                Tablet: 0.5, 1, 2 mg
   B. Dosage
      1. Anxiety and sedation:
         a. Infants and children: Oral, IV: Usual: 0.05 mg/kg/dose (range: 0.02–0.09 mg/kg) q4–8h
         b. Adults: Oral: 1–10 mg/day in 2–3 divided doses; usual dose: 2–5 mg/day in divided doses
      2. Preoperative: Adults
         a. IM: 0.05 mg/kg administered 2 hr before surgery; maximum: 4 mg/dose
         b. IV: 0.044 mg/kg 15–20 min before surgery; usual maximum: 2 mg/dose
      3. Status epilepticus: Slow IV
         a. Neonates: 0.05 mg/kg over 2–5 min; can repeat in 10–15 min
         b. Infants and children: 0.1 mg/kg IV over 2–5 min; do not exceed 4 mg/single dose; can repeat second dose of 0.05 mg/kg IV in 10–15 min if needed
         c. Adolescents: 0.07 mg/kg IV over 2–5 min; maximum: 4 mg/dose; can repeat in 10–15 min
CXLIII. Lypressin
   A. Available in solution: 185 µg/ml—8-ml squeeze btl
   B. Dosage: 1–2 nasal sprays qid and at bedtime
CXLIV. Magnesium citrate
   A. Available in solution: 10-oz btl
   B. Dosage: 2–4 ml/kg (to a maximum of 200 ml)/dose; can repeat q4–6h until liquid stool results
   C. Caution: Contraindicated in renal failure
CXLV. Magnesium gluconate
   A. Available in tablet: 500 mg
   B. Dosage: 3–6 mg/kg/day; maximum: 400 mg/24 hr divided into 3–4 doses
   C. Contains: 27 mg elemental magnesium per tablet
CXLVI. Magnesium hydroxide
   A. Available in suspension: 15 ml and 30 ml units/day, and 480-ml btl
   B. Dosage: 0.5 ml/kg/dose
   C. Caution: Can change rate of absorption of orally administered drugs
CXLVII. Magnesium sulfate
   A. Available preparations: Injection: 500 mg/ml—2-ml vial (= 4 mEq/ml)
                                Powder: 8 mEq m/g
   B. Dosage
      1. Hypomagnesemia: Parenteral, IV or IM: 25–50 mg/kg/dose 4–6 times a day for 3–4 doses; can repeat if hypomagnesemia persists
      2. Anticonvulsant: Parenteral, IV or IM: 20–40 mg/kg/dose
      3. Cathartic: Oral: 250 mg/kg/dose 4–6 times a day
   C. Caution: Contraindicated in renal failure
CXLVIII. Malt soup extract (Maltsupex)
   A. Available preparations: Powder: 16-oz btl
                                Solution: 5.3 g/5 ml—16-oz jar
   B. Dosage
      1. Infants, bottle fed: ½–2 heaping tbsp/day mixed in formula
      2. Breast-fed: 1–2 tsp in 2–4 oz water or juice 1–2 times a day
      3. Children: 1–2 tbsp in 8 oz liquid 1–2 times a day
CIL. Mannitol
   A. Available as injection: 20, 25%—50-ml vial
   B. Dosage
      1. Anuria or oliguria (test dose): 500–1,000 mg/kg/dose over 3–5 min
      2. Acute intracranial hypertension (cerebral edema): 250 mg/kg IV push over 3–5 min as needed; response is better if furosemide is given concurrently with or 5 min before the first dose; dose can be increased to 1 g/kg/dose

CL. Mebendazole
  A. Available as chewable tablet: 100 mg
  B. Dosage
    1. Pinworms: 100 mg once; repeat in 2 wk if not cured
    2. Roundworms, whipworms, hookworms: 100 mg bid for 3 days; repeat in 3 wk if infestation persists
    3. Caution: Dosing guidelines are for patients ≥2 yr of age
CLI. Menadiol sodium diphosphate
  A. Available in tablet: 5 mg
  B. Dosage: 2.5–10.0 mg qd
CLII. Meperidine
  A. Available preparations: Injection: 25, 50, 100 mg/ml
      Syrup: 50 mg/5 ml
      Tablet: 50 mg
  B. Dosage: 1.0–1.5 mg/kg/dose q3–4h as needed; maximum: 100 mg/dose. See also Table 1–1
  C. Caution
    1. Approximately 25% of an oral dose is absorbed
    2. When given IV can precipitate seizures in patients with seizure disorders
CLIII. Mephobarbital
  A. Available preparation: Tablet: 32, 50, 100 mg
  B. Dosage: 6–12 mg/kg/day ÷ bid–qid
  C. Caution: Follow plasma phenobarbital level
CLIV. Metaproterenol
  A. Available preparations: Inhalant solution: 5%—10-ml drop btl
      Aerosol: 0.65 mg/dose—150-mg inhaler
      Solution: 10 mg/5 ml
      Tablet: 10, 20 mg
  B. Dosage
    1. PO: <6 yr: 1.3–2.6 mg/kg/24 hr in 3–4 divided doses
      6–9 yr and <27 kg: 10 mg tid–qid
      >27 kg: 20 mg tid–qid
    2. Inhalation: 2 puffs q3–4h
CLV. Metaraminol bitartrate
  A. Available as injection: 10 mg/ml—1-ml ampul
  B. Dosage: IM: 0.1 mg/kg/dose as needed
      IV bolus: 0.01 mg/kg as needed
      IV drip: Begin with 5 µg/kg/min
CLVI. Methadone
  A. Available preparations: Injection: 10 mg/ml
      Solution: 1 mg/ml
      Tablet: 5 mg
  B. Dosage: Analgesia: IV/IM or oral: 0.1–0.15 mg/kg/dose given q4h
CLVII. Methenamine mandelate
  A. Available preparations: Tablet: 500 mg
      Suspension: 250 mg/5 ml—16-oz btl
  B. Dosage
    1. <5 yr: 50 mg/kg/24 hr in 4 divided doses to a maximum of 250 mg/dose
    2. 6–12 yr: 500 mg qid
  C. Caution: Acid urine (pH ≤ 5.5) is essential for antibacterial action. Ascorbic acid can be used to achieve urine acidification
CLVIII. Methimazole
  A. Available in tablet: 5 mg
  B. Dosage
    1. *Initial:* <6 yr: 12.0–17.5 mg/m^2/day in 3 divided doses
      >6 yr: 0.4 mg/kg/24 hr in 3 divided doses
    2. *Maintenance:* 0.2 mg/kg/24 hr in 3 divided doses, beginning when patient is euthyroid
  C. Caution: Adjust dose according to individual response

CLIX. Methyldopa
  A. Available preparations: Injection: 50 mg/ml—5-ml vial
  Suspension: 250 mg/5 ml—16-oz btl
  Tablet: 125, 250 mg
  B. Dosage
   1. Parenteral, IV: 5–10 mg/kg/dose q6–8h to a total dose of 20–40 mg/kg/24 hr
   2. Oral
    a. *Initial:* 10 mg/kg/24 hr in 2–4 divided doses
    b. *Increment:* 5–10 mg/kg/24 hr at intervals of 2–7 days
    c. *Maximum:* 40 mg/kg/24 hr in 2–4 divided doses
  C. Caution: Monitor hepatic function
CLX. Methylene blue
  A. Available as injection: 1%—10-ml ampul
  B. Caution: Methemoglobinemia: 1–2 mg/kg/dose IV, slowly over 5–10 min; can repeat in 1 hr if needed
  C. Caution
   1. Contraindicated in glucose 6-phosphate dehydrogenase (G6PD) deficiency
   2. Can discolor urine and feces
CLXI. Methylphenidate
  A. Available preparations: Sustained-release tablet: 20 mg
  Tablet: 5, 10 mg
  B. Dosage: >6 yr: Attention deficit disorder
   1. Oral: Initial: 0.3 mg/kg/dose or 2.5005 mg/dose given before breakfast and lunch
   2. Increase by 0.1 mg/kg/dose or by 5–10 mg/day at weekly intervals; usual dose: 0.5–1.0 mg/kg/day; maximum dose: 2 mg/kg/day or 60 mg/day
CLXII. Methylprednisolone
  A. Available preparations: Injection: 40-, 125-, 500-mg vial
  Tablet: 4, 16 mg
  B. Dosage
   1. Anti-inflammatory or immunosuppressive: 0.16–0.8 mg/kg/24 hr in 2–4 divided doses
   2. Status asthmaticus: *Initial:* 1–2 mg/kg/dose
    Maintenance: 0.5–1.0 mg/kg/dose qid
CLXIII. Metoclopramide
  A. Available preparations: Injection: 5 mg/ml
  Solution: 5 mg/5 ml
  Tablet: 10 mg
  B. Dosage
   1. Parenteral, **antiemetic:** 0.5–2.0 mg/kg/dose 30 min before chemotherapy and repeated 2 hr for 2 doses, then q3h for 3 doses
   2. Oral, for gastroesophageal reflux: 0.1 mg/kg/dose up to qid
  C. Caution: Extrapyramidal symptoms can occur
CLXIV. Metronidazole
  A. Available preparations: Injection: 5 mg/ml—100-ml vial
  Tablet: 250 mg
  B. Dosage
   1. Anaerobic bacterial infection: *Loading dose:* 15 mg/kg; then 30 mg/kg/24 hr in 4 divided doses
   2. Amebiasis: 35–50 mg/kg/24 hr in 3 divided doses for 10 days
   3. *Clostridium difficile colitis:* 20–30 mg/kg/24 hr in 4 divided doses for 7 days
   4. *Helicobacter pylori infection:* 20–30 mg/kg/day in 4 divided doses (maximum 500 mg/dose) for 14 days
  C. Caution
   1. Injectable dosage form contains 24 mEq sodium per gram
   2. No alcohol should be ingested for 24 hr after the dose
CLXV. Mezlocillin

    A. Available as injection: 4-g vial

    B. Dosage: Newborns: <1 wk: 150 mg/kg/24 hr in 2 divided doses

        Newborns: >1 wk: 225 mg/kg/24 hr in 3 divided doses

        Infants and children: >300 mg/kg/24 hr in 4 divided doses

    C. Contains: 1.85 mEq sodium per gram

CLXVI. Miconazole

    A. Available preparations: Injection: 10 mg/ml

        Topical: 2% cream, powder

    B. Dosage: IV: 20–40 mg/kg/day divided q8h

        Topical: Apply bid

CLXVII. Midazolam hydrochloride

    A. Available preparation: Injection: 1, 5 mg/ml

    B. Dosage: Conscious sedation: IV: 0.1–0.2 mg/kg; follow loading dose with a 2-µg/kg/min continuous infusion; titrate to desired effect using 0.4–6.0 µg/kg/min

CLXVIII. Morphine sulfate

    A. Available preparations: Injection: 2, 5, 10 mg/ml

        Oral solution: 10 mg/5 ml

    B. IM or SC: 0.1–0.2 mg/kg/dose repeated q4h as needed

CLXIX. Mupirocin

    A. Available preparation: 2% ointment

    B. Dosage: Apply tid

CLXX. Nadolol

    A. Available preparation: Tablet: 40, 80 mg

    B. Dosage: 1–2 mg/kg/24 hr in 1 dose

    C. Caution: Adjust dose in renally impaired patients

CLXXI. Naloxone hydrochloride

    A. Available preparation as injection: 200 µg/ml, 400 µg/ml, 1 mg/ml

    B. Dosage: Neonates: IM, IV, SC: 0.01–0.1 mg/kg

        Children: 0.1–0.3 mg/kg

    C. Caution: Repeat dose in 2–3 min as needed. If no improvement after 3 doses, a nonopioid drug should be suspected

CLXXII. Naproxen

    A. Available preparations: Tablet: 250 mg

    Suspension: 25 mg/ml

    B. Dosage: 5–10 mg/kg/dose q12h

    C. Caution: A daily dose > 1 g should be avoided

CLXXIII. Nedocromil

    A. Available in metered-dose inhaler: 1.75 mg/puff

    B. Dosage: 2 puffs qid

CLXXIV. Neomycin

    A. Available preparations: Oral solution: 125 mg/5 ml—16-oz btl

        Tablet: 500 mg

    B. Dosage: 50–100 mg/kg/24 hr in 4–6 divided doses. Maximum dose: 12 g/day

CLXXV. Neostigmine

    A. Available as injection: 250-µg/ml ampul; 1 mg/ml—10-ml vial

    B. Dosage: **Myasthenia gravis test dose:** IM: 0.04 mg/kg/dose once

CLXXVI. Neutra-Phos*

    A. Available preparations: Capsule: combination product

        Powder: 64-g btl

    B. Dosage: <4 yr: Begin at 60 ml qid

        >4 yr: Begin at 75 ml (or 1 capsule) qid; do not exceed 600 ml/24 hr

    C. Caution: Do not swallow whole capsule. Empty contents of 1 capsule in 75 ml water. The resulting solution contains: phosphorus, 8 mmole; sodium, 7.125 mEq; potassium, 7.125 mEq

CLXXVII. Nifedipine
    A. Available preparations: Capsule: 10 mg
                                      Sustained-release tablet: 30 mg
    B. Dosage: Oral, sublingual: 1–2 mg/kg/day ÷ qid

CLXXVIII. Nitrofurantoin
    A. Available preparations: Capsule: 50 mg
                                        Suspension: 25 mg/5 ml—16-oz btl
                                        Tablet: 50 mg
    B. Dosage: 5–7 mg/kg/24 hr in 4 divided doses; reduce to 2.5–5.0 mg/kg/24 hr after 10–14 days
    C. Caution
        1. Administer with meals
        2. Avoid usage in neonates < 1 wk old
        3. Avoid in renal failure

CLXXIX. Nitroprusside
    A. Available as injection: 50-mg vial
    B. 0.5–5.0 µg/kg/min as a constant infusion
    C. Caution
        1. Wrap solution bottle in aluminum foil; discard after 24 hr
        2. Monitor serum cyanide levels and acid-base balance

CLXXX. Norepinephrine bitartrate
    A. Available as injection: 1 mg/ml—4-ml ampul
    B. Dosage: Begin at 2.0 µg/kg/min; titrate to desired blood pressure; maximum dosage: 6 µg/kg/min
    C. Caution
        1. Each milliliter of solution contains 1 mg base
        2. Avoid extravasation; administer into large catheterized vein

CLXXXI. Nystatin
    A. Available preparations: Cream: 100,000 units/g—15-g tube
                                         Ointment: 100,000 units/g—15-g tube
                                         Powder: 100,000 units/g—15-g squeeze btl
                                         Suppository: 100,000 units
                                         Suspension: 100,000 units/ml—60-ml drop btl and 16-oz btl
                                         Tablet: 500,000 units
    B. Dosage
        1. Oral: Infants, premature: 50,000 units (0.5 ml) PO qid
                     Infants: 100,000 units (1 ml) PO qid
                     Children: 200,000–300,000 (2–3 ml) PO qid
        2. Topical: Apply tid–qid

CLXXXII. Omeprazole
    A. Available in capsules: 20 mg

CLXXXIII. Ondansetron
    A. Available preparations: IV solution: 2 mg/ml
                                         Tablet: 4, 8 mg
    B. Dosage
        1. IV: 0.15 mg/kg 30 min before chemotherapy, then repeated at 4 and 8 hr after chemotherapy
        2. PO: 4 mg/dose scheduled as above

CLXXXIV. Opium, tincture (opium, deodorized)
    A. Available in tincture: 16-oz btl
    B. Dosage: Analgesia: 0.01–0.02 ml/kg/dose q3–4h
                     Diarrhea: 0.005–0.01 ml/kg/dose q2–4h; do not exceed 6 doses/24 hr
    C. Contains: 10 mg/ml anhydrous morphine

CLXXXV. Oxacillin
    A. Available as injection: 1-g vial
    B. Dosage: Neonates < 1 wk: 100 mg/kg/24 hr in 2 divided doses
                     >1 wk: 200 mg/kg/24 hr in 4 divided doses
                     Infants and children: 150–200 mg/kg/24 hr in 6 divided doses

CLXXXVI. Oxybutynin
  A. Available preparations: Solution: 1 mg/ml
  Tablet: 5 mg
  B. Dosage: 1–5 yr: 0.2 mg/kg/dose bid–qid
  >5 yr: 5 mg bid–tid
CLXXXVII. Oxycodone
  A. Dosage: 0.5–1.5 mg/kg PO q3–4h
CLXXXVIII. Oxymetazoline
  A. Available preparations: Solution: 0.05%
  Pediatric solution: 0.025%
  Spray: 0.05%
  B. Dosage: 2–5 yr: 2–3 drops of pediatric solution in each nostril bid
  >6 yr: 2–3 drops or 1–2 sprays each nostril bid
  C. Caution
    1. Rebound rhinitis is common
    2. Do not use longer than 3–5 days
CLXXXIX. Pancrelipase
  A. Available in capsules: Combination product: Pancrease
  Pancrease MT-4
  Pancrease MT-10
  Pancrease MT-16
  B. Dosage: <1 yr: 2,000 units of lipase with meals
  1–6 yr: 4,000–8,000 units of lipase with meals and 4,000 units with snacks
  7–12 yr: 4,000–12,000 units of lipase with meals and snacks
  C. Contains:

	Lipase (units)	Protease (units)	Amytase (units)
Enteric-coated microspheres* Pancrease	4,000	25,000	20,000
Enteric-coated microtablets MT-4	4,000	12,000	12,000
MT-10	10,000	30,000	30,000
MT-16	16,000	48,000	48,000

*To protect enteric coating, microspheres should **not** be crushed or chewed

CXC. Paraldehyde
  A. Available in liquid: 1 g/ml
  B. Dosage: Oral, rectal
    1. Sedative: 0.15 ml/kg/dose
    2. Hypnotic or anticonvulsant: 0.3 ml/kg/dose
  C. Caution
    1. Avoid IV administration
    2. For rectal use, dilute 2 : 1 with oil
    3. Dilute oral solution well
CXCI. Paramethadione
  A. Available preparations: Solution: 300 mg/ml
  Capsule: 300 mg
  B. Dosage: <2 yr: 300 mg/24 hr
  2–6 yr: 600 mg/24 hr
  >6 yr: 900 mg/24 hr
  C. Caution
    1. Adjust subsequent doses by response
    2. Divide into 3–4 doses/day
CXCII. Pemoline
  A. Available in tablet: 18.75, 37.5 mg
  B. Dosage: >6 yr: *Initial:* 37.5 mg as a single dose in the morning; dose can

be increased by 18.75 mg/24 hr at weekly intervals until a desired clinical response is achieved; dosage in children should not exceed 112.5 mg/24 hr
   C. Special considerations: Beneficial effects may not become evident until the third or fourth week of therapy
CXCIII. **Penicillamine**
   A. Available in tablet: 250 mg
   B. Dosage: ≤30 mg/kg/24 hr
      1. *Rheumatoid arthritis:* Initial: 3 mg/kg/day (≤250 mg/day) for 3 mo, then 6 mg/kg/day (≤500 mg/day) in divided doses bid for 3 mo; maximum: 10 mg/kg/day in 3–4 divided doses
      2. *Wilson's disease:* 20 mg/kg/day in 4 divided doses
      3. *Cystinuria:* 30 mg/kg/day in 4 divided doses
      4. *Lead poisoning:* 10–30 mg/kg/day in 2–3 divided doses
CXCIV. **Penicillin G, benzathine**
   A. Available, as injection: 600,000 units/ml—1-, 2-ml cartridge
   B. Dosage: Newborn, IM: 50,000 units/kg/24 hr once
      Infants and children, <30 kg, IM: 600,000 units once
      >30 kg, IM: 1.2 million units once
CXCV. **Penicillin G potassium**
   A. Available preparations: Injection: 1,000,000-, 5,000,000-unit vial
      Tablet: 200,000 units
   B. Dosage
      1. **Infection:** Newborn, <1 wk: 50,000 units/kg/24 hr in 2–3 divided doses
         Infants: 75,000 units/kg/24 hr in 3 divided doses
         Children: 25,000–100,000 units/kg/24 hr in 4–6 divided doses
      2. **Meningitis:** Newborn, <1 wk: 200,000–300,000 units/kg/24 hr in 2–3 divided doses
         Infants: 200,000–300,000 units/kg/24 hr in 4 divided doses
         Children: 200,000–400,000 units/kg/24 hr in 6 divided doses
CXCVI. **Penicillin G procaine**
   A. Available as injection: 600,000 units/ml—1-, 2-ml cartridge, and 4-ml syringe
   B. Dosage: Newborn, IM: 50,000 units/kg/24 hr daily
      Children, IM: 100,000–600,000 units/24 hr in 1–2 divided doses
   C. Special considerations: When used to treat gonorrhea, simultaneously dose with probenecid (25 mg/kg)
CXCVII. **Penicillin G sodium**
   A. Available as injection: 5,000,000-unit vial
   B. Dosage: **See Penicillin G potassium**
CXCVIII. **Penicillin V**
   A. Available preparations: Solution: 125 mg/5 ml—200-ml btl; 250 mg/5 ml—200-ml btl
      Tablet: 250 mg
   B. Dosage: 25–50 mg/kg/24 hr in 3–4 divided doses
   C. Caution: Administer on empty stomach 1 hr before or 2 hr after meals
CIC. **Pentamidine**
   A. Available preparations: Injection: 300 mg/vial, in single-dose vials
      Inhalation solution: 300 mg/vial in single-dose vials
   B. Dosage
      1. *Pneumocystis carinii* pneumonia treatment in patients who are unresponsive to, are allergic to, or cannot tolerate trimethoprim sulfamethoxazole. Parenteral dosage:
         a. Adults: 4 mg/kg IM, or IV infused over 1–2 hr, once a day for 14–21 days
         b. Children: 150 mg/m^2 IM, or IV infused over 1–2 hr, once a day for 5 days, then 100 mg/m^2 for the remainder of therapy
      2. *Pneumocystis carinii* pneumonia primary prophylaxis in HIV-positive patients with CD4 counts < 200 cells/mm
         a. Nebulized dosage: Adults: 300 mg nebulized once q4 wk or 150 mg q2 wk via nebulizer, until the nebulizer chamber is empty. Nebulizer flow

rate should be 5–7 liters/min from 40–50 PSO oxygen or air source. Treatments last 30–45 min
  b. Parenteral dosage: Adults: 4 mg/kg IM, or IV infused over no less than 60 min, once every month
  C. Special considerations
  1. Inhalation administration
    a. Use sterile water for injection only. Sodium chloride injection can cause precipitation
    b. Reconstitute 300 mg for inhalation with 6 ml sterile water for injection
    c. Administer the solution via nebulization
  2. Aerosolized therapy with pentamidine has been shown to be inferior to systemic prophylaxis with either oral co-trimoxazole or oral dapsone.
  3. Parenteral pentamidine causes several serious adverse reactions.
CC. Phenazopyridine
  A. Available in tablet: 100, 200 mg
  B. Dosage: 6–9 yr: 12 mg/kg/24 hr in 2–3 divided doses
        9–12 yr: 100 mg tid
  C. Special consideration: Phenazopyridine is an azo dye and produces an orange to red color in urine
CCI. Phenobarbital
  A. Available preparations: Injection: 65 mg/ml
          Solution: 20 mg/5 ml
          Tablet: 15, 30, 100 mg
  B. Dosage: IV, oral
    1. Sedative: 2 mg/kg tid
    2. Anticonvulsant: 3–5 mg/kg/dose
  C. Caution: Therapeutic serum level = 10–20 µg/ml
CCII. Phenytoin
  A. Available preparations: Chewable tablet: 50 mg
          Capsule: 30, 100 mg
          Injection: 50 mg/1 ml
          Suspension: 30 mg/5 ml, 125 mg/5 ml
  B. Dosage
    1. *Status epilepticus: IV*
      a. Loading dose: Neonates: 15–20 mg/kg in a single or divided dose
            Infants, children, adults: 15–18 mg/kg in a single or divided dose
      b. Maintenance anticonvulsant: Neonates and infants: 5–8 mg/kg/day in 2 divided doses
            Children: 4–7 mg/kg/day in a single dose or in 2 divided doses
    2. *Anticonvulsant: Oral*
      a. Loading dose: 20 mg/kg; based on phenytoin serum concentrations and if no doses had been administered in the previous 24 hr; on the average, for every 1 mg/kg administered, serum level will increase by 1 µg/ml
      b. Maintenance dose: Neonates: 5 mg/kg/day in divided doses q12h
            >10 days to ≤3 yr: 8–10 mg/kg/day in divided doses q8–12h
            ≥4 yr: 5–8 mg/kg/day in divided doses q12–24h
    3. *Arrhythmias*
      a. Loading dose: IV push: 1.25 mg/kg q5 min for 12 doses; total loading dose: 15 mg/kg
      b. Maintenance dose: Children: Oral: IV: 2–5 mg/kg/day in 2 divided doses
            Adults: Oral: 250 mg qid for 1 day, 250 mg bid for 2 days, then 300–400 mg/day in divided doses 1–4 times a day
  C. Special considerations

    1. Ideal serum concentration is 10–20 µg/ml

    2. Select a blood sample at steady state (6–12 hr after dose)

    3. Clinically significant interactions can occur when other drugs are administered with phenytoin

    4. Suspension must be shaken before each dose

CCIII. Physostigmine salicylate

    A. Available as injection: 1 mg/ml—2-ml ampul

    B. Dosage: **Anticholinergic poisoning:** 0.01–0.03 mg/kg/dose. Can repeat after 15–20 min

    C. Caution

        1. Consult Poison Control Center

        2. IV rate not to exceed 0.5 mg/min

CCIV. Phytonadione

    A. Available preparations: Injection: 2 mg/ml—0.5-ml ampul, 10 mg/ml—1-ml ampul

                Tablet: 5 mg

    B. Dosage: **Hemorrhagic disease of newborn**

        1. **Prophylaxis**, IM or SC: 0.5–1.0 mg within 1 hr of birth

        2. **Treatment**, IM or SC: 1 mg

        3. **Oral anticoagulant-induced hypoprothrombinemia:** 2.5–10.0 mg PO; repeat in 12–48 hr if needed

    C. Caution: Avoid IV route whenever possible

CCV. Piperacillin

    A. Available in powder: 2, 3, 4 g

        Dosage: Neonates: 200 mg/kg/day divided bid

                Infants/children: 200–300 mg/kg/day divided q4–6h to a maximum of 24 g/day

CCVI. Potassium chloride

    A. Available preparations: Tablet: 750 mg

                          Injection: 2 mEq/ml—10-ml vial

                          Oral powder: 20-mEq pkt

                          Solution: 5, 10, 15, 20, 30 mEq units/day; 5 mEq/ 5 ml— 120-ml btl

    B. Dosage

        1. *Maintenance:* 1–3 mEq/kg/24 hr

        2. *Replacement:* Up to maximum of 4 mEq/kg/24 hr; replace over 3–7 days to avoid hyperkalemia

    C. Caution

        1. Maximum concentration of 40 mEq/liter when infused into peripheral vein

        2. Can give higher concentrations via central line **with caution**

CCVII. Potassium iodide

    A. Available in solution: 1 g/ml—30-ml drop btl

    B. Dosage: 1 drop per year of age tid

    C. Caution

        1. Give with food or milk after meals

        2. Dilute 1 : 10 (100 mg/ml) before administering

CCVIII. Potassium phosphate

    A. Available as injection: 5-ml vial

    B. Dosage: *Maintenance* or **hypophosphatemia**: 0.5–1.5 mmole/kg/24 hr

    C. Each ml contains: potassium, 4.4 mEq; phosphorus, 3 mmole

CCIX. Prednisolone

    A. Available preparations: Injection: 20 mg/ml

                          Liquid, oral: 3 mg/ml

    B. Dosage: See Prednisone

CCX. Prednisone

    A. Available in tablet: 1, 5, 20, 50 mg

    B. Dosage: See text for specific dosage up to 2 mg/kg/24 hr

    C. Caution: History of varicella susceptibility should be obtained

CCXI. Primidone
  A. Available preparations: Suspension: 250 mg/5 ml—8-oz btl
       Tablet: 50, 250 mg
  B. Dosage: <8 yr: 10–25 mg/kg/day ÷ bid–qid
       >8 yr: 750–1,500 mg/day ÷ tid–qid
  C. Special considerations
     1. Select a blood sample at steady state between doses after 24 hr
     2. Therapeutic levels: 7–15 µg/ml as primidone or 15–40 µg/ml as phenobarbital

CCXII. Probenecid
  A. Available in tablet: 500 mg
  B. Dosage: **uricosuric**
     1. <2 yr: not recommended
     2. 2–14 yr: *Initial:* 25 mg/kg for 1 dose
        Maintenance: 40 mg/kg/24 hr in 4 divided doses

CCXIII. Procainamide
  A. Available preparations: Capsule: 250, 375, 500 mg
       Prolonged-release tablet: 250, 500, 750 mg
       Injection: 100-mg/ml vial
  B. Dosage: See Chap. 10 (Cardiac Disorders)
  C. Caution: Monitor Q-T interval and blood pressure closely

CCXIV. Prochlorperazine
  A. Available preparations: Injection: 5 mg/ml—2-ml ampul
       Solution: 5 mg/5 ml—120-ml btl
       Suppository: 2.5, 5, 25 mg
       Tablet: 5 mg
  B. Dosage
     1. Parenteral, IM: Children, > 10 kg: 0.2 mg/kg/24 hr in 3–4 divided doses
     2. Oral or rectal: Children, > 10 kg: 0.4 mg/kg/24 hr in 3–4 divided doses
  C. Caution
     1. Not recommended for use in children <2 yr of age or weight <10 kg.
     2. Children seem prone to development of extrapyramidal reactions, even on moderate doses; therefore, use lowest effective dose
     3. **Do not use IV**

CCXV. Promethazine
  A. Available preparations: Injection: 25 mg/ml—16-oz btl
       Suppository: 12.5, 25, 50 mg
       Tablet: 12.5, 25 mg
       Syrup: 1.25 mg/ml
  B. Dosage
     1. **Antihistamine:** 0.1 mg/kg/dose q6h during the day and 0.5 mg/kg/dose at bedtime
     2. **Motion sickness:** 0.5 mg/kg/dose, 30–60 min before departure, q12h
     3. **Nausea and vomiting:** 0.25–0.5 mg/kg/dose q4–6h as needed
     4. **Sedative or preop:** 0.5–1.0 mg/kg/dose q6h as needed

CCXVI. Propranolol
  A. Available preparations: Injection: 1 mg/ml—1-ml ampul
       Tablet: 10, 20, 40 mg
  B. Dosage: See text for specific dosage

CCXVII. Propylthiouracil
  A. Available in tablet: 50 mg
  B. Dosage: *Initial:* 5–7 mg/kg/24 hr in 3 divided doses
       Maintenance: ⅓–⅔ of initial dose, beginning when patient is euthyroid
  C. Caution: Follow thryroid function

CCXVIII. Pseudoephedrine
  A. Available preparations: Solution: 30 mg/5 ml—120-, 473-ml btl
       Tablet: 30, 60 mg

B. Dosage: 5 mg/kg/24 hr in 4 divided doses

CCXIX. Pyridostigmine bromide
- **A.** Available preparations: Syrup: 12 mg/ml
  - Tablet: 60 mg
  - Sustained-release tablet: 180 mg
- **B.** Dosage: **Myasthenia gravis:** Oral: 7 mg/kg/24 hr in 4–6 divided doses

CCXX. Pyridoxine
- **A.** Available preparations: Injection: 100 mg/ml—10-ml vial
  - Tablet: 25, 50 mg
- **B.** Dosage: **Neuritis,** treatment: 10–50 mg qd
  - **Prophylaxis:** 1–2 mg/kg daily

CCXXI. Pyrimethamine
- **A.** Available in tablet: 25 mg
- **B.** Dosage
  1. **Malaria (chloroquine-resistant):** <10 kg: 6.25 mg qd for 3 days
     - 10–20 kg: 12.5 mg qd for 3 days
     - 20–40 kg: 25 mg qd for 3 days
     - >40 kg: 25 mg bid for 3 days
  2. **Toxoplasmosis:** *Loading dose:* 2 mg/kg/dose qd for 3 days
     - *Maintenance:* Consult infectious disease specialist

CCXXII. Quinidine gluconate
- **A.** Available preparations: Sustained-release tablet: 324 mg
  - Injection: 80 mg/ml—20-ml vial
- **B.** Dosage: Parenteral, IV: 2–10 mg/kg/dose q3–6h as needed
  - Oral: 15–60 mg/kg/24 hr in 3 divided doses
- **C.** Caution
  1. See text
  2. If used with digoxin, reduce digoxin dose by ½
  3. IV use not recommended; use only if drug cannot be given orally

CCXXIII. Quinidine sulfate
- **A.** Available in tablet: 200 mg
- **B.** Dosage: Oral: 15–60 mg/kg/24 hr in 4 divided doses
- **C.** Caution: If used with digoxin, reduce digoxin dose by ½

CCXXIV. Quinine sulfate
- **A.** Available in capsule: 325 mg
- **B.** Dosage: **Malaria, uncomplicated attack (chloroquine-resistant):** 25 mg/kg/24 hr in 3 divided doses for 3 days
- **C.** Caution: For severe malaria attack IV therapy is recommended; however, IV dosage form is unavailable commercially in the United States except from the Centers for Disease Control (CDC)

CCXXV. Rabies immune globulin
- **A.** Available preparation: 150 units/ml—2-ml vial
- **B.** Dosage: Parenteral, IM: 20 units/kg
- **C.** Caution
  1. Indicated for all persons suspected of having been exposed to rabies, except those previously immunized with vaccine
  2. Should be given as promptly as possibly after exposure, but can be administered up to 8 days after first dose of vaccine
  3. Should be administered in conjunction with vaccine
  4. Give ½ dose IM; other ½ should be infiltrated around site of bite

CCXXVI. Rabies vaccine (human)
- **A.** Available as injection: 1 pack
- **B.** Dosage: *Postexposure dose,* IM: 5 doses of 1 ml each; the first dose should be administered as soon as possible after exposure in conjunction with rabies immune globulin; an additional dose should be given on each of days 3, 7, 14, and 28 after the first dose
- **C.** Caution: The World Health Organization (WHO) currently recommends a sixth dose 90 days after the first dose

CCXXVII. Ranitidine hydrochloride
  A. Available preparations: Injection: 25 mg/ml
                             Solution: 75 mg/ml
                             Tablet: 150 mg
  B. Dosage: Oral: 2–3 mg/kg/dose q12h
             IV: 1 mg/kg/dose q8h
CCXXVIII. Ribavirin
  A. Available as inhalation solution: 6 g sterile lyophilized ribavirin powder for reconstitution, in a 100-ml vial
  B. Dosage: Respiratory syncytial virus (RSV) infection
    1. Children: A concentration of 20 mg/ml (6 g reconstituted with 300 ml sterile water without preservatives) is placed in the SPAG-2 aerosol generator. A mist containing 190 µg/liter of air is then delivered to the patient via the SPAG-2 aerosol generator and an oxygen hood, face mask, or oxygen tent at a rate of about 12.5 liters of mist per minute continuously for 12–18h daily for 3–7 days. Alternatively, deliver the mist at a rate of about 15 liters/min when using an oxygen hood or tent or about 12 liters/min when using a face mask. *Note:* Prolonged or repeated therapy may be necessary in infants with preexisting cardiac or respiratory disease or in immunocompromised infants
    2. Adults: Dose has not been established
  C. Special considerations
    1. Only the SPAG-2 aerosol generator should be used
    2. Using sterile technique, add sterile water for injection or inhalation. Water must be preservative and additive free
    3. Nonmechanically ventilated infants: Administer via an infant oxygen hood using the SPAG-2 aerosol generator. If hood cannot be used, ribavirin can be administered by face mask or oxygen tent.
    4. Mechanically ventilated infants
    A. Administer using the SPAG-2 aerosol generator in conjunction with either a pressure or volume cycle ventilator
    B. Endotracheal tubes should be suctioned q1–2h and pulmonary pressures measured every 2–4 hr
CCXXIX. Riboflavin (vitamin B$_2$)
  A. Available in tablet: 10 mg
  B. Dosage: 5–10 mg daily
CCXXX. Rifampin
  A. Available preparations: Capsule: 150, 300 mg
                             Injection: 600-mg vial
  B. Dosage
    1. **Meningococcal disease prophylaxis:** 10–20 mg/kg/24 hr in 2 divided doses to a maximum of 600 mg/24 hr for 2 days (4 doses)
    2. *Haemophilus influenzae type b prophylaxis:* 20 mg/kg/24 hr as a single dose to a maximum of 600 mg/24 hr for 4 days
    3. **Tuberculosis:** 10–20 mg/kg/24 hr qd
  C. Caution
    1. Administer 1 hr before or 2 hr after meals
    2. Stains urine orange
    3. Stains soft contact lenses
    4. Interferes with oral contraceptives
    5. Not used during pregnancy
CCXXXI. Salmeterol
  A. Available in metered dose inhaler: 25 µg/dose in 6.5- and 13-g aerosol containers
  B. Dosage
    1. Asthma prevention: Oral inhalation dosage: Adults: 42 µg (2 inhalations) salmeterol base PO bid
    2. Exercised-induced bronchospasm prevention: Oral inhalation dosage: Adults: 42 µg (2 inhalations) salmeterol base PO at least 30–60 min before

exercise. *Note:* Additional doses should not be used. Patients receiving salmeterol bid as maintenance therapy should not use an additional dose to prevent exercise-induced bronchospasm

C. Special considerations
   1. Because of its relatively slow onset, salmeterol should never be used to treat an acute asthmatic attack.
   2. Shake the canister well before administering. Place the mouthpiece between open lips, past the teeth. Close lips firmly around the mouthpiece. Press down on the canister while breathing in deeply and slowly. Remove canister from the mouth, hold breath for at least 10 seconds, and then exhale. If additional doses are required, wait 1 min between inhalations, shake the inhaler again, and repeat above procedure
   3. A tube spacer extension may be beneficial in children
   4. Following administration, instruct patient to rinse mouth with water to minimize dry mouth

CCXXXII. Selenium sulfide lotion
A. Available in suspension: 2.5%—120-ml btl
B. Dosage
   1. As shampoo: Massage 5–10 ml into wet scalp, leave on scalp 2–3 min, rinse thoroughly and repeat; shampoo twice a week for 2 wk, then every week for 2 wk
   2. As lotion (for tinea versicolor): Leave on for 10 min, then rinse; use daily for 7 days

CCXXXIII. Senna fruit
A. Available preparations: Granules: 110 mg/g—170-g can
   Solution: 218 mg/5 ml—8-oz btl
   Suppository: 652 mg
   Tablet: 187 mg
B. Dosage: Solution: 1 mo–1 yr: 1.25–2.5 ml bid
   1–5 yr: 2.5–5.0 ml bid
   5–15 yr: 5–10 ml bid
   Tablet: Children, > 35 kg: 1 tablet bid

CCXXXIV. Sodium bicarbonate
A. Available preparations: Injection: 1 mEq/ml—10-ml, 50-ml syringe, and 50-ml vial
   Oral solution: 1 mEq/ml—128-oz btl (special prep)
   Tablet: 300 mg
B. Dosage: **Cardiac arrest:** Infants and children: 1–2 mEq/kg initially, then as indicated by blood gases
C. Caution: See text for specific usage

CCXXXV. Sodium fluoride
A. Available preparations: Chewable tablet: 2.2 mg
   Gel: 1.1% 60-g tube
   Solution: 5.5 mg/ml (0.125 mg/drop—30-ml drop btl)
B. Dosage
   1. Based on fluoride (f) concentration in drinking water, <0.3 ppm f
      a. 6 mo–3 yr: 0.25 mg qd
      b. 3–6 yr: 0.5 mg qd
      c. 6–12 yr: 1 mg qd
   2. 0.3–0.7 ppm f: ½ the above dose; >0.7 ppm f: fluoride supplements contraindicated
C. Contains: Each 2.2-mg sodium fluoride is equivalent to 1 mg elemental fluoride (on which the doses are based)

CCXXXVI. Sodium polystyrene sulfonate (Kayexalate)
A. Available preparations: Powder: 454-g btl
   Suspension: 15 g/60 ml—16-oz btl
B. Dosage: Oral: 1 g/kg/dose qid
   Rectal: 1 g/kg/dose q2–6h
C. Caution

   1. Effective exchange rate = approximately 1 mEq potassium/g resin
   2. Rectal route is less effective than oral
CCXXXVII. Spectinomycin hydrochloride
   A. Available as injection: 4-g vial
   B. Dosage: IM: 40 mg/kg/dose once
CCXXXVIII. Spironolactone
   A. Available in tablet: 25 mg
   B.   Dose at 1.5–3.0

wt (kg)	mg/kg/24 hr
<5	6.25 mg daily or every other day
5–10	12.5 mg daily or every other day
10–20	12.5 mg bid
>20	25 mg qd

   C. Special considerations
   1. Tablets are scored
   2. Monitor for hyperkalemia
CCXXXIX. Streptomycin
   A. Available as injection: 1-g vial
   B. Dosage: Newborn, IM: 20–30 mg/kg/24 hr in 2 divided doses for 10 days
   Children, IM: 20–40 mg/kg/24 hr in 2 divided doses for 10 days
   Maximum dose: 2 g/24 hr
CCXL. Succimer
   A. Available in capsule: 100 mg
   B. Dosage: Oral: 30 mg/kg/day for 5 days followed by 20 mg/kg/day for 14 days
   C. Caution: Treatment of lead poisoning in children with blood levels > 45
   µg/dl. It is not indicated for prophylaxis of lead poisoning in a lead-contained environment
CCXLI. Sucralfate
   A. Available preparations: Tablet: 1 g
   Suspension: 1 g/10 ml
   B. Dosage
   1. Duodenal ulcer, acute treatment: Adults: 1 g PO qid, given 1 hr before
   meals, and at bedtime for 4–8 wk or less if healing has been effectively
   demonstrated
   2. Duodenal ulcer, maintenance
   a. Adults: 1 g PO bid on an empty stomach
   b. Children: Safety and efficacy have not been established
   3. Gastric ulcer and esophagitis associated with gastroesophageal reflux
   disease (GERD)
   a. Adults: 1 g PO qid given 1 hr before meals and at bedtime
   b. Children: 500 mg PO qid given 1 hr before meals and at bedtime
   C. Special considerations
   1. Take on an empty stomach at least 1 hr before a meal and at bedtime. If
   antacids are being administered, do not give them within 30 min to 1 hr after sucralfate
   2. Tablets: Do not crush or chew
   3. Suspension: Shake well before administration.
   4. Should not be given concomitantly with other agents that contain aluminum (e.g., aluminum-containing antacids) because the total body burden
   of aluminum can increase
CCXLII. Sulfadiazine
   A. Available in tablet: 500 mg
   B. Dosage
   1. Bacterial infection: Newborn: **not recommended**
   Children: *Loading dose:* 75 mg/kg/dose once; then
   150 mg/kg/24 hr in 4 divided doses to a maximum of
   4 g/24 hr
   2. Malaria (chloroquine-resistant): 100–200 mg/kg/24 hr in 4 divided doses
   to a maximum of 2 g/24 hr for 5 days

3. Toxoplasmosis: 25 mg/kg qid for 3–4 wk given with pyrimethamine, 2 mg/kg/day for 3 days, then 1 mg/kg/day for 3–4 wk
  C. Special considerations: Used together with pyrimethamine and quinine for chloroquine-resistant strains of *Plasmodium falciparum*

CCXLIII. Sulfasalazine
  A. Available in tablet: 500 mg
  B. Dosage: *Initial:* 40–60 mg/kg/24 hr in 3–6 divided doses
        Maintenance: 20–30 mg/kg/24 hr in 4 divided doses
        Maximum dose: 2 g/day
  C. Caution: Can cause orange-yellow discoloration of urine and skin

CCXLIV. Sulfisoxazole
  A. Available preparations: Suspension: 500 mg/5 ml
        Tablet: 500 mg
  B. Dosage: Oral: Newborn: **not recommended**
        >2 mo: 120–150 mg/kg/24 hr in 4 divided doses to a maximum of 6 g/24 hr

CCXLV. Terbutaline
  A. Available preparations: Injection: 1 mg/ml—1-ml ampul
        Tablet: 2.5, 5 mg
        Aerosol, oral: 0.2 mg/activation (10.5 g)
  B. Dosage
    1. Oral
      a. <12 yr: *Initial:* 0.05 mg/kg/dose tid, increased gradually as required; max: 0.1 mg/kg/dose tid or total of 5 mg/24 hr
      b. >12 yr: *Initial:* 2.5 mg tid
        Maintenance: Usually 5 mg or 0.075 mg/kg/dose tid
    2. Subcutaneous
      a. <12 yr: 0.01 mg/kg/dose to a maximum of 0.3 mg/dose q15–20 min for 3 doses
      b. >12 yr: 0.25 mg/dose, repeated in 15–30 min if needed once only; a total dose of 0.5 mg should not be exceeded within a 4-hr period
    3. Intravenous: bolus 2 µg/kg over 5 min, followed by 0.08 µg/kg/min. Titrate infusion by 0.02-µg/kg/min increments to keep heart rate less than 200/min
    4. Inhalation: 2 q4–6h

CCXLVI. Terfenadine
  A. Available in tablet: 60 mg
  B. Dosage: Oral: ≤12 yr: 15–30 mg/dose bid
        >12 yr: 60 mg bid
  C. Caution: should not be used with macrolides, ketoconazole, or itraconazole

CCXLVII. Tetracycline
  A. Available preparations: Capsule: 100, 250, 500 mg
        Suspension/syrup: 125 mg/5 ml
  B. Dosage: Oral: >8 yr: 25–50 mg/kg/24 hr in 4 divided doses not to exceed 3 g/day
        Adult: 250–500 mg/dose qid
  C. Caution
    1. Use of tetracycline in childhood (to 8 yr of age) **can cause permanent discoloration and enamel hypoplasia of the teeth**
    2. Give 1 hr before or 2 hr after meals
    3. Do not give with dairy products or antacid
    4. Can cause photosenitivity

CCXLVIII. Theophylline
  A. Available preparations: Solution: 5.3 mg/ml
        Capsule: 60, 126, 250 mg
        Sustained-release capsule: 50, 100, 300 mg
        Sustained-release capsule: 75 mg (sprinkle)
        Sustained-release tablet: 100, 200, 300 mg
        See Table 16–4

B. Dosage: **Asthma:** <9 yr: 12–24 mg/kg/24 hr
  9–12 yr: 12–20 mg/kg/24 hr
  12–16 yr: 10–18 mg/kg/24 hr
  >16 yr: 10–13 mg/kg/24 hr
  See Table 16–5

C. Caution
  1. Therapeutic levels: **bronchial asthma,** 10–20 µg/ml; **status asthmaticus,** maintain at 16–20 µg/ml; **neonatal apnea,** 7–23 µg/ml
  2. Slo-Phyllin Gyrocaps frequently require q6h dosing in children
  3. Drug interactions: calcium-channel blockers, carbamazepine, cimetidine, macrolides, propranolol, phenobarbital, or phenytoin

CCIL. Thiamine
  A. Available preparations: Injection: 100 mg/ml—10-ml vial
    Tablet: 10, 100 mg
  B. Dosage: dietary supplement
    1. Thiamine deficiency: IM, IV (if critically ill): 10–25 mg/dose daily; PO: 10–30 mg/day for 2 wk
    2. Maintenance: Oral: 5–10 mg/day for 1 mo

CCL. Thioridazine
  A. Available preparations: Concentrated solution: 30, 100 mg/ml
    Tablet: 10, 15, 25, 50, 100, 150, 200 mg
  B. Dosage: >2 yr: Oral initially: 0.5–1.0 mg/kg/24 hr in 3–4 divided doses individualized to patient (at minimum of 3 mg/kg/24 hr)

CCLI. Ticarcillin
  A. Available as injection: vial
  B. Dosage
    1. <1 wk, <2 kg: 150 mg/kg/24 hr in 2 divided doses; >2 kg: 200 mg/kg/24 hr in 3 divided doses
    2. >1 wk, <2 kg: 200 mg/kg/24 hr in 3 divided doses; >2 kg: 300 mg/kg/24 hr in 3 divided doses
    3. Neonates, children: 200–300 mg/kg/24 hr in 6 divided doses
  C. Contains: 5.2–6.5 mEq sodium per gram

CCLII. Tobramycin
  A. Available preparations: Injection: 40 mg/ml—2-ml vial, and 60-, 80-mg syringe
    Ophthalmic ointment: 0.3%—3.5-g tube
  B. Dosage: Neonates, <1 wk: 5 mg/kg/24 hr in 2 divided doses; >1 wk: 7.5 mg/kg/24 hr in 3 divided dosesChildren, <5 yr: 7.5 mg/kg/24 hr in 3 divided doses
    5–10 yr: 6 mg/kg/24 hr in 3 divided doses
    >10 yr: 4.5 mg/kg/24 hr in 3 divided doses
    1. Children with cystic fibrosis: Usual dose: 7.5 mg/kg/day in 3 divided doses; range: 6–10 mg/kg/day in 3 divided doses
    2. Ophthalmic ointment: Apply bid–tid
  C. Caution: Allowable predose level (trough): 0.5–2.0 µg/ml; allowable 1-hr postdose range (peak): 4–8 µg/ml

CCLIII. Tolazoline
  A. Available as injection: 25-mg/ml vial
  B. Dosage: **Neonatal pulmonary hypertension:** Parenteral, IV
    1. Loading dose: 1–2 mg/kg over 10 min
    2. Maintenance: 1–2 mg/kg/hr

CCLIV. Tolmetin
  A. Available in tablet: 200 mg
  B. Dosage: >2 yr: *Initial:* 15 mg/kg/24 hr in 3 divided doses; increase in increments of 5 mg/kg/24 hr at intervals of 1 wk until therapeutic effect or adverse reaction is noted. *Maximum:* 2 g/day
  C. Caution: Administer with meals or milk to minimize GI side effects

CCLV. Triamterene
  A. Available in capsule: 50, 100 mg
  B. Dosage: 2–4 mg/kg/24 hr in 1–2 divided doses

C. Caution: Monitor for hyperkalemia

CCLVI. **Trifluoperazine (Stelazine)**
  A. Available in tablet: 1, 2, 5 mg
  B. Dosage: 6–12 yr: Psychoses: Hospitalized or well supervised: 0.2–0.5 mg/kg/24 hr in 2 divided doses
  C. Contains: 100 mg chlorpromazine = 10 mg trifluoperazine

CCLVII. **Trihexyphenidyl**
  A. Available preparations: Solution: 2 mg/ml
    Tablet: 2, 5 mg
  B. Dosage: **Drug-induced extrapyramidal disorders:** 1–15 mg/24 hr in 1–4 divided doses
  C. Caution: Contraindicated in children <3 yr

CCLVIII. **Trimethadione**
  A. Available preparations: Solution: 40 mg/ml
    Capsule: 300 mg
    Chewable tablet: 150 mg
  B. Dosage: 40 mg/kg/24 hr in 3–4 divided doses to a maximum of 2.4 g/day

CCLIX. **Trimethobenzamide (Tigan)**
  A. Available preparations: Capsule: 100, 250 mg
    Suppository: 100, 200 mg
  B. Dosage
    1. Oral: 13–40 kg: 100–200 mg tid–qid
    2. Rectal: Children < 13 kg: 15–20 mg/kg/day ÷ tid–qid
      Children ≥ 14 kg: 100–200 mg qid-tid

CCLX. **Trimethoprim (TMP)-sulfamethoxazole**
  A. Available preparations: Injection: 5-ml vial
    Suspension: 2.5 ml, 5 ml units/day, and 100-, 473-ml btl
    Tablet: combination product
  B. Dosage: Not recommended for newborns. Children > 2 mo: 8 mg TMP/kg/24 hr in 2 divided doses
    1. **Serious gram-negative infection or** *P. carinii:* 20 mg TMP/kg 24 hr in 3–4 divided doses
    2. *P. carinii* **prophylaxis:** 150 mg TMP/m^2/day ÷ bid on 3 consecutive days/wk
  C. Contains: Concentrations: trimethoprim, 80 mg/5 ml injection, 40 mg/5 ml suspension, 80 mg/tablet; sulfamethoxazole, 400 mg/5 ml injection; 200 mg/5 ml suspension, 400 mg/tablet. Also known as co-trimoxazole

CCLXI. **Tromthamine (Tham)**
  A. Available as injection: 0.3 M solution
  B. Dosage
    1. Depends on buffer base deficit
      a. When deficit is known: tromethamine ml of 0.3 M solution = body weight (kg) × base deficit (mEq/liter)
      b. When base deficit is not known: 2–4 ml/kg/dose IV
    2. Metabolic acidosis with cardiac arrest: IV: 3.5–6.0 ml/kg into large peripheral vein
  C. Caution
    1. Administer through central vein whenever possible
    2. Must not be given for period > 24 hr
    3. **Contraindicated** in anuria, uremia, chronic respiratory acidosis, and salicylate intoxication

CCLXII. **Valproic acid**
  A. Available preparations: Capsule—sprinkle: 125 mg
    Tablet: 125, 250, 500 mg
    Solution: 250 mg/5 ml—16-oz btl
  B. Dosage: 15 mg/kg/24 hr in 1–3 divided doses; increased in weekly intervals by 5–10 mg/kg/24 hr; maximum dose: 60 mg/kg/24 hr
  C. Caution

      1. Dose divided bid is preferable
      2. Monitor for hepatotoxicity

CCLXIII. **Vancomycin**
    A. Available preparations: Injection: 500-mg vial
                                Oral solution: 250 mg/5 ml (special prep)
                                  Capsules: 125, 250 mg
    B. Dosage
      1. Parenteral, IV: Neonates, <1 wk: 30 mg/kg/24 hr in 2 divided doses
                       Infants and children: 40–60 mg/kg/24 hr in 4 divided doses
      2. Oral: 10–50 mg/kg/day in 3–4 divided doses not to exceed 2 g/day
    C. Caution
      1. Check serum levels
      2. Therapeutic range: 50–100 µg/ml

CCLXIV. **Varicella-zoster immune globulin**
    A. Available as injection: 125-units vial
    B. Dosage:

Wt (kg)	Dose (units)	No. of vials
0–10	125	1
10–20	250	2
20–30	375	3
30–40	500	4
40–50	625	5

    C. Caution
      1. Administer by deep IM injection only
      2. Use within 72 hr of exposure

CCLXV. **Vasopressin, aqueous**
    A. Available as injection (aqueous): 20-units/ml ampul
    B. Dosage
      1. *Diabetes insipidus:* IM, SC: highly variable dosage
                       Children: 2.5–5.0 units bid–qid
      2. *GI hemorrhage:* IV continuous infusion: Initial: 0.1–0.3 units/min, then titrate dose as needed
    C. Caution
      1. Do not confuse with injection in oil
      2. Titrate dose based on serum and urine osmolality in addition to fluid balance

CCLXVI. **Vasopressin tannate, in oil**
    A. Available as injection in oil: 5-units/ml ampul
    B. Dosage: 1.25–2.5 units q1–3 days
    C. Caution
      1. Do not confuse with aqueous injection
      2. Titrate dose to achieve desired control of excessive thirst and urination

CCLXVII. **Verapamil**
    A. Available preparations: Injection: 5 mg/2 ml
                                    Tablet: 80, 120 mg
    B. Dosage
      1. Parenteral, IV: 0.1 mg/kg/dose (maximum 5 mg) IV push over 2 min; can be repeated 3 times
      2. Oral: 4–15 mg/kg/24 hr in 3 divided doses
    C. Caution
      1. Contraindicated in children <1 yr of age
      2. IV use contraindicated in patients taking beta blockers or quinidine

CCLXVIII. **Vidarabine**
    A. Available in ophthalmic ointment: 3%—3.5-g tube
    B. Dosage: Apply 1 cm ointment 5 times a day at 3-hr intervals; continue application for 5–7 days after healing seems to be complete

CCLXIX. **Vitamin A**
    A. Available preparations: Capsule: 10,000, 25,000, 50,000 units
                                        Injection: 50,000 units/ml—2-ml vial

B. Dosage
1. Deficiency
    a. <1 yr: 10,000 units/kg/day for 5 days, then 7,500–15,000 units/day for 10 days
    b. 1–8 yr: 5,000–10,000 units/kg/day for 5 days, then 17,000–35,000 units/day for 10 days
    c. >8 yr and adults: 100,000 units/day for 3 days, then 50,000 units/day for 14 days
2. Malabsorption syndrome (prophylaxis): >8 yr and adults: 10,000–50,000 units/day
3. Dietary supplement: Infants up to 6 mo: 1,500 units/day
    6 mo–3 yr: 1,500–2,000 units/day
    4–6 yr: 2,500 units/day
    7–10 yr: 3,300–3,500 units/day
    >10 yr and adults: 4,000–5,000 units/day
C. Caution: 3 drops = 0.1 ml

CCLXX. Vitamin B complex
A. Available preparations: Capsule: multiple combinations
    Injection: 2-ml ampul
    Solution: 12-oz btl
B. Dosage: 1 capsule daily
C. Contains: 1 capsule = 10 ml solution

CCLXXI. Vitamin E
A. Available preparations: Capsule: 100, 200, 400 units

Solution: 50 units/ml—30-ml drop btl
B. Dosage: Vitamin E deficiency
1. Treatment
    a. Neonates, premature and low birth weight: 25 units/day results in normal levels within 1 wk
    b. Children with malabsorption syndrome: 1 unit/kg/day water-miscible vitamin E to raise plasma tocopherol concentrations to the normal range within 2 mo
    c. Adults: 60–70 units/day
2. Prevention
    a. Neonates, low birth weight: 5 units/day; if full term: 5 units/liter formula
    b. Adults: 30 units/day
    c. Cystic fibrosis, beta-thalassemia, sickle cell anemia may require higher daily maintenance doses: Cystic fibrosis: 100–400 units/day
        Sickle cell: 450 units/day
        Beta-thalassemia: 750 units/day

CCLXXII. Warfarin
A. Available in tablet: 1, 2, 2.5, 5, 7.5, 10 mg
B. Dosage
1. Infants and children: 0.1 mg/kg/day; range 0.05–0.34 mg/kg/day; adjust dose to achieve the desired prothrombin time
2. Infants < 12 mo may require doses near high end of range

CCLXXIII. Zinc sulfate
A. Available in capsule: 220 mg
B. Dosage: Zinc deficiency: 0.5–1.0 mg/kg/24 hr elemental zinc divided 1–3 times/day
C. Contains: 55 mg elemental zinc per 220-mg capsule
D. Caution: Administer with food or milk

Index